# Bayesianism

# Bayesianism

Guest Editors

**Carlos Alberto de Bragança Pereira**
**Paulo Canas Rodrigues**
**Mark Andrew Gannon**

Basel • Beijing • Wuhan • Barcelona • Belgrade • Novi Sad • Cluj • Manchester

*Guest Editors*
Carlos Alberto de Bragança Pereira
Institute of Mathematics and Statistics
University of São Paulo
São Paulo
Brazil

Paulo Canas Rodrigues
Department of Statistics
Federal University of Bahia
Salvador
Brazil

Mark Andrew Gannon
Independent Researcher
São Paulo
Brazil

*Editorial Office*
MDPI AG
Grosspeteranlage 5
4052 Basel, Switzerland

This is a reprint of the Special Issue, published open access by the journal *Entropy* (ISSN 1099-4300), freely accessible at: https://www.mdpi.com/journal/entropy/special_issues/4LGZ41C88T.

For citation purposes, cite each article independently as indicated on the article page online and as indicated below:

Lastname, A.A.; Lastname, B.B. Article Title. *Journal Name* **Year**, *Volume Number*, Page Range.

**ISBN 978-3-7258-4791-4 (Hbk)**
**ISBN 978-3-7258-4792-1 (PDF)**
**https://doi.org/10.3390/books978-3-7258-4792-1**

# Contents

# About the Editors

**Carlos Alberto de Bragança Pereira**

Carlos Alberto de Bragança Pereira was born on 7/1/1946. His first job was as a quality-control technician at General Electric in Rio de Janeiro from 1964 to 1966. He was then a teaching assistant in statistics at the public health education foundation FENSP of the Oswaldo Cruz Institute. He graduated in Statistics in 1968 from the National School of Statistical Sciences (ENCE) and was hired as an assistant instructor by the University of São Paulo (USP) in May of 1969. He obtained a master's degree in Statistics from USP in 1971 and became an assistant professor at USP's Institute of Mathematics and Statistics (IME-USP). He also obtained an M.Sc. in 1978 and a Ph.D. in 1980, both in statistics, from Florida State University. In 1986-87, he was a Visiting Research Engineer at the University of California, Berkeley. He holds the title of Livre Docente, obtained from the IME-USP in 1984, and was appointed as an associate professor in 1988, a full professor in 1990, and a senior lecturer in 2016. He was a visiting professor in 2018-20 at UFMS, the Federal University of Mato Grosso do Sul. He has experience in probability and statistics, with emphasis on fundamentals of inference, mainly in medical, biological, and financial applications. His favorite subjects are Bayesian prediction, hypothesis testing, and bioinformatics. He was elected and served as the head of the statistics department of the IME-USP three times, as the director of the USP Bioinformatics Lab, and as director of the IME-USP in 1994-98. He has served on numerous committees for master's and doctoral defenses and academic-career competitions. He supervised 29 master's dissertations and 30 doctoral theses. He has been an observer for the Organization of American States (OAS) in elections in Nicaragua, El Salvador, Haiti, and Paraguay. He is an ad hoc consultant for grant-giving agencies CNPq, CAPES, and FAPESP. His work has been cited over 9,800 times, with over 150 of his published works cited more than nine times each.

**Paulo Canas Rodrigues**

Paulo Canas Rodrigues is more than a statistician — he is a global explorer, academic leader, and cultural enthusiast. With roots in Portugal and a home in Brazil, Paulo's journey has taken him through the academic corridors of Indonesia and Australia, the highlands of Ethiopia, and the reefs of the Philippines. At every step, he bridges rigorous data science with lived experience. He is a Professor at the Federal University of Bahia (UFBA) and Director of the Statistical Learning Laboratory (SaLLy), where he leads cutting-edge research in artificial intelligence, statistical learning, time series forecasting, and high-dimensional data analysis. Among other activities, he serves as President of the International Society for Business and Industrial Statistics (ISBIS), President-Elect of the International Association for Statistical Computing (IASC), Council member of the International Statistical Institute (ISI), and Member of the Representative Council of the International Biometric Society (IBS), helping shape the global future of statistics and data science.

But Paulo's story extends far beyond papers and conferences. He has taught and inspired minds at the African Institute for Mathematical Sciences in Cameroon, led workshops across Southeast Asia, and contributed to academic communities from Finland to Chile. His path is marked by deep curiosity, cultural connection, and a quiet optimism that fuels purposeful action. He chases the world not just to see it, but to understand it: in code, in rhythm, in silence, and in waves.

A man of precision, but also of soul. A mentor, a mover, and a mind in motion.

**Mark Andrew Gannon**

Mark Andrew Gannon holds a bachelor's degree in physics from the University of Chicago, a master's degree and Ph.D. in physics from the University of California, Santa Barbara, and a D.Sc. in statistics from the University of São Paulo. He has participated in research in a wide variety of fields, including theoretical condensed-matter physics, polymer physics, biological physics, biochemistry, mathematical physics, stochastic processes, theoretical statistics, statistical modeling, and projection of sports-player performance.

*entropy*

MDPI

*Editorial*

# A Snapshot of Bayesianism

**Mark A. Gannon**

Independent Researcher, São Paulo 05508-090, SP, Brazil; mark.a.gannon@gmail.com

Students are told in basic probability classes that there are two main "schools" of statistics, the frequentist and the Bayesian, and that those different views of how to approach statistical inference problems arise from two different views of the meaning of probability. Practicing scientists know things are not that simple.

First, statisticians as a group cannot be divided so simply into two schools. There are other approaches, such as likelihoodism. Additionally, the schools are not mutually exclusive. All three of the invited academic editors of this special edition of *Entropy* have published work that could be classified as using a frequentist approach and work that could be classified as using a Bayesian approach. There are even articles in our publication history that report on methods that blend Bayesian and frequentist approaches to inference problems, and this is not as unusual as teachers of basic probability courses would have us believe. It is not uncommon for researchers who use one of the two major approaches to statistics in much of their work to occasionally use a concept, tool, or procedure from another "school" of statistics to solve an otherwise intractable problem.

Additionally, even among those using Bayesian approaches to parametric inference, there are differing views on how to choose prior distributions for the parameters of interest. Conjugate priors are useful for theoretical work, because they facilitate closed-form analytic results, but sometimes there is no choice of hyperparameters that can make a given conjugate prior reflect what experts expect of the distribution of the parameters. Among the statisticians with a more "subjectivist" approach, elicitation of priors is a way of translating expert knowledge into a mathematical starting point for inference. Those with a more "objectivist" approach attempt to reduce the influence of subjective choices made by human beings, with all of our flaws and biases.

Subjectivist and objectivist Bayesians adopt concepts from each other, so the division between those approaches to Bayesian inference also tends not to be clearly defined. The father of modern subjectivist Bayesian statistics, Bruno de Finetti, treated probability as a degree of belief in his work, and that view has been adopted by many Bayesians, regardless of their views on how to choose prior distributions. Objectivist Bayesians tend to think of probability as a degree of rational belief like subjectivists do, but they start with priors meant to represent "neutral" knowledge rather than an initial individual or group belief. Subjectivist Bayesians occasionally use "non-informative" priors that are defined using the methods of objectivist Bayesian inference. While the classification of approaches to statistics into "schools" and the classification of Bayesian approaches as objectivist or subjectivist do not define clear partitions, they are still useful for understanding approaches to a given problem, the differences between them, and their relative strengths and weaknesses.

The present Special Issue of *Entropy* was conceived as an attempt to provide a "snapshot" of Bayesian thought and Bayesian inference in 2024. And while 16 articles cannot do justice to the breadth and depth of the theoretical work, simulation studies, and real-world data analysis using Bayesian ideas and methods worldwide, we feel that the content of this Special Issue provides a representative sample of the wide variety of current directions in Bayesian-inference-based research and applications.

Despite the fact that *Entropy* does not usually publish "perspective" articles, the invited academic editors of this Special Issue consider the subject of the article "Statistics as a Social Activity: Attitudes toward Amalgamating Evidence" [contribution 1] sufficiently important to such an immensely broad range of activities, and the approach taken to the subject sufficiently unique, forward-thinking, and broadly applicable, that it was worth arguing for an exception to be made. That article makes this Special Issue a snapshot of much more than just Bayesianism, bringing all of statistics, science, and all the potential applications of descriptive statistics and inference into the picture by treating some of the most fundamental issues in data analysis.

Among the major applications of statistics in the mid-2020s is "machine learning", where "supervised machine learning"—the variety that is appearing frequently in news reports—refers to algorithms for making various types of regression models, with classification being an important subclass of regression models with small, discrete ranges. The article entitled "Probabilistic Nearest Neighbors Classification" [contribution 2] takes a Bayesian approach to delving into a widely used classification technique, developing a theoretical understanding of its computational complexity, and using that knowledge to produce a practical real-world result: a new model that performs as well for classification tasks as the previous algorithm, but with more manageable computational cost. Statisticians naturally have important roles to play in machine learning, and this article is an example of advances in machine learning algorithms made possible by a Bayesian approach.

One of the editors of the present Special Issue is the creator of the idea behind the Full Bayesian Significance Test (FBST) [1–3], a Bayesian replacement for the familiar and oft-abused Neyman–Pearson hypothesis tests and Fisher significance tests, with the "*e*-value" playing a similar role to the more familiar *p*-value, a measure of the compatibility of observed data with a null hypothesis. The FBST has been used in a variety of fields, and researchers around the world have analyzed, explored, and extended it with further theoretical work (see, for example, [4–11], and references cited in section 4 of [3]). A common issue in parametric statistics is how to handle inferences about some of a given model's parameters in the presence of "nuisance parameters", the name given to the model's other parameters—the ones about which inferences are *not* being drawn. As its title suggests, the article "Objective Priors for Invariant e-Values in the Presence of Nuisance Parameters" [contribution 3] takes an objectivist-Bayesian approach to exploring properties of the FBST in cases with nuisance parameters. Such work is important because advances in our understanding of existing inferential tools like the FBST and their properties contribute to the maturation of those tools and potentially guide the development of new ones.

Poisson distributions are widely used to model counts of infrequent occurrences in fixed time intervals. In 1960, the possibility of an observer not noticing a single occurrence in a given time interval was considered, allowing for an interval in which there was actually one occurrence being recorded as having none, leading to the "misrecorded Poisson distribution" or "Cohen–Poisson distribution", which is studied further in the article "Linear Bayesian Estimation of Misrecorded Poisson Distribution" [contribution 4] in the present Special Issue. The authors propose and show the advantages of a linear Bayesian estimation procedure for the parameters of the misrecorded Poisson distribution, including demonstrating, via numerical studies and specific examples using real-world data, that the performance of the linear-Bayesian approach to estimating those parameters is superior to that of maximum-likelihood estimation. This article represents a Bayesian approach to one way of handling the possibility of misrecorded count data.

Because the elicitation of expert knowledge frequently does not yield a unique possible prior distribution, much Bayesian research, especially in the last two decades of the 20th

Century and the first decade of the 21st Century, focused on the issue of robustness, defined as the insensitivity of inferential results to the inputs of the inferential process, including the choice of a prior. One-sample and two-sample $t$-tests have been used for over a century, with both frequentist and Bayesian versions devised in the early 20th Century. "An Objective and Robust Bayes Factor for the Hypothesis Test One Sample and Two Population Means" [contribution 5] takes an objectivist-Bayesian approach to two classic hypothesis testing problems. The authors propose an objective and robust Bayes factor and use it to analyze real-world data and show the finite-sample consistency of these tools. The authors also develop a modified version of the Bayesian information criterion for comparing sample means and find that, in practice, their approaches to two-sample comparisons tend to yield similar results to each other, including support for the null hypothesis in the case of data generated from distributions with equal means and variances. This article represents theoretical statistics work to develop tools for researchers in a wide range of fields of study, the continued updating of objectivist Bayesian methods of statistical inference, and specifically, the refinement of robust-analysis objectivist Bayesianism.

"On the Nuisance Parameter Elimination Principle in Hypothesis Testing" [contribution 6] treats inference in the presence of nuisance parameters in the specific case of hypothesis testing. It does so by developing a form of Berger and Wolpert's non-informative nuisance parameter principle (NNPP) that is appropriate for hypothesis tests, exploring the compatibility of that form of the principle with both Bayesian and non-Bayesian views and methods, and treating a specific example by showing that a class of hypothesis tests that mix elements from the Bayesian and frequentist paradigms, proposed and developed by Pereira and collaborators [12,13], adheres to the NNPP when the sample space is discrete and the parameter space finite and variation-independent. The authors further show that the adherence of those tests to the NNPP can facilitate calculations and reduce the computing cost of performing the mixed-paradigm tests. In this article, we can see a Bayesian approach to a fundamental issue in theoretical statistics yielding practical results, facilitating the real-world use of a relatively new inferential tool.

"Stochastic Volatility Models with Skewness Selection" [contribution 7] extends the stochastic volatility models that have been successful at modeling asset returns in financial time series, doing so in a way that permits dynamic skewness but does not require it. The authors employ a data-driven sparsity scheme for their model's parameters, similar in concept to the shrinkage in LASSO regression, but based on a Bayesian approach, that chooses from three possibilities based on the data: dynamic skewness, static skewness, and zero skewness. They then apply their new models to financial time series, showing examples that result in dynamic skewness and zero skewness, with implications for some of the biggest issues in econometrics, finance, and even monetary policy. This article is an example of a Bayesian approach to asset-return modeling yielding a more flexible extension of previously existing models that can deepen our understanding of the behavior of asset returns and financial markets.

Extreme value theory seeks to provide inferences for rare events, that is, those found in the tails of probability distributions. "Peaks-over-threshold" approaches use the subset of points that are peaks of periods of a time series that are above a threshold value as a way of selecting the most extreme events in the available time series. Theoretical results such as the Pickands–Balkema–De Haan Theorem then allow the peaks-over-threshold subset to be used for inferences about very rare events, and this can have important applications in risk assessment for extreme climate and weather events, financial market crashes, and other situations in which rare and extreme events can have wide-ranging impacts. "Bayesian Non-Parametric Inference for Multivariate Peaks-over-Threshold Models" [contribution 8] starts with the Pareto process, a generalization to infinite dimensionality of the generalized

Pareto distribution that arises in univariate peaks-over-threshold extreme value analysis, shows how the Pareto process can be decomposed into radial and angular components, with the angular component containing information about the dependence structure of the random vector, and proposes a novel non-parametric Bayesian approach to modeling the angular component. The technique is applied to synthetic data and to using real-world integrated vapor transport data to estimate the extremal dependence structure for a measure of water vapor flow in the atmosphere. The advances reported in the article are set up as steps on the way to detailed modeling of atmospheric events that lead to storm activity. The article brings the important area of extreme value theory and its applications into our snapshot of the applications of Bayesian methods in 2024.

"Bayesian Spatio-Temporal Modeling of the Dynamics of COVID-19 Deaths in Peru" [contribution 9] brings an example of spatio-temporal data analysis and Bayesian spatio-temporal modeling, applied to understanding public health data on COVID-19 in Peru. The study models the count of COVID-19 deaths as the response variable, with covariates including the total number of COVID-19 cases and the counts of first, second, third, and fourth doses of vaccines administered, all measured 14 days before the corresponding COVID-19 death count. Their analysis of Peruvian public health data shows, for example, that higher coverage of the first two doses of COVID-19 vaccines reduced the number of deaths in the period studied, with third-dose coverage having an even stronger effect. This article demonstrates the flexibility of Bayesian methodologies in modeling real-world data, particularly spatio-temporal data. The authors show how these methods allow them to reach conclusions that could inform decisions by public health authorities and legislators regarding health policy and interventions.

"A Metric Based on the Efficient Determination Criterion" [contribution 10] uses a generalization of the Bayesian information criterion (BIC) to extend a BIC-based metric that has been indispensable for estimating minimal partitions in research involving partition Markov models, including models of viral genetic sequences, Huffman coding, and data compression. The BIC-based metric allows for strong consistency in estimating a minimal partition, which in turn allows for more efficient estimation of the model's transition probabilities. The authors introduce the efficient determination criterion (EDC), a generalization of the BIC, and prove that it can serve as the basis of a metric similar to the BIC-based metric, but with different possible terms to penalize higher numbers of model parameters. They show that strong consistency can be maintained with a penalty term of the form $\ln(\ln(n))$, where $n$ is the number of parameters in the model. The authors then apply their new metric to a specific application, modeling three genetic sequences of dengue virus type 3, the return of which to Brazil could have serious public health implications, as the population is expected not to have immunity due to the length of time the virus has been nearly absent.

Copulas are used to model the dependence between random variables. "Likelihood Inference for Factor Copula Models with Asymmetric Tail Dependence" [contribution 11] addresses a limitation of copulas and proposes a Bayesian solution. Multivariate non-Gaussian factor-copula inference tends to be dominated by central data, and as a result, fitted models might not yield accurate model-based estimates of tail dependence parameters or reliable joint tail inference. When plots of data and likelihood analysis suggest asymmetric tail dependence, the authors propose a Bayesian approach that incorporates previous information about tail dependence to construct a prior, which can be used with the likelihood for extreme-value inference based on joint upper tails and joint lower tails. A real-world example and a simulation study show that this approach improves extreme value inference by giving more weight to the joint tails. Here we see an example of researchers applying Bayesian methods to improve inference in cases that arise in research using non-Bayesian methods.

Point patterns in geographic spaces, such as the pattern of locations of cases of an infectious disease or the coordinates of plants infected by a pest, may be interpreted as realizations of spatial point processes—stochastic processes that produce locations in their respective spaces. "Bayesian Modeling for Nonstationary Spatial Point Process via Spatial Deformations" [contribution 12] seeks to treat cases in which the potentially simplifying assumptions of isotropy and stationarity are unrealistic. The authors propose a point process analysis model that incorporates anisotropy and nonstationarity via a multidimensional Gaussian deformation process. Their approach uses Bayesian inference via MCMC (specifically, HMC) to estimate the intensity function and is shown to outperform approaches that do not permit anisotropy and nonstationarity, both for synthetic and real-world data. In the case of data on infestation of corn plants by an insect pest, the new approach identifies anisotropy that should be expected due to the way corn is planted in rows. The flexibility of Bayesian methods allows important complicating factors such as anisotropy and nonstationarity to be included in the modeling, leading to more accurate estimates of infestation levels, which in turn allow for targeted pesticide use, potentially yielding environmental and consumer health benefits.

Bayesian inference has had a major impact on how medical studies are conducted. The use of Bayesian techniques has enabled more ethical and more efficient medical studies, while simultaneously providing methods that are more reliable and harder to manipulate or "hack" than the deeply flawed Neyman–Pearson hypothesis tests involved in so many of the highly publicized, non-reproducible results in science, including medical science. "Dose Finding in Oncology Trials Guided by Ordinal Toxicity Grades Using Continuous Dose Levels" [contribution 13] is an example of applying Bayesian techniques to medical studies, specifically in first-in-humans dose-finding trials for cancer treatments. Doses for the next cohort are set by controlling the posterior probability of a patient receiving a dose above the maximum tolerated dose. The methodology made possible the first phase-1 human trial with continuous dose levels that considers grade-2 toxicity in addition to the usual binary dose-limiting toxicity, demonstrating how the adaptability of Bayesian inference continues to support innovation in medical studies while fulfilling all the ethical requirements for human trials.

There are several different common approaches to statistical inference, each with one or more underlying theories of inference. "Relative Belief Inferences from Decision Theory" [contribution 14] contains a new addition to the author's ongoing program of developing a theory of inference that starts with a clear definition of statistical evidence—something mentioned in all theories but clearly defined in few—along with a few *desiderata*, such as reparametrization invariance. The theory is distinctly Bayesian, using Bayes's theorem to update prior distributions with experimental data to obtain posterior distributions, from which inferences can be made, and these inferences have been shown to have certain optimality properties. The contribution to relative-belief inference theory presented in this Special Issue shows how inferences in relative belief theory can arise in a decision-theoretic context.

The authors of "A Bayesian Approach for Modeling and Forecasting Solar Photovoltaic Power Generation" [contribution 15] present data on solar power generation recorded at 71 moments each day over 19 days at a photovoltaic plant installed on a university campus. They develop a Bayesian kriging (Gaussian-process regression) scheme to use the available history of power generation at $k$ recording moments per day over $N$ days to predict power generation on the $(N+1)^{\text{th}}$ day. The article adds to the variety of Bayesian techniques applied in the present Special Issue and provides a further example of how the flexibility of Bayesian techniques facilitates new analysis.

"Bayesian Assessment of Corrosion-Related Failures in Steel Pipelines" [contribution 16] presents a real-world example in which the limitations of the available historical data are mitigated by the use of expert knowledge, making it a perfect opportunity for the application of Bayesian techniques. The authors describe how they transform the knowledge of gas-distribution-pipe engineers and technicians into prior distributions and how they use these priors in Bayesian analysis to understand the roles of multiple types of corrosion in the failure of gas pipes. They also demonstrate how this analysis informs practical recommendations in both the design and maintenance phases of gas distribution networks.

Sixteen articles, of course, cannot come close to covering the immense breadth and depth of current directions in Bayesian research. However, our selection includes theoretical advances and novel practical applications, subjectivist-Bayesian and objectivist-Bayesian parametric inference, Bayesian non-parametic inference and Bayesian kriging, Bayesian model selection tools, prior elicitation, Bayesian robustness, Bayesian spatial and spatio-temporal modeling, Bayesian extreme value theory, Bayesian analysis of inference in the presence of nuisance parameters, Bayesian techniques applied to problems in research involving non-Bayesian inference, and a Bayesian philosophy-of-science approach to some of the most fundamental issues in all endeavors that involve data. Additionally, the Special Issue includes applications of Bayesian analysis in machine learning, finance, macroeconomics, genetics, epidemiology, medical trials, industry, and public policy. Like an actual photographic snapshot, our Special Issue, as a "snapshot" of the state of Bayesian inference in 2024, cannot capture the entire scope of the field but offers a glimpse of its key subjects. This snapshot provides insight into a variety of current research directions and practical applications of Bayesian inference in real-world problems.

**Acknowledgments:** The invited editors of this special issue would like to thank in-house editors for her invaluable guidance and support.

**Conflicts of Interest:** The author declares no conflicts of interest.

## List of Contributions

1. Gelman, A.; O'Rourke, K. Statistics as a Social Activity: Attitudes toward Amalgamating Evidence. *Entropy* **2024**, *26*, 652. https://doi.org/10.3390/e26080652.
2. Fava, B.; F., P.C.M.; Lopes, H.F. Probabilistic Nearest Neighbors Classification. *Entropy* **2024**, *26*, 39. https://doi.org/10.3390/e26010039.
3. Bortolato, E.; Ventura, L. Objective Priors for Invariant e-Values in the Presence of Nuisance Parameters. *Entropy* **2024**, *26*, 58. https://doi.org/10.3390/e26010058.
4. Gao, H.; Chen, Z.; Li, F. Linear Bayesian Estimation of Misrecorded Poisson Distribution. *Entropy* **2024**, *26*, 62. https://doi.org/10.3390/e26010062.
5. Almodóvar-Rivera, I.A.; Pericchi-Guerra, L.R. An Objective and Robust Bayes Factor for the Hypothesis Test One Sample and Two Population Means. *Entropy* **2024**, *26*, 88. https://doi.org/10.3390/e26010088.
6. Flórez Rivera, A.F.; Esteves, L.G.; Fossaluza, V.; de Bragança Pereira, C.A. On the Nuisance Parameter Elimination Principle in Hypothesis Testing. *Entropy* **2024**, *26*, 117. https://doi.org/10.3390/e26020117.
7. Martins, I.; Freitas Lopes, H. Stochastic Volatility Models with Skewness Selection. *Entropy* **2024**, *26*, 142. https://doi.org/10.3390/e26020142.
8. Trubey, P.; Sansó, B. Bayesian Non-Parametric Inference for Multivariate Peaks-over-Threshold Models. *Entropy* **2024**, *26*, 335. https://doi.org/10.3390/e26040335.
9. Galarza, C.R.C.; Sánchez, O.N.D.; Pimentel, J.S.; Bulhões, R.; López-Gonzales, J.L.; Rodrigues, P.C. Bayesian Spatio-Temporal Modeling of the Dynamics of COVID-19 Deaths in Peru. *Entropy* **2024**, *26*, 474. https://doi.org/10.3390/e26060474.

10. García, J.E.; González-López, V.A.; Gomez Sanchez, J.I. A Metric Based on the Efficient Determination Criterion. *Entropy* **2024**, *26*, 526. https://doi.org/10.3390/e26060526.
11. Joe, H.; Li, X. Likelihood Inference for Factor Copula Models with Asymmetric Tail Dependence. *Entropy* **2024**, *26*, 610. https://doi.org/10.3390/e26070610.
12. Gamerman, D.; Quintana, M.d.S.B.; Alves, M.B. Bayesian Modeling for Nonstationary Spatial Point Process via Spatial Deformations. *Entropy* **2024**, *26*, 678. https://doi.org/10.3390/e26080678.
13. Tighiouart, M.; Rogatko, A. Dose Finding in Oncology Trials Guided by Ordinal Toxicity Grades Using Continuous Dose Levels. *Entropy* **2024**, *26*, 687. https://doi.org/10.3390/e26080687.
14. Evans, M.; Jang, G.H. Relative Belief Inferences from Decision Theory. *Entropy* **2024**, *26*, 786. https://doi.org/10.3390/e26090786.
15. Flesch, M.V.; de Bragança Pereira, C.A.; Saraiva, E.F. A Bayesian Approach for Modeling and Forecasting Solar Photovoltaic Power Generation. *Entropy* **2024**, *26*, 824. https://doi.org/10.3390/e26100824.
16. Ruggeri, F.; Cagno, E.; Caron, F.; Mancini, M.; Pievatolo, A. Bayesian Assessment of Corrosion-Related Failures in Steel Pipelines. *Entropy* **2024**, *26*, 1111. https://doi.org/10.3390/e26121111.

## References


1. Pereira, C.; Stern, J. Evidence and Credibility: Full Bayesian Significance Test for Precise Hypotheses. *Entropy* **1999**, *1*, 99. [CrossRef]
2. Pereira, C.; Stern, J.; Wechsler, S. Can a significance test be genuinely Bayesian? *Bayesian Anal.* **2008**, *3*, 79. [CrossRef]
3. Pereira, C.; Stern, J. The *e*-value: A fully Bayesian significance measure for precise statistical hypotheses and its research program. *São Paulo J. Math. Sci.* **2022**, *16*, 566. [CrossRef]
4. Andrade, P.; Rifo, L.L.R.; Torres, S.; Torres-Avilés, F. Bayesian Inference on the Memory Parameter for Gamma-Modulated Regression Models. *Entropy* **2015** , *17*, 6576. [CrossRef]
5. Cerezetti, F.V.; Stern, J.M. Non-arbitrage in Financial Markets: A Bayesian Approach for Verification. *AIP Conf. Proc.* **2012**, *1490*, 87. [CrossRef]
6. Chaiboonsri, C.; Wannapan, S.; Saosaovaphak, A. Economic and Business Cycle of India: Evidence from ICT Sector. In *Advances in Panel Data Analysis in Applied Economic Research*; Tsouris, N., Vlachvei, A., Eds.; Springer Nature: Cham, Switzerland, 2018; pp. 29–43. [CrossRef]
7. Chakrabarty, D. A New Bayesian Test to Test for the Intractability-Countering Hypothesis. *J. Am. Stat. Assoc.* **2017**, *112*, 561. [CrossRef]
8. Chen, C.W.S.; Lee, S. A local unit root test in mean for financial time series. *J. Stat. Comput. Simul.* **2015**, *86*, 788. [CrossRef]
9. García, J.E.; González-López, V.; Nelsen, R.B. The Structure of the Class of Maximum Tsallis-Havrda-Chavat Entropy Copulas. *Entropy* **2016**, *18*, 264. [CrossRef]
10. Maranhao, V.d.L.; Lauretto, M.d.S.; Stern, J.M. FBST for Covariance Structures of Generalized Gompertz Models. *AIP Conf. Proc.* **2012**, *1490*, 202. [CrossRef]
11. Kelter, R. The evidence interval and the Bayesian evidence value: On a unified theory for Bayesian hypothesis testing and interval estimation. *Br. J. Math. Stat. Psychol.* **2022**, *75*, 550. [CrossRef] [PubMed]
12. Gannon, M.A.; Pereira, C.A.d.B.; Polpo, A. Blending Bayesian and Classical Tools to Define Optimal Sample-Size-Dependent Significance Levels. *Am. Stat.* **2019**, *73* (Supp. S1), 213. [CrossRef]
13. Pereira, C.A.d.B.; Nakano, E.Y.; Fossaluza, V.; Esteves, L.G.; Gannon, M.A.; Polpo, A. Hypothesis Tests for Bernoulli Experiments: Ordering the Sample Space by Bayes Factors and Using Adaptive Significance Levels for Decisions. *Entropy* **2017** *19*, 696. [CrossRef]

*entropy*

MDPI

*Article*

# Probabilistic Nearest Neighbors Classification

**Bruno Fava [1], Paulo C. Marques F. [2,*] and Hedibert F. Lopes [2]**

[1] Department of Economics, Northwestern University, Evanston, IL 60208, USA; brunofava@u.northwestern.edu

[2] Insper Institute of Education and Research, Rua Quatá 300, São Paulo 04546-042, Brazil; hedibertfl@insper.edu.br

* Correspondence: paulocmf1@insper.edu.br

**Abstract:** Analysis of the currently established Bayesian nearest neighbors classification model points to a connection between the computation of its normalizing constant and issues of NP-completeness. An alternative predictive model constructed by aggregating the predictive distributions of simpler nonlocal models is proposed, and analytic expressions for the normalizing constants of these nonlocal models are derived, ensuring polynomial time computation without approximations. Experiments with synthetic and real datasets showcase the predictive performance of the proposed predictive model.

**Keywords:** probabilistic machine learning; nearest neighbors classification; NP-completeness

## 1. Introduction

The now classic nearest neighbors classification algorithm, introduced in a 1951 technical report by Fix and Hodges (reprinted in [1]), marked one of the early successes of machine learning research. The basic idea is that, given some notion of proximity between pairs of observations, the class of a new sample unit is determined by majority voting among its $k$ nearest neighbors in the training sample [2,3]. A natural question is whether it is possible to develop a probabilistic model that captures the essence of the mechanism contained in the classic nearest neighbors algorithm while adding proper uncertainty quantification of predictions made by the model. In a pioneering paper, Holmes and Adams [4] defined a probabilistic nearest neighbors model specifying a set of conditional distributions. A few years later, Cucala et al. [5] pointed out the incompatibility of the conditional distributions specified by Holmes and Adams, which do not define a proper joint model distribution. As an alternative, Cucala et al. developed their own nearest neighbors classification model, defining directly a proper, Boltzmann-like joint distribution. A major difficulty with the Cucala et al. model is the fact that its likelihood function involves a seemingly intractable normalizing constant. Consequently, in order to perform a Bayesian analysis of their model, the authors engaged in a *tour de force* of Monte Carlo techniques, with varied computational complexity and approximation quality.

In this paper, we introduce an alternative probabilistic nearest neighbors predictive model constructed from an aggregation of simpler models whose normalizing constants can be exactly summed in polynomial time. We begin by reviewing the Cucala et al. model in Section 2, showing by an elementary argument that the computational complexity of the exact summation of its normalizing constant is directly tied to the concept of NP-completeness [6]. The necessary concepts from the theory of computational complexity are briefly reviewed. Section 3 introduces a family of nonlocal models, whose joint distributions take into account only the interactions between each sample unit and its $r$-th nearest neighbor. For each nonlocal model, we derive an analytic expression for its normalizing constant, which can be computed exactly in polynomial time. The nonlocal models are combined in Section 4, yielding a predictive distribution that does not rely on costly Monte

Carlo approximations. We run experiments with synthetic and real datasets, showing that our model achieves the predictive performance of the Cucala et al. model, with a more manageable computational cost. We present our conclusions in Section 5.

## 2. A Case of Intractable Normalization

This section sets the environment for the general classification problem discussed in this paper. We begin in Section 2.1 with the definition of the Cucala et al. Bayesian nearest neighbors classification model, whose normalizing constant requires an exponential number of operations for brute force calculation. We indicate the Monte Carlo techniques used by the authors to sample from the model posterior distribution, as well as the approximations made to circumvent the computational complexity issues. Section 2.2 reviews briefly the fundamental concepts of the theory of computational complexity, ending up with the characterization of NP-complete decision problems, which are considered intractable. Section 2.3 establishes by an elementary argument a connection between the summation of the normalizing constant appearing on the likelihood of the Cucala et al. model and one of the classical NP-complete problems. In a nutshell, we show that the availability of an algorithm to exactly compute the normalizing constant of the Cucala et al. model in polynomial time in an ordinary computer would imply that all so-called NP problems could also be solved in polynomial time under equivalent conditions.

### 2.1. The Cucala et al. Model

Suppose that we have a size $n$ training sample such that for each sample unit we know the value of a vector $x_i \in \mathbb{R}^p$ of predictor variables and a response variable $y_i$ belonging to a set of class labels $\mathscr{L} = \{1, 2, \dots, L\}$. Some notion of proximity between training sample units is given in terms of the corresponding vectors of predictors. For example, we may use the Euclidean distance between the vectors of predictors of every pair of training sample units to establish a notion of neighborhood in the training sample. Given this neighborhood structure, let the brackets $[i]_r$ denote the index of the sample unit in the training sample that is the $r$-th nearest neighbor of the $i$-th sample unit, for $i = 1, \dots, n$, and $r = 1, \dots, n-1$.

Introducing the notations $x = (x_1, \dots, x_n)$ and $y = (y_1, \dots, y_n)$, the Cucala et al. model [5] is defined by the joint distribution

$$p(y \mid x, \beta, k) = \frac{1}{Z(\beta, k)} \exp\left( \frac{\beta}{k} \sum_{i=1}^{n} \sum_{r=1}^{k} \mathbb{I}(y_i = y_{[i]_r}) \right),$$

in which $\beta > 0$ and $k = 1, \dots, n-1$ are model parameters and $\mathbb{I}(\,\cdot\,)$ denotes an indicator function. Notice that dependence on the predictors occurs through the neighborhood brackets $[i]_r$, which are determined by the $x_i$'s. The model normalizing constant is given by

$$Z(\beta, k) = \sum_{y \in \mathscr{L}^n} \exp\left( \frac{\beta}{k} \sum_{i=1}^{n} \sum_{r=1}^{k} \mathbb{I}(y_i = y_{[i]_r}) \right).$$

From this definition, we see that direct (brute force) summation of $Z(\beta, k)$ would involve an exponential number of operations ($\mathcal{O}(L^n)$). The much more subtle question about the possible existence of an algorithm that would allow us to exactly compute $Z(\beta, k)$ in polynomial time is addressed in Section 2.3.

In their paper [5], the authors relied on a series of techniques to implement Markov Chain Monte Carlo (MCMC) frameworks in the presence of the seemingly intractable model normalizing constant $Z(\beta, k)$. They developed solutions based on pseudo-likelihood [7], path sampling [8,9] (which essentially approximates $Z(\beta, k)$ using a computationally intensive process, for each value of the pair $(\beta, k)$ appearing in the iterations of the underlying MCMC procedure) and the Møller et al. auxiliary variable method [10]. Although there is currently no publicly available source code for further experimentation, at the end of Section 3.4 the authors report computation times ranging from twenty minutes to more than one week for the different methods using compiled code. We refer the reader to [5] for the technical details.

### 2.2. Computational Complexity

Informally, by a deterministic computer we mean a device or process that executes the instructions in a given algorithm one at a time in a single-threaded fashion. A decision problem is one whose computation ends with a "yes" or "no" output after a certain number of steps, which is referred to as the running time of the algorithm. The class of all decision problems, with the input size measured by a positive integer $n$, for which there exists an algorithm whose running time on a deterministic computer is bounded by a polynomial in $n$, is denoted by P. We think of P as the class of computationally "easy" or tractable decision problems. Notable P problems are the decision version of linear programming and the problem of determining if a number is prime.

A nondeterministic computer is an idealized device whose programs are allowed to branch the computation at each step into an *arbitrary* number of parallel threads. The class of nondeterministic polynomial (NP) decision problems contains all decision problems for which there is an algorithm or program that runs in polynomial time on a nondeterministic computer. An alternative and equivalent view is that NP problems are those decision problems whose solution is difficult to find but easy to verify. We think of NP problems as the class of computationally "hard" or intractable decision problems. Notable NP problems are the Boolean satisfiability (SAT) problem and the travelling salesman problem. Every problem in P is obviously in NP. In principle, for any NP problem, it could be possible to find an algorithm solving the problem in polynomial time on a deterministic computer. However, a proof for a single NP problem that there is no algorithm running on a deterministic computer that could solve it in polynomial time would establish that the classes P and NP are not equal. The problem of whether P is or is not equal to NP is the most famous open question of theoretical computer science.

Two given decision problems can be connected by the device of polynomial reduction. Informally, suppose that there is a subroutine that solves the first problem. We say that the first problem is polynomial time reducible to the second if both the time required to transform the first problem into the second and the number of times the subroutine is called are bounded by a polynomial in $n$.

In 1971, Stephen Cook [11] proved that all NP problems are polynomial-time-reducible to SAT, meaning that 1) no NP problem is harder than SAT and 2) a polynomial time algorithm that solves SAT on a deterministic computer would give a polynomial time algorithm solving every other NP problem on a deterministic computer, ultimately implying that P is equal to NP. In general terms, a problem is said to be NP-complete if it is NP and all other NP problems can be polynomial-time reduced to it, and SAT was the first ever problem proven to be NP-complete. In a sense, each NP-complete problem encodes the quintessence of intractability.

### 2.3. $Z(\beta, k)$ and NP Completeness

Let $G = (V, E)$ be an undirected graph, in which $V$ is a set of vertices and $E$ is a set of edges $e = \{v, v'\}$, with $v, v' \in V$. Given a function $w : E \to \mathbb{Z}_+$, we refer to $w(e)$ as the weight of the edge $e \in E$. A cut of $G$ is a partition of $V$ into disjoint sets $V_0$ and $V_1$. The size of the cut is the sum of the weights of the edges in $E$ with one endpoint in $V_0$ and one endpoint in $V_1$. The decision problem known as the *maximum cut* can be stated as follows: for a given integer $m$, is there a cut of $G$ with size at least $m$? Karp [12] proved that the general maximum cut problem is NP-complete. In what follows, we point to an elementary link between the exact summation of the normalizing constant $Z(\beta, k)$ of the Cucala et al. model and the decision of an associated maximum cut problem.

Without a loss of generality, suppose that we are dealing with a binary classification problem in which the response variable $y_i \in \{0, 1\}$, for $i = 1, \ldots, n$. Define the $n \times n$ matrix $A = (a_{ij})$ by $a_{ij} = 1$ if $j$ is one of the $k$ nearest neighbors of $i$, and $a_{ij} = 0$ otherwise.

Letting $B = (b_{ij}) = A + A^\top$, this is the adjacency matrix of a weighted undirected graph $G$, whose vertices represent the training sample units, and the edges connecting these vertices may have weights zero, one, or two, based on whether the corresponding training sample units do not belong to each other's $k$-neighborhoods, just one belongs to the other's $k$-neighborhood, or both are part of each other's $k$-neighborhoods, respectively. The double sum in the exponent of $Z(\beta, k)$ can be rewritten as

$$T(y) = \sum_{i=1}^{n} \sum_{r=1}^{k} \mathbb{I}(y_i = y_{[i]_r}) = \sum_{i,j=1}^{n} a_{ij}\, \mathbb{I}(y_i = y_j) = \frac{1}{2} \sum_{i,j=1}^{n} b_{ij}\, \mathbb{I}(y_i = y_j),$$

for every $y \in \{0,1\}^n$. Furthermore, each $y \in \{0,1\}^n$ corresponds to a cut of the graph $G$ if we define the disjoint sets of vertices $V_0 = \{i \in E : y_i = 0\}$ and $V_1 = \{i \in E : y_i = 1\}$. The respective cut size is given by:

$$\texttt{cut-size}(y) = \frac{1}{2} \sum_{i,j=1}^{n} b_{ij}\, \mathbb{I}(y_i \neq y_j).$$

Since for every $y \in \{0,1\}^n$ we have that

$$\sum_{i,j=1}^{n} b_{ij} = \sum_{i,j=1}^{n} b_{ij}\, \mathbb{I}(y_i = y_j) + \sum_{i,j=1}^{n} b_{ij}\, \mathbb{I}(y_i \neq y_j),$$

it follows that

$$\texttt{cut-size}(y) = \left( \frac{1}{2} \sum_{i,j=1}^{n} b_{ij} \right) - T(y). \qquad (*)$$

Figure 1 gives an example for a specific neighborhood structure involving the three nearest neighbors with respect to Euclidean distance.

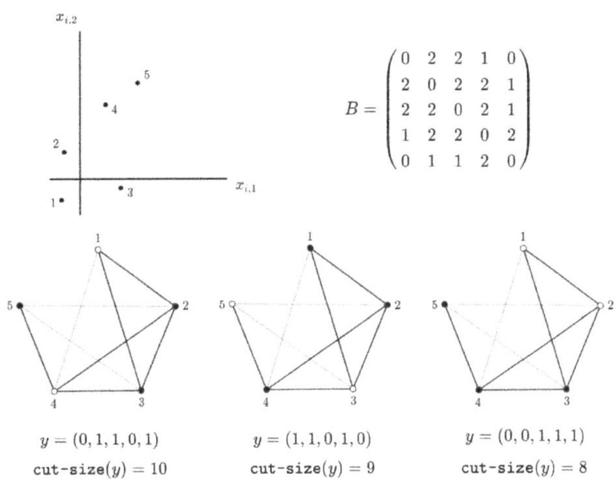


**Figure 1.** Weighted undirected nonplanar graphs associated with a specific neighborhood structure, determined by the three nearest neighbors according to Euclidean distance, and the sizes of three different cuts, obtained by summing the weights of all edges linking two vertices of different colors. On each graph, light gray and black edges have weights with values one and two, respectively, according to the adjacency matrix $B$. Black and white vertices correspond to class labels being equal to one and zero, respectively.

By grouping each possible value of $T(y)$ in the sum over $y \in \{0,1\}^n$ appearing in the definition of $Z(\beta, k)$, we obtain the alternative polynomial representation

$$Z(\beta, k) = \sum_{t=0}^{nk} d_t z^t,$$

in which $z = e^{\beta/k}$ and $d_t = \sum_{y\in\{0,1\}^n} \mathbb{I}(T(y) = t)$, for $t = 0, 1, \ldots, nk$. Note that $d_t$ is the number of vectors $y \in \{0,1\}^n$ such that $T(y) = t$, and from $(*)$ we have that $d_t$ is also the number of possible cuts of the graph $G$ with size $\left(\frac{1}{2}\sum_{i,j=1}^{n} b_{ij}\right) - t$.

Suppose that we have found a way to sum $Z(\beta, k)$ in polynomial time on a deterministic computer, for every possible value of $\beta$ and $k$ and any specified neighborhood structure. By polynomial interpolation (see [13]), we would be able to compute the value of each coefficient $d_t$ in polynomial time, thus determining the number of cuts of $G$ with all possible sizes, thereby solving any maximum cut decision problem associated with the graph $G$. In other words: the existence of a polynomial time algorithm to sum $Z(\beta, k)$ *for an arbitrary neighborhood structure* on a deterministic computer would imply that P is equal to NP.

## 3. Nonlocal Models Are Tractable

This section introduces a family of models that are related to the Cucala et al. model but differ in two significant ways. First, making use of a physical analogy, while the likelihood function of the Cucala et al. model is such that each sampling unit "interacts" with all of its $k$ nearest neighbors, for the models introduced in this section each sampling unit interacts only with its $r$-th nearest neighbor, for some $r = 1, \ldots, n-1$. Keeping up with the physical analogy, we say that we a have a family of nonlocal models (for the sake of simplicity, we are abusing terminology a little bit here, since the model with $r = 1$ is perfectly "local"). Second, the nice fact about the nonlocal models is that their normalizing constants are tractable; the main result of this section being an explicit analytic expression for the normalizing constant of a nonlocal model that is computable in polynomial time. The purpose of these nonlocal models is to work as building blocks for our final aggregated probabilistic predictive model in Section 4.

For $r = 1, \ldots, n-1$, the likelihood of the $r$-th nonlocal model is defined as

$$p_r(y \mid x, \beta_r) = \frac{1}{Z_r(\beta_r)} \exp\left(\beta_r \sum_{i=1}^{n} \mathbb{I}(y_i = y_{[i]_r})\right),$$

in which the normalizing constant is given by

$$Z_r(\beta_r) = \sum_{y\in\mathscr{L}^n} \exp\left(\beta_r \sum_{i=1}^{n} \mathbb{I}(y_i = y_{[i]_r})\right),$$

with parameter $\beta_r \geq 0$.

In line with what was pointed out in our discussion of the normalizing constant $Z(\beta, k)$ of the Cucala et al. model, brute force computation of $Z_r(\beta_r)$ is also hopeless for the nonlocal models, requiring the summation of an exponential number of terms ($\mathcal{O}(L^n)$). However, the much simpler topology associated with the neighborhood structure of a nonlocal model can be exploited to give us a path to sum $Z_r(\beta_r)$ analytically, resulting in an expression that can be computed exactly in polynomial time on an ordinary computer.

Throughout the remainder of this section, our goal is to derive a tractable closed form for the normalizing constant $Z_r(\beta_r)$. For the $r$-th nonlocal model, consider the directed graph $G = (V, E)$ representing the associated neighborhood structure of a given training sample. For $i = 1, \ldots, n$, each vertex $i \in V$ corresponds to one training sample unit, and the existence of an oriented edge $(i, j) \in E$, represented pictorially by an arrow pointing from $i$ to $j$, means that the $j$-th sample unit is the $r$-th nearest neighbor of the $i$-th sample unit.

An example is given in Figure 2 for the nonlocal models with $r = 1$ and $r = 2$. We see that in general $G$ can be decomposed into totally disconnected subgraphs $G' = (V', E'), G'' = (V'', E''), \ldots$, meaning that vertices in one subgraph have no arrows pointing to vertices in the other subgraphs. If $V' = \{i_1, \ldots, i_k\}$, we use the notation for the multiple sum

$$\sum_{\substack{y_i=1\\ i\in V'}}^{L} := \sum_{y_{i_1}=1}^{L} \cdots \sum_{y_{i_k}=1}^{L}.$$

Since

$$\sum_{y\in\mathscr{L}^n} := \sum_{y_1=1}^{L}\sum_{y_2=1}^{L}\cdots\sum_{y_n=1}^{L},$$

the normalizing constant $Z_r(\beta_r)$ can be factored as a product of summations involving only the $y_i$'s associated with each subgraph:

$$Z_r(\beta_r) = \left(\sum_{\substack{y_i=1\\ i\in V'}}^{L} \exp\left(\beta_r \sum_{i=1}^{n} \mathbb{I}(y_i = y_{[i]_r})\right)\right) \times \left(\sum_{\substack{y_i=1\\ i\in V''}}^{L} \exp\left(\beta_r \sum_{i=1}^{n} \mathbb{I}(y_i = y_{[i]_r})\right)\right) \times \cdots.$$

For each subgraph, starting at some vertex and following the arrows pointing to each subsequent vertex, if we return to the first vertex after $m$ steps, we say that the subgraph has a simple cycle of size $m$. The outdegree of a vertex is the number of arrows pointing from it to other vertices; the indegree of a vertex is defined analogously. Figure 3 depicts the fact that each subgraph has exactly one simple cycle: in a subgraph without simple cycles, there would be at least one vertex with outdegree equal to zero. Moreover, a subgraph with more than one simple cycle would have at least one vertex in one of the simple cycles pointing to a vertex in another simple cycle, implying that such a vertex would have outdegree equal to two. Both cases contradict the fact that every vertex of each subgraph has outdegree equal to one, since each sample unit has exactly one $r$-th nearest neighbor.

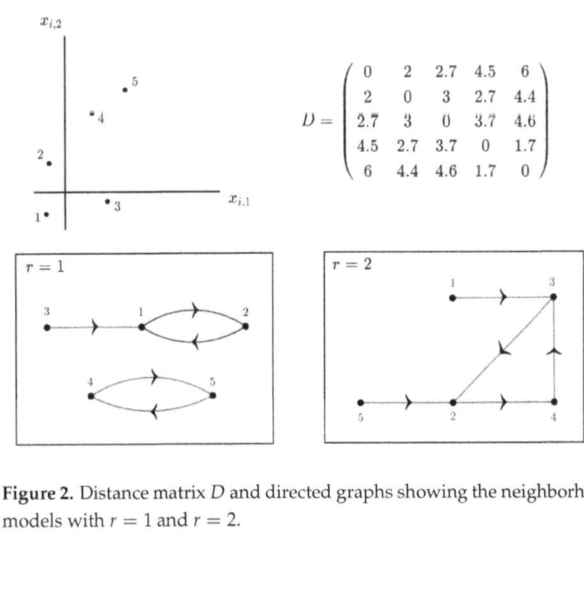


**Figure 2.** Distance matrix $D$ and directed graphs showing the neighborhood structure for the nonlocal models with $r = 1$ and $r = 2$.

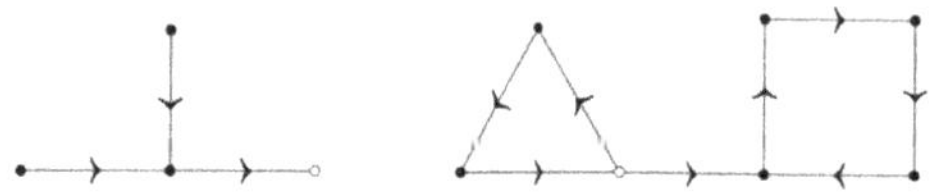

**Figure 3.** Two impossible directed graphs for a nonlocal model. On the left graph, the white vertex has outdegree equal to zero. On the right graph, the white vertex has outdegree equal to two. Both graphs contradict the fact that each training sample unit has exactly one $r$-th nearest neighbor. The conclusion is that in a directed graph describing the neighborhood structure of a nonlocal model each subgraph contains exactly one simple cycle.

Figure 4 portrays the reduction process used to perform the summations for one subgraph. For each vertex with indegree equal to zero, we sum over the correspondent $y_i$ and remove the vertex from the graph. We repeat this process until we are left with a summation over the vertices forming the simple cycle. The summation for each vertex $i$ with indegree equal to zero in this reduction process gives the factor

$$\sum_{y_i=1}^{L} \exp(\beta_r \mathbb{I}(y_i = y_{[i]_r})) = e^{\beta_r} + L - 1,$$

because—and this is a crucial aspect of the reduction process—in this sum the indicator is equal to one just for a single term, and it is equal to zero for all the remaining $L-1$ terms, *whatever the value of* $y_{[i]_r}$. Summation over the vertices forming the simple cycle is performed as follows. Relabeling the indexes of the sample units if necessary, suppose that the vertices forming a simple cycle of size $m$ are labeled as $1, 2, \ldots, m$. Defining the matrix $S = (s_{a,b})$ by $s_{a,b} = \exp(\beta_r \mathbb{I}(a = b))$, we have

$$\begin{aligned}
&\sum_{y_1=1}^{L} \sum_{y_2=1}^{L} \cdots \sum_{y_m=1}^{L} \exp(\beta_r \mathbb{I}(y_1 = y_2)) \times \exp(\beta_r \mathbb{I}(y_2 = y_3)) \times \cdots \times \exp(\beta_r \mathbb{I}(y_m = y_1)) \\
&\quad = \sum_{y_1=1}^{L} \sum_{y_2=1}^{L} \cdots \sum_{y_m=1}^{L} s_{y_1,y_2} \times s_{y_2,y_3} \times \cdots \times s_{y_m,y_1} = \sum_{y_1=1}^{L} (S^m)_{y_1,y_1} = \operatorname{Tr}(S^m).
\end{aligned}$$

By the spectral decomposition [14], we have that $S = Q\Lambda Q^\top$, with $QQ^\top = Q^\top Q = I$. Therefore, $S^m = Q\Lambda^m Q^\top$, implying that $\operatorname{Tr}(S^m) = \operatorname{Tr}(\Lambda^m Q^\top Q) = \operatorname{Tr}(\Lambda^m) = \sum_{\ell=1}^{L} \lambda_\ell^m$, in which we used the cyclic property of the trace, and the $\lambda_\ell$'s are the eigenvalues of $S$, which are easy to compute: the characteristic polynomial of $S$ is

$$\det(S - \lambda I) = (e^{\beta_r} - 1 - \lambda)^{L-1}(e^{\beta_r} + L - 1 - \lambda) = 0,$$

yielding

$$\lambda_1 = \lambda_2 = \cdots = \lambda_{L-1} = e^{\beta_r} - 1, \text{ and } \lambda_L = e^{\beta_r} + L - 1.$$

For the $r$-th nonlocal model, let $c_m^{(r)}$ be the number of simple cycles of size $m$, considering all the associated subgraphs. Algorithm 1 shows how to compute $c_m^{(r)}$, for $r = 1, \ldots, n-1$ and $m = 2, \ldots, n$, in polynomial time. Taking into account all the subgraphs, and multiplying all the factors, we arrive at the final expression:

$$Z_r(\beta_r) = (e^{\beta_r} + L - 1)^{n - \sum_{m=2}^{n} m \times c_m^{(r)}} \times \prod_{m=2}^{n} \left( (e^{\beta_r} + L - 1)^m + (L-1)(e^{\beta_r} - 1)^m \right)^{c_m^{(r)}}.$$

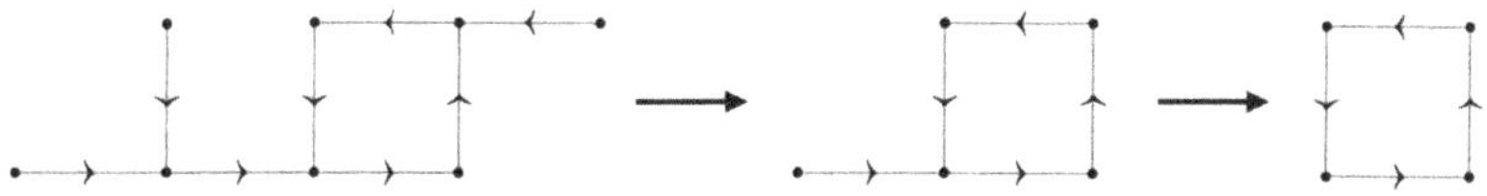

**Figure 4.** Example of the reduction process for the summation on each subgraph.

**Algorithm 1** Count the occurrences of simple cycles of different sizes on the directed subgraphs representing the neighborhood structures of all nonlocal models

**Require:** Neighborhood brackets $\{[i]_r : i = 1, \ldots, n; r = 1, \ldots, n-1\}$.

```
function COUNT_SIMPLE_CYCLES({[i]_r : i = 1,...,n; r = 1,...,n-1})
    c_m^(r) ← 0 for (r, m) ∈ {1,...,n-1} × {2,...,n}
    for r ← 1 to n-1 do
        visited ← ∅
        for j ← 1 to n do
            next if j ∈ visited
            i ← j
            walk ← empty stack
            while i ∉ visited do
                visited ← visited ∪ {i}
                push i into walk
                i ← [i]_r
            end while
            m ← 1
            while walk not empty do
                delete top element from walk
                if top element of walk = i then
                    c_m^(r) ← c_m^(r) + 1
                    break
                end if
                m ← m + 1
            end while
        end for
    end for
    return {c_m^(r) : r = 1,...,n-1; m = 2,...,n}
end function
```

## 4. Predictive Model

The nonlocal models developed in Section 3 will be the building blocks of our probabilistic nearest neighbors classification model. Introducing a hyperparameter $k = 1, \ldots, n-1$, the first $k$ nonlocal models can be combined; the heuristic being that a "superposition" of nonlocal models could work as a model whose neighborhood structure takes into account the sets of $k$ nearest neighbors of each sample unit. Section 4.1 explains the aggregation procedure leading to the predictive distribution of the combined model. The results in Section 4.2 showcase the computational cost and the predictive performance of the new model, examining the same synthetic and real datasets explored in [5].

### 4.1. Aggregating the Predictions of the Nonlocal Models

For the $r$-th nonlocal model, with $r = 1, \ldots, n-1$, using the information in the training sample and the analytic expression obtained for $Z_r(\beta_r)$ in Section 3, we construct an estimate $\hat{\beta}_r$ for the parameter $\beta_r$ by maximizing the corresponding likelihood function:

$$\hat{\beta}_r = \arg\max_{\beta_r \geq 0} p_r(y \mid x, \beta_r) = \arg\max_{\beta_r \geq 0} \left( \frac{1}{Z_r(\beta_r)} \exp\left( \beta_r \sum_{i=1}^{n} \mathbb{I}(y_i = y_{[i]_r}) \right) \right).$$

Using this estimate, we define the predictive distribution of the $r$-th nonlocal model as

$$p_r(y_{n+1} \mid x_{n+1}, x, y) := p_r(y_{n+1} \mid x_{n+1}, x, y, \hat{\beta}_r) \\ \propto \exp\left( \hat{\beta}_r \left( \mathbb{I}(y_{n+1} = y_{[n+1]_r}) + \sum_{i=1}^{n} \mathbb{I}(y_i = y_{n+1}, [i]_r = n+1) \right) \right),$$

with $\sum_{y_{n+1}=1}^{L} p_r(y_{n+1} \mid x_{n+1}, x, y) = 1$.

Finally, we aggregate the predictive distributions of the nonlocal models, introducing a hyperparameter $k = 1, \ldots, n-1$ and defining

$$p_{(k)}(y_{n+1} \mid x_{n+1}, x, y) := \frac{1}{k} \sum_{r=1}^{k} p_r(y_{n+1} \mid x_{n+1}, x, y).$$

The value of the hyperparameter $k$ is chosen using leave-one-out cross validation [15] on the training sample. From now on, we refer to this predictive model as the probabilistic nearest neighbors classification model (`pnnclass`, for short).

An open source software library implementing the predictive model described in this section is publicly available at https://github.com/paulocmarquesf/pnnclass (access on 29 December 2023). It is an R [16] library, having internal routines written in C++ [17] with the help of Rcpp [18].

### 4.2. Experiments with Synthetic and Real Datasets

The first example examined in [5] was the simulated dataset proposed by Ripley in his classic book [19]. It consists of training and testing samples with sizes 250 and 1 000, respectively. The response variable is binary, and we have two generic real-valued predictor variables. The `pnnclass` predictive model achieves a testing error rate of 8.4%, which is the same as the best error rate reported in [5] for this dataset. Doing 100 replications, the median running time using the `pnnclass` library was 124.45 milliseconds, on a standard notebook with an Intel i7-11390H processor. Figure 5 shows the training sample and a heatmap representing the probabilities produced by the `pnnclass` predictive model. Figure 6 reports the classifier ROC curve obtained using the testing sample. The annotated summaries correspond to the probability threshold maximizing the sum of the classifier sensitivity and specificity.

The second example examined in [5] was the Pima Indian women diabetes dataset, available in the MASS R library [20], with training and test samples of sizes 200 and 332, respectively. In this dataset, for each sample unit we have the values of seven numerical predictors, and the response variable is again binary, indicating the result of the diabetes diagnosis for the corresponding sample unit. The `pnnclass` predictive model achieves a testing error rate of 21.99%, which is close to the best error rate reported in [5] for this dataset (20.9%). Performing 100 replications, the median running time using the `pnnclass` library was 59.04 milliseconds. The ROC curve and summaries for the Pima Indian dataset are given in Figure 6.

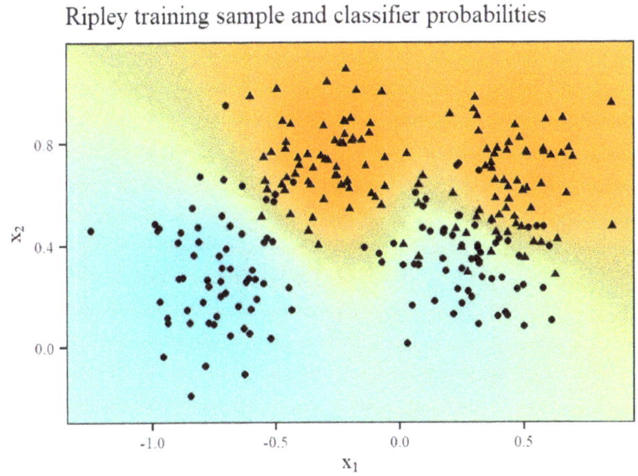


**Figure 5.** Training sample for the Ripley synthetic dataset. Circles and triangles indicate the two possible values of the response variable. The heatmap represents the probabilities of class "triangle" given by the predictive model `pnnclass`, ranging from pure cyan (probability zero) to pure orange (probability one).

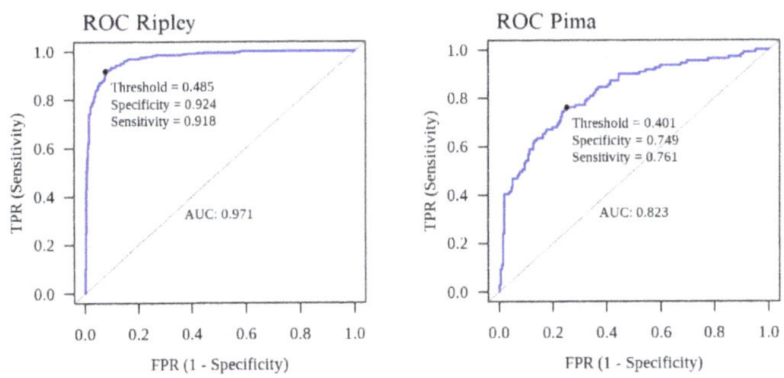


**Figure 6.** ROC curves for the Ripley and the Pima Indian datasets. Annotated summaries correspond to the probability threshold maximizing the sum of the classifier sensitivity and specificity.

The third and final example considered in [5] was the multiclass Forensic Glass fragments dataset described in [19]. In this dataset, we have nine numerical predictors, and the response variable was coalesced into four classes. With randomly split training and testing samples of sizes 89 and 96, respectively, the `pnnclass` predictive model achieves a testing error rate of 28.04%, which is better than the error rate of 29% reported in [5] for this dataset. Performing 100 replications, the median running time using the `pnnclass` library was 9.15 milliseconds. Since in this dataset the predictor space is nine-dimensional, in Figure 7 we use Principal Component Analysis (PCA) as a visualization tool to depict the predictive performance on the the testing sample (PCA played no role in the modeling process). The confusion matrix for the Forensic Glass testing sample is given in Table 1. Table 2 gives more detailed summaries for the running times on the three datasets. Table 3 summarizes the predictive performance comparison between the `pnnclass` and the Cucala et al. models for the three datasets. For comparison, we added the test errors of a Random Forest [21,22] constructed by bootstrap aggregating 500 classification trees.

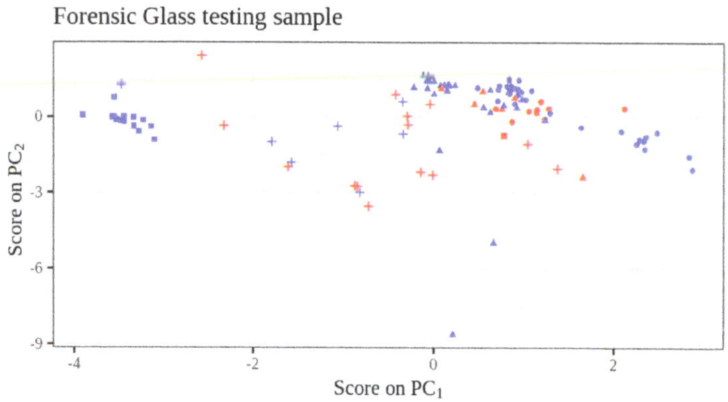


**Figure 7.** Testing sample scores on the first two principal components of the predictors in the Forensic Glass dataset. The different shapes indicate the four possible values of the response variable. The colors blue or red mean, respectively, that the corresponding testing sample units were classified correctly or incorrectly.

**Table 1.** Confusion matrix for the Forensic Glass testing sample.

| | | | | **Observed Class** | |
|---|---|---|---|---|---|
| | | **0** | **1** | **2** | **3** |
| Predicted class | **0** | 29 | 2 | 0 | 5 |
| | **1** | 2 | 27 | 1 | 7 |
| | **2** | 0 | 1 | 14 | 2 |
| | **3** | 7 | 3 | 0 | 7 |

**Table 2.** Descriptive summaries for the running times in milliseconds of the `pnnclass` predictive model library based on 100 replications.

| **Dataset** | **Median (ms)** | **Min (ms)** | **Max (ms)** |
|---|---|---|---|
| Ripley | 124.45 | 118.83 | 182.34 |
| Pima Indian | 59.04 | 52.68 | 114.97 |
| Forensic Glass | 9.15 | 8.80 | 16.38 |

**Table 3.** Testing errors for the three datasets. In the third column, we report the smallest errors achieved in [5] considering all Monte Carlo approximations implemented by the authors.

| **Dataset** | `pnnclass` | **Cucala et al.** | **Random Forest** |
|---|---|---|---|
| Ripley | 8.4% | 8.4% | [illegible] |
| Pima Indian | 21.99% | 20.9% | 24.1% |
| Forensic Glass | 28.04% | 29% | 24.3% |

## 5. Concluding Remarks

This work can be seen as the construction of a probabilistic predictive model based on the concept of nearest neighbors, wherein we shifted the algorithmic complexity of the solution from an intractable class into the realm of polynomial time computation. It would be interesting to explore how the ideas discussed in this paper could be adapted to assist in the analysis of spatial data models or models with graph-type data in general, since these models may pose similar challenges related to the presence of intractable normalizing constants in the corresponding likelihood functions.

**Author Contributions:** Conceptualization, B.F., P.C.M.F. and H.F.L.; Methodology, B.F., P.C.M.F. and H.F.L.; Software, B.F., P.C.M.F. and H.F.L. All authors have read and agreed to the published version of the manuscript.

**Funding:** Hedibert F. Lopes and Paulo C. Marques F. receive support from FAPESP (Fundação de Amparo à Pesquisa do Estado de São Paulo) through projects 2018/04654-9 and 2023/02538-0.

**Data Availability Statement:** The data used in the paper is available through the software library developed by the authors.

**Conflicts of Interest:** The authors declare no conflicts of interest.

## References

1. Fix, E.; Hodges, J.L. Discriminatory analysis—Nonparametric discrimination: Consistency properties. *Int. Stat. Rev.* **1989**, *57*, 238–247. [CrossRef]
2. Devroye, L.; Györfi, L.; Lugosi, G. *A Probabilistic Theory of Pattern Recognition*; Springer: Berlin, Germany, 2013; Volume 31.
3. Biau, G.; Devroye, L. *Lectures on the Nearest Neighbor Method*; Springer: Berlin, Germany, 2015; Volume 246.
4. Holmes, C.; Adams, N. A probabilistic nearest neighbour method for statistical pattern recognition. *J. R. Stat. Soc. B Stat. Methodol.* **2002**, *64*, 295–306. [CrossRef]
5. Cucala, L.; Marin, J.M.; Robert, C.P.; Titterington, D.M. A Bayesian Reassessment of Nearest-Neighbor Classification. *J. Am. Stat. Assoc.* **2009**, *104*, 263–273. [CrossRef]
6. Garey, M.R.; Johnson, D.S. *Computers and Intractability: A Guide to the Theory of NP-Completeness*; W. H. Freeman: New York, NY, USA, 1979.
7. Besag, J. Spatial Interaction and the Statistical Analysis of Lattice Systems. *J. R. Stat. Soc. B Stat. Methodol.* **1974**, *36*, 192–236. [CrossRef]
8. Ogata, Y. A Monte Carlo method for high dimensional integration. *Numer. Math.* **1989**, *55*, 137–157. [CrossRef]
9. Gelman, A.; Meng, X.L. Simulating Normalizing Constants: From Importance Sampling to Bridge Sampling to Path Sampling. *Stat. Sci.* **1998**, *13*, 163–185. [CrossRef]
10. Møller, J.; Pettitt, A.N.; Reeves, R.; Berthelsen, K.K. An Efficient Markov Chain Monte Carlo Method for Distributions with Intractable Normalising Constants. *Biometrika* **2006**, *93*, 451–458. [CrossRef]
11. Cook, S.A. The Complexity of Theorem-Proving Procedures. In Proceedings of the STOC '71: Third Annual ACM Symposium on Theory of Computing, Shaker Heights, OH, USA, 3–May 1971; Association for Computing Machinery: New York, NY, USA, 1971; pp. 151–158. [CrossRef]
12. Karp, R. Reducibility Among Combinatorial Problems. In *Complexity of Computer Computations*; Miller, R., Thatcher, J., Eds.; Plenum Press: New York, NY, USA, 1972; pp. 85–103.
13. Rivlin, T. *An Introduction to the Approximation of Functions*; Blaisdell Publishing Company: Waltham, MA, USA, 1969.
14. Strang, G. *Linear Algebra and Its Applications*; Thomson, Brooks/Cole: Pacific Grove, CA, USA, 2006.
15. Hastie, T.; Tibshirani, R.; Friedman, J. *The Elements of Statistical Learning: Data Mining, Inference, and Prediction*, 2nd ed.; Springer: Berlin, Germany, 2009.
16. R Core Team. *R: A Language and Environment for Statistical Computing*; R Foundation for Statistical Computing: Vienna, Austria, 2017.
17. Stroustrup, B. *The C++ Programming Language*, 4th ed.; Addison-Wesley Professional: Reading, MA, USA, 2013.
18. Eddelbuettel, D. *Seamless R and C++ Integration with Rcpp*; Springer: Berlin, Germany, 2013.
19. Ripley, B.D. *Pattern Recognition and Neural Networks*; Cambridge University Press: Cambridge, UK, 1996. [CrossRef]
20. Venables, W.N.; Ripley, B.D. *Modern Applied Statistics with S*, 4th ed.; Springer: New York, NY, USA, 2002; ISBN 0-387-95457-0.
21. Breiman, L. Random Forests. *Mach. Learn.* **2001**, *45*, 5–32. [CrossRef]
22. Marques F., P.C. Confidence intervals for the random forest generalization error. *Pattern Recognit. Lett.* **2022**, *158*, 171–175. [CrossRef]

*entropy*

*Article*

# Objective Priors for Invariant *e*-Values in the Presence of Nuisance Parameters

**Elena Bortolato † and Laura Ventura *,†**

Department of Statistical Sciences, University of Padova, 35121 Padova, Italy; elena.bortolato@unipd.it
* Correspondence: ventura@stat.unipd.it
† These authors contributed equally to this work.

**Abstract:** This paper aims to contribute to refining the *e*-values for testing precise hypotheses, especially when dealing with nuisance parameters, leveraging the effectiveness of asymptotic expansions of the posterior. The proposed approach offers the advantage of bypassing the need for elicitation of priors and reference functions for the nuisance parameters and the multidimensional integration step. For this purpose, starting from a Laplace approximation, a posterior distribution for the parameter of interest is only considered and then a suitable objective matching prior is introduced, ensuring that the posterior mode aligns with an equivariant frequentist estimator. Consequently, both Highest Probability Density credible sets and the *e*-value remain invariant. Some targeted and challenging examples are discussed.

**Keywords:** asymptotic expansions; adjusted score function; bias reduction; evidence; Full Bayesian Significance Test; higher-order asymptotics; matching priors; median bias reduction

## 1. Introduction

In this article, we discuss an objective matching prior that maintains the invariance of the posterior mode when testing specific hypotheses for parametric models, especially in the presence of nuisance parameters. These parameters are often introduced to establish flexible and realistic models, although the primary focus of inference is typically limited to a parameter of interest. The proposed approach offers the advantage of eliminating the need for eliciting information on the nuisance components and for conducting multidimensional integration, and it produces invariant *e*-values in the presence of nuisance parameters.

The parametric framework that we consider can be described as follows. Consider a random sample $y = (y_1, \ldots, y_n)$ of size $n$ from a random variable $Y$ with parametric model $f(y;\theta)$, indexed by a paramater $\theta$, with $\theta \in \Theta \subseteq \mathbb{R}^d$. Given a prior $\pi(\theta)$ on $\theta$, Bayesian inference for $\theta$ is based on the posterior density

$$\pi(\theta|y) \propto \pi(\theta)L(\theta), \tag{1}$$

where $L(\theta)$ represents the likelihood function based on $f(y;\theta)$. Interest is, in particular, in the situation in which $\theta = (\psi, \lambda)$, where $\psi$ is a scalar parameter for which inference is required, and $\lambda$ represents the remaining $(d-1)$ nuisance parameters. In such case, Bayesian inference for $\psi$ is based on the marginal posterior density

$$\pi_m(\psi|y) = \int \pi(\psi,\lambda|y)\, d\lambda \propto \int \pi(\psi,\lambda)L(\psi,\lambda)\, d\lambda, \tag{2}$$

which for its computation requires both elicitation on the nuisance parameter $\lambda$ and multidimensional integration.

Asymptotic arguments are widely used in Bayesian inference through (1) and (2), based on developments of so-called higher-order asymptotics (see, e.g., [1–3]). Indeed, the theory of asymptotic expansions provides very accurate approximations to posterior distributions, and to various summary quantities of interest, including tail areas, credible regions and for the Full Bayesian Significance Test (see, e.g., [4,5]). Moreover, they are particularly useful for sensitivity analyses (see [6,7]) and also for the derivation of matching priors (see [8], and references therein). For instance, focusing on the presence of nuisance parameters, the Laplace approximation to (2) provides

$$\pi_m(\psi|y) \doteq \frac{1}{\sqrt{2\pi}}|j_p(\hat{\psi})|^{1/2}\exp\{\ell_p(\psi)-\ell_p(\hat{\psi})\}\frac{|j_{\lambda\lambda}(\hat{\psi},\hat{\lambda})|^{1/2}}{|j_{\lambda\lambda}(\psi,\hat{\lambda}_\psi)|^{1/2}}\frac{\pi(\psi,\hat{\lambda}_\psi)}{\pi(\hat{\psi},\hat{\lambda})}, \tag{3}$$

where $\ell_p(\psi) = \log L_p(\psi) = \log L(\psi, \hat{\lambda}_\psi)$ is the profile log-likelihood for $\psi$, with $\hat{\lambda}_\psi$ the constrained maximum likelihood estimate (MLE) of $\lambda$ given $\psi$, $(\hat{\psi}, \hat{\lambda})$ is the full MLE, and $j_p(\psi) = -\partial^2\ell_p(\psi)/\partial\psi^2$ is the profile observed information. Moreover, $j_{\lambda\lambda}(\psi,\lambda)$ is the $(\lambda,\lambda)$-block of the observed information from the full log-likelihood $\ell(\psi,\lambda) = \log L(\psi,\lambda)$, and the notation $\doteq$ indicates that the approximation is accurate to order $O(n^{-3/2})$ in moderate deviation regions (see, e.g., [9], Chapter 2). One appealing feature of higher-order approximations like (3) is that they may routinely be applied in practical Bayesian inference, since they require little more than standard likelihood quantities for their implementation, and hence, they may be available at little additional computational cost over simple first-order approximations.

In the presence of nuisance parameters, starting from approximation (3), it is possible to define a general posterior distribution for $\psi$ of the form

$$\pi^*(\psi|y) \propto \pi^*(\psi)L_p(\psi), \tag{4}$$

where $\pi^*(\psi)$ is now a prior distribution on $\psi$ only. Bayesian inference based on pseudo-likelihood functions—i.e., functions of $\psi$ only and of the data $y$ with properties similar to those of a genuine likelihood function, such as the profile likelihood—have been widely used and discussed in the recent statistical literature. Moreover, it has been theoretically motivated in several papers (see, for instance, [10–12], and references therein), also focusing on the derivation of suitable objective priors. Especially when the dimension of $\lambda$ is large, there are two advantages in using (4) instead of the marginal posterior distribution (2). First, the elicitation over $\lambda$ is not necessary, and second, the computation of the integrals in (2) is circumvented.

Focusing on (4), in this paper, it is of interest to test the precise (or sharp) null hypothesis

$$H_0 : \psi = \psi_0 \quad \text{against} \quad H_1 : \psi \neq \psi_0 \tag{5}$$

using the measure of evidence for the Full Bayesian Significance Test (see, e.g., [4,5]). The Full Bayesian Significance Test (FBST) quantifies evidence by considering the posterior probability associated with the least probable points in the parameter space under $H_0$. Higher-order asymptotic computation of the FBST for precise null hypotheses in the presence of nuisance parameters has been discussed in [13].

The original measure of evidence for the FBST is not invariant under suitable transformations of the parameter, a property which has, however, been reached in the more recent definition of the $e$-value (see [14,15], and references therein). Neverthless, when working on a scalar parameter of interest, in the presence of nuisance parameters, the $e$-value is not invariant with respect to marginalizations of the nuisance parameter, and it must be used in the full dimensionality of the parameter space. This requires elicitation on the complete parameters, numerical optimization and numerical integration, that can be computationally heavy, especially when the dimension of $\lambda$ is large.

The aim of this paper is to consider the $e$-value in the context of the pseudo-posterior distribution $\pi^*(\psi|y)$, suggesting in this respect a suitable objective prior $\pi^*(\psi)$ to be used in (4). More precisely, focus is on a particular matching prior, which ensures the invariance of the posterior mode of the pseudo-posterior distribution. As a consequence, Highest Probability Density credible (HPD) sets are also invariant, as well as the $e$-value.

This paper is organized as follows. Section 2 provides a short review on the FBST for testing precise null hypotheses and also illustrates asymptotic approximations for the $e$-value, extending results of [13]. Section 3 discusses the derivation of the objective matching prior for the parameter of interest only, called median matching prior, that produces invariant $e$-values. Also, several targeted and challenging examples are discussed. Finally, Section 4 closes with some concluding remarks.

## 2. The FBST Measure of Evidence

Suppose that we need to decide between two hypotheses: the null $H_0$ and the alternative $H_1$. The usual Bayesian testing procedure is based on the well-known Bayes factor (BF), defined as the ratio of the posterior odds to the prior odds in favor of the null hypothesis. A high BF or its logarithm suggests evidence in favor of $H_0$. However, it is well known that, when improper priors are used, the BF can be undetermined, and when the null hypothesis is precise (as specified in (5)), the BF can lead to the so-called Jeffreys–Lindley's paradox (see, e.g., [16]). Moreover, the BF is not calibrated, i.e., its finite sampling distribution is unknown and it may depend on the nuisance parameter.

To avoid these drawbacks, in recent years, an alternative Bayesian procedure, called FBST, has been introduced by [5] in case of sharp hypothesis $H_0$ identified by the null set $\Theta_0$, a submanifold of $\Theta$ of lower dimension. The FBST quantifies evidence by considering the posterior probability associated with the least probable points in the parameter space $\Theta_0$. When this probability is high, it favors the null hypothesis, providing a clear and interpretable measure of support for $H_0$ (see, e.g., [4,15,17], and references therein). The FBST is based on a specific loss function, and thus, the decision made under this procedure is the action that minimizes the corresponding posterior risk.

The FBST operates by determining the $e$-value, a representation of Bayesian evidence associated to $H_0$. To construct the $e$-value, the authors introduced the *posterior surprise function* and its supremum given, respectively, by

$$\pi_s(\theta|y) = \frac{\pi(\theta|y)}{r(\theta)} \quad \text{and} \quad s^* = \pi_s(\theta^*|y) = \sup_{\theta \in \Theta_0} \pi_s(\theta|y),$$

where $r(\theta)$ is a suitable *reference function* to be chosen. The surprise function was introduced in the context of statistical inference also by [18] (see [15], and references therein). Then, they introduce the *tangential set* $T_y(\theta^*)$ defined as the set of parameter values for which the posterior surprise function exceeds the supremum $s^*$, that is

$$T_y(\theta^*) = \{\theta \in \Theta : \pi_s(\theta|y) > s^*\}.$$

This set, often referred to as the Highest Relative Surprise Set, includes parameter values with higher surprise than those within the null set $\Theta_0$. The $e$-value is then computed as

$$ev = 1 - \int_{T_y(\theta^*)} \pi_s(\theta|y)\, d\theta,$$

and $H_0$ is rejected for *small* values of $ev$.

The original FBST, as proposed by [5,19], relies on a flat reference function $r(\theta) \propto 1$, so that this first version involved the determination of the tangential set $T_y(\theta)$ starting only from the posterior distribution $\pi(\theta|y)$. However, this initial version lacked invariance under reparameterizations. Subsequent refinements of the FBST introduced the importance of reference density functions, making the $e$-value explicitly invariant under appropriate transformations of the parameter. Common choices for the reference function include uninformative priors, like the uniform distribution, maximum entropy densities, or Jeffreys' invariant prior. In [20], the use of the Jeffreys' prior, $\pi(\theta) \propto |i(\theta)|^{1/2}$, where $i(\theta)$ is the Fisher information derived from $L(\theta)$, is discussed as the reference function to derive invariant HPD sets and Maximum A Posteriori (MAP) estimators that are invariant under reparameterizations. Note that the $ev$ uses the full dimensionality of the parameter space. Moreover, this measure is not invariant with respect to transformations of the nuisance parameters, and the use of high posterior densities to construct credible sets may produce inconsistencies.

Concerning the asymptotic behavior of the $ev$, it can be proven that, under suitable regularity conditions as the sample size increases, with $\theta_0$ representing the true parameter value (see [15]), it holds:

- If $H_0$ is false, i.e., $\theta_0 \notin H_0$ , then $ev$ converges in probability to 1.
- If $H_0$ is true, i.e., $\theta_0 \in H_0$ , then, denoting by $V(c) = Pr(ev \leq c)$ the cumulative distribution function of $ev$, we have that $V(c) \approx Q(d-h, Q^{-1}(d,c))$, with $d = dim(\Theta)$, $h = dim(\Theta_0)$ and $Q(k,x)$ the cumulative chi-square distribution with $k$ degrees of freedom.

In practice, the computation of $ev$ is performed in two steps: (a) a numerical optimization and (b) a numerical integration. The numerical optimization step consists of finding the maximizer $\theta^*$ of $\pi_s(\theta|y)$ under the null hypothesis. The numerical integration step consists of integrating the posterior surprise function over the region where it is greater than $\pi_s(\theta^*|y)$, to obtain the $e$-value. These computational steps make the FBST a computationally intensive procedure. Despite efficient computational algorithms for local and global optimization, as well as numerical integration, obtaining precise results for hypotheses like (5) is highly demanding, especially with large nuisance parameter dimensions. Numerical integration can be tackled by resorting to higher-order tail area approximations, as reviewed in the Bayesian framework in [3]. An application of asymptotic approximation to the FBST in its first formulation, i.e., with reference function $r(\theta) \propto 1$, has been discussed in [13].

*Asymptotic Approximations for the e-Value*

A first-order approximation for the $e$-value, when testing (5), is simply given by (see, e.g., [21,22])

$$ev \doteq 2\left(1 - \Phi\left(\left|\frac{\psi_0 - \hat{\psi}}{\sqrt{j_p(\hat{\psi})^{-1}}}\right|\right)\right), \tag{6}$$

where the symbol "$\doteq$" indicates that the approximation is accurate to $O(n^{-1/2})$, and $\Phi(\cdot)$ is the standard normal distribution function. Thus, to first-order, $ev$ agrees with the $p$-value based on the profile Wald statistic

$$w_p(\psi) = \frac{(\hat{\psi} - \psi_0)}{\sqrt{j_p(\hat{\psi})^{-1}}}. \tag{7}$$

In practice, the approximation (6) of $ev$ may be inaccurate, in particular when the dimension of $\lambda$ is large with respect to the sample size, because it forces the marginal posterior distribution to be symmetric.

The practical computation of $ev$ requires the evaluation of integrals of the marginal posterior distribution. In order to have more accurate evaluations of $ev$, it may be useful to resort to higher-order asymptotics based on tail area approximations (see, e.g., [2, 3], and references therein). Indeed, the measure of evidence involves integrals of the marginal surprise posterior density $\pi_{ms}(\psi|y)$. In particular, extending the application of the tail area argument to the marginal surprise posterior density, we can derive a $O(n^{-3/2})$ approximation to the marginal surprise posterior tail area probability, given by

$$\int_{\psi_0}^{\infty} \pi_{ms}(\psi|y)\, d\psi \doteq \Phi(r_B^*(\psi_0)), \tag{8}$$

where

$$r_B^*(\psi) = r_p(\psi) + \frac{1}{r_p(\psi)} \log \frac{q_B(\psi)}{r_p(\psi)},$$

with

$$r_p(\psi) = \text{sign}(\hat{\psi} - \psi)[2(\ell_p(\hat{\psi}) - \ell_p(\psi))]^{1/2}$$

profile likelihood root and

$$q_B(\psi) = \ell_p'(\psi)|j_p(\hat{\psi})|^{-1/2} \frac{|j_{\lambda\lambda}(\psi, \hat{\lambda}_\psi)|^{1/2}}{|j_{\lambda\lambda}(\hat{\psi}, \hat{\lambda})|^{1/2}} \frac{\pi(\hat{\psi}, \hat{\lambda})}{\pi(\psi, \hat{\lambda}_\psi)} \frac{r(\psi, \hat{\lambda}_\psi)}{r(\hat{\psi}, \hat{\lambda})}.$$

In the expression of $q_B(\psi)$, $\ell_p'(\psi) = \partial\ell_p(\psi)/\partial\psi$ is the profile score function.

Using the tail area approximation (8), a third-order approximation of the measure of evidence $ev$ can be derived. The approximation, assuming without loss of generality that $\psi_0$ is smaller than the MAP of $\pi_{ms}(\psi|y)$, is given by

$$ev(\psi) \doteq 1 - \Phi(r_B^*(\psi_0)) + \Phi(r_B^*(\psi_0^*)), \tag{9}$$

with $\psi_0^*$ the value of the parameter such that $\pi_{ms}(\psi_0^*|y) = \pi_{ms}(\psi_0|y)$. Note that

$$\Phi(r_B^*(\psi_0)) - \Phi(r_B^*(\psi_0^*)) \doteq \int_{\psi_0^*}^{\psi_0} \pi_{ms}(\psi|y)\, d\psi = 1 - ev$$

in (9) gives the posterior probability of the HPD credible interval $(\psi_0, \psi_0^*)$. Note also that the higher-order approximation (9) does not call for any condition on the prior $\pi(\psi, \lambda)$, i.e., it can be also improper. Finally, when $\pi_{ms}(\psi|y)$ is symmetric, Equation (9) reduces to $ev \doteq 2(1 - \Phi(r_B^*(\psi_0)))$.

While tail area approximations require little more than standard likelihood quantities for their implementation and, in this respect, they are available at little additional computational cost over the first-order approximation, they require elicitation on the complete parameter $\theta$ and to choose the reference function $r(\theta)$.

## 3. An Invariant Objective Prior

The aim of this section is to derive a default prior $\pi^*(\psi)$ to be used in (4). To this end, following [8], we use the shrinkage argument, which is a crucial procedure in the development of matching priors, i.e., priors that ensure, up to the desired order of asymptotics, an agreement between Bayesian and frequentist procedures. Examples of matching priors are (see [8]) for posterior quantiles, for credible regions and for prediction. Here, we focus on a specific matching prior that ensures the invariance of the posterior mode in the posterior distribution (4). As a consequence, the invariance extends to HPDs, as well as the $e$-value, achieved incorporating the reference function within the prior.

The proposed choice of the prior $\pi^*(\psi)$, which makes the MAP and thus also HPDs and the $e$-value invariant under 1-1 reparameterization, will depend on the log likelihood $\ell(\theta)$ and on its derivatives. In regular parametric estimation problems, both the MLE and the score-estimating function exhibit an asymptotically symmetric distribution centered at the true parameter value and at zero, respectively. However, these asymptotic behaviors may poorly reflect exact sampling distributions, particularly in cases with small or moderate sample information, sparse data, or complex models. Several proposals have been developed to correct the estimate or the estimating function. Most available methods are aimed at approximate bias adjustment, either of the MLE or of the profile score function, also when nuisance parameters are present (see [23] for a review of bias reduction for the MLE and [24] and subsequent literature for bias correction of the profile score). Lack of equivariance impacts the so-called implicit bias reduction methods, which achieve first-order bias correction by modifying the score equation (see [23,25]). To avoid this drawback, in this paper we focus on the median modification of the score, or profile score equation, whose solution respects equivariance under monotone reparameterizations ([26]). Similar to Firth's implicit method ([25]), the median modification of the score, or profile score, does not rely on finiteness of the MLE, thereby effectively preventing infinite estimates.

In practice, to derive the median matching prior $\pi^*(\psi)$, we impose that the MAP of $\pi^*(\psi|y)$ coincides with a refined version of the MLE, obtained as the solution of the median modified score function ([26]). To introduce this new invariant prior, we initially explore the scenario without nuisance parameters and then the situation in which nuisance parameters are present.

### 3.1. No Nuisance Parameters

Let us explore first the scenario where $\theta$ is scalar. In order to obtain median bias reduction of the MLE, it is possible to resort to a modified version of the score function of the form

$$t(\theta) = \ell_\theta(\theta) + m(\theta), \tag{10}$$

where $\ell_\theta(\theta) = \ell_\theta(\theta; y) = \partial\ell(\theta; y)/\partial\theta$ is the score function, and $m(\theta)$ is a suitable correction term of order $O(1)$. In particular, the median modified score function assumes for $m(\theta)$ the expression

$$m(\theta) = -\frac{E(\ell_\theta(\theta)^3)}{6\,i(\theta)}.$$

The solution $\tilde{\theta}$ to the equation $t(\theta) = 0$ not only upholds equivariance under componentwise monotone reparameterizations, but also approximates median unbiasedness ([26]). Note that likelihood inference based on (10) does not depend explicitely on the MLE. Indeed, the modified score function has been found to overcome infinite estimate problems. Likewise, the MLE and also $\tilde{\theta}$ is asymptotically $N(\theta, i(\theta)^{-1})$, so that the Wald-type statistics only differ in location.

Since Bayes' theorem is a statement of adittivity on the log scale $\log\pi(\theta|y) = \log\pi(\theta) + \log L(\theta) +$ constant, we observe that in the Bayesian framework, $m(\theta)$ can be interpreted as the derivative of the logarithm of a prior, that is, $m(\theta) = \partial\log\pi(\theta)/\partial\theta$. We are thus looking for a matching prior $\pi^*(\theta)$ such that

$$\frac{\partial\log\pi^*(\theta)}{\partial\theta} = -\frac{E(\ell_\theta(\theta)^3)}{6\,i(\theta)}.$$

In the scalar parameter case, it is straightforward to show that the proposed *median matching prior* takes the form

$$\begin{aligned}\pi^*(\theta) &\propto \exp\left(-\frac{1}{6}\int i(\theta)^{-1}E(\ell_\theta(\theta)^3)\,d\theta\right)\\ &\propto \exp\left(\frac{1}{6}\int i(\theta)^{-1}(3E(\ell_{\theta\theta}(\theta)\ell_\theta(\theta)) + E(\ell_{\theta\theta\theta}(\theta)))\,d\theta\right),\end{aligned}$$

with $\ell_{\theta\theta}(\theta) = \partial\ell_\theta(\theta)/\partial\theta$ and $\ell_{\theta\theta\theta}(\theta) = \partial\ell_{\theta\theta}(\theta)/\partial\theta$, where the second expression for $\pi^*(\theta)$ follows from the Bartlett's identities. The posterior based on the median matching prior is thus

$$\pi^*(\theta|y) \propto \exp\left(\ell(\theta) - \frac{1}{6}\int i(\theta)^{-1}E(\ell_\theta(\theta)^3)\,d\theta\right).$$

A first-order approximation for the $e$-value, when testing $H_0 : \theta = \theta_0$, is simply given by

$$ev \doteq 2\left(1 - \Phi\left(\left|\frac{\theta_0 - \tilde{\theta}}{\sqrt{i(\theta_0)^{-1}}}\right|\right)\right), \tag{11}$$

which differs in location with respect to the classical first-order approximation for the $e$-value based on the MLE. A second approximation for the $e$-value, when testing $H_0 : \theta = \theta_0$, can be obtained from the asymptotic distribution of the modified score function (10), that is

$$ev \doteq 2\left(1 - \Phi\left(\left|\frac{t(\theta_0)}{\sqrt{i(\theta_0)}}\right|\right)\right). \tag{12}$$

Although the first-order equivalence between (11) and (12), note that (11) is based on an easily understandable comparison between estimated value and hypothetical value, taking estimation error into account, and is widely used in applications but does not satisfy the principle of parameterization invariance. On the other hand, $t(\theta)/\sqrt{i(\theta)}$ is parameterization invariant.

Note that, when using a *predictive matching prior*, i.e., a prior ensuring asymptotic equivalence of higher-order frequentist and Bayesian predictive densities (see, e.g., [8]), the term $m(\theta)$ in (10) corresponds to the Firth's adjustment ([25])

$$m_F(\theta) = -\frac{(E(\ell_\theta(\theta)^3) + E(\ell_{\theta\theta}(\theta)\ell_\theta(\theta)))}{2i(\theta)}.$$

In view of this, for general regular models, Firth's estimate coincides with the mode of the posterior distribution obtained using the default predictive matching prior. However, lack of invariance affects this kind of adjustment ([23]), unless dealing with linear transformations.

**Example 1 (One parameter exponential family).** *For a one-parameter exponential family with canonical parameter $\theta$, i.e., with density*

$$f(y;\theta) = \exp\{\theta a(y) - K(\theta)\}b(y),$$

*the median modified score function has the form*

$$t(\theta) = \ell_\theta(\theta) + \frac{K_{\theta\theta\theta}}{6K_{\theta\theta}},$$

*where $K_{\theta\theta\theta} = \partial^3 K(\theta)/\partial\theta^3$ and $K_{\theta\theta} = \partial^2 K(\theta)/\partial\theta^2 = i(\theta)$. In this parameterization, $t(\theta)$ can be seen as the first derivative of the log-posterior*

$$\log \pi(\theta|y) = \ell(\theta) + \log i(\theta)/6.$$

*On the other hand, Firth's modified score takes the form $t_F(\theta) = \ell_\theta(\theta) + K_{\theta\theta\theta}/(2K_{\theta\theta})$. The effect of the median modification is to consider the median matching prior $\pi^*(\theta) \propto i(\theta)^{1/6}$, while $t_F(\theta)$ implies a Jeffreys' prior $\pi_J(\theta) \propto i(\theta)^{1/2}$. Note that, for a one-parameter exponential family with canonical parameter $\theta$, both $\pi^*(\theta)$ and $\pi_J(\theta)$ belong to the family of invariant priors discussed in [27,28].*

**Example 2 (Scale model).** *Consider the scale model $f(y;\theta) = (1/\theta)p_0(y/\theta)$, where $p_0(\cdot)$ is a given function. Let $g(\cdot) = -\log p_0(\cdot)$. We have $E(\ell_\theta^3) = c_1/\theta^3$, $E(\ell_\theta^3\ell_\theta) = c_2/\theta^3$ and $i(\theta) = c_3/\theta^2$, with $c_1 = \int(y^3 g'''(y) + 6y^2 g''(y) + 6yg'(y) - 2)p_0(y)dy$, $c_2 = \int(3yg'(y) + y^2 g''(y) - 2y^2 g'(y)^2 - y^3 g'(y)g''(y) - 1)p_0(y)dy$ and $c_3 = \int(2yg'(y) + y^2 g''(y) - 1)p_0(y)dy$. The median matching prior is thus $\pi^*(\theta) \propto \theta^{-c_1/6c_3}$, while the Jeffreys' prior for a one-parameter scale model is $\pi_J(\theta) \propto \theta^{-1}$ and the prior associated to the Firth's adjustment is $\pi_F(\theta) \propto \theta^{-(c_1+c_2)/2c_3}$.*

**Example 3 (Skew–normal distribution).** *Consider a skew-normal distribution with shape parameter $\theta \in \mathbb{R}$, with density $f(y;\theta) = 2\phi(y)\Phi(y\theta)$, where $\phi(\cdot)$ is the standard normal density* *function. The median correction term for the score function associated to the median matching prior is (see [26,29])*

$$m(\theta) = \frac{E(y^3\phi(y\theta)^3/\Phi(y\theta)^3)}{6E(y^2\phi(y\theta)^2/\Phi(y\theta)^2)}.$$

*Numerical integration must be performed to obtain the expected values involved in* $m(\theta)$.

*In order to illustrate the proposed prior, we consider draws from the skew–normal model with true parameter* $\theta_0 = 3$ *and increasing sample sizes* $n = 20, 30, 50, 200$ *(Figure 1). The posterior distributions are obtained with the method by [30], i.e., drawing* $10^5$ *values and accepting the best 5%. The e-values associated to the null (true) hypothesis* $H_0 : \theta = 3$ *and the (false) hypothesis* $H_0 : \theta = 4$ *are reported in Table 1. For comparison, the Jeffreys' prior ([31]), the predictive matching prior ([29]) and the flat prior, with uniform reference function, are also considered. Progressive agreement among evidence values obtained with the proposed median matching prior and the other priors for larger sample size is shown. Also, as expected, when progressively increasing* $n$*, the evidence values indicate agreement with the true hypothesis* $H_0 : \theta_0 = 3$ *and disagreement with* $H_0 : \theta_0 = 4$ *for all the priors used. Anyway, note that the posterior distribution obtained with a flat prior and a uniform reference function is proportional to the likelihood function that can be monotone. In view of this, while the MAPs of the posterior based on the default priors are always finite, in some samples the MAP of the posterior with the non-informative prior may be infinite. An example of this effect is illustrated in Figure 2.*

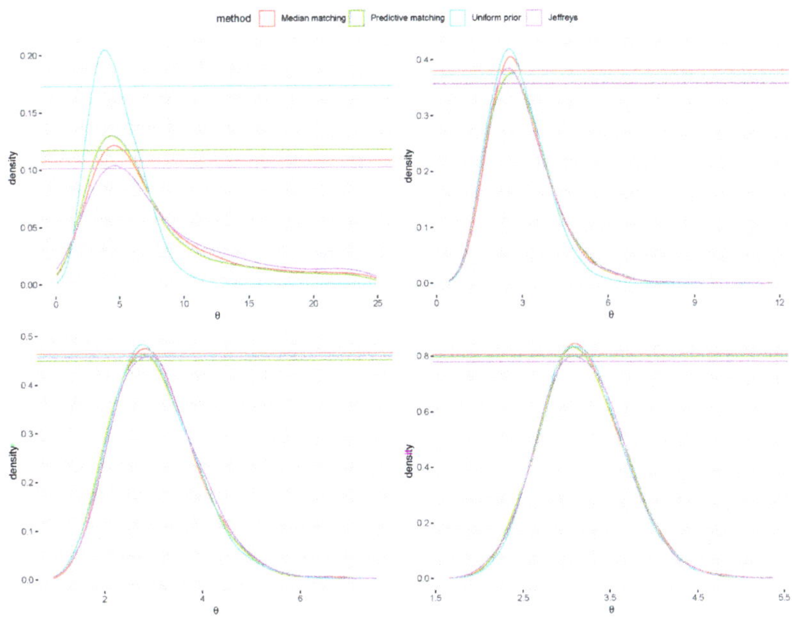


**Figure 1.** Inference for the scalar parameter $\theta$ of the skew-normal model with sample sizes $n = 20, 30, 50, 200$ (**top-left**, **top-right**, **bottom-left** and **bottom-right** panels, respectively). The red line is used for the posterior obtained from the median matching prior, the green one for the predictive matching prior, the violet one for the Jeffreys' prior and the blue one from an improper flat prior. The horizontal lines identify the corresponding tangential sets associated to the hypothesis $H_0 : \theta = 3$.

**Table 1.** Skew-normal: *e*-values associated to the hypotheses $H_0 : \theta = 3$ and $H_0 : \theta = 4$.

| Hypothesis $H_0$ | $n$ | Flat Prior | Median Matching Prior | Predictive Matching Prior | Jeffreys' Prior |
|---|---|---|---|---|---|
| $\theta = 3$ | 20 | 0.59 | 0.62 | 0.56 | 0.65 |
| | 30 | 0.65 | 0.70 | 0.73 | 0.64 |
| | 50 | 0.81 | 0.84 | 0.82 | 0.91 |
| | 200 | 0.79 | 0.79 | 0.81 | 0.82 |
| $\theta = 4$ | 20 | 0.82 | 0.91 | 0.98 | 0.84 |
| | 30 | 0.17 | 0.22 | 0.22 | 0.22 |
| | 50 | 0.20 | 0.20 | 0.20 | 0.21 |
| | 200 | 0.07 | 0.08 | 0.08 | 0.09 |

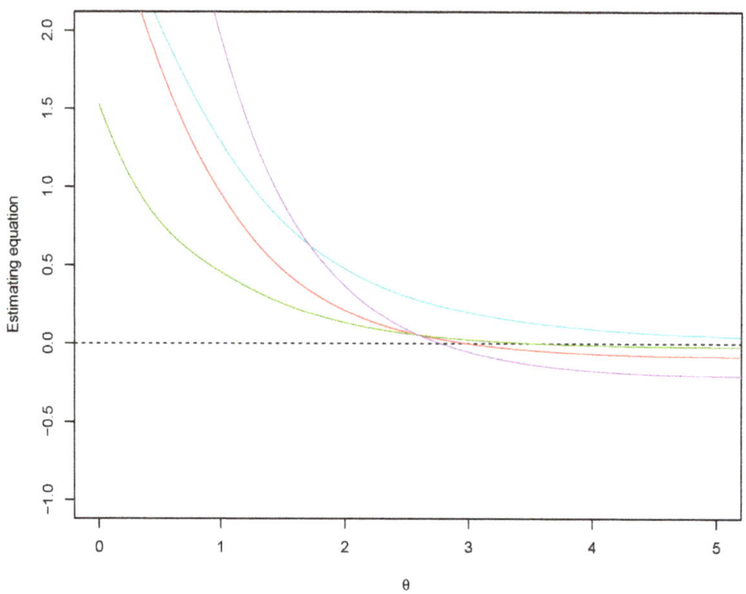


**Figure 2.** Skew-normal model: An example of $\partial \log \pi(\theta|y)/\partial\theta$ (estimating equation) with a flat prior (blue line), the median matching prior (red line) the predictive matching prior (green line) and the Jeffreys' prior (violet line) in a sample where all the observations are positive.

*The properties of first-order approximations of the e-values have been investigated by a simulation study, with sample sizes n* $= 20, 30, 50, 200$. *Results are displayed in Figure 3. Distributions of the e-value from the posterior based on the median matching prior are better, both for small and moderate sample sizes, in terms of convergence to the uniform distribution. Moreover, score-type e-values (12) are also preferable over Wald-type e-values (11). For the results with the posterior distribution obtained with a flat prior, we found* 4.3%, 4.2%, 0.9%, 0% *of infinite estimates for the sample sizes considered in the simulation study, and in these cases the e-value was considered as 0.*

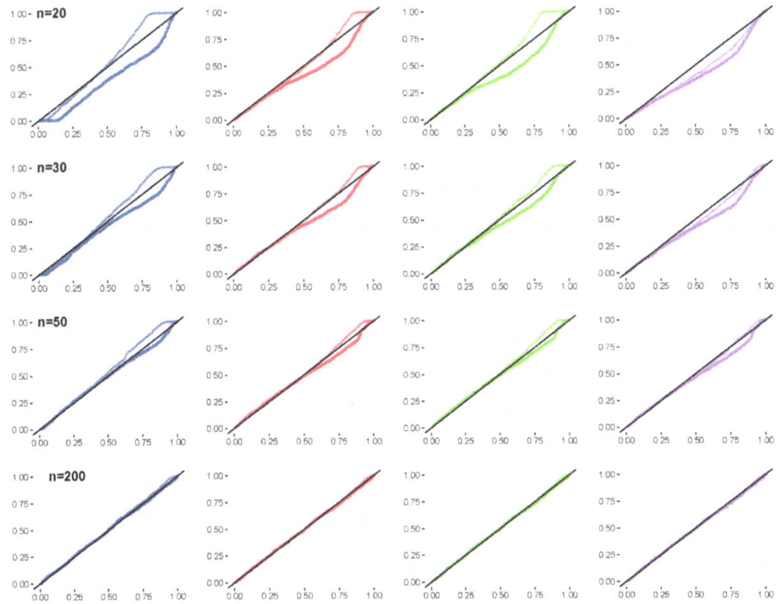

**Figure 3.** Skew-normal model: Distributions of *e*-values from a simulation study under the null hypothesis $H_0 : \theta = 3$, using a flat prior (blue line), the median matching prior (red line), the predictive matching prior (green line), and the Jeffreys' prior (violet line). The darker line is used for the approximation (11), while the lighter is for that based on (12).

### *3.2. Presence of Nuisance Parameters*

In the presence of nuisance parameters, in order to obtain median bias reduction of the MLE, it is possible to resort to a modified version of the profile score function of the form

$$t_p(\psi) = \ell_p'(\psi) + m(\psi, \hat{\lambda}_\psi), \tag{13}$$

where $m(\psi, \lambda)$ is a suitable correction term of order $O(1)$. In particular, for the median modified profile score function, the adjustment $m(\psi, \lambda)$ assumes the expression

$$m(\psi, \lambda) = -\kappa_{1\psi} + \frac{\kappa_{3\psi}}{6\kappa_{2\psi}},$$

where $\kappa_{1\psi}$, $\kappa_{2\psi}$ and $\kappa_{3\psi}$ are the first three cumulants of $\ell_p'(\psi)$ (see [26], Section 2.2, for their expression). For the estimator $\tilde{\psi}_p$, defined as the solution of $t_p(\psi) = 0$, parameterization equivariance holds under interest respecting reparameterizations ([26]).

Note that, also in the context of nuisance parameters, we are in the situation in which the proposed prior $\pi^*(\psi)$ is known through its first derivative; this is typically the situation with matching priors (see, e.g., [8]). Since the parameter of interest is scalar, the posterior based on the median matching prior can be written as

$$\pi^*(\psi|y) \propto \exp\left(\ell_p(\psi) + \int m(\psi, \hat{\lambda}_\psi)\, d\psi\right). \tag{14}$$

A simple analytical way of approximating to first-order the posterior distribution (14) based on the median matching prior is to resort to a quadratic form of $t_p(\psi)$. In particular, the approximate posterior distribution for $\psi$ takes the form

$$\pi^*(\psi|y) \,\dot{\propto}\, \exp\left(-\frac{1}{2}s_p(\psi;y)\right), \tag{15}$$

where $s_p(\psi) = t_p(\psi)^2 j_p(\psi)^{-1}$ is a Rao score-type statistic based on (13), and the symbol "$\dot{\propto}$" means asymptotic proportionality to first-order. In this case, a first-order approximation of the $e$-value, when testing $H_0 : \psi = \psi_0$, is given by

$$ev \doteq 2\left(1 - \Phi\left(\left|\frac{t_p(\psi_0)}{\sqrt{j_p(\psi_0)}}\right|\right)\right). \tag{16}$$

In this case, an higher-order approximation via (3) would be impractical since a closed-form prior is not available. As an alternative, simulation-based approaches may be used to derive the implied posterior distribution (14) based on the median matching prior. The first one relies on Approximate Bayesian Computation (ABC) techniques, using $\tilde{\psi}_p$ or the modified profile score function $t_p(\psi)$ as summary statistics; see [32] for the modification of the algorithm of [30] by using a profile estimating equation. This first method introduces an approximation at the level of the posterior estimation. The second one still relies on (13) but considers use of Manifold MCMC methods (see, e.g., [33]) to conditioning exactly on the profile equation and not up to a tolerance level, as in ABC (see [34,35]). The algorithm moves on the constrained space $\{(y,\psi) \in \mathcal{Y} \times \Theta | t_p(\tilde{\psi}_p) = 0\}$, where $\tilde{\psi}_p$ is the solution of the estimating equation on the original data. For the latter method, we need minimal regularity assumptions on $m(\psi,\lambda)$, which is assumed to be continuous, differentiable and available in closed form expression. Note, for instance, that in the skew-normal example in Section 3.1 these conditions are not met.

**Example 4 (Exponential family).** *If $f(y;\theta)$ is an exponential family of order $d$ with canonical parameter $(\psi,\lambda)$, i.e., $f(y;\psi,\lambda) = \exp\{\psi t(y) + \lambda^T s(y) - K(\psi,\lambda)\}h(y)$, quantities involved in $m(\psi,\lambda)$ are simply obtained from derivatives of $K(\psi,\lambda)$ ([26]). Note that, in this framework, $\ell_p'(\psi) - \kappa_{1\psi}$ is an approximation with error of order $O(n^{-1})$ of the score for $\psi$ in the conditional model given $s(y)$ (see e.g., [36], Section 10.2). Then, in the continuous case, the MAP $\tilde{\psi}_p$ is an approximation of the optimal conditional median unbiased estimator, and $\pi^*(\psi|y)$ is related to the conditional likelihood for $\psi$ given by $L_c(\psi) = \exp(\psi t(y) - K_s(\psi))$; see [37] for a Bayesian interpretation of such pseudo-likelihoods.*

**Example 5 (Multivariate regression model).** *Consider a regression model of the form*

$$Y_{ij} = \beta_0 + \beta_1 x_{i1} + \beta_2 x_{i2} + \epsilon_{ij}, \quad i = 1,\ldots,n, \quad j = 1,2,$$

*where it is assumed that $\epsilon_i \sim N_2(0,\Sigma)$, with $\Sigma = \sigma^2\begin{pmatrix}1 & \rho\\ \rho & 1\end{pmatrix}$ positive definite matrix, and $(\beta_0,\beta_1,\beta_2,\sigma^2,\rho)$ are unknown parameters. This model is widely used for instance in time series analysis, in which as regression covariates the past of the observables $y$ are used. We focus on the problem of testing hypothesis on the correlation coefficient $\rho$.*

*Consider a draw with true parameter $\rho_0 = 0.95$ and $n = 20$. For obtaining the proposed posterior (14) for $\rho$, we first compute the MAPs with the median matching prior and also, for comparison, with the predictive matching prior, which are, respectively, 0.953 and 0.92. Note that the expression of the predictive matching prior for $(\psi,\lambda)$ corresponds to the Firth's adjustment to the score function. The expressions of the modified profile estimating functions $t_p(\psi)$ and $t_F(\psi)$ are obtained from [38] and are available in closed form expressions. Hence, the Manifold MCMC* *method can be used to obtain the implied posteriors, whose approximation is comparable to that of any MCMC sampler. In particular we used 20,000 iterations.*

*We compare the posterior distribution based on the proposed median matching prior, with those obtained with the predictive matching prior and with an inverse-Wishart prior for the covariance matrix $\Sigma$ with one degree of freedom and identity position, and uniform prior on the regression parameters. The posterior distributions are displayed in Figure 4. The hypothesis of interest is $H_0 : \rho = 0.9$, and a smaller e-value indicating disagreement with the hypothesis should be preferable. The e-values are 0.25 with the median matching prior, 0.36 for the predictive matching prior and 0.60 with the inverse-Wishart prior. Note that the e-value based on the inverse-Wishart prior involves the constrained maximization and multidimensional integration and thus is not directly readable in Figure 4. Indeed, one crucial difference is that the original e-value formulation links the evidence of the null hypothesis to the evidence of a more refined hypothesis, choosing the MAP under the null hypothesis for all the nuisance parameters, while in the alternative (tangential) set, all values are used, and integration is performed on the full dimensionality of the space. On the contrary, in the proposed posterior based on the median matching prior, the maximizer of nuisance parameters are taken both in the null and non-null sets.*

*Finally, for the posterior based on the inverse-Wishart prior, we also computed the e-value based on the high-order tail area approximation (9) of the marginal surprise posterior, which is equal to 0.27. This procedure still avoids the multidimensional integration, but the result is not invariant to changes in parametrization.*

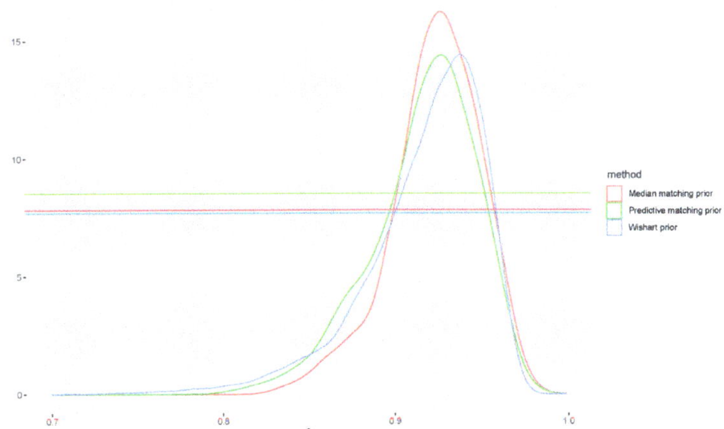


**Figure 4.** Posterior distributions for the correlation parameter $\rho$ of the bivariate regression model obtained from MCMC draws and the three different priors.

**Example 6 (Logistic regression model).** *Let $y_i$, $i = 1, \ldots, n$, be independent realizations of binary random variables with probability $\pi_i$, where $\log(\pi_i/(1-\pi_i)) = \eta_i = x_i\beta$ and $x_i = (x_{i1}, \ldots, x_{ip})$ is a row vector of covariates. We assume that a generic scalar component of $\beta$ is of interest, and we treat the remaining components as nuisance parameters.*

*As an example, we consider the* endometrial cancer grade *dataset analyzed, among others, in [39]. The aim of the clinical study was to evaluate the relationship between the histology of the endometrium (HG), the binary response variable, of $n = 79$ patients and three risk factors: 1. Neovascularization (NV), that indicates the presence or extent of new blood vessel formation; 2. Pulsatility Index (PI), that measures blood flow resistance in the endometrium, 3. Endometrium Height (EH), that indicates the thickness or height of the endometrium. A logistic model for HG, including an intercept and using all the covariates (NV, PI, EH), has been fitted, but a maximum likelihood leads to the infinite MLE of the coefficient $\beta_2$ related to NV, due to quasi-complete separation. This phenomenon prohibits the use of diffuse priors for $\beta_2$, since the* *corresponding posterior would not concentrate. Moreover, the e-value with non-informative priors cannot be obtained also for any hypothesis concerning parameters different from* $\beta_2$.

*If we consider* $\beta_2$ *as the parameter of interest, while the remaining regression coefficients are treated as nuisance parameters, the analysis with the median matching prior allows us to obtain a global proper posterior, with MAP equal to 3.86, open to interpretation both in the original scale and in terms of odds ratios. Similarly, the posterior based on the predictive matching prior, which in this model coincides with Jeffreys' prior* $\pi(\beta) \propto |i(\beta)|^{1/2}$ *is proper, with the MAP set at 2.92. The latter suffers from a lack of interpretability on different scales, since a different parametrization in the estimation phase would affect the results.*

*If we consider* $\beta_3$ *as the parameter of interest, related to the risk factor PI, the MAPs are* $-0.038$ *when using the median matching prior and* $-0.035$ *when using the predictive matching prior. The e-values for the hypothesis* $\mathcal{H}_0 : \beta_3 = 0$ *are 0.60 and 0.55, respectively (see Figure 5). Likewise, the interpretation of e-values remains consistent and independent of parametrization solely in the first case.*

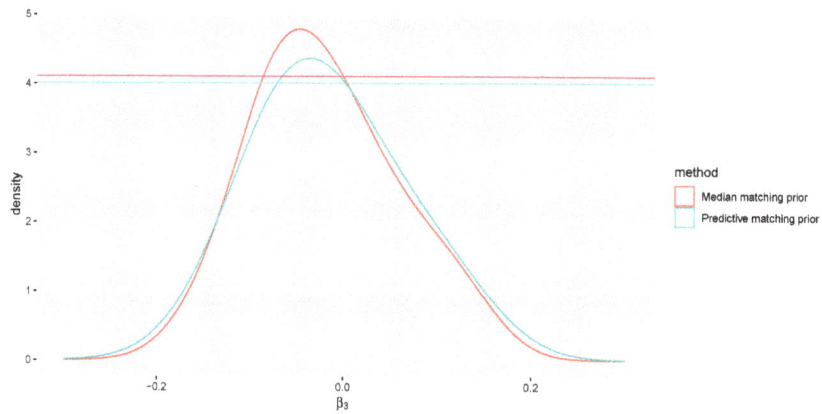


**Figure 5.** Median matching posterior distribution and predictive matching posterior distributions for $\beta_3$ in the logistic regression model.

## 4. Conclusions

Although (14) cannot always be considered as orthodox in a Bayesian setting, the use of alternative likelihoods is nowadays widely shared, and several papers focus on the Bayesian application of some well-known pseudo-likelihoods. In particular, the proposed posterior $\pi^*(\psi|y)$ has the advantages of avoiding the elicitation on the nuisance parameter $\lambda$ and of the computation of multidimensional integrations. Moreover, it provides invariant MAPs, HPDs and *e*-values, without the adoption of a reference function. Finally, we remark that frequentist properties of the MAP of the posterior based off the proposed median matching prior in comparison with the MAP of the posterior based of the predictive matching prior have been investigated in [28,38] for some of the examples discussed in this paper.

For inference on a full vector parameter $\theta$, with $d > 1$ components, a direct extension of the rationale leading to (10) does not seem to be practicable due to lack of a manageable definition of the multivariate median. Actually, in [26,40], it is shown how the method can be extended to a vector parameter of interest in the presence of nuisance parameters by simultaneously solving median bias-corrected score equations for all parameter components. This leads to componentwise third-order median unbiasedness and parameterization equivariance. Moreover, the use of default priors involving all parameter components, also the nuisance, becomes necessary to regularize likelihoods in case of monotonicity. We note that among the possible objective priors that ensures invariance of the posterior, we did not focus on the Jeffreys' in the multidimensional case, since it often exhibits poor convergence properties. Conversely, the default matching priors considered in this paper are easily generalizable to the multidimensional case [40] preserving good convergence properties.

As a final remark, we highlight that this paper opens several topics of future research. In particular, from a computational point of view, it could be of interest:

- To develop a library of computational routines exploring the methods proposed in this paper for a wide range of statistical models of interest;
- To develop semi-automated procedures for further expanding this library, as is done for point estimation for Generalized Linear Models in the `R` package `brglm2` [41].

Moreover, from a theoretical point of view, it could be of interest:

- To further explore the theoretical connections between the *e*-value invariance properties and matching priors;
- To explore the existence of similar connections in other classes of pseudo-likelihoods, in particular in the context of empirical and profile empirical likelihoods, with a large number of nuisance parameters ([42]),
- To apply and extend the methodology to consider other objective priors used in Bayesian inference, such as those obtained from scoring rules, as proposed in [10], that are expressed as solutions of differential equations.

**Author Contributions:** Conceptualization, E.B. and L.V.; methodology, E.B. and L.V.; software, E.B.; validation, E.B. and L.V.; formal analysis, E.B. and L.V.; investigation, E.B. and L.V.; resources, E.B. and L.V.; data curation, E.B.; writing—original draft preparation, E.B. and L.V.; writing—review and editing, E.B. and L.V.; visualization, E.B. and L.V.; supervision, E.B. and L.V.; project administration, E.B. and L.V.; funding acquisition, L.V. All authors have read and agreed to the published version of the manuscript.

**Funding:** This research received no external funding.

**Data Availability Statement:** Data and code used in the examples are available in https://github.com/elenabortolato/invariant_evalues (accessed on 28 November 2023).

**Conflicts of Interest:** The authors declare no conflict of interest.

## Abbreviations

The following abbreviations are used in this manuscript:

| | |
|---|---|
| ABC | Approximate Bayesian Computation |
| BF | Bayes Factor |
| FBST | Full Bayesian Significance Test |
| HPD | Highest Probability Density |
| MAP | Maximum A Posteriori |
| MLE | Maximum Likelihood Estimator |

## References

1. Brazzale, A.R.; Davison, A.C.; Reid, N. *Applied Asymptotics. Case-Studies in Small Sample Statistics*; Cambridge University Press: Cambridge, UK, 2007.
2. Reid, N. The 2000 Wald memorial lectures: Asymptotics and the theory of inference. *Ann. Stat.* **2003**, *31*, 1695–1731. [CrossRef]
3. Ventura, L.; Reid, N. Approximate Bayesian computation with modified loglikelihood ratios. *Metron* **2014**, *7*, 231–245. [CrossRef]
4. Madruga, M.; Pereira, C.; Stern, J. Bayesian evidence test for precise hypotheses. *J. Stat. Plan. Inference* **2003**, *117*, 185–198. [CrossRef]
5. Pereira, C.; Stern, J.M. Evidence and Credibility: Full Bayesian Significance Test for Precise Hypotheses. *Entropy* **1999**, *1*, 99–110. [CrossRef]
6. Kass, R.E.; Tierney, L.; Kadane, J. Approximate methods for assessing influence and sensitivity in Bayesian analysis. *Biometrika* **1989**, *76*, 663–674. [CrossRef]
7. Reid, N.; Sun, Y. Assessing sensitivity to priors using higher order approximations. *Commun. Stat. Theory Methods* **2010**, *39*, 1373–1386. [CrossRef]
8. Datta, G.S.; Mukerjee, R. *Probability Matching Priors: Higher-Order Asymptotics*; Lecture Notes in Statistics; Springer: Berlin/Heidelberg, Germany, 2004.

9. Severini, T.A. *Likelihood Methods in Statistics*; Oxford University Press: Oxford, UK, 2000.
10. Leisen, F.; Villa, C.; Walker, S.G. On a class of objective priors from scoring rules (with discussion). *Bayesian Anal.* **2020**, *15*, 1345–1423. [CrossRef]
11. Miller, J.W. Asymptotic normality, concentration, and coverage of generalized posteriors. *J. Mach. Learn. Res.* **2021**, *22*, 1.
12. Ventura, L.; Racugno, W. Pseudo-likelihoods for Bayesian inference. In *Topics on Methodological and Applied Statistical Inference*; Studies in Theoretical and Applied Statistics; Springer: Cham, Switzerland, 2016; pp. 205–220. ISBN 978-3-319-44093-4.
13. Cabras, S.; Racugno, W.; Ventura, L. Higher-order asymptotic computation of Bayesian significance tests for precise null hypotheses in the presence of nuisance parameters. *J. Stat. Comput. Simul.* **2015**, *85*, 2989–3001. [CrossRef]
14. Diniz, M.B.; Pereira, C.; Stern, J.M. Cointegration and unit root tests: A fully Bayesian approach. *Entropy* **2020** *22*, 968. [CrossRef]
15. Pereira, C.; Stern, J.M. The $e-$value: A fully Bayesian significance measure for precise statistical hypotheses and its research program. *Sao Paulo J. Math. Sci.* **2022**, *16*, 566–584. [CrossRef]
16. Robert, C.P. On the Jeffreys Lindley paradox. *Philos. Sci.* **2014**, *81*, 216–232. [CrossRef]
17. Madruga, M.R.; Esteves, L.G.; Wechsler, S. On the bayesianity of pereira-stern tests. *Test* **2001**, *10*, 291–299. [CrossRef]
18. Evans, M. Bayesian inference procedures derived via the concept of relative surprise. *Commun. Stat. – Theory Methods* **1997**, *26*, 1125–1143. [CrossRef]
19. Pereira, C.; Stern, J.M. Model Selection: Full Bayesian Approach. *Environmetrics* **2001**, *12*, 559–568. [CrossRef]
20. Druilhet, P.; Marin, J.M. Invariant HPD credible sets and MAP estimators. *Bayesian Anal.* **2007**, *2*, 681–692. [CrossRef]
21. Pereira, C.; Stern, J.M.; Wechsler, S. Can a significance test be genuinely Bayesian? *Bayesian Anal.* **2008**, 79–100. [CrossRef]
22. Diniz, M.A.; Pereira, C.; Polpo, A.; Stern, J.M.; Wechsler, S. Relationship between Bayesian and frequentist significance indices. *Int. J. Uncertain. Quantif.* **2012**, *2*, 161–172. [CrossRef]
23. Kosmidis, I. Bias in parametric estimation: Reduction and useful side effects. *Wiley Interdiscip. Rev. Comput. Stat.* **2014**, *6*, 185–196. [CrossRef]
24. Stern, S.E. A second-order adjustment to the profile likelihood in the case of a multidimensional parameter of interest. *J. R. Stat. Ser. B* **1997**, *59*, 653–665. [CrossRef]
25. Firth, D. Bias reduction of maximum likelihood estimates. *Biometrika* **1993**, *80*, 27–38. [CrossRef]
26. Kenne Pagui, E.C.; Salvan, A.; Sartori, N. Median bias reduction of maximum likelihood estimates. *Biometrika* **2017**, *104*, 923–938. [CrossRef]
27. Hartigan, J.A. Invariant prior densities. *Ann. Math. Statist.* **1964**, *35*, 836–845. [CrossRef]
28. Hartigan, J.A. The asymptotically unbiased density. *Ann. Math. Statist.* **1965**, *36*, 1137–1152. [CrossRef]
29. Sartori, N. Bias prevention of maximum likelihood estimates for scalar skew normal and skew t distributions. *J. Stat. Plan. Inference* **2006**, *136*, 4259–4275. [CrossRef]
30. Ruli, E.; Sartori, N.; Ventura, L. Robust approximate Bayesian inference. *J. Stat. Plan. Inference* **2020**, *205*, 10–22. [CrossRef]
31. Liseo, B.; Loperfido, N. A note on reference priors for the scalar skew-normal distribution. *J. Stat. Plan. Inference* **2006**, *136*, 373–389. [CrossRef]
32. Bortolato, E.; Ventura, L. On approximate robust confidence distributions. *Econom. Stat.* **2023**. [CrossRef]
33. Brubaker, M.; Salzmann, M.; Urtasun, R. A family of MCMC methods on implicitly defined manifolds. *Artif. Intell. Stat.* **2012**, *22*, 161–172.
34. Lewis, J.R.; MacEachern, S.N.; Lee, Y. Bayesian restricted likelihood methods: Conditioning on insufficient statistics in Bayesian regression (with discussion). *Bayesian Anal.* **2021**, *104*, 1393–1462. [CrossRef]
35. Graham, M.; Storkey, A. Asymptotically exact inference in differentiable generative models. *Artif. Intell. Stat.* **2017**, 499–508. [CrossRef]
36. Pace, L.; Salvan, A. *Principles of Statistical Inference*; World Scientific: Singapore, 1997.
37. Severini, T.A. On the relationship between Bayesian and non-Bayesian elimination of nuisance parameters. *Stat. Sin.* **1999**, *9*, 713–724.
38. Bortolato, E.; Kenne Pagui, E.C. Bias reduction and robustness in gaussian longitudinal data analysis. *J. Stat. Comput. Simul.* **2023**, 1–16. [CrossRef]
39. Agresti, A. *Foundations of Linear and Generalized Linear Models*; John Wiley & Sons: New York, NY, USA, 2015.
40. Kosmidis, I.; Kenne Pagui, E.C.; Sartori, N. Mean and median bias reduction in generalized linear models. *Stat. Comput.* **2020**, *30*, 43–59. [CrossRef]
41. Kosmidis, I. brglm2: Bias Reduction in Generalized Linear Models. R Package Version 0.9.2. 2023. Available online: https://CRAN.R-project.org/package=brglm2 (accessed on 28 November 2023).
42. Bedoui, A.; Lazar, N.A. Bayesian empirical likelihood for ridge and lasso regressions. *Comput. Stat. Data Anal.* **2020**, *145*, 106917. [CrossRef]

*entropy*

*Article*

# Linear Bayesian Estimation of Misrecorded Poisson Distribution

**Huiqing Gao [1], Zhanshou Chen [1,2,*] and Fuxiao Li [3]**

1 School of Mathematics and Statistic, Qinghai Normal University, Xining 810008, China; huiqinggao0820@outlook.com
2 The State Key Laboratory of Tibetan Intelligent Information Processing and Application, Xining 810008, China
3 Faculty of Science, Xi'an University of Technology, Xi'an 710048, China; lifuxiao@xaut.edu.cn
* Correspondence: chenzhsh@qhnu.edu.cn

**Abstract:** Parameter estimation is an important component of statistical inference, and how to improve the accuracy of parameter estimation is a key issue in research. This paper proposes a linear Bayesian estimation for estimating parameters in a misrecorded Poisson distribution. The linear Bayesian estimation method not only adopts prior information but also avoids the cumbersome calculation of posterior expectations. On the premise of ensuring the accuracy and stability of computational results, we derived the explicit solution of the linear Bayesian estimation. Its superiority was verified through numerical simulations and illustrative examples.

**Keywords:** misrecorded Poisson distribution; linear Bayesian estimation; bootstrap

## 1. Introduction

Count data, which are typically characterized as data points that cannot be collected consecutively or are represented as 0 or natural numbers like 1, 2, 3, etc., are commonly encountered in various aspects of daily life. These data points are often effectively approximated by binomial or Poisson distributions. However, certain challenges may emerge during the actual counting process. When determining the number of defects per unit or item, there is a possibility that the recorder may inaccurately classify some units that actually contain one defect as perfect or defect-free while accurately recording other values. More specifically, some observations with a value of 1 are misclassified and reported as 0, while others, such as 2, 3, and 4, are correctly recorded. For this type of data containing erroneous records, direct modeling with a Poisson distribution is not appropriate. Instead, it can be approximated using a misrecorded Poisson distribution.

The misrecorded Poisson distribution, first proposed by Cohen [1], is often denoted as the Cohen–Poisson (CP) or MSR-Poisson distribution. Since then, many authors have studied this distribution and its various forms. For surveys, Dorris and Foote [2] provided a comprehensive survey and analysis of the impact of inspection errors on statistical quality control procedures. They discuss their effects on various aspects of statistical quality control procedures, including control charts, sample size, and inspection efficiency. Subsequently, the article introduces methods for estimating error probabilities and adjusting parameters in Poisson distributions, along with strategies for designing compensatory plans to mitigate the impact of inspection errors. All these efforts are grounded in Cohen's seminal work, which developed multiple estimators for error probability assessment and parameter recalibration in Poisson distributions, thereby establishing a significant theoretical framework. Gupta et al. [3] studied when the observed frequency of zeros is significantly higher or lower than predicted by the model; the adjusted random variable can be described as a mixture of two Poisson distributions. This distribution can be regarded as a mixture of two distributions, one of which is degenerate at zero. Zhang et al. [4] study the zero-and-one inflated Poisson (ZOIP) distribution, develop likelihood-based inference methods, and provide simulations and real data examples to illustrate the proposed methods. The key properties of the ZOIP distribution are established, including five equivalent stochastic representations and other important distributional properties. Maximum likelihood estimates of parameters are obtained through Fisher scoring and the expectation–maximization algorithm, and bootstrap confidence intervals and hypothesis testing methods are provided for parameters in large samples. Liu [5] et al. introduce a new multivariate ZAP distribution, building on the traditional multivariate Poisson distribution. A key feature of this distribution is its ability to model count vectors that are zero-truncated, zero-deflated, or zero-inflated with a more flexible dependency structure. This means that correlation coefficients between components can be both positive and negative. They introduce an expectation–maximization (EM) algorithm for calculating the maximum likelihood estimates (MLEs) and posterior modes of parameters. Bagui and Mehra [6] gave a historical background for the Poisson distribution and also described some of its applications in the early days and more. Additionally, they introduced a new ratio method that demonstrates convergence to the normal distribution, which may attract attention. In the context of Poisson processes, considering the swift progress in current industrial and technological spheres, statistical models must advance to keep up with the times, adapting to handle data with higher frequencies and greater complexity.

The Hawkes process model, noted for its self-excitation and time-dependence, serves as an extension to the Poisson process. This extension offers more sophisticated and adaptable tools for analyzing and forecasting error patterns in ever-changing environments. For relevant research results, refer to Zhang et al. [7] and Wang and Zhang [8]. Lamprinakou et al. [9] proposed a new epidemiological model using the Hawkes process to study the spread of COVID-19. It focuses on estimating unobserved infection cases, offering insights into the disease's transmission dynamics.

Furthermore, numerous monographs and doctoral dissertations have investigated the misrecorded Poisson distribution and its various forms. Xu [10] studied the statistical properties of a Poisson generalized inverse Gaussian distribution, a negative binomial distribution, a Poisson inverse Gaussian distribution, and a Poisson inverse gamma distribution. The model they studied is similar to the model studied in this article, which is very helpful for the study of properties and parameter derivation methods in this article. Johnson [11] has effectively synthesized the findings from various studies on the misrecorded Poisson distribution and its parameter estimation, encompassing research conducted by Cohen as well as contributions from other researchers in the field. Djuraš [12] discussed the one-displaced misrecorded Poisson and size-biased misrecorded Poisson distributions, deriving their parameter estimators. Tuwei [13] derived the probability density function from the probability generating function and provided expressions for the mean, the variance, and the relationship between parameters based on this probability density function.

While the majority of previous studies have focused on classical estimation methods, Angers and Biswas [14] employ Bayesian methods for parameter estimation and prediction. Specifically, they contemplate a zero-inflated generalized Poisson model, which encompasses three parameters: the zero-inflation parameter, the dispersion parameter of the generalized Poisson distribution, and the mean parameter. For the purpose of Bayesian estimation, the article utilizes appropriate prior distributions and employs a Monte Carlo integration technique via importance sampling to obtain the posterior distributions. Subsequently, the expected values of the posterior distributions are computed, serving as the Bayesian estimates of the parameters. Rodrigues [15] studied the zero-inflated distributions from a Bayesian point of view using a data augmentation algorithm. Wang [16] considered a 0–1 expansion Poisson regression model with covariates and proposed a Bayesian estimation of the model parameters.

Compared to traditional Bayesian estimation methods, it is worth noting that the linear Bayesian method, initially proposed by Hartigan [17], has gained popularity as a simple Bayesian approach for parameter estimation. Rao [18] studied the linear Bayesian method from the perspective of linear optimization and argued that this method better considers the prior uncertainty and uses this "incomplete" information to construct linear Bayesian parameter estimates. LaMotte [19] introduced a linear Bayesian estimator that has the smallest total mean square error among all linear estimators. Hesselager [20] demonstrated that if the average risk of an empirical linear Bayesian estimate converges to the risk of the corresponding linear Bayesian estimate, then it is asymptotically optimal in the usual sense. Goldstein [21] adeptly modified the linear Bayesian estimator, specifically designed for estimating the mean of a distribution whose form is unknown, by incorporating the use of an estimate derived from sample variance. Hoffmann [22] applied the linear Bayesian method to estimate an unknown parameter vector in the linear regression model with ellipsoidal parameter constraints. The conditions under which certain linear empirical Bayesian estimators are superior to the standard estimator for an arbitrary $k \geq 1$ are given by Samaniego and Vestrup [23]. Wei and Zhang [24] verified under the Predictive Pitman Closeness criterion and Posterior Pitman Closeness that the linear Bayesian method outperforms the generalized least squares method for linear models. More recently, Lin [25] employed Monte Carlo simulations and empirical computations to compare the outcomes of constrained least-squares estimation and constrained linear Bayesian estimation, as well as their distances from the Bayesian estimates. This approach serves to validate the superiority of constrained linear Bayesian estimation over constrained least-squares estimation. Tao [26] provided an empirical linear Bayesian approach, conducting an empirical analysis using a Bayesian model for multiple insurance contracts with Pareto distributions. This method does not rely on any prior distribution information. Liu [27] studied the parameter estimation problem of singular linear models with equality constraints and concluded that the higher the degree of singularity of the model, the more obvious the superiority of the best homogeneous linear Bayesian unbiased estimation over the least-squares estimation. Chen [28] introduces a linear Bayesian method for estimating parameters in extreme value distributions from Type II censored samples. This approach, which combines Bayesian and optimization techniques, offers a straightforward and practical solution, overcoming the complexity often associated with classical Bayesian estimation. The method's advantages, particularly for small or heavily censored samples, are validated through numerical experiments, demonstrating its effectiveness when compared to maximum likelihood and unbiased estimations. The models, parameter estimation methods, and criteria for assessing their effectiveness used in the aforementioned work have significantly contributed to the research presented in this paper. These models, encompassing a range of statistical, probabilistic, and computational approaches, form the fundamental basis of our analysis. They provide a structured and systematic framework that aids in the coherent understanding and interpretation of the complex data sets we are dealing with. The selection of a particular model is heavily dependent on the specific nature of the data under study and the overarching research question, with each model introducing its own set of assumptions and perspectives to the analysis.

Parameter estimation methods are a key component in refining and fine-tuning these models. These methods are instrumental in extracting significant insights from the data, as they focus on determining the values of the model parameters that most accurately represent the observed data. Depending on the model's nature and the data's characteristics, various techniques like maximum likelihood estimation, Bayesian inference, or least-squares fitting are utilized. The precision and reliability of these methods are paramount, as they have a direct bearing on the validity and credibility of our research findings. Therefore, the judicious selection and application of these methods are critical.

Given the notable advantages of linear Bayesian estimators, this paper specifically focuses on parameter estimation for the misrecorded Poisson distribution using linear functions derived from sample data. We employ the criterion of minimizing the mean square error to formulate linear Bayesian estimation expressions for the distribution's parameters. To our knowledge, no existing studies have explored linear Bayesian estimation specifically for parameters within the misrecorded Poisson distribution. Traditional methods often fall short in addressing the unique challenges posed by misrecorded data, such as biased estimates or increased error variance. Therefore, our method fills a significant gap in the statistical methodology by providing a tailored solution for this specific distribution. Furthermore, we use the criterion of minimizing the mean square error to formulate linear Bayesian estimation expressions for the distribution's parameters. This criterion ensures that the estimations are not only accurate but also consistent by minimizing the average of the squares of the errors—the difference between the estimator and what is estimated. This approach optimizes the balance between bias and variance in the estimations, leading to more reliable results.

Our work stands out not only for its innovative approach to handling the misrecorded Poisson distribution but also for its potential wide-ranging applications in various fields. In areas where misrecorded count data are common, such as epidemiology, environmental studies, and quality control in manufacturing, the implications of this research are substantial. By introducing new insights and techniques for managing such distributions, our study promises to enhance the accuracy and reliability of data analysis in these fields, leading to more informed and dependable conclusions. This could mark a significant advancement in statistical methods, opening doors to more robust and sophisticated data analysis techniques in these critical areas of study.

The rest of this paper is structured as follows: Section 2 offers a detailed examination of the misrecorded Poisson distribution and delves into its maximum likelihood estimation. In Section 3, we introduce and elaborate on a linear Bayesian estimation method, highlighting its superior estimation results, primarily based on the principle of the mean square error matrix. Section 4 presents numerical simulations and example analyses. Lastly, in Section 5, we summarize the entire study, provide our conclusions, point out the shortcomings of the article, and suggest future research directions

## 2. Misrecorded Poisson Distribution

The probability mass function of the misrecorded Poisson distribution is

$$P(X=x)=\begin{cases} e^{-\lambda}(1+\lambda\phi) & x=0 \\ e^{-\lambda}\lambda(1-\phi) & x=1 \\ e^{-\lambda}\frac{\lambda^x}{x!} & x=2,3,\ldots \end{cases}, \tag{1}$$

where $\lambda > 0, 0 < \phi < 1$. $\phi$ is the probability of misclassification or the proportion of ones that are reported as zeros. The misrecorded Poisson distribution is reduced to a Poisson distribution when $\phi = 0$. Also, all the observations falling in class one will be reported as zero when $\phi = 1$; thus, it is a zero–one modified distribution. We can say that the misrecorded Poisson distribution is zero-inflated (there is an excess of zeros) and one-deflated (there are fewer ones than expected). If $\phi_0 = \lambda\phi e^{-\lambda} > 0$, then the Poisson's zero probability is increased (zero inflation), while the Poisson's one probability is decreased for $\phi_1 = -\lambda\phi e^{-\lambda} < 0$.

The corresponding probability generating function, the mean, the variance, and the second, third, and fourth moments are given as, respectively,

$$G_X(s) = e^{-\lambda}(1+\lambda\phi) + \lambda e^{-\lambda}(1-\phi)s + \sum_{x=2}^{\infty}\frac{(\lambda s)^x e^{-\lambda}}{x!}$$

$$= e^{-\lambda}(1+\lambda\phi) + \lambda s e^{-\lambda}(1-\phi) + \left\{e^{-\lambda(s-1)} - \lambda s e^{-\lambda} - e^{-\lambda}\right\}$$

$$= e^{-\lambda} + \lambda\phi e^{-\lambda} + \lambda s e^{-\lambda} - \lambda\phi s e^{-\lambda} + e^{-\lambda(s-1)} - \lambda s e^{-\lambda} - e^{-\lambda}$$

$$= \lambda\phi e^{-\lambda} - \lambda\phi s e^{-\lambda} + e^{-\lambda(s-1)},$$

$$E(X) = \mu = \lambda(1-\phi e^{-\lambda}),$$

$$Var(X) = C_2(0) = \sigma_X^2 = \lambda^2 + (1+\phi e^{-\lambda})(1-\lambda(\phi e^{-\lambda})),$$

$$E(X^2) = \mu_{(0)} = \lambda^2 + \lambda(1 - \phi e^{-\lambda}),$$
$$E(X^3) = \mu_{(0,0)} = \lambda^3 + 3\lambda^2 + (1 - \phi e^{-\lambda}),$$
$$E(X^4) = \mu_{(0,0,0)} = \lambda^4 + 6\lambda^3 + 7\lambda^2 + (1 - \phi e^{-\lambda}).$$

assuming that the random variables $x_1, x_2, \ldots\ldots, x_N$ are samples consisting of $N$ observations from the misrecorded Poisson distribution, with $n_0$ denoting the number of zero observations and $n_1$ denoting the number of one observations. The likelihood function is

$$L(x_1, x_2, \cdots x_N; \lambda, \phi) = [e^{-\lambda}(1 + \phi\lambda)]^{n_0}[(1 - \phi)\lambda e^{-\lambda}]^{n_1}\prod * e^{-\lambda}\lambda^{x_i}/x_i$$
$$= e^{-N\lambda}(1 + \phi\lambda)^{n_0}(1 - \phi)^{n_1}\lambda^{\sum_{i=1}^{N} x_i}\left[\prod * x_i!\right]^{-1}, \quad (2)$$

where $\prod *$ is the product of $x_1, x_2, \ldots\ldots, x_N$ that are neither zero nor one. Taking the logarithms of Equation (2) and letting its partial derivatives with respect to $\lambda$ and $\phi$, respectively, equal zero, we obtain the following equation:

$$\partial \log L/\partial\lambda = -N + n_0\phi/(1 + \phi\lambda) + \sum_{i=1}^{N} x_i/\lambda = 0.$$

$$\partial \log L/\partial\phi = n_0\lambda(1 + \phi\lambda) - n_1/(1 - \phi) = 0,$$

and then we have:

$$\lambda^2 - (\overline{x} - 1 + n_0/N)\lambda - (\overline{x} - n_1/N) = 0, \quad (3)$$
$$\phi = [n_0 - n_1/\lambda]/(n_0 + n_1), \quad (4)$$

where $\overline{x} = \sum_{i=1}^{N} x_i/N$ is the mean of the sample. Solving the above equation yields the maximum likelihood estimates $\hat{\lambda}_{MLE}$ and $\hat{\phi}_{MLE}$ for $\lambda$ and $\phi$:

$$\hat{\lambda}_{MLE} = \left[(\overline{x} - 1 + n_0/N) + \sqrt{(\overline{x} - 1 + n_0/N)^2 + 4(\overline{x} - n_1/N)}\right]/2, \quad (5)$$

$$\hat{\phi}_{MLE} = (n_0 - n_1/\hat{\lambda}_{MLE})/(n_0 + n_1). \quad (6)$$

Translating the solution of this estimate into matrix form to express it, we have

$$\hat{\theta}_{MLE} = (\hat{\lambda}_{MLE}, \hat{\phi}_{MLE})' = \begin{pmatrix} 1/2 & 0 \\ 0 & \frac{1}{n_0+n_1} \end{pmatrix}\begin{pmatrix} t_1 \\ t_2 \end{pmatrix} \triangleq AT, \quad (7)$$

where

$$A = \begin{pmatrix} 1/2 & 0 \\ 0 & \frac{1}{n_0+n_1} \end{pmatrix}, T = \begin{pmatrix} t_1 \\ t_2 \end{pmatrix}. \quad (8)$$

## 3. Linear Bayesian Estimation

### 3.1. The Expressions of Linear Bayesian Estimation

**Definition 1.** *Assume that the prior distribution function, $\pi(\theta)$ of $\theta = (\lambda, \phi)'$, satisfies the family of prior distributions:*

$$\xi = \left\{\pi(\theta) : E\|\theta\|^2 < \infty\right\}. \quad (9)$$

Let $\hat{\theta}_{LB} = BT + b$ be a linear estimate of the parameter $\theta$ under the statistic $T$, in which $B$ and $b$ are $2 \times 2$- and $2 \times 1$-dimensional unknown matrices, respectively. Then, $\hat{\theta}_{LB}$ is called the linear Bayesian estimate of $\theta$ if $\hat{\theta}_{LB}$ satisfies the following conditions:

$$E_{(T,\theta)}(\hat{\theta}_{LB} - \theta) = 0, \tag{10}$$

$$R(\hat{\theta}_{LB}, \theta) = \min_{B,b} E_{(T,\theta)} L(\hat{\theta} - \theta), \tag{11}$$

where $E_{(T,\theta)}$ denotes the expectation of the joint distribution of $T$ and $\theta$.

The function

$$L(\hat{\theta}_{LB}, \theta) = (\hat{\theta}_{LB}, \theta)' D(\hat{\theta}_{LB}, \theta), \tag{12}$$

where $D$ is a $2 \times 2$ positive definite matrix, is called the squared loss function. Minimizing the squared loss, we can obtain the expressions of $B$ and $b$, which are given in the following theorem.

**Theorem 1.** *Suppose that the prior distribution, $\pi(\theta)$, of the parameter vector $\theta = (\lambda, \varphi)'$ in the misrecorded Poisson distribution (1) satisfies the family of prior distributions (9). Then, under the squared loss function, the linear Bayesian estimate, $\hat{\theta}_{LB}$, of $\theta$ is*

$$\hat{\theta}_{LB} = (A - AWM)T + AWMA^{-1}E\theta, \tag{13}$$

$$b = (I - B)E(\theta) = (I - B)\mu, \tag{14}$$

*where*

$$W = E[Cov(T, \theta)], \tag{15}$$

$$M = \left[W + A^{-1}Cov(\theta)(A^{-1})'\right]^{-1}. \tag{16}$$

**Proof.**

According to the condition in Equation (10), we have

$$0 = E[E(\hat{\theta}_{LB} - \theta|\theta)] = E[E(BT + b) - \theta],$$

so

$$BE_{(T,\theta)}(T) + b = E\theta,$$

$$b = E\theta - BA^{-1}E\theta. \tag{17}$$

According to the condition in Equation (11), we have

$$E_{(T,\theta)}L(\hat{\theta}, \theta) = E_{(Y,\theta)}\{[BT + b - \theta]'D[BT + b - \theta]\}$$

$$= E_{(T,\theta)}L(\hat{\theta}, \theta)$$

$$= E_{(T,\theta)}\left\{[BT + E\theta - BA^{-1}E\theta - \theta]'D[BT + E\theta - BA^{-1}E\theta - \theta]\right\}.$$

$$E_{(T,\theta)}\left\{tr(D[BT + E\theta - BA^{-1}E\theta - \theta][BT + E\theta - BA^{-1}E\theta - \theta]')\right\}$$

$$= E_{(T,\theta)}\left\{tr(D[B(T - A^{-1}E\theta) - (\theta - E\theta)][B(T - A^{-1}E\theta) - (\theta - E\theta)]')\right\}$$

$$= tr(DE_{(T,\theta)}\left\{[B(T - A^{-1}E\theta) - (\theta - E\theta)][B(T - A^{-1}E\theta) - (\theta - E\theta)]'\right\})$$

$$= tr(DE_{(T,\theta)}\left\{B(T - A^{-1}E\theta)(T - A^{-1}E\theta)'B' - B(T - A^{-1}E\theta)(\theta - E\theta)'\right.$$

$$\left. - (\theta - E\theta)(T - A^{-1}E\theta)'B' + (\theta - E\theta)(\theta - E\theta)'\right\})$$

$$= tr(BDE_{(T,\theta)}[(T - A^{-1}E\theta)(T - A^{-1}E\theta)']B') - tr(DBA^{-1}Cov(\theta))$$
$$-tr(DCov(\theta)(A^{-1})'B') + tr(DCov(\theta)). \quad (18)$$

In the above equation,

$$E_{(T,\theta)}[(T - A^{-1}E\theta)(T - A^{-1}E\theta)']$$
$$= E_{(T,\theta)}[TT' - T(A^{-1}E\theta)' - A^{-1}E\theta T' + A^{-1}E\theta(A^{-1}E\theta)']$$
$$= E_{(T,\theta)}TT' + A^{-1}E\theta(A^{-1}E\theta)' - E_{(T,\theta)}T(A^{-1}E\theta)' - (A^{-1}E\theta)E_{(T,\theta)}T']$$
$$= E_{(T,\theta)}TT' + A^{-1}E\theta(A^{-1}E\theta)' - A^{-1}E\theta(A^{-1}E\theta)' - A^{-1}E\theta(A^{-1}E\theta)'$$
$$= E_{(T,\theta)}TT' - A^{-1}E\theta(A^{-1}E\theta)'$$
$$= E[E(TT'\big|\theta)] - A^{-1}E\theta(A^{-1}E\theta)'$$
$$= E\Big\{E[(T - A^{-1}\theta + A^{-1}\theta)(T - A^{-1}\theta + A^{-1}\theta)'\big|\theta]\Big\} - A^{-1}E\theta(A^{-1}E\theta)'$$
$$= E\Big\{E[A^{-1}\theta(A^{-1}\theta)' + (T - A^{-1}\theta)(T - A^{-1}\theta)' + (T - A^{-1}\theta)(A^{-1}\theta)'$$
$$+(A^{-1}\theta)(T - A^{-1}\theta)'\big|\theta]\Big\} - A^{-1}E\theta(A^{-1}E\theta)'$$
$$= E\Big\{A^{-1}\theta(A^{-1}\theta)' + E[(T - A^{-1}\theta)(T - A^{-1}\theta)'] + E\Big[(T - A^{-1}\theta)(A^{-1}\theta)'\Big]$$
$$= E[A^{-1}\theta(A^{-1}\theta)' + E((T - A^{-1}\theta)(T - A^{-1}\theta)')] - A^{-1}E\theta(A^{-1}E\theta)'$$
$$+E(A^{-1}\theta(A^{-1}\theta)')\Big\} - A^{-1}E\theta(A^{-1}E\theta)'$$
$$= E[A^{-1}\theta(A^{-1}\theta)'] + E(Cov(T\big|\theta)) - A^{-1}E\theta(A^{-1}E\theta)'$$
$$= E(Cov(T\big|\theta)) + A^{-1}[E(\theta\theta') - E(\theta)E(\theta)'](A^{-1})$$
$$= W + A^{-1}Cov(\theta)(A^{-1})'.$$

Therefore,

$$E_{(T,\theta)}L(\hat{\theta},\theta) = tr(DB(W + A^{-1}Cov(\theta)(A^{-1})')B') - tr(DBA^{-1}Cov(\theta))$$
$$-tr(DCov(\theta)(A^{-1})'B') + tr(DCov(\theta)).$$

By taking a partial derivative of the matrix $B$ in the above equation, we have

$$\frac{\partial R(\hat{\theta},\theta)}{\partial B} = 2DB[W + A^{-1}Cov(\theta)(A^{-1})'] - 2DCov(\theta)(A^{-1}) = 0,$$
$$B = A - AW[W + A^{-1}Cov(\theta)(A^{-1})']^{-1} = A - AWM, \quad (19)$$

where

$$W = E[Cov(T,\theta)]$$
$$= E[(T - A^{-1}\theta)(T - A^{-1}\theta)'\big|\theta]$$
$$= E\left\{E\left[\begin{pmatrix} t_1 \\ t_2 \end{pmatrix} - \begin{pmatrix} 2 & 0 \\ 0 & \frac{1}{n_0+n_1} \end{pmatrix}\begin{pmatrix} \lambda \\ \phi \end{pmatrix}\right]\left[\begin{pmatrix} t_1 \\ t_2 \end{pmatrix} - \begin{pmatrix} 2 & 0 \\ 0 & \frac{1}{n_0+n_1} \end{pmatrix}\begin{pmatrix} \lambda \\ \phi \end{pmatrix}\right]' |\theta\right\}$$
$$= \begin{bmatrix} E(t_1 - 2\lambda)^2 & 0 \\ 0 & E(t_2 - (n_0 + n_1)\lambda)^2 \end{bmatrix}$$

$$= \begin{bmatrix} Var(t_1) & 0 \\ 0 & Var(t_2) \end{bmatrix}. \tag{20}$$

Theorem 1 proved. □

An expression for linear Bayesian estimation, as detailed in the previously stated Theorem 1, has been constructed. This expression is derived while adhering to the constraints of unbiasedness and focused on the minimization of risk.

### 3.2. The Superiority of Linear Bayesian Estimation

In this subsection, we focus on examining the superiority of linear Bayesian estimation. To evaluate the effectiveness of this estimator, we utilize the mean square error (MSE), a well-regarded measure for assessing how closely an estimator approximates the actual parameter it seeks to estimate. Additionally, for a more careful comparison, we also consider the mean square error matrix (MSEM). To assess the superiority of $\hat{\theta}_{LB}$ according to the MSEM criterion, let us start by defining the MSEM.

**Definition 2.** *Let $\hat{\theta}$ be an estimator of the parameter vector $\theta$. The MSE of $\hat{\theta}$ is defined as*

$$MSE(\theta) = E[(\hat{\theta} - \theta)'(\hat{\theta} - \theta)], \tag{21}$$

*and the MSEM of $\hat{\theta}$ is defined as*

$$MSEM(\theta) = E[(\hat{\theta} - \theta)(\hat{\theta} - \theta)']. \tag{22}$$

Let the parameter vector $\theta$ be estimated in two different ways as $\hat{\theta}_1$ and $\hat{\theta}_2$. If

$$MSEM(\hat{\theta}_2) - MSEM(\hat{\theta}_1) \geq 0,$$

or

$$(MSEM(\hat{\theta}_2) - MSEM(\hat{\theta}_1) \geq 0), \tag{23}$$

then $\hat{\theta}_1$ is said to be better than $\hat{\theta}_2$ under the MSEM or MSE criterion, and it is clear that the MSEM criterion is stronger than the MSE criterion.

From the previous section, the maximum likelihood estimation, $\hat{\theta}_{MLE}$, can be expressed as the product of the statistic $T$ and the matrix $A$, and the linear Bayesian estimation, $\hat{\theta}_{LB}$, is also constructed from the statistic $T$. Therefore, in this section, the MSEM criterion is applied to compare $\hat{\theta}_{LB}$ and $\hat{\theta}_{MLE}$.

**Theorem 2.** *The linear Bayesian estimation, $\hat{\theta}_{LB}$, defined in (7) is preferred to the maximum likelihood estimation, $\hat{\theta}_{MLE}$, defined in (13) under the MSEM criterion, i.e.,*

$$MSEM(\hat{\theta}_{LB}) \leq MSEM(\hat{\theta}_{MLE})$$

**Proof.**

$$\begin{aligned} MSEM(\hat{\theta}_{LB}) &= E_{(T,\theta)}[(\hat{\theta}_{LB} - \theta)(\hat{\theta}_{LB} - \theta)'] \\ &= E[Cov(\hat{\theta}_{LB} - \theta|\theta)] + Cov[E(\hat{\theta}_{LB} - \theta|\theta)] \\ &= E[Cov(\hat{\theta}_{LB}|\theta)] + Cov[E(\hat{\theta}_{LB} - \theta|\theta)] \\ &= E[Cov(A - AWM)T + AWMA^{-1}E\theta\Big|\theta)] \\ &+Cov[E(AT - AWM(T - A^{-1}E\theta\Big) - \theta\Big|\theta)] \\ &= (A - AWM)E(Cov(T|\theta)(A - AWM)') \end{aligned}$$

$$
\begin{aligned}
&+Cov[E(AT|\theta) - E(AWM(T - A^{-1}E\theta|\theta) - \theta)] \\
&= (A - AWM)W(A - AWM)' + Cov(-AWME(T - A^{-1}E\theta|\theta)) \\
&= (A - AWM)W(A - AWM)' + Cov(AWMA^{-1}E[AT - E\theta|\theta]) \\
&= A[(I - WM)W(I - WM) + WMA^{-1}Cov(\theta)(A^{-1})'MW]A' \\
&= A[W - 2WMW + WM(W + A^{-1}Cov(\theta)(A^{-1})')MW]A' \\
&= A[W - WMW]A'.
\end{aligned}
$$

However,

$$
\begin{aligned}
MSEM(\hat{\theta}_{MLE}) &= E_{(T,\theta)}[(\hat{\theta} - \theta)(\hat{\theta} - \theta)'] \\
&= E\{E[(\hat{\theta} - \theta)(\hat{\theta} - \theta)'|\theta]\} \\
&= E\{E[(AT - \theta)(AT - \theta)'|\theta]\} \\
&= AWA'.
\end{aligned}
$$

According to the defining equation of $W$, we can easily find that $W$ is positive and definite, and because of the definition of the matrix $M$, both $A^{-1}$ and $(A^{-1})'$ are positive definite matrices. Thus, Theorem 2 is proved. □

## 4. Numerical Simulation and Empirical Application

### 4.1. Numerical Simulation

In this section, we evaluate the performance superiority of classical and linear Bayesian estimation methods for the misrecorded Poisson distribution using numerical simulations. By choosing a range of different parameter values, we compute the mean square error (MSE) for both classical and linear Bayesian estimations relative to these values. A smaller error indicates a more accurate estimation. The procedures for these numerical simulations are detailed in the following steps.

1. Generate a dataset that accurately follows the characteristics of the misrecorded Poisson distribution, ensuring to use the predefined true parameter values as a foundational reference.

2. Proceed to calculate and derive parameter estimates, utilizing and comparing different established estimation methods for the analysis.

3. Calculate the mean and variance of the statistic $T$ defined in Equation (20) using the bootstrap sampling method, and then use these values in the computation.

4. Repeat the above steps $J$ times to obtain the mean of the estimate and give the MSE.

We set the sample size to $N$ = 200 and 800 and set the parameters in the misrecorded Poisson distribution (1) to very between $\lambda = 0.7$ and $\phi = 0.7$; $\lambda = 0.7$ and $\phi = 0.9$; $\lambda = 0.9$ and $\phi = 0.7$; and $\lambda = 0.9$ and $\phi = 0.9$. All the simulations are performed via $J = 100$ repetitions. The results are listed in Tables 1 and 2. In these two tables, $\hat{\lambda}_{LB}$ and $\hat{\phi}_{LB}$ represent the linear Bayesian estimates of $\lambda$ and $\phi$, $\hat{\theta}_{MLEMSE}$ denotes the MSE for the maximum likelihood estimation, $\hat{\theta}_{LBMSE}$ denotes the MSE of the linear Bayesian estimation, and $||\hat{\theta}_{MLEMSE} - \hat{\theta}_{LBMSE}||_2$ is the Euclidean distance between $\hat{\theta}_{MLEMSE}$ and $\hat{\theta}_{LBMSE}$.

**Table 1.** Estimation results.

| | $\lambda$ | $\phi$ | $\hat{\lambda}_{MLE}$ | $\hat{\phi}_{MLE}$ | $\hat{\lambda}_{LB}$ | $\hat{\phi}_{LB}$ |
|---|---|---|---|---|---|---|
| $N = 200$ | 0.7 | 0.7 | 0.704053 | 0.694272 | 0.703608 | 0.694273 |
| | | 0.9 | 0.712559 | 0.893031 | 0.711961 | 0.893031 |
| | 0.9 | 0.7 | 0.89567 | 0.692927 | 0.895587 | 0.692927 |
| | | 0.9 | 0.897774 | 0.89222 | 0.897602 | 0.89222 |
| $N = 800$ | 0.7 | 0.7 | 0.702591 | 0.699152 | 0.702557 | 0.699152 |
| | | 0.9 | 0.69286 | 0.89726 | 0.692883 | 0.89726 |
| | 0.3 | 0.8 | 0.294824 | 0.795203 | 0.294818 | 0.795203 |
| | 0.8 | 0.3 | 0.794149 | 0.294536 | 0.794162 | 0.294536 |

**Table 2.** The MSE and distance from the true value.

| | $\lambda$ | $\phi$ | $\hat{\theta}_{MLEMSE}$ | $\hat{\theta}_{LBMSE}$ | $\|\|\hat{\theta}_{MLEMSE} - \hat{\theta}_{LBMSE}\|\|_2$ |
|---|---|---|---|---|---|
| $N = 200$ | 0.7 | 0.7 | 0.007665 | 0.007364 | 0.001971974 |
| | | 0.9 | 0.00576 | 0.005474 | 0.002007057 |
| | 0.9 | 0.7 | 0.005215 | 0.005035 | 0.001461555 |
| | | 0.9 | 0.006006 | 0.005752 | 0.001724022 |
| $N = 800$ | 0.7 | 0.7 | 0.00149 | 0.001474 | 0.000222702 |
| | | 0.9 | 0.001428 | 0.001411 | 0.000225155 |
| | 0.3 | 0.8 | 0.001506 | 0.001492 | 0.000243135 |
| | 0.8 | 0.3 | 0.003181 | 0.003162 | 0.000233711 |

From Table 1, we can see that all the estimates are close to the true values regardless of the values of $\lambda$ and $\phi$. Importantly, our analysis reveals a key trend: as the sample size increases, all the estimates progressively converge towards their true values. This pattern is evident for both the maximum likelihood estimation and the linear Bayesian estimation, underscoring their consistency as estimators. The reliability of these approaches is evidenced in Table 2, which presents a noteworthy distinction in the mean square error (MSE) values between them. Specifically, the MSE for the linear Bayesian estimation is lower than that for maximum likelihood estimation. Remarkably, the Euclidean distance between $\hat{\theta}_{MLEMSE}$ and $\hat{\theta}_{LBMSE}$ diminishes as the sample size increases, suggesting that the advantage of linear Bayesian estimation becomes more pronounced in smaller sample sizes.

### 4.2. Empirical Application

In this section, we illustrate our proposed method using two sets of real data.

#### 4.2.1. Empirical Application 1

The first dataset for our research originates from Ladislaus Bortkiewicz's acclaimed book '*Das Gesetz der Kleinen Zahlen*', published in 1898 [29]. This particular data set gained historical significance when Cohen introduced the misrecorded Poisson distribution model for the first time. It comprises a collection of statistical records detailing the annual fatalities among Prussian soldiers due to horse-related incidents from 1875 to 1884. The data encompass detailed records from 14 distinct regiments and one guard unit, providing a diverse and comprehensive dataset for the analysis. The nature of these incidents inherently suggests the suitability of a Poisson distribution for modeling the frequency and patterns of these rare events. In an effort to validate and corroborate the findings discussed in this paper, we undertook some modifications to the original dataset. Specifically, we adjusted 20 entries that were originally noted as having a value of 1, revising them to 0. This adjustment is carefully documented in Table 3, allowing for a more accurate analysis in line with our study objectives.

**Table 3.** Soldiers who were kicked to death by horses between 1875 and 1984.

| Number per Deaths of Army Corps per Year | Number of Observations | |
|---|---|---|
| | Original Data | Altered Data |
| 0 | 109 | 129 |
| 1 | 65 | 45 |
| 2 | 22 | 22 |
| 3 | 3 | 3 |
| 4 | 1 | 1 |
| 5 | 0 | 0 |

We now fit a misrecorded Poisson distribution to this modified dataset using both maximum likelihood estimation and linear Bayesian estimation. From Table 3, we have $N = 200$, $n_0 = 129$, $n_1 = 45$, $\bar{x} = 102/200 = 0.51$, $n_0/N = 0.645$, and $n_1/N = 0.225$. Substituting these values into the maximum likelihood estimation, as shown in Equations (5) and (6), we have

$$\hat{\lambda}_{MLE} = \left[ (\bar{x} - 1 + n_0/N) + \sqrt{(\bar{x} - 1 + n_0/N)^2 + 4(\bar{x} - n_1/N)} \right] /2$$

$$= \left[ (0.51 - 1 + 0.645) + \sqrt{(0.51 - 1 + 0.645)^2 + 4 \times (0.51 - 0.225)} \right] /2$$

$$= 0.61695.$$

$$\hat{\varphi}_{MLE} = (n_0 - n_1/\hat{\lambda})/(n_0 + n_1)$$

$$= ((129 - 45)/\hat{\lambda})/(129 + 45)$$

$$= 0.322187.$$

From the unchanged raw data [29], we have that $\lambda = 0.610$ and $\varphi = 20/65 = 0.308$, which is the proportion of ones that were misclassified in the process of altering the original data for this illustration. The specific proof process can be found in Appendix A. Utilizing linear Bayesian estimation (13), we obtain $\hat{\lambda}_{LB} = 0.6167831$ and $\hat{\varphi}_{LB} = 0.3221758$. Subsequently, we can compute the MSE by comparing the true values of the two parameters with the combined estimations from above: $MSE(\hat{\theta}_{MLE}) = 0.0001247861$ and $MSE(\hat{\theta}_{LB}) = 0.0001235136$, so $MSE(\hat{\theta}_{LB}) \leq MSE(\hat{\theta}_{MLE})$. This indicates that the linear Bayesian estimation has better performance than the maximum likelihood estimation.

#### 4.2.2. Empirical Application 2

The second dataset for our research, originating from Yang [30], is presented in Table 4. The frequent occurrence of accidents at intersections in the area increases the probability of traffic accidents due to the vehicle type, traffic volume, and linear congestion. People can analyze data to discover the changes and distribution patterns of traffic volume over time and space. These findings help develop effective traffic control measures and reduce accident rates under different traffic conditions.

**Table 4.** Traffic volume at intersection C.

| The Number of Passes for Small-Sized Cars | Number of Observations | |
|---|---|---|
| | Original Data | Altered Data |
| 0 | 15 | 18 |
| 1 | 5 | 2 |
| 2 | 9 | 9 |
| 3 | 6 | 6 |
| 4 | 7 | 7 |
| 5 | 1 | 1 |
| 6 | 2 | 2 |

The investigation was conducted at the T-shaped intersection of West Ring Road outside the University City and Xingguang Road under the University City in Guangzhou Province. The survey focuses on the traffic volume of motor vehicles at this intersection, which was collected through manual monitoring.

According to Table 4, we can calculate from the original data that $\lambda = 1.911$ and $\phi = 3/5 = 0.6$. Substituting these values into the maximum likelihood estimation, as shown in Equations (5) and (6), we have $\hat{\lambda}_{MLE} = 2.101127$ and $\hat{\phi}_{MLE} = 0.8524065$. Utilizing linear Bayesian estimation (13), we obtain $\hat{\lambda}_{LB} = 1.817069$ and $\hat{\phi}_{LB} = 0.852164$. Therefore, similarly to the previous example, we can obtain $MSE(\hat{\theta}_{MLE}) = 0.7400561$, $MSE(\hat{\theta}_{LB}) = 0.4422734$, and $MSE(\hat{\theta}_{LB}) \leq MSE(\hat{\theta}_{MLE})$. This still indicates that the linear Bayesian estimation is superior to the maximum likelihood estimation.

## 5. Conclusions

This research study primarily focuses on an in-depth examination of the unique characteristics and distinct properties of linear Bayesian estimation, specifically applied to the misrecorded Poisson distribution. A key aspect of this study is providing robust empirical evidence that demonstrates the enhanced performance of linear Bayesian estimation when compared to maximum likelihood estimation, particularly within the framework of this distribution. Moreover, to reinforce these theoretical insights, the study employs a comprehensive approach, encompassing both rigorous validation through a series of detailed numerical simulations and the use of illustrative examples to further elucidate these findings. This multifaceted approach not only solidifies the theoretical underpinnings but also showcases the practical applicability of linear Bayesian estimation in real-world scenarios.

The method employed in this paper may not capture all dynamic characteristics when dealing with complex real-world situations. Due to the development of big data and advanced statistical methods and the need for more complex models in recent years, we consider extending the traditional framework of the Poisson distribution with the Hawkes process, thereby providing more effective tools and methodologies for solving practical problems.

**Author Contributions:** Writing—original draft, H.G.; Writing—review & editing, Z.C. and F.L. All authors have read and agreed to the published version of the manuscript.

**Funding:** This work was supported by the Natural Science Foundation of China (No. 12161072) and the Natural Science Foundation of Qinghai Province (No. 2019-ZJ-920).

**Data Availability Statement:** The data presented in this study are available on request from the corresponding author.

**Conflicts of Interest:** The authors declare no conflict of interest.

## Appendix A

1. Proof process in Empirical Application 1

According to Definition 1, $\theta = (\lambda, \phi)'$, we define $MES(\hat{\theta}_{MLE}) = \frac{1}{2}((\hat{\lambda}_{MLE} - \lambda)^2 + (\hat{\phi}_{MLE} - \phi)^2)$ and $MES(\hat{\theta}_{LB}) = \frac{1}{2}((\hat{\lambda}_{LB} - \lambda)^2 + (\hat{\phi}_{\mathrm{LB}} - \phi)^2)$ to represent the mean square errors of the population for both parameters in the two estimation methods. The true values in this example are $\lambda = 0.610$ and $\phi = 0.308$, where $\lambda = \frac{\Sigma(x_i \times f_i)}{N}$. $f_i$ represents the observed frequency of each event occurrence and $\phi$ is the probability of misclassification or the proportion of ones that are reported as zeros. The estimated values calculated based on the maximum likelihood estimation are $\hat{\lambda}_{MLE} = 0.61695$ and $\hat{\phi}_{MLE} = 0.322187$, and those obtained from the linear Bayesian estimation are $\hat{\lambda}_{LB} = 0.6167831$ and $\hat{\phi}_{LB} = 0.3221758$. Hence, we have two parameters with the combined estimations $MSE(\hat{\theta}_{MLE}) = 0.0001247861$ and $MSE(\hat{\theta}_{LB}) = 0.0001235136$. Therefore, it follows that $MSE(\hat{\theta}_{LB}) \leq MSE(\hat{\theta}_{MLE})$. Proof completed.

## References


1. Cohen, J.R.; Clifford, A. Estimating the parameters of a modified Poisson distribution. *J. Am. Stat. Assoc.* **1960**, *55*, 139–143. [CrossRef]
2. Dorris, A.L.; Foote, B.L. Inspection errors and statistical quality control: A survey. *AIIE Trans.* **1978**, *10*, 184–192. [CrossRef]
3. Gupta, P.L.; Gupta, R.C.; Tripathi, R.C. Analysis of zero-adjusted count data. *Comput. Stat. Data Anal.* **1996**, *23*, 207–218. [CrossRef]
4. Zhang, C.; Tian, G.L.; Ng, K.W. Properties of the zero-and-one inflated Poisson distribution and likelihood-based inference methods. *Stat. Its Interface* **2016**, *9*, 11–32. [CrossRef]
5. Liu, Y.; Tian, G.L.; Tang, M.L. A new multivariate zero-adjusted Poisson model with applications to biomedicine. *Biom. J.* **2019**, *61*, 1340–1370. [CrossRef] [PubMed]
6. Bagui, S.C.; Mehra, K.L. The Poisson Distribution and Its Convergence to the Normal Distribution. *Int. J. Stat. Sci.* **2020**, *36*, 37–56.
7. Zhang, Q.; Lipani, A.; Kirnap, O.; Yilmaz, E. Self-Attentive Hawkes Process. In Proceedings of the 37th International Conference on Machine Learning, Virtual, 13–18 July 2020; Volume 119, pp. 11183–11193.
8. Wang, L.W.; Zhang, L. *Hawkes Processes for Understanding Heterogeneity in Information Propagation on Twitter*; School of Science, Beijing University of Posts and Telecommunications: Beijing, China, 2022.
9. Lamprinakou, S.; Gandy, A.; McCoy, E. Using a latent Hawkes process for epidemiological modelling. *PLoS ONE* **2023**, *18*, e0281370. [CrossRef] [PubMed]
10. Xu, J. Study on a Class of Mixed Poisson and Its Zero-Inflated Distribution. Master's Thesis, Chang'an University, Chang'an, China, 2022.
11. Johnson, N.L. *Univariate Discrete Distributions*; John Wiley and Sons: Hoboken, NJ, USA, 2004.
12. Djuraš, G. *Generalized Poisson Models for Word Length Frequencies in Texts of Slavic Languages*; Graz University of Technology Press: Graz, Austria, 2012.
13. Tuwei, K.E. *Power Series Distribution Sand Zero-Inflated Models*; University of Nairobi Press: Nairobi, Kenya, 2014.
14. Angers, J.F.; Biswas, A. A Bayesian analysis of zero-inflated generalized Poisson model. *Comput. Stat. Data Anal.* **2003**, *42*, 37–46. [CrossRef]
15. Rodrigues, J. Bayesian Analysis of Zero-Inflated Distributions. *Commun. Stat.—Theory Methods* **2003**, *32*, 281–289. [CrossRef]
16. Wang, Y.Q. Bayesian Estimation Based on Zero-and-One-Inflated Poisson Regression Model. Master's Thesis, Central China Normal University, Wuhan, China, 2022.
17. Hartigan, J.A. Linear Bayesian Methods. *J. R. Stat. Soc. Ser. B Methodol.* **1969**, *31*, 446–454. [CrossRef]
18. Rao, C.R. *Linear Statistical Inference and Its Applications*, 2nd ed.; John Wiley and Sons: Hoboken, NJ, USA, 1973.
19. LaMotte, L.R. Bayes linear estimators. *Technometrics* **1978**, *20*, 281–290. [CrossRef]
20. Hesselager, O. Rates of risk convergence of empirical linear Bayes estimators. *Scand. Actuar. J.* **1992**, *1*, 88–94. [CrossRef]
21. Goldstein, M. General Variance Modifications for Linear Bayes Estimators. *J. Am. Stat. Assoc.* **1983**, *78*, 616–618. [CrossRef]
22. Hoffmann, K. A subclass of Bayes linear estimators that are minimax. *Acta Appl. Math.* **1996**, *43*, 87–95. [CrossRef]
23. Samaniego, J.F.; Vestrup, V.E. On improving standard estimators via linear empirical Bayes methods. *Stat. Probab. Lett.* **1999**, *44*, 309–318. [CrossRef]
24. Wei, L.S.; Zhang, W.P. The superiorities of Bayes Linear Minimum Risk Estimation in Linear Model. *Commun. Stat. Theory Methods* **2007**, *36*, 917–926. [CrossRef]
25. Lin, P.P. Linear Bayesian Estimation under Constraint Conditions. Master's Thesis, Beijing Jiaotong University, Beijing, China, 2018.
26. Tao, R.F. Linear Bayesian Estimation of Parameters in Pareto Distribution. Master's Thesis, Jiangxi Normal University, Beijing, China, 2019.
27. Liu, X.H. Linear Bayes Estimators in Singular Linear Model. Master's Thesis, Beijing Jiaotong University, Beijing, China, 2022.
28. Chen, T. Linear Bayes Estimator of the Extreme Value Distribution Based on Type II Censored Samples. Master's Thesis, Beijing Jiaotong University, Beijing, China, 2021.
29. von Bortkiewicz, L. *Das Gesetz der Kleinen Zahlen*; Teubner Press: Leipzig, Germany, 1898.
30. Yang, C.Q. Investigation and Analysis of Traffic Flow in Urban Road Intersection. Master's Thesis, Guangzhou University, Guangzhou, China, 2018.

*entropy*

MDPI

*Article*

# An Objective and Robust Bayes Factor for the Hypothesis Test One Sample and Two Population Means

**Israel A. Almodóvar-Rivera [1,*] and Luis R. Pericchi-Guerra [2]**

[1] Department of Mathematical Sciences, University of Puerto Rico at Mayagüez, Mayagüez, PR 00680, USA
[2] Department of Mathematics, University of Puerto Rico at Rio Piedras, San Juan, PR 00930, USA; luis.pericchi@upr.edu
* Correspondence: israel.almodovar@upr.edu

**Abstract:** It has been over 100 years since the discovery of one of the most fundamental statistical tests: the Student's $t$ test. However, reliable conventional and objective Bayesian procedures are still essential for routine practice. In this work, we proposed an objective and robust Bayesian approach for hypothesis testing for one-sample and two-sample mean comparisons when the assumption of equal variances holds. The newly proposed Bayes factors are based on the intrinsic and Berger robust prior. Additionally, we introduced a corrected version of the Bayesian Information Criterion (BIC), denoted BIC-TESS, which is based on the effective sample size (TESS), for comparing two population means. We studied our developed Bayes factors in several simulation experiments for hypothesis testing. Our methodologies consistently provided strong evidence in favor of the null hypothesis in the case of equal means and variances. Finally, we applied the methodology to the original Gosset sleep data, concluding strong evidence favoring the hypothesis that the average sleep hours differed between the two treatments. These methodologies exhibit finite sample consistency and demonstrate consistent qualitative behavior, proving reasonably close to each other in practice, particularly for moderate to large sample sizes.

**Keywords:** student's $t$ test; Bayes factors; intrinsic priors; robust prior

## 1. Introduction

One of the fundamental topics in statistics revolves around the one-sample population means and the comparison of two-sample means. The go-to method for addressing this question is typically the Student's $t$ test [1]. Conducting a hypothesis test for the population mean holds significant importance in the scientific research community and various fields where making inferences about population parameters is pivotal. Frequentists heavily rely on $p$-values to determine whether to reject or not reject the null hypothesis [2]. However, $p$-values, along with significance testing based on fixed $\alpha$-levels, tend to exaggerate evidence against null hypotheses for large sample sizes and lack the operational meaning of a probability [3–5]. While the Bayesian approach has gained attention in hypothesis testing and model selection [6,7], its application in essential statistics topics remains somewhat limited [8]. This raises the question: Why is a Bayesian Student's $t$ test necessary? We argue for two main reasons. Firstly, Bayesian tests provide evidence for a hypothesis of interest that naturally adapts to any sample size. Secondly, the Bayes factor can be easily converted to posterior model probabilities and support one of the testing frameworks. Another crucial consideration is that scientific questions often have a Bayesian nature, such as, "What is the probability that these two treatments differ?".

Bayesian hypothesis testing and model selection have been undergoing extensive development because of recent advances in the creation of "default" Bayes factors that can be used in the absence of substantial subjective prior information [5,9–11]. The study in [12] proposed some arguments for the choice of the prior, such as (i) the fact that it is located around zero, (ii) the scale parameter $\sigma$, (iii) the fact that it is symmetric, and (iv) that it should have no moments. Bayes factors are attractive in terms of interpretation as odds, and the direct probability of the posterior model is readily understandable by general users of statistics [13]. Methods based on conjugate priors for the Student's $t$ test have a long history. Perhaps the most transparent approach for the two-sample Student's $t$ is in [14]. However, natural conjugate priors do not lead to robust procedures; they have tails that are typically of the same form as the likelihood function and will hence remain influential when the likelihood function is concentrated in the prior tails, which can lead to inconsistency [15]. This conjugate Bayes factor for comparing two samples based on the Student's $t$ is finite sample-inconsistent, i.e., it does not go to zero when the estimates go to infinity.

In this work, we proposed an objective and robust Bayes factor for testing the hypothesis of one-sample and two-sample means based on the $t$-statistic. Our Bayes factors can be easily implemented, allowing researchers to determine support for a particular hypothesis. This manuscript proceeds as follows. In Section 2, we derive these objectives and robust Bayes factors for one-sample and two-sample scenarios and demonstrate their finite sample consistency. In Section 3, we compare our Bayes factors with existing methodologies under several experimental frameworks. In Section 4, we apply our methodologies to real-life datasets such as the original Gosset sleep data and to comparisons of changes in blood pressure in mice according to their assigned diet. We conclude this work with a discussion in Section 5.

## 2. Methodology

Statistical inference for the mean (one or two samples) has an important rule in statistics and several fields. For instance, it is very common to test in terms of the average or population mean. Suppose that we are comparing two hypotheses, $H_0 : \boldsymbol{\theta}_0 \in \Theta$ vs. $H_1 : \boldsymbol{\theta}_1 \in \Theta$. Suppose that we have available prior densities $\pi_i, i = 1, 2$ for each hypothesis and let $f_i(\boldsymbol{x}|\boldsymbol{\theta}_i)$ be the probability density function under the $i$th hypothesis. Define the marginal or predictive densities for each hypothesis of interest (or model),

$$m_i(\boldsymbol{x}) = \int f_i(\boldsymbol{x}|\boldsymbol{\theta}_i)\pi_i(\boldsymbol{\theta}_i)d\boldsymbol{\theta}_i, \tag{1}$$

which are sometimes called the evidence of the $i$th hypothesis or model. The Bayes factor for comparing $H_0$ to $H_1$ is then given by

$$B_{01} = \frac{m_0(\boldsymbol{x})}{m_1(\boldsymbol{x})} = \frac{\int f_0(\boldsymbol{x}|\boldsymbol{\theta}_0)\pi_0(\boldsymbol{\theta}_0)d\boldsymbol{\theta}_0}{\int f_1(\boldsymbol{x}|\boldsymbol{\theta}_1)\pi_1(\boldsymbol{\theta}_1)d\boldsymbol{\theta}_1}. \tag{2}$$

The interpretation of the Bayes factor proceeds as follows. If $B_{01} > 1$, then the evidence is in favor of the null hypothesis, while $B_{01} < 1$ gives evidence in favor of the alternative hypothesis. If prior probabilities $P(H_i)$ $i = 0, 1$ of the hypotheses are available, then one can compute the posterior probabilities of it from the Bayes factors. The posterior probability of $H_0$, given the data $\boldsymbol{x}$, is

$$\mathbb{P}(H_0|\boldsymbol{x}) = \frac{m_0(\boldsymbol{x})P(H_0)}{\sum_{j=0}^{1} m_j(\boldsymbol{x})P(H_j)} = \frac{1}{1 + \frac{P(H_1)}{P(H_0)}B_{10}}; \tag{3}$$

where $B_{10} = 1/B_{01}$.

### 2.1. One-Sample Mean Hypothesis Testing

A one-sample hypothesis test for the population mean is one of the most fundamental statistics topics, either as an introductory topic or to address research questions. Suppose we have a random sample from a normal distribution, i.e., $X_1, \ldots, X_n \sim N(\mu, \sigma^2)$, with an unknown standard deviation $\sigma > 0$. We are interested in testing for the population mean $\mu$

$$H_0 : \mu = \mu_0 \text{ vs. } H_1 : \mu \neq \mu_0. \tag{4}$$

A Bayesian approach to test this hypothesis is based on the theory of intrinsic priors [16,17]. The authors begin with the noninformative priors for the null and alternative hypotheses, $\pi_0^N(\sigma) = 1/\sigma$ and $\pi_1^N(\mu, \sigma) = 1/\sigma^2$. After some calculations, the authors showed that the conditional proper intrinsic prior under the alternative Hypothesis $H_1$ is given by

$$\pi^I(\mu|\sigma) = \frac{1}{2\sqrt{\pi}\sigma} \frac{1 - e^{-\mu^2/\sigma^2}}{(\mu^2/\sigma^2)}.$$

One can express $\pi^I(\mu, \sigma) = \pi(\mu|\sigma)\pi(\sigma)$. The resulting intrinsic prior under $H_1$ is defined as

$$\pi_1^I(\mu, \sigma) = \pi_1^I(\mu|\sigma)/\sigma = \frac{1}{2\sqrt{\pi}} \frac{1 - e^{-\mu^2/\sigma^2}}{\mu^2}.$$

The approximate Bayes factors based on the intrinsic prior ($B_{01}^{IP}$) for a one-sample population mean are

$$B_{01}^{IP} \approx B_{01}^{N} \cdot \frac{\pi_1^N(\hat{\mu}, \hat{\sigma})}{\pi_1^I(\hat{\mu}, \hat{\sigma})}(1 + o(1)).$$

Here, $\hat{\mu}$ and $\hat{\sigma}$ are the Maximum Likelihood Estimators (MLEs) under $H_1$. The resulting Bayes factor for the hypothesis in (4) is

$$B_{01}^{IP} \approx \sqrt{2n}\left(1 + \frac{t^2}{n-1}\right)^{-n/2} \frac{t^2/(n-1)}{1 - e^{-t^2/(n-1)}}; \tag{5}$$

where $t = (\bar{x} - \mu_0)/s/\sqrt{n}$, where $\bar{x}$ is the sample mean and $s$ is the sample standard deviation. Larges values of $B_{01}$ give evidence in favor of the null hypothesis. Also, we can transform these Bayes factors using the natural logarithm scale ($2 \log B_{01}$), and values above 3 give some evidence in favor of the null hypothesis, while values above 10 give stronger evidence in favor of the null hypothesis; see [13].

This Bayes factor satisfies the finite sample consistency principle. Suppose that we are comparing the alternative hypothesis with the null hypothesis, $H_0 : \boldsymbol{\beta} = \mathbf{0}$. As the least squares estimate $\widehat{\boldsymbol{\beta}}$ (and the noncentrality parameter) goes to infinity, so that one becomes sure that $H_0$ is wrong, the Bayes factor of $H_0$ to $H_1$ goes to zero.

**Theorem 1.** *For a fixed sample size $n \geq 2$, the Bayes factor based on the intrinsic prior ($B_{01}^{IP}$) for the one-sample mean $\mu$ is finite sample-consistent.*

**Proof.** For a fixed sample, $n \geq 2$, and letting $t^2 \to \infty$ or equivalently $|t| \to \infty$, the Bayes factor based on the intrinsic prior goes to 0, i.e.,

$$\lim_{|t| \to \infty} B_{01}^{IP} \to 0; \text{ or equivalently } \lim_{|t| \to \infty} \mathbb{P}(H_0|\boldsymbol{x}) \to 0.$$

The Bayes Factor based on the intrinsic prior $B_{01}^{IP}$ is finite sample consistent. □

Robust Bayes Factor for the One-Sample Test for the Mean

Even though the Bayes Factor constructed using the intrinsic prior is finite sample-consistent, it is only an approximation. Evidence has been found that priors with flatter tails than those of the likelihood function tend to be fairly robust, [18,19]. The robust prior proposed here is developed by [20]; we call it the Berger robust prior. This prior is hierarchical; by such a choice, we can obtain robustness while keeping the calculations relatively simple, and the computations are exact. The definition of this robust prior, denoted $\pi^R(\xi)$, can be defined as follows:

1. $\xi|\lambda \sim \mathcal{N}_p(\boldsymbol{\mu}, \mathbf{B}(\lambda))$, where $\mathbf{B}(\lambda) = \rho\lambda^{-1}(b+d) - d$ and $\rho = \frac{p+1}{p+3}$.
2. $\lambda$ has a density $\pi(\lambda) = \frac{1}{2}\lambda^{-1/2}$ on $(0,1)$.

where $p$ is the rank of the design matrix. Recall that we are interested in testing (4); therefore, under the null hypothesis, the likelihood is in the form

$$f_0(\mathbf{x}|\mu_0,\sigma) = (2\pi)^{-n/2}\sigma^{-n}\exp\left\{-\frac{\sum_{i=1}^{n}(x_i-\mu_0)^2}{2\sigma^2}\right\}.$$

The noninformative prior under the null hypothesis is $\pi^N(\sigma) = 1/\sigma$. The marginal density $m(\mathbf{x})$ under the null hypothesis is given by

$$\begin{aligned} m_0(\mathbf{x}) &= \int f_0(\mathbf{x}|\sigma)\pi^N(\sigma)d\sigma = \int_0^\infty (2\pi)^{-n}\sigma^{-n}e^{-\frac{SS_0^2}{2\sigma^2}}\sigma^{-1}d\sigma \\ &= (2\pi)^{-n/2}(SS_0^2)^{-n/2}\Gamma\left(\frac{n}{2}\right); \end{aligned} \tag{6}$$

where $SS_0^2 = \sum_{i=1}^{n}(x_i-\mu_0)^2$, the sums of squares under $H_0$ and $\Gamma(\cdot)$ is the gamma function. Similarly, we can obtain an alternative likelihood under the alternative Hypothesis $H_1$:

$$f_1(\mathbf{x}|\mu,\sigma) = (2\pi)^{-n/2}\sigma^{-n}\exp\left\{-\frac{SS_1^2}{2\sigma^2} - \frac{n(\mu-\bar{x})^2}{2\sigma^2}\right\}.$$

Here, $\bar{x} = n^{-1}\sum_{i=1}^{n}x_i$ is the sample mean and $SS_1^2 = \sum_{i=1}^{n}(x_i-\bar{x})^2$ is the sum of squares under the alternative. The Berger robust prior will be considered under the alternative hypothesis $\pi_1(\mu,\sigma) = \pi^R(\mu|\sigma)/\sigma$. The marginal density under $H_1$ is

$$\begin{aligned} m_1(\mathbf{x}) &= \int f_1(\mathbf{x}|\mu,\sigma)\pi_1(\mu,\sigma)d\mu d\sigma = \int f_1(\mathbf{x}|\mu,\sigma)\pi^R(\mu|\sigma)\frac{1}{\sigma}d\mu d\sigma \\ &= \frac{(2\pi)^{-n/2}}{n\cdot(\bar{x}-\mu_0)^2}\sqrt{\frac{n+1}{2}}\left(\frac{\Gamma((n-2)/2)}{2(\frac{s^2}{2})^{(n-2)/2}} - \frac{\Gamma((n-2)/2)}{2(\frac{s^2}{2}+\frac{(\bar{x}-\mu_0)^2}{(n+1)/n})^{(n-2)/2}}\right). \end{aligned} \tag{7}$$

Computing the ratio of the marginals from (6) and (7), the Bayes factor based on the Berger robust prior is given by

$$B_{01}^R = \sqrt{\frac{2}{n+1}\frac{n-2}{n-1}t^2}\left(1+\frac{t^2}{n-2}\right)^{-n/2}\left(1-\left(1+\frac{2t^2}{n^2-1}\right)^{-(n-2)/2}\right)^{-1}. \tag{8}$$

Here, $t = (\bar{x}-\mu_0)/(s/\sqrt{n})$ is the usual $t$-statistic with $n-1$ degrees of freedom, where $\bar{x}$ and $s$ are the sample mean and sample standard deviation, respectively.

**Theorem 2.** *For a fixed sample size $n \geq 3$, the Bayes factor based on the Berger robust prior ($B_{01}^R$) for the one-sample mean $\mu$ is finite sample-consistent.*

**Proof.** For a fixed sample, $n \geq 3$, and letting $t^2 \to \infty$, or equivalently $|t| \to \infty$, the Bayes factor based on the Berger robust prior goes to 0, i.e.,

$$\lim_{|t|\to\infty} B_{01}^R \to 0; \text{ or equivalently } \lim_{|t|\to\infty} \mathbb{P}(H_0|x) \to 0.$$

The Bayes factor based on the Berger robust prior $B_{01}^R$ is finite sample-consistent. □

Unlike the Bayes factor derived with the intrinsic prior, this robust Bayes factor has a closed form. We conclude the derivations for the Bayesian approach based on the intrinsic and robust prior that are finite sample consistent. We now extend the objective and robust Bayesian approach to the two-sample scenarios.

### 2.2. Two-Sample Mean Hypothesis Test

Another fundamental research question of interest is whether or not the two groups are similar. This problem is usually addressed in the two-sample Student's $t$ test to compare if these groups differ in means. Let $X_1,\ldots,X_{n_1} \sim N(\mu_1,\sigma^2)$ and let $Y_1,\ldots,Y_{n_2} \sim N(\mu_2,\sigma^2)$ independent of $X$ with $\sigma > 0$ unknown. At first, we noticed that we were assuming that these two samples arise from a normal distribution with different means but equal variances. It is common interest to determine if these two samples are equal, or at least that they do not differ in location. To answer this, a hypothesis test for comparing two-sample means is performed, i.e., $H_0 : \mu_1 = \mu_2$ against $H_1 : \mu_1 \neq \mu_2$. To answer this question, Ref. [14] proposed the conjugate Bayes factor. This Bayes factor is based on the conjugate prior: $(\mu_1-\mu_2)/\sigma = \delta/\sigma|\sigma \sim N(\lambda,\sigma_\delta^2)$. Centering the prior assessment on the null hypothesis, i.e., making $\lambda = 0$, is usually a very reasonable choice. Then, the conjugate Bayes factor is simplified as $B_{01}^C = \left[\frac{1+t_\nu^2/\nu}{1+t_\nu^2/(\nu(1+n_\delta\sigma_\delta^2))}\right]^{-(\nu+1)/2}\sqrt{1+n_\delta\sigma_\delta^2}$. However, this Bayes factor is not finite sample-consistent, as $|t| \to \infty$, or $t^2 \to \infty$; the $B_{01}^C$ does not go to zero, or equivalently, the posterior probability of the null hypothesis $\mathbb{P}(H_0|data)$ does not go to zero. In fact, as $|t| \to \infty$, then $B_{01}^C \to \left(1+n_\delta\sigma_\delta^2\right)^{-\nu/2} > 0$, where $n_\delta = 1/(1/n_1+1/n_2)$ and $\nu = n_1+n_2-2$ are the degrees of freedom.

#### 2.2.1. Intrinsic Bayes Factor for Two-Sample Means

To address the limitation of the conjugate prior, our first approach is based on the theory of intrinsic priors introduced in [16,17]. Similar to the one-sample case, the method is to dig out a prior that yields, for moderate to large sample sizes, results equivalent to an established method for scaling the intrinsic Bayes factors. The resulting set of equations typically has solutions, at least in the nested hypothesis scenario, which is our case, and has been successfully applied coupled with the intrinsic Bayes factor method. Consider the hypotheses tests for the comparison of two populations means with unknown and equal variance $\sigma^2 > 0$, $H_0 : \mu_1 = \mu_2$ vs. $H_1 : \mu_1 \neq \mu_2$. Let $\delta_0 = (\mu_1+\mu_2)/2$ and $\delta_1 = (\mu_1-\mu_2)/2$, then $\mu_1 = \delta_0+\delta_1$ and $\mu_2 = \delta_0-\delta_1$. This transformation leads us to the following design matrix $\mathbf{X}$ based on the training samples:

$$\mathbf{X}\mu = \begin{bmatrix} \mathbf{1}_{2\times 1} & \mathbf{0}_{2\times 1} \\ \mathbf{0}_{2\times 1} & \mathbf{1}_{2\times 1} \end{bmatrix}\begin{bmatrix} \mu_1 \\ \mu_2 \end{bmatrix} = \begin{bmatrix} \mathbf{1}_{4\times 1} | & \begin{bmatrix} \mathbf{1}_{2\times 1} \\ -\mathbf{1}_{2\times 1} \end{bmatrix} \end{bmatrix}\begin{bmatrix} \delta_0 \\ \delta_1 \end{bmatrix} = [\mathbf{X}_0(l) : \ \mathbf{X}_1(l)]\delta;$$

where $\mathbf{1}_{k\times 1}$ and $\mathbf{0}_{k\times 1}$ are vectors of 1's and 0's of length $k$. The parameter of non-centrality can be computed as

$$\begin{aligned} \lambda(l) &= \sigma^{-2}\delta_1^t\mathbf{X}_1^t(l)\left(\mathbf{I}-\mathbf{X}_0(l)\left[\mathbf{X}_0^t(l)\mathbf{X}_0(l)\right]^{-1}\mathbf{X}_0^t\right)\mathbf{X}_1(l)\delta_1 \\ &= \sigma^{-2}\left(\frac{\mu_1-\mu_2}{2}\right)^2\cdot 4 = \frac{(\mu_1-\mu_2)^2}{\sigma^2}; \end{aligned} \tag{9}$$

which becomes, in the comparison of two means, $\lambda(l) = (\mu_1-\mu_2)^2/\sigma^2$. Following the general theory of the intrinsic Bayes factor for linear models [16,17], we have that an intrinsic prior is of the following form:

$$\pi^I(\lambda(l)|\sigma) = \frac{1}{\sqrt{2\pi}\sigma}\frac{(1-e^{-\lambda(l)/2})}{\lambda(l)}.$$

Substitution from $\lambda(l)$ using the non-centrality parameter of (9), then the transformation to the conditional of the parameter under the simple test, is $H_0: \delta_1 = 0$ vs. $H_1: \delta_1 \neq 0$. The conditional intrinsic prior for the hypothesis test is

$$\pi_1^I(\delta_1|\sigma) = \frac{1 - e^{-8\delta_1^2/\sigma^2}}{4\sqrt{2\pi}(\delta_1^2/\sigma)}. \tag{10}$$

This conditional prior is proper, i.e., $\int \pi_1^I(\delta_1|\sigma)d\delta_1 = 1$ and it satisfies the condition discussed by [12]. The intrinsic prior, under the alternative Hypothesis $H_1$, is of the form $\pi_1^I(\delta_1, \delta_0, \sigma) = \pi_1^I(\delta_1|\delta_0, \sigma) \cdot \pi_1^I(\delta_0, \sigma)$, where $\pi_1^I(\delta_0, \sigma) = 1/\sigma$, i.e.,

$$\pi_1^I(\delta_0, \delta_1, \sigma) = \frac{1}{\sigma} \cdot \frac{1 - e^{-8\delta_1^2/\sigma^2}}{4\sqrt{2\pi}\delta_1^2/\sigma} = \frac{1 - e^{-8\delta_1^2/\sigma^2}}{4\sqrt{2\pi}\delta_1^2}. \tag{11}$$

Setting up this framework, we can derive the intrinsic Bayes factor to compare two-sample means. We will first obtain the marginal density under the null hypothesis $m_0(\mathbf{x}, \mathbf{y})$. First, consider the joint likelihood function of the two samples under the null Hypothesis $H_0$:

$$f_0(\mathbf{x}, \mathbf{y}|\delta_0, \sigma) = (2\pi)^{-n/2}\sigma^{-n} \exp\left\{ -\frac{S_x^2 + S_y^2 + n_1(\bar{x} - \delta_0)^2 + n_2(\bar{y} - \delta_0)^2}{2\sigma^2} \right\}.$$

Here, $\bar{x}$ is the sample mean of the first group, $\bar{y}$ is the sample mean of the first group, and $S_x^2 = \sum_{i=1}^{n_1}(x_i - \bar{x})^2$, $S_y^2 = \sum_{i=1}^{n_2}(y_i - \bar{y})^2$ are the sums of squares under the null hypothesis. The marginal density using the non-informative prior $\pi^N(\delta_0, \sigma) = 1/\sigma$ is computed as

$$\begin{aligned} m_0(\mathbf{x}, \mathbf{y}) &= \int\int f_0(\mathbf{x}, \mathbf{y}|\delta_0, \sigma)\pi(\delta_0, \sigma)\mathrm{d}\delta_0\mathrm{d}\sigma \\ &= \frac{2^{(n-3)/2}\Gamma\left(\frac{n-1}{2}\right)(S_x^2 + S_y^2)^{-(n-1)/2}\left(1 + \frac{t^2}{n-2}\right)^{-(n-1)/2}}{\sqrt{n}}, \end{aligned} \tag{12}$$

where $t = (\bar{x} - \bar{y})/(S_p\sqrt{n_\delta})$, where $n = n_1 + n_2$, $S_p$ is the pooled standard deviation, i.e., $S_p^2 = (S_x^2 + S_y^2)/(n-2)$ and $n_\delta = 1/n_1 + 1/n_2$. Similarly, the joint likelihood function of the two samples under the alternative Hypothesis $H_1$ is given by

$$f_1(\mathbf{x}, \mathbf{y}|\delta_0, \delta_1, \sigma) = (2\pi)^{-n/2}\sigma^{-n} \exp\left\{ -\frac{S_x^2 + S_y^2 + n_1(\bar{x} - (\delta_0 + \delta_1))^2 + n_2(\bar{y} - (\delta_0 - \delta_1))^2}{2\sigma^2} \right\}.$$

The marginal density using the intrinsic prior $\pi^I(\delta_0, \delta_1, \sigma)$ defined in (11) is given by

$$m_1(\mathbf{x}, \mathbf{y}) = \int\int\int f_1(\mathbf{x}, \mathbf{y}|\delta_0, \delta_1, \sigma)\pi^I(\delta_0, \delta_1, \sigma)\mathrm{d}\delta_0\mathrm{d}\delta_1\mathrm{d}\sigma. \tag{13}$$

As in the one-sample framework, this Bayes factor can be approximated using the non-informative prior $\pi^N(\delta_0, \delta_1, \sigma) = 1/\sigma^2$ in the asymptotic result as

$$\begin{aligned} m_1(\mathbf{x}, \mathbf{y}) &\approx m_1^N(\mathbf{x}, \mathbf{y})\frac{\pi^I(\hat{\delta}_0, \hat{\delta}_1, \hat{\sigma})}{\pi^N(\hat{\delta}_0, \hat{\delta}_1, \hat{\sigma})} \\ &= \int\int\int f_1(\mathbf{x}, \mathbf{y}|\delta_0, \delta_1, \sigma)\pi^N(\delta_0, \delta_1, \sigma)\mathrm{d}\delta_0\mathrm{d}\delta_1\mathrm{d}\sigma\frac{\pi^I(\hat{\delta}_0, \hat{\delta}_1, \hat{\sigma})}{\pi^N(\hat{\delta}_0, \hat{\delta}_1, \hat{\sigma})} \\ &= \frac{\sqrt{\pi}2^{(n-3)/2-1/2}\Gamma\left(\frac{n-1}{2}\right)(S_x^2 + S_y^2)^{-(n-1)/2}}{\sqrt{n_1 n_2}}. \end{aligned} \tag{14}$$

Using (12) and (14), we can compute $B_{01}^N$:

$$B_{01}^N = \frac{m_0^N(\mathbf{x},\mathbf{y})}{m_1^N(\mathbf{x},\mathbf{y})} = \sqrt{\frac{2}{\pi n_\delta}}\left(1+\frac{t^2}{n-2}\right)^{-(n-1)/2}; \tag{15}$$

where $t^2 = (\bar{x}-\bar{y})^2/(S_p n_\delta)$, $S_p$ is the pooled estimate of the variance, $S_p^2 = (S_x^2+S_y^2)/(n-2)$ and $n_\delta = (1/n_1+1/n_2)$. Let $\hat{\delta}_1$ and $\hat{\sigma}^2$ be the corresponding maximum likelihood estimator (MLE). Let $\hat{\delta}_1 = (\bar{x}-\bar{y})/2$ and $\hat{\sigma}^2 = (S_x^2+S_y^2)/n = (n-2)/nS_p^2$; where $S_p^2$ is the variance pooled estimates and $n = n_1+n_2$. We can express the $\hat{\delta}_1^2/\hat{\sigma}^2 = n_\delta n t^2/(n-2)$ in terms of the $t$-statistic. Then, the approximate intrinsic Bayes factor $B_{01}^{IP}$ can be obtained by

$$\begin{aligned} B_{01}^{IP} \approx B_{01}^N \frac{\pi^N(\hat{\delta}_0,\hat{\delta}_1,\hat{\sigma})}{\pi^I(\hat{\delta}_0,\hat{\delta}_1,\hat{\sigma})} &= \sqrt{\frac{2}{\pi n_\delta}}\left(1+\frac{t^2}{n-2}\right)^{-(n-1)/2} \frac{\hat{\delta}_1^2/\hat{\sigma}^2}{\frac{1-e^{-8\hat{\delta}_1^2/\hat{\sigma}^2}}{4\sqrt{2\pi}}} \\ &= \frac{\sqrt{n_\delta}nt^2}{n-2}\left(1+\frac{t^2}{n-2}\right)^{-(n-1)/2}\left(1+\coth\left(\frac{n_\delta n t^2}{n-2}\right)\right). \end{aligned} \tag{16}$$

Here, $t = (\bar{x}-\bar{y})/(Sp\sqrt{n_\delta})$ and $\coth(\cdot)$ is the hyperbolic cotangent function defined as $\coth(x) = (e^{2x}+1)/(e^{2x}-1)$.

**Theorem 3.** *For a fixed sample size $n \geq 4$, the Bayes factor based on the intrinsic prior ($B_{01}^{IP}$) for the comparison of two population means is finite sample-consistent.*

**Proof.** For a fixed sample, $n \geq 4$, and letting $t^2 \to \infty$, or equivalently $|t| \to \infty$, the Bayes factor based on the intrinsic prior goes to 0, i.e.,

$$\lim_{|t|\to\infty} B_{01}^{IP} \to 0; \text{ or equivalently } \lim_{|t|\to\infty} \mathbb{P}(H_0|x) \to 0.$$

The Bayes factor based on the intrinsic prior $B_{01}^{IP}$ is finite sample-consistent. □

2.2.2. Robust Bayes Factor for the Comparison of Two-Sample Means

Consider observations of a random sample from group 1 and group 2 of size $n_1$ and $n_2$, respectively. We assume these groups have common variance ($\sigma_1^2 = \sigma_2^2 = \sigma^2$), respectively. The model of interest in this case, $y_{ij} = \mu + \alpha_i + \varepsilon_{ij}$, with $\varepsilon_{ij} \sim N(0,\sigma^2)$, for $i = 1,2$ and $j = 1,\ldots,n_i$. We want to compare $H_0 : \alpha_1 = \alpha_2$ against $H_0 : \alpha_1 \neq \alpha_2$. Further, consider the constraint that $\alpha_1 + \alpha_2 = 0$; then, the design matrix $\mathbf{X}$ can be written as

$$\mathbf{X} = \left[\mathbf{1}_{n\times 1} \quad \left| \begin{bmatrix} 1/n_1\mathbf{1}_{n_1\times 1} \\ -1/n_2\mathbf{1}_{n_2\times 1}\end{bmatrix}\right.\right];$$

This leads us to consider the following hypothesis, $H_0 : \alpha_1 = 0$ vs. $H_1 : \alpha_1 \neq 0$. The reference's priors, under the null hypothesis $H_0$ and alternative hypothesis $H_1$: $\pi_0^N(\mu,\sigma) = 1/\sigma$ and $\pi_1^N(\mu,\alpha_1,\sigma) = 1/\sigma$. First, we proceed to find the marginal density under $H_0$. Consider the joint likelihood function under the null Hypothesis $H_0$:

$$f_0(\mathbf{y}_1,\mathbf{y}_2|\mu,\sigma) = (2\pi)^{-n/2}\sigma^{-n}\exp\left\{-\frac{SS_0^2 + n_1(\bar{y}_{1.}-\mu)^2 + n_2(\bar{y}_{2.}-\mu)^2}{2\sigma^2}\right\}.$$

Here, $\mathbf{y}_1 = (y_{11},\ldots,y_{1n_1})$ and $\mathbf{y}_2 = (y_{21},\ldots,y_{2n_2})$, $\bar{y}_{i.}$ is the sample mean of the $i$th group, and $SS_0^2$ is the sum of squares under the null hypothesis. The marginal density under the null hypothesis $m_0(\mathbf{y}_1,\mathbf{y}_2)$ is given by

$$m_0(\mathbf{y}_1,\mathbf{y}_2) = \int\int f_0(\mathbf{y}|\mu,\sigma)\sigma^{-1}\, d\mu d\sigma$$
$$= \frac{\Gamma((n-1)/2)}{\sqrt{n}} \frac{(\pi)^{-(n-1)/2}}{2} (SS_0^2)^{-(n-1)/2} \left(1+\frac{t^2}{n-2}\right)^{-(n-1)/2}. \quad (17)$$

where $t^2 = (\bar{y}_{1.} - \bar{y}_{2.})^2/(S_p n_\delta)$. Here, $S_p$ is the sample pooled estimate of the variance, $S_p^2 = (S_1^2 + S_2^2)/(n-2)$, and $n_\delta = (1/n_1 + 1/n_2)$. For the alternative Hypothesis $H_1$, we first consider the joint likelihood of group 1 and group 2:

$$f_1(\mathbf{y}_1,\mathbf{y}_2|\mu,\alpha,\sigma) = (2\pi)^{-n/2}\sigma^{-n} \exp\left\{\frac{(S_1^2 + S_2^2 + n_1(\bar{y}_{1.} - (\mu+\alpha))^2 + n_2(\bar{y}_{2.} - (\mu-\alpha))^2)}{2\sigma^2}\right\}.$$

The marginal density $m_1(\mathbf{y}_1,\mathbf{y}_2)$ is given by

$$m_1(\mathbf{y}_1,\mathbf{y}_2) = \int\int\int f_1(\mathbf{y}|\mu,\alpha,\sigma) \times \sigma^{-1}\pi^R(\alpha)\, d\mu d\alpha d\sigma$$
$$= \sqrt{\frac{n_\delta(b+d)}{(2\pi)^{(n-2)}}} \frac{\Gamma((n-3)/2)}{4\sqrt{\pi}n\hat{\alpha}^2} \left[\left(\frac{S_1^2+S_2^2}{2}\right)^{-(n-3)/2} - \left(\frac{S_1^2+S_2^2}{2} + \frac{\hat{\alpha}^2}{b+d}\right)^{-(n-3)/2}\right]. \quad (18)$$

Here, $\hat{\alpha} = (\bar{y}_{1.} - \bar{y}_{2.})/2$. The robust Bayes factor is obtained by computing the ratio of the marginal densities of (17) and (18):

$$B_{01}^R = \sqrt{\frac{8n_\delta}{b+d}} \left(\frac{t^2(n-3)}{4(n-2)}\right) \left(1+\frac{t^2}{n-2}\right)^{-(n-1)/2} \left(1 - \left(1+\frac{t^2 n_\delta}{2(n-2)(b+d)}\right)^{-(n-3)/2}\right)^{-1}. \quad (19)$$

To finish the calculation of the robust Bayes factor $B_{01}^R$, the term $b+d$ has to be defined. Therefore, we propose using the effective sample size (TESS) $n_o^e$ of [21]. The first factor $d = 0.25n_\delta \cdot \sigma^2$, and the second factor $b$ is $b = n_o^e \cdot d = 0.25\sigma^2 \left(\max\left\{\left|\frac{1}{n_1}\right|, \left|-\frac{1}{n_2}\right|\right\}\right)^{-2}$; then, $b+d = 0.25\sigma^2 \times \left[n_\delta + \left(\max\left\{\left|\frac{1}{n_1}\right|, \left|-\frac{1}{n_2}\right|\right\}\right)^{-2}\right] = 0.25\sigma^2 \times (d^* + b^*)$. Derivation of TESS is displayed in Appendix A.1.

**Theorem 4.** *For a fixed sample size $n \geq 4$, the Bayes factor based on the robust prior ($B_{01}^R$) for the comparison of two populations means is finite sample-consistent.*

**Proof.** For a fixed sample, $n \geq 4$, and letting $t^2 \to \infty$, or equivalently $|t| \to \infty$, the Bayes factor based on the Berger robust prior goes to 0, i.e.,

$$\lim_{|t|\to\infty} B_{01}^R \to 0; \text{ or equivalently } \lim_{|t|\to\infty} \mathbb{P}(H_0|\boldsymbol{x}) \to 0.$$

The Bayes factor based on the Berger robust prior $B_{01}^R$ is finite sample-consistent. □

The Berger robust prior yields the following (exact) expression for the correction of the main term (for group $i$):

$$\pi^R(\xi_i|d_i,b_i) = \frac{1}{\sqrt{2\pi(d_i+b_i)}} \frac{[1-\exp(-\frac{\xi_i^2}{(d_i+b_i)})]}{\sqrt{2}\xi_i^2/(d_i+b_i)}.$$

Making the change of variables $\xi_i = \sqrt{8(d_i+b_i)}\ \ \beta^*/\sigma$ and $\eta = \sigma$ then taking the Jacobian,

$$|J| = \begin{vmatrix} \frac{\sqrt{8(d_i+b_i)}}{\sigma} & \frac{-\sqrt{8(d_i+b_i)}\beta^*}{\sigma^2} \\ 0 & 1 \end{vmatrix} = \left|\frac{\sqrt{8(d_i+b_i)}}{\sigma}\right|.$$

the conditional intrinsic prior of Equation (10) is exactly recovered; $\pi^I(\beta^*|\sigma) = \pi^R(\xi_i|d_i, b_i)|J|$. This established a correspondence between the intrinsic and Berger's robust priors for the Student's $t$ test.

### 2.2.3. The Effective Sample Size Bayesian Information Criterion (BIC-TESS)

Our final Bayes factor for comparing two-sample means is a variation of the Bayesian Information Criterion (BIC) of [22]. The BIC is a popular method to determine the best model in a set of competing models. However, in comparing the two-sample means, the BIC does not consider the information available in both groups but rather the entire sample. Here, we proposed replacing the sample size $n$ with TESS. This may be used to form what may be claimed to be the corrected BIC or BIC-TESS. It can be demonstrated that BIC with TESS is:

$$B_{01}^{TESS} = \sqrt{n_0^e}\left(1 + \frac{t^2}{n-2}\right)^{-n/2}, \tag{20}$$

where $n_0^e$ is defined by [11]. Derivation of TESS is in Appendix A.1. If we have a balanced situation, where $n_1 = n_2$, the BIC-TESS is similar to the regular BIC. If the situation is unbalanced, the BIC-TESS is stabilized, since as $n_2 \to \infty$, the $B_{01}^{TESS} \to \sqrt{n_1}$.

**Theorem 5.** *For a fixed sample size $n \geq 3$, the corrected BIC ($B_{01}^{TESS}$) for the two-sample mean $\mu$ is finite sample-consistent.*

**Proof.** For a fixed sample, $n \geq 3$, and letting $t^2 \to \infty$, or equivalently $|t| \to \infty$, the Bayesian Information Criterion constructed with TESS goes to 0, i.e.,

$$\lim_{|t|\to\infty} B_{01}^{TESS} \to 0; \text{ or equivalently } \lim_{|t|\to\infty} \mathbb{P}(H_0|\boldsymbol{x}) \to 0.$$

The corrected Bayesian Information Criterion is $B_{01}^{TESS}$ is finite sample-consistent. □

In Figure 1, we compare the asymptotic behavior of the Bayes factors and the posterior probability of the null hypothesis when the samples are balanced ($n_1 \approx n_2$) and unbalanced ($n_1 << n_2$). The Bayes factor, based on the Berger robust prior (dark red), is very close in the range of evidence to the intrinsic Bayes factor (green) and the BIC-TESS (light orange). The robust Bayes factor, the intrinsic Bayes factor, and the BIC-TESS are relatively closed when the situation is balanced. In the unbalanced scenario, the robust Bayes factor and the BIC-TESS remain relatively close, while the intrinsic Bayes factor slightly increases. The conjugate Bayes factor (blue) is represented with different values of the prior variance $\sigma_\delta^2$; darker color means higher values for the prior variance. Recall that the conjugate Bayes factor is not finite sample-consistent, and its behavior depends on the choice of $\sigma_\delta^2$.

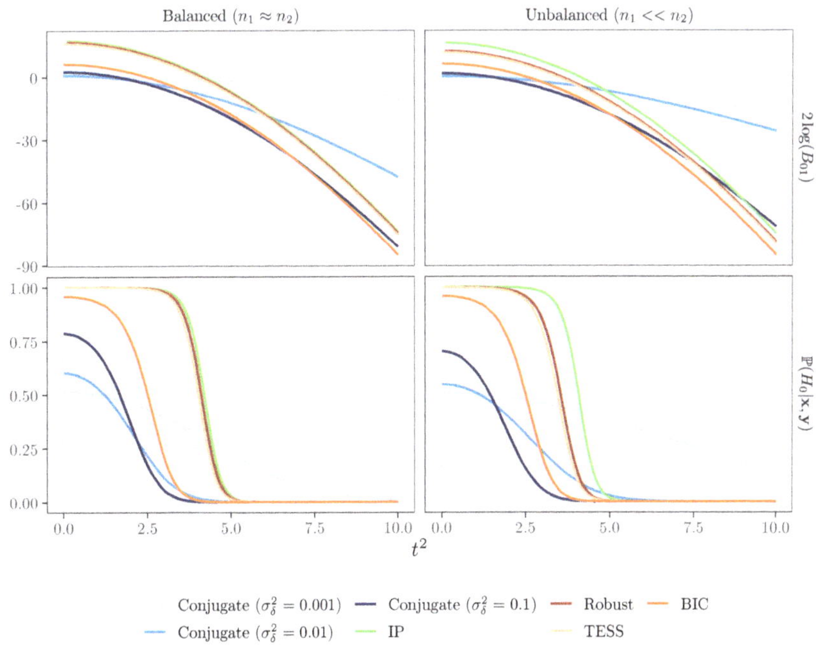


**Figure 1.** Results in terms of $2\log(B_{01})$ and posterior probability for the finite sample consistency.

## 3. Simulation Experiments

*Experiments for the One- and Two-Sample Mean Comparisons*

We generated 500 datasets from random samples taken from a normal distribution, Student's $t$ distribution with one degree of freedom, and gamma distribution. For each of these distributions, the mean and standard deviation values were set to $\mu_1 = 5$ and $\sigma_1 = 3$. The second group was created with a combination of several parameters for the location; the mean values were $\mu_2 \in \{\mu_1, 1.5\mu_1, 2\mu_1\}$, and for the standard deviation of the second group, $\sigma_2 \in \{\sigma_1, 2\sigma_1, 3\sigma_1\}$. In the case of the Student's $t$ distribution, both groups were simulated with $\nu = 1$ degrees of freedom. The simulated gamma samples were obtained using the method of moments for the shape parameter, with $\alpha_i = \mu_i^2/\sigma_i^2$, and the scale parameter, with $\beta_i = \sigma_i^2/\mu_i$, for $i = 1, 2$.

We compared our methodologies with several Bayes factors used when comparing two population means, displayed in Table 1. $B_{01}^S$ is the classical Bayesian Information Criterion (BIC) of [22], ($B_{01}^{ZS}$) is based on the Zellner and Siow prior [23], the two-sample Student's $t$ Bayes factor of [14] is based on the conjugate prior with $\sigma_\delta^2 = 1/3$, the arithmetic Bayes factor ($B_{10}^{EIA}$) of [24], and [12]'s Bayes Factor ($B_{01}^J$) for the comparison of two-sample means with equal variances. One set of these Bayes factors—the BIC of Schwartz and the Zellner and Siow Bayes factors—depends only on the sample size $n$. The other set, based on the conjugate prior, intrinsic, Berger's (here called robust), and finally, the modified Jeffrey's prior, depends on the term $n_\delta = 1/n_1 + 1/n_2$. In our experiments, we do not consider the constant $2/5$ for $B_{01}^J$, since we believe it satisfies the condition that the samples arise from the same distribution; for more details about the use of the constant $2/5$, see [12]. We also studied these Bayes factors in unbalanced situations. Heavily unbalanced samples are interesting not only from a theoretical point of view but also because they are often observed in practice in observational studies; the results of these are displayed in Figures A1–A3.

Performance was compared using the twice natural base logarithm Bayes factors ($2\log(B_{01})$) for comparing the null hypothesis ($\mu_1 = \mu_2$) against the alternative ($\mu_1 \neq \mu_2$). This transformation allows the interpretation to be on the same scale as the deviance and likelihood ratio test statistics, as discussed in [13].

**Table 1.** **Bayes factors based on the one- and two-sample means based on the Student's $t$ test. The third column applies only to the two-sample comparison and is limiting when $t^2 \to 0$ and $n_2 \to \infty$.**

| | | | |
|---|---|---|---|
| One Sample | $B_{01}^{IP} \approx$ | $\sqrt{2n}\left(1+\frac{t^2}{n-1}\right)^{-\frac{n}{2}} \frac{t^2}{n-1}(1-e^{-t^2/(n-1)})^{-1}$ | - |
| | $B_{01}^{R} =$ | $\sqrt{\frac{2}{n+1}\frac{n-2}{n-1}t^2}\left(1+\frac{t^2}{n-1}\right)^{-\frac{n}{2}}\left(1-\left(1+\frac{2t^2}{n^2-1}\right)^{-\frac{n-2}{2}}\right)^{-1}$ | - |
| Two Samples | $B_{01}^{IP} \approx$ | $\frac{\sqrt{n_\delta}nt^2}{n-2}\left(1+\frac{t^2}{n-2}\right)^{-(n-1)/2}\left(1+\coth\left(\frac{n_\delta nt^2}{n-2}\right)\right)$ | $\sqrt{n_1}$ |
| | $B_{01}^{R} =$ | $\sqrt{\frac{8n_\delta}{b+d}\left(\frac{t^2(n-3)}{4(n-2)}\right)}\left(1+\frac{t^2}{n-2}\right)^{-(n-1)/2}\left(1-\left(1+\frac{t^2n_\delta}{2(n-2)(b+d)}\right)^{-(n-3)/2}\right)^{-1}$ | $\sqrt{2(1+n_1^3)}$ |
| | $B_{01}^{TESS} =$ | $\sqrt{n_o^e}\left(1+\frac{t^2}{n-2}\right)^{-n/2}$ | $\sqrt{n_1}$ |
| | $B_{01}^{J} \approx$ | $\frac{2}{5}\sqrt{\frac{\pi n_\delta}{2}}\left(1+\frac{t^2}{n-2}\right)^{-(n-1)/2}$ | $\frac{2}{5}\sqrt{\frac{\pi n_1}{2}}$ |
| | $B_{01}^{C*} =$ | $\left[\frac{1+t^2/(n-2)}{1+t^2/((n-2))(1+\sigma_\delta^2 n_\delta))}\right]^{-(n-1)/2}\sqrt{1+\sigma_\delta^2 n_\delta}$ | $\sqrt{1+n_1\sigma_\delta^2}$ |
| | $B_{01}^{S} \approx$ | $\sqrt{n}\left(1+\frac{t^2}{n-2}\right)^{-n/2}$ | $\infty$ |
| | $B_{01}^{ZS} \approx$ | $\sqrt{\frac{\pi(n-2)}{2}}\left(1+\frac{t^2}{n-2}\right)^{-(n-3)/2}$ | $\infty$ |
| | $B_{01}^{EIA**} \approx$ | $\pi^{-1}\sqrt{n_\delta/(3\hat{\eta})}S^{(n-1)/2}(S_1^2+S_2^2)^{-(n-2)/2}\frac{\Gamma((n-2)/2)}{\Gamma((n-1)/2)} \times \int_0^1(1-x)^{-1/2}e^{-\hat{\delta}/2x}dx$ | - |

* Ref. [14] defines $n_\delta = (1/n_1 + 1/n_2)^{-1}$. ** Ref. [24] defines $\hat{\eta} = (S_1^2 + S_2^2)/n$ and $\hat{\delta} = 2/3(\bar{y}_{1.} - \bar{y}_{2.})^2/\hat{\eta}$, and $S$ is the sum of square of the two samples combined.

Figure 2 displays the results for the evidence based on the normal distributions when testing whether two-sample means are equal ($\mu_1 = \mu_2$). The red line represents the cut-off for 10 (strong evidence), the yellow line for 6 (positive evidence), and the green for 2 (weak evidence). In the actual case when the means are equal, the Bayes factors based on the intrinsic prior and robust prior show strong evidence in favor of the null hypothesis. The average $2\log(B_{01})$ based on the intrinsic prior shows strong evidence in favor of the null hypothesis ($11.3 \pm 1.59$), while the Bayes factor based on the robust prior gives strong evidence in favor of the true case ($10.61 \pm 1.59$), all above the red line. BIC-TESS also strongly supports the true case ($9.9 \pm 1.61$). The other Bayes factors provide positive evidence for the true case, with averages ranging from 2.54 to 3.93. Even when the means were equal, and the samples had larger variance ($\sigma_2 = 3\sigma_1$), our objectives and robust Bayes factors provided strong evidence in favor of the true case, with the average above 10. The intrinsic Bayes factor and the robust prior were above 90%, showing either strong or very strong evidence in favor of the null hypothesis when the means were equal; see Table A2 for a detailed comparison.

In the Student's $t$ random samples, when testing whether two-sample means are equal ($\mu_1 = \mu_2$), we can observe in Figure 3 the results when the means are equal. The Bayes Factors based on the intrinsic prior and robust prior show strong evidence in favor of the null hypothesis. The average $2\log(B_{01})$ based on the intrinsic prior, robust prior, and BIC-TESS shows strong evidence in favor of the null hypothesis (averages above 10), with values of $11.41, 10.72$, and $10.02$; dispersion was relatively low, ranging from 1.01 to 1.03. The competing Bayes factors provide slightly positive evidence for the true case, with averages ranging from 2.65 to 4.04. It is interesting to see that in the case of $\mu_2 = 2\mu_1$, our Bayes factor gave positive evidence above the yellow line but was very variable; the sample standard deviation ranged from 4.98 to 5.03. Finally, in the case of gamma samples, our Bayes factors gave strong evidence only when the means and the variances were equal. Departing from any of these conditions gave strong evidence that the means were unequal; see Figure 4. For more details about the simulation results' numerical performance, see Table A1.

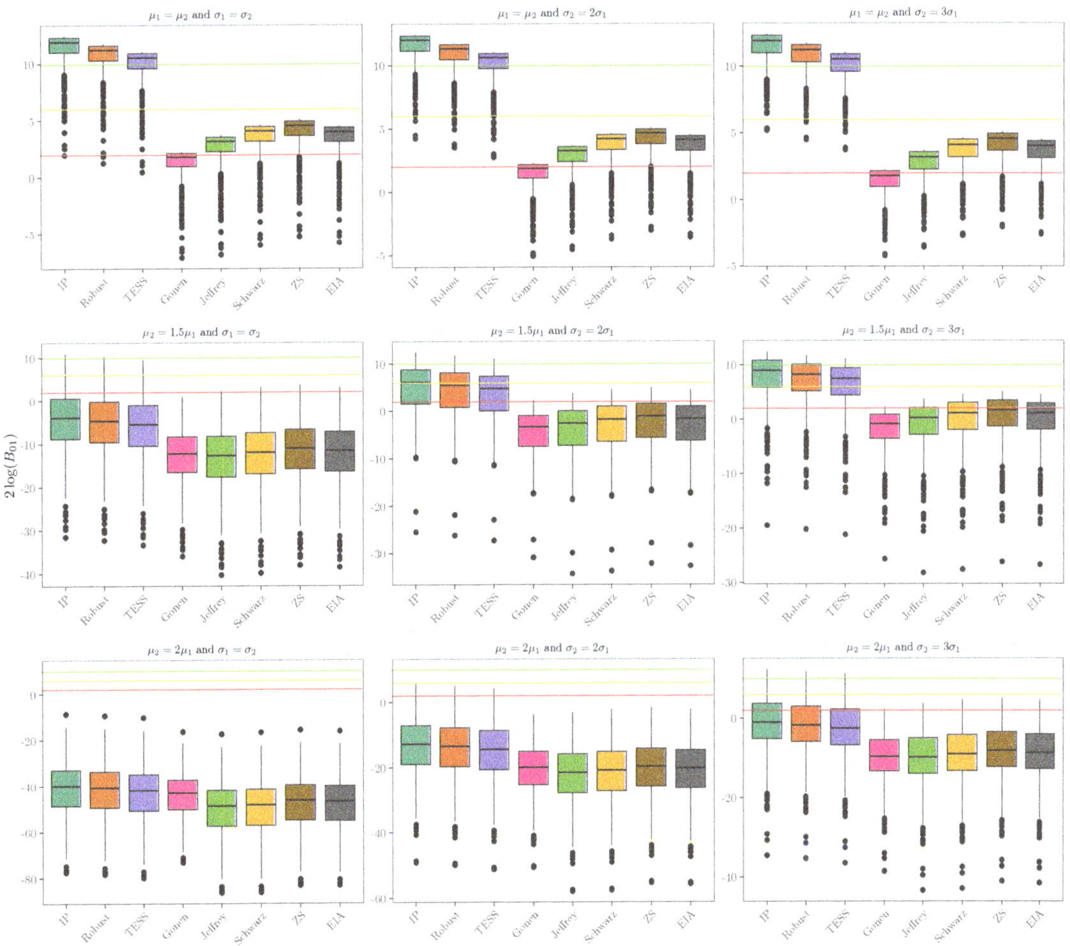


**Figure 2.** Evidence in the $2\log(B_{01})$ scale when comparing the population means of two samples that arise from a normal distribution with several means and variances with equal sizes $n_1 = n_2 = 50$.

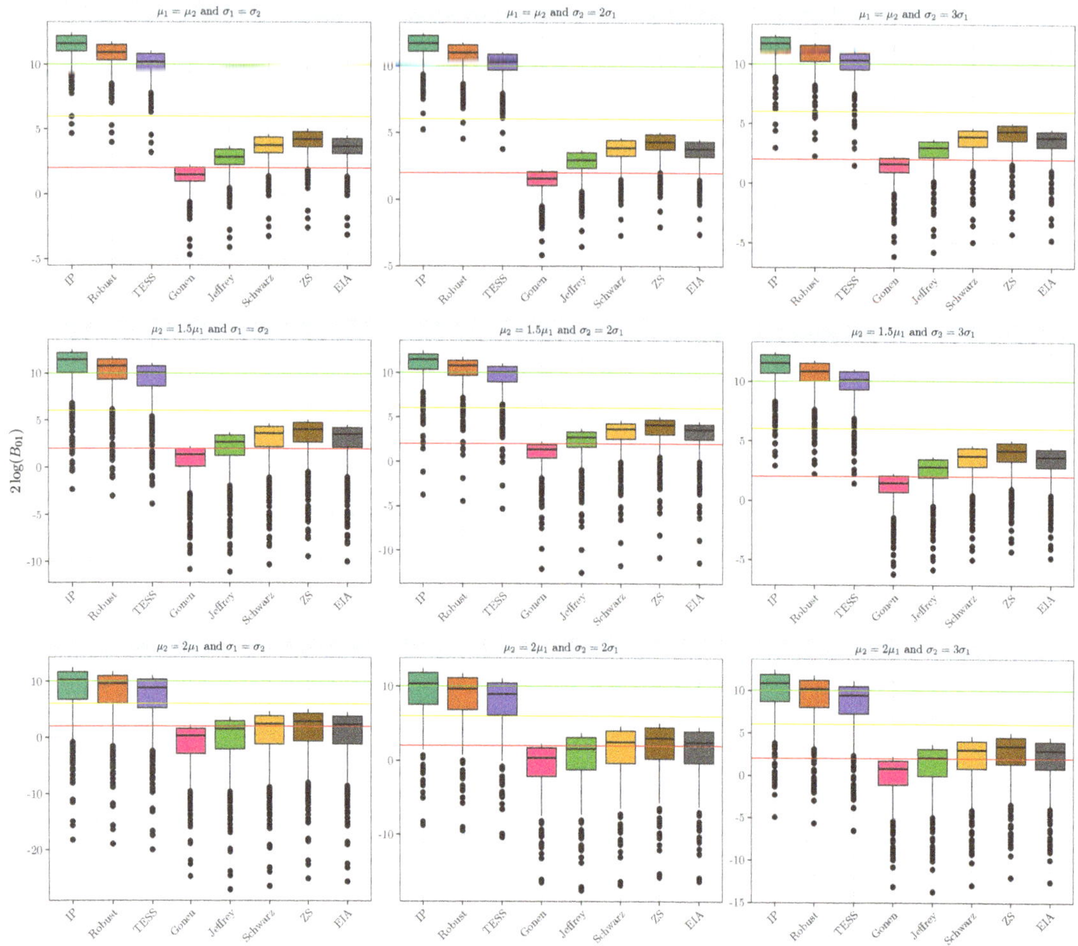


**Figure 3.** Evidence in the $2\log(B_{01})$ scale when comparing the population means of two samples that arise from a Student's $t$ with one degree of freedom with several means and variances with equal sizes $n_1 = n_2 = 50$.

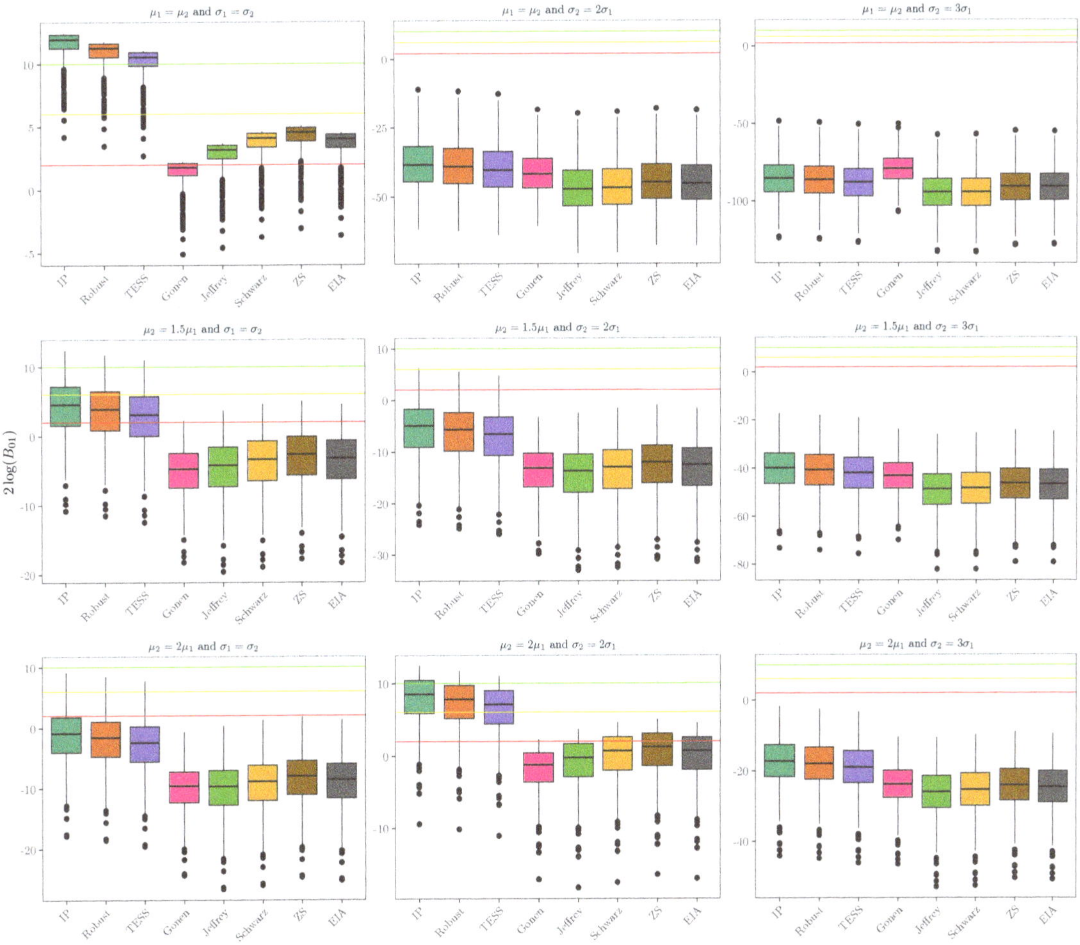

**Figure 4.** Evidence in the $2\log(B_{01})$ scale when comparing the population means of two samples that arise from a gamma distribution with several shapes and scales with equal sizes $n_1 = n_2 = 50$.

## 4. Application in Real Dataset

In this section, we applied the proposed one and two Bayes factors based on the intrinsic, Berger, and robust priors, and BIC-TESS based on the Student's $t$ statistic.

### 4.1. Gosset Original Dataset

We first consider the century-long original Student's $t$ sleep data from [1,25] that still raise interesting discussion; see [26,27]. In this study, the number of hours of sleep under both drugs (Dextro and Laevo) was recorded for each patient. The difference in hours was recorded to determine effectiveness, and the average number of hours of sleep gained by using each drug (Dextro and Laevo) was measured. The authors concluded that, in usual doses, Laevo was soporific, but Dextro was not. This analysis is treated as a paired sample, since it compares the sleep hours between treatments. Paired samples lead us to the one sample. The hypothesis of interest is $H_0 : \mu_d = 0$ versus $H_1 : \mu_d \neq 0$; the test statistic is $t = -4.06$ with a $p$-value of 0.002. At the 5% significance level, we can conclude that there is a difference in the average sleep hours between Laevo and Dextro.

However, the Gosset original dataset has not been addressed using an objective and robust Bayesian approach. The value of the test statistics is the same as before, with $n = 10$. The $(2\log(B_{10}))$ was computed for the intrinsic and robust Bayes factor, along with the associated posterior probabilities $(\mathbb{P}(H_1|data))$. The $2\log(B_{10}^{IP}) = 5.858$ and $2\log(B_{10}^{R}) = 5.988$ are positive, indicating strong evidence that the average sleep hours are different. Further, the posterior probability based on the intrinsic prior is 0.949, and the posterior probability based on the Berger robust prior is 0.952. Both posterior probabilities are above 90%, suggesting strong evidence favoring the average sleep difference.

This dataset is considered as a paired sample, since the recorded number of sleep hours belongs to the same participant. However, the treatments, Dextro and Laevo, might need to be considered independently. If these are considered independently, then a two-sample framework arises. We are interested in determining the sleep hours when receiving Laevo versus when receiving Dextro. Assuming equal variances between Laevo and Dextro, the hypothesis of interest is $H_0 : \mu_L = \mu_D$ versus $H_1 : \mu_L \neq \mu_D$, where $\mu_L$ is the average sleep hours when receiving Laevo and $\mu_D$ is the average sleep hours when receiving Dextro. The two-sample test statistic is $t = -1.86$ with a $p$-value of 0.079. At the 5% significance level, we can conclude that there is no difference in the average sleep hours when using Laevo versus Dextro. In our Bayesian approach, $2\log(B_{10}^{IP}) = -4.33$ and $2\log(B_{10}^{R}) = -3.57$, indicating weak evidence that the average number of sleep hours differs between Laevo and Dextro. Both posterior probabilities are above 15%, suggesting weak evidence that the average number of sleep hours differs when using Laevo and Dextro.

### 4.2. Induced Hypertension on Mice According to Diet

Our first application consists of the data from [28], but they were analyzed in a Bayesian framework using intrinsic priors by [24]. In this study, the researchers were interested in how intermittent feeding affected the blood pressure of rats. The treatment group consisted of eight rats fed intermittently for weeks, and at the final period, the rats' blood pressure measurements were taken. The blood pressure measurements of a second group of seven rats fed the usual way were defined as a control group. The hypothesis of interest is that the average blood pressure is different when the rats have intermittent fasting compared to those with their usual diet, i.e., $H_0 : \mu_1 = \mu_2$ versus $H_1 : \mu_1 \neq \mu_2$. At the 5% significance level, with a $p$-value $= 0.044$, one can conclude that there exists a difference in the mean blood pressure level according to their feeding style.

The study in Ref. [24] computed the expected arithmetic Bayes factor that favors the alternative hypothesis $B_{10}^{EAI} = 2.035$ with $\mathbb{P}(H_1|(\mathbf{x},\mathbf{y})) = 0.671$, providing support that the average blood pressure measurements differ based on diet. Notably, the Bayes factors based on the intrinsic priors and robust priors yield negative values, $2\log(B_{10}^{IP}) = -2.412$ and $2\log(B_{10}^{R}) = -1.414$, respectively, indicating evidence against $H_1$. However, the corresponding posterior probabilities $(\mathbb{P}(H_1|\mathbf{x},\mathbf{y}))$ are 0.23 and 0.33, suggesting weak evidence for the alternative hypothesis that the means are different. The corrected BICTESS suggests weaker evidence against $H_1$ with a $2\log(B_{10}^{TESS}) = -0.3634$ and a posterior probability of $\mathbb{P}(H_1|\mathbf{x},\mathbf{y}) = 0.155$. In contrast, the conjugate $2\log(B_{10}^{C}) = 1.517$ and $2\log(B_{10}^{EAI}) = 1.421$, indicating very weak evidence in favor of $H_1$. The associated posterior probability is 0.681.

The extreme observation in the intermittent group (115) was removed. The $2\log(B_{10}^{IP*}) = 2.347$, suggesting evidence in favor of $H_1$, while the posterior probability of $\mathbb{P}(H_1|(\mathbf{x}^*,\mathbf{y}^*)) = 0.764$ indicates a moderate level of confidence in this conclusion. The Bayes factor constructed with the Berger robust prior exhibits a higher $2\log(B_{10}^{R*}) = 3.535$, along with the posterior probability of $\mathbb{P}(H_1|(\mathbf{x}^*,\mathbf{y}^*)) = 0.854$, indicating stronger support that the average of blood pressure differs by type of fasting. TESS models present even higher $2\log(B_{10}^{TESS*}) = 5.041$, respectively, with corresponding posterior probabilities of 0.926, indicating substantial evidence for $H_1$.

## 5. Discussion

In this work, we proposed the objective and robust Bayes factors for the one-sample and two-sample comparisons. These newly proposed Bayes factors are finite sample-consistent. Both the exact and approximate forms of the Bayes factors can be easily implemented using any open-source or commercial software. Another advantage of using Bayes factors is that the posterior probabilities of the hypothesis test are easily interpretable. We reanalyzed the original study by [1] and the comparison of blood pressure in rats according to different feeding types. Our objective and robust Bayes factors showed strong evidence that the average number of hours differed between Laevo and Dextro in the mouse application. When removing potential extreme values, we concluded that there is strong evidence that the means differed. However, we reported weak evidence with the complete dataset that these averages differed according to their diet. This might occur, since the assumption of equal variances might not hold. Even though the samples might have equal means, departing from the assumption of equal variances can lead in favor of the wrong hypothesis. Although we have made a significant contribution, an aspect that might alleviate this issue is deriving an objective and robust Bayes factor for the Behrens–Fisher problem, i.e., unequal variances for both groups. Also, the Bayes factor based on the intrinsic prior depends on the maximum likelihood estimate (MLE); perhaps robust estimates can be considered, although a modified test statistic might arise. Another possible extension is to develop an objective Bayes factor for the hypothesis of several equal means; this will be an analysis of variance (ANOVA) approach in the frequentist approach.

**Author Contributions:** Conceptualization, I.A.A.-R. and L.R.P.-G.; methodology, I.A.A.-R. and L.R.P.-G.; software, I.A.A.-R.; validation, I.A.A.-R. and L.R.P.-G.; formal analysis, I.A.A.-R. and L.R.P.-G.; writing—original draft preparation, I.A.A.-R. and L.R.P.-G. All authors have read and agreed with the published version of the manuscript.

**Funding:** This research received no external funding.

**Data Availability Statement:** The data presented in this study are available in [1,24].

**Acknowledgments:** The second author thanks Jim Berger for the fundamental discussions about the subject of this article.

**Conflicts of Interest:** The authors declare no conflict of interest.

### Abbreviations

The following abbreviations are used in this manuscript:

| | |
|---|---|
| TESS | The effective sample size |
| BIC | Bayesian Information Criterion |
| $B_{01}^{IP}$ | Bayes Factor based on the intrinsic prior for measuring $H_0$ vs. $H_1$ |
| $B_{01}^{R}$ | Bayes Factor based on the Berger's Robust prior for measuring $H_0$ vs. $H_1$ |
| $B_{01}^{TESS}$ | Corrected BIC using the effective sample size for measuring $H_0$ vs. $H_1$ |
| $B_{01}^{J}$ | Bayes Factor based on Jeffreys's prior for measuring $H_0$ vs. $H_1$ |
| $B_{01}^{C}$ | Bayes Factor based on the conjugate prior for measuring $H_0$ vs. $H_1$ |
| $B_{01}^{ZS}$ | Bayes Factor based on the Zellner and Siow prior for measuring $H_0$ vs. $H_1$ |
| $B_{01}^{EIA}$ | Bayes Factor expected arithmetic intrinsic prior for measuring $H_0$ vs. $H_1$ |

## Appendix A.

### *Appendix A.1. Calculation of the Effective Sample Size*

We suggest using the effective sample size of [21] to define the robust Bayes factor and BIC-Tess. The effective sample size for the parameter $\boldsymbol{\alpha}$, $n_0^e = C^{-1}(\mathbf{X}'\Gamma^{-1}\mathbf{X})C^{-1}$. Let $\mathbf{X}$ be the design matrix:

$$\mathbf{X} = \left[\mathbf{1}_{n\times 1} \quad \Big| \begin{bmatrix} 1/n_1 \mathbf{1}_{n_1\times 1} \\ -1/n_2 \mathbf{1}_{n_2\times 1} \end{bmatrix}\right];$$

where $n = n_1 + n_2$. Let $\mathbf{X}_1$ be the second column of the design matrix $\mathbf{X}_1 = \begin{bmatrix} 1/n_1 \mathbf{1}_{n_1 \times 1} \\ -1/n_2 \mathbf{1}_{n_2 \times 1} \end{bmatrix}$, and let $C_1 = \max\left\{ \left|\frac{1}{n_1 \sigma}\right|, \left|-\frac{1}{n_2 \sigma}\right| \right\}$. Further, let $\mathbf{\Gamma}^{-1} = \sigma^{-2} \mathbf{I}_{n \times n}$, where $\mathbf{I}_{n \times n}$ is an identity matrix of size $n$. It follows from the definition of the effective sample size for the original $\boldsymbol{\alpha}$ that

$$
\begin{aligned}
n_o^e &= C_1^{-1} (\mathbf{X}_1^t \mathbf{\Gamma}^{-1} \mathbf{X}_1) C_1^{-1} \\
&= C_1^{-2} \left[ \frac{\sigma^{-2}}{n_1}, \ldots, \frac{\sigma^{-2}}{n_1}, -\frac{\sigma^{-2}}{n_2}, \ldots, -\frac{\sigma^{-2}}{n_2} \right] \mathbf{X} \\
&= \frac{1}{C_1^2} \left[ \frac{\sigma^{-2}}{n_1^2} n_1 + \frac{\sigma^{-2}}{n_2^2} n_2 \right] \\
&= \sigma^{-2} \cdot \left( \max\left\{ \left|\frac{1}{n_1 \sigma}\right|, \left|-\frac{1}{n_2 \sigma}\right| \right\} \right)^{-2} \left( \frac{1}{n_1} + \frac{1}{n_2} \right) \\
&= \sigma^{-2} \cdot \left( \max\left\{ \left|\frac{1}{n_1 \sigma}\right|, \left|-\frac{1}{n_2 \sigma}\right| \right\} \right)^{-2} n_\delta \\
&= \left( \max\left\{ \left|\frac{1}{n_1}\right|, \left|-\frac{1}{n_2}\right| \right\} \right)^{-2} n_\delta .
\end{aligned} \tag{A1}
$$

Since $\sigma > 0$, $\max\left\{ \left|\frac{1}{n_1 \sigma}\right|, \left|-\frac{1}{n_2 \sigma}\right| \right\} = \frac{1}{\sigma} \max\left\{ \left|\frac{1}{n_1}\right|, \left|-\frac{1}{n_2}\right| \right\}$. Then, the final expression of the effective sample size is obtained. The definition of the unit information is $d = 0.25 n_\delta \cdot \sigma^2$ and for $b$,

$$
b = n_o^e \cdot d = 0.25\sigma^2 \cdot \left( \max\left\{ \left|\frac{1}{n_1}\right|, \left|-\frac{1}{n_2}\right| \right\} \right)^{-2} . \tag{A2}
$$

The factors $b$ and $d$ will be defined as

$$
b + d = 0.25\sigma^2 \left[ n_\delta + \left( \max\left\{ \left|\frac{1}{n_1}\right|, \left|-\frac{1}{n_2}\right| \right\} \right)^{-2} \right] = 0.25\sigma^2 (b^* + d^*). \tag{A3}
$$

This last calculation defines the factors $b$ and $d$ for the Robust Bayesian Student's $t$ test, $B_{01}^R$.

*Appendix A.2. Simulation Experiments*

In the two-sample framework, we generated 500 datasets from a random sample from a normal distribution with parameters $\mu_1 = 5, \sigma_1 = 3$; the second group was created with a combination of several parameters for the location. The mean values were $\mu_2 \in \{\mu_1, 1.5\mu_1, 2\mu_1\}$ for the standard deviation $\sigma_2 \in \{\sigma_1, 2\sigma_1, 3\sigma_1\}$. In the case of the Student's $t$ with $\nu = 1$ degrees of freedom, the gamma distribution was simulated using the methods of moments for the shape parameter $\alpha_i = \mu_i^2 / \sigma_i^2$ and scale parameter $\beta_i = \sigma_i^2 / \mu_i$ for $i = 1, 2$. We reported the twice natural base logarithm Bayes factors ($2\log(B_{01})$) for comparing the null hypothesis ($\mu_1 = \mu_2$) against the alternative ($\mu_1 \neq \mu_2$). This transformation allows the interpretation to be on the same scale as deviance and likelihood ratio test statistics; see Ref. [13] for a deeper discussion.

**Table A1.** Summary statistics (means ± standard deviation) for the balanced sample ($n_1 = n_2 = 50$) of the $2\log(B_{01})$ simulation experiments for the intrinsic priors (IP), Berger robust prior (Robust), BIC based on the effective sample size (TESS), conjugate, Jeffrey's, Schwarz, Zellner and Siow (ZS), and the expected arithmetic intrinsic prior of [24].

| | | $\mu_1 = \mu_2$ | | | $\mu_2 = 1.5\mu_1$ | | | $\mu_2 = 2\mu_1$ | | |
|---|---|---|---|---|---|---|---|---|---|---|
| | | $\sigma_1 = \sigma_2$ | $\sigma_2 = 2\sigma_1$ | $\sigma_2 = 3\sigma_1$ | $\sigma_1 = \sigma_2$ | $\sigma_2 = 2\sigma_1$ | $\sigma_2 = 3\sigma_1$ | $\sigma_1 = \sigma_2$ | $\sigma_2 = 2\sigma_1$ | $\sigma_2 = 3\sigma_1$ |
| Normal | IP | 11.3 ± 1.59 | 11.44 ± 1.37 | 11.42 ± 1.24 | −4.85 ± 7.44 | 4.85 ± 5.29 | 7.85 ± 4.18 | −41.19 ± 11.66 | −13.18 ± 8.77 | −1.53 ± 7.19 |
| | Robust | 10.61 ± 1.59 | 10.75 ± 1.38 | 10.73 ± 1.25 | −5.55 ± 7.45 | 4.15 ± 5.29 | 7.15 ± 4.18 | −41.94 ± 11.68 | −13.9 ± 8.78 | −2.23 ± 7.19 |
| | TESS | 9.9 ± 1.61 | 10.04 ± 1.39 | 10.03 ± 1.26 | −6.42 ± 7.53 | 3.38 ± 5.35 | 6.41 ± 4.22 | −43.18 ± 11.8 | −14.85 ± 8.87 | −3.07 ± 7.27 |
| | Conjugate | 1.23 ± 1.42 | 1.35 ± 1.23 | 1.34 ± 1.11 | −13.02 ± 6.5 | −4.5 ± 4.67 | −1.84 ± 3.7 | −43.99 ± 9.64 | −20.27 ± 7.57 | −10.11 ± 6.29 |
| | Jeffrey's | 2.54 ± 1.59 | 2.68 ± 1.38 | 2.66 ± 1.25 | −13.62 ± 7.45 | −3.92 ± 5.29 | −0.91 ± 4.18 | −50.01 ± 11.68 | −21.97 ± 8.78 | −10.3 ± 7.19 |
| | Schwarz's | 3.47 ± 1.61 | 3.61 ± 1.39 | 3.59 ± 1.26 | −12.86 ± 7.53 | −3.06 ± 5.35 | −0.02 ± 4.22 | −49.62 ± 11.8 | −21.29 ± 8.87 | −9.5 ± 7.27 |
| | ZS | 3.93 ± 1.56 | 4.07 ± 1.35 | 4.05 ± 1.22 | −11.9 ± 7.3 | −2.4 ± 5.19 | 0.55 ± 4.1 | −47.56 ± 11.44 | −20.08 ± 8.61 | −8.65 ± 7.05 |
| | EIA | 3.4 ± 1.57 | 3.53 ± 1.35 | 3.51 ± 1.22 | −12.45 ± 7.3 | −2.94 ± 5.19 | 0 ± 4.1 | −47.97 ± 11.36 | −20.62 ± 8.59 | −9.2 ± 7.04 |
| Student-$t(1)$ | IP | 11.41 ± 1.01 | 11.46 ± 1.04 | 11.4 ± 1.22 | 10.55 ± 2.42 | 10.83 ± 2.01 | 11.09 ± 1.61 | 8.32 ± 4.98 | 9.05 ± 3.76 | 9.79 ± 2.97 |
| | Robust | 10.72 ± 1.01 | 10.77 ± 1.04 | 10.7 ± 1.22 | 9.85 ± 2.42 | 10.13 ± 2.02 | 10.39 ± 1.62 | 7.62 ± 4.98 | 8.36 ± 3.77 | 9.09 ± 2.97 |
| | TESS | 10.02 ± 1.03 | 10.06 ± 1.05 | 10 ± 1.23 | 9.14 ± 2.44 | 9.42 ± 2.04 | 9.69 ± 1.63 | 6.89 ± 5.03 | 7.63 ± 3.81 | 8.37 ± 3 |
| | Conjugate | 1.33 ± 0.9 | 1.37 ± 0.93 | 1.31 ± 1.08 | 0.56 ± 2.15 | 0.81 ± 1.79 | 1.04 ± 1.44 | −1.42 ± 4.4 | −0.77 ± 3.34 | −0.12 ± 2.63 |
| | Jeffrey's | 2.65 ± 1.01 | 2.7 ± 1.04 | 2.64 ± 1.22 | 1.79 ± 2.42 | 2.07 ± 2.02 | 2.33 ± 1.62 | −0.44 ± 4.98 | 0.29 ± 3.77 | 1.03 ± 2.97 |
| | Schwarz's | 3.58 ± 1.03 | 3.63 ± 1.05 | 3.56 ± 1.23 | 2.7 ± 2.44 | 2.99 ± 2.04 | 3.25 ± 1.63 | 0.45 ± 5.03 | 1.19 ± 3.81 | 1.94 ± 3 |
| | ZS | 4.04 ± 0.99 | 4.09 ± 1.02 | 4.03 ± 1.19 | 3.19 ± 2.37 | 3.47 ± 1.98 | 3.72 ± 1.58 | 1.01 ± 4.88 | 1.73 ± 3.69 | 2.45 ± 2.91 |
| | EIA | 3.5 ± 1 | 3.55 ± 1.02 | 3.49 ± 1.19 | 2.65 ± 2.37 | 2.93 ± 1.98 | 3.18 ± 1.59 | 0.47 ± 4.88 | 1.19 ± 3.7 | 1.91 ± 2.91 |
| Gamma | IP | 11.48 ± 1.26 | −38.13 ± 9.19 | −85.57 ± 13.22 | 4.16 ± 4.16 | −5.59 ± 5.51 | −40.51 ± 9.69 | −1.33 ± 4.72 | 7.9 ± 3.41 | −17.76 ± 7.26 |
| | Robust | 10.79 ± 1.26 | −38.87 ± 9.21 | −86.4 ± 13.25 | 3.46 ± 4.16 | −6.3 ± 5.52 | −41.26 ± 9.7 | −2.04 ± 4.73 | 7.2 ± 3.41 | −18.48 ± 7.27 |
| | TESS | 10.08 ± 1.27 | −40.08 ± 9.3 | −88.08 ± 13.38 | 2.68 ± 4.21 | −7.18 ± 5.57 | −42.49 ± 9.8 | −2.87 ± 4.77 | 6.46 ± 3.44 | −19.48 ± 7.34 |
| | Conjugate | 1.39 ± 1.12 | −41.48 ± 7.68 | −79.22 ± 9.99 | −5.11 ± 3.68 | −13.69 ± 4.81 | −43.46 ± 8.02 | −9.96 ± 4.15 | −1.8 ± 3.02 | −24.24 ± 6.23 |
| | Jeffrey's | 2.72 ± 1.26 | −46.94 ± 9.21 | −94.46 ± 13.25 | −4.6 ± 4.16 | −14.37 ± 5.52 | −49.33 ± 9.7 | −10.1 ± 4.73 | −0.86 ± 3.41 | −26.55 ± 7.27 |
| | Schwarz | 3.64 ± 1.27 | −46.52 ± 9.3 | −94.52 ± 13.38 | −3.75 ± 4.21 | −13.61 ± 5.57 | −48.93 ± 9.8 | −9.31 ± 4.77 | 0.02 ± 3.44 | −25.92 ± 7.34 |
| | ZS | 4.1 ± 1.23 | −44.55 ± 9.02 | −91.12 ± 12.98 | −3.07 ± 4.08 | −12.64 ± 5.4 | −46.89 ± 9.51 | −8.46 ± 4.63 | 0.59 ± 3.34 | −24.57 ± 7.12 |
| | EIA | 3.57 ± 1.24 | −44.99 ± 8.97 | −91.11 ± 12.83 | −3.62 ± 4.08 | −13.18 ± 5.4 | −47.32 ± 9.44 | −9.01 ± 4.63 | 0.05 ± 3.35 | −25.1 ± 7.1 |

**Table A2.** Frequency distribution for the balanced framework ($n_1 = n_2 = 50$) in the normal random variables of the $2\log(B_{01})$ based on the scale proposed by [13]. Intrinsic priors (IP), Berger robust prior (Robust), BIC based on the effective sample size (TESS), conjugate, Jeffrey's, Schwarz, Zellner and Siow (ZS), and the expected arithmetic intrinsic prior of [24].

| | $\mu_1 = \mu_2$ | | | | | | | | | | | | | | |
|---|---|---|---|---|---|---|---|---|---|---|---|---|---|---|---|
| | $\sigma_1 = \sigma_2$ | | | | | $\sigma_2 = 2\sigma_1$ | | | | | $\sigma_2 = 3\sigma_1$ | | | | |
| | **Very Strong** | **Strong** | **Positive** | **Weak** | **Negative** | **Very Strong** | **Strong** | **Positive** | **Weak** | **Negative** | **Very Strong** | **Strong** | **Positive** | **Weak** | **Negative** |
| IP | 434 (86.8%) | 56 (11.2%) | 9 (1.8%) | 1 (0.2%) | 0 (0%) | 439 (87.8%) | 57 (11.4%) | 4 (0.8%) | 0 (0%) | 0 (0%) | 438 (87.6%) | 60 (12%) | 2 (0.4%) | 0 (0%) | 0 (0%) |
| Robust | 400 (80%) | 85 (17%) | 13 (2.6%) | 2 (0.4%) | 0 (0%) | 407 (81.4%) | 85 (17%) | 8 (1.6%) | 0 (0%) | 0 (0%) | 402 (80.4%) | 93 (18.6%) | 5 (1%) | 0 (0%) | 0 (0%) |
| TESS | 339 (67.8%) | 141 (28.2%) | 17 (3.4%) | 3 (0.6%) | 0 (0%) | 344 (68.8%) | 144 (28.8%) | 12 (2.4%) | 0 (0%) | 0 (0%) | 329 (65.8%) | 164 (32.8%) | 7 (1.4%) | 0 (0%) | 0 (0%) |
| Conjugate | 0 (0%) | 0 (0%) | 171 (34.2%) | [illegible] (52.8%) | 65 (13%) | 0 (0%) | 0 (0%) | 200 (40%) | 241 (48.2%) | 59 (11.8%) | 0 (0%) | 0 (0%) | 182 (36.4%) | 261 (52.2%) | 57 (11.4%) |
| Jeffrey | 0 (0%) | 0 (0%) | 392 (78.4%) | [illegible] (14.6%) | 35 (7%) | 0 (0%) | 0 (0%) | 402 (80.4%) | 68 (13.6%) | 30 (6%) | 0 (0%) | 0 (0%) | 396 (79.2%) | 78 (15.6%) | 26 (5.2%) |
| Schwarz | 0 (0%) | 0 (0%) | 437 (87.4%) | [illegible] (8%) | 23 (4.6%) | 0 (0%) | 0 (0%) | 444 (88.8%) | 39 (7.8%) | 17 (3.4%) | 0 (0%) | 0 (0%) | 445 (89%) | 45 (9%) | 10 (2%) |
| ZS | 0 (0%) | 0 (0%) | 452 (90.4%) | [illegible] (5%) | 18 (3.6%) | 0 (0%) | 0 (0%) | 458 (91.6%) | 31 (6.2%) | 11 (2.2%) | 0 (0%) | 0 (0%) | 459 (91.8%) | 34 (6.8%) | 7 (1.4%) |
| EIA | 0 (0%) | 0 (0%) | 435 (87%) | [illegible] (3.4%) | 23 (4.6%) | 0 (0%) | 0 (0%) | 444 (88.8%) | 39 (7.8%) | 17 (3.4%) | 0 (0%) | 0 (0%) | 444 (88.8%) | 46 (9.2%) | 10 (2%) |
| | $\mu_2 = 1.5\mu_1$ | | | | | | | | | | | | | | |
| | $\sigma_1 = \sigma_2$ | | | | | $\sigma_2 = 2\sigma_1$ | | | | | $\sigma_2 = 3\sigma_1$ | | | | |
| | Very Strong | Strong | Positive | Weak | Negative | Very Strong | Strong | Positive | Weak | Negative | Very Strong | Strong | Positive | Weak | Negative |
| IP | 2 (0.4%) | 19 (3.8%) | 67 (13.4%) | 43 [illegible] | 364 (72.8%) | 69 (13.8%) | 184 (36.8%) | 110 (22%) | 54 (10.8%) | 83 (16.6%) | 176 (35.2%) | 195 (39%) | 87 (17.4%) | 21 (4.2%) | 21 (4.2%) |
| Robust | 1 (0.2%) | 12 (2.4%) | 60 (12%) | 4[illegible] | 382 (76.4%) | 50 (10%) | 176 (35.2%) | 122 (24.4%) | 52 (10.4%) | 100 (20%) | 137 (27.4%) | 214 (42.8%) | 97 (19.4%) | 23 (4.6%) | 29 (5.8%) |
| TESS | 0 (0%) | 11 (2.2%) | 45 (9%) | 4[illegible] | 399 (79.8%) | 24 (4.8%) | 167 (33.4%) | 137 (27.4%) | 46 (9.2%) | 126 (25.2%) | 76 (15.2%) | 248 (49.6%) | 116 (23.2%) | 26 (5.2%) | 34 (6.8%) |
| Conjugate | 0 (0%) | 0 (0%) | 0 (0%) | 2 [illegible] | 498 (99.6%) | 0 (0%) | 0 (0%) | 8 (1.6%) | 63 (12.6%) | 429 (85.8%) | 0 (0%) | 0 (0%) | 36 (7.2%) | 147 (29.4%) | 317 (63.4%) |
| Jeffrey | 0 (0%) | 0 (0%) | 1 (0.2%) | 5 [illegible] | 494 (98.8%) | 0 (0%) | 0 (0%) | 50 (10%) | 77 (15.4%) | 373 (74.6%) | 0 (0%) | 0 (0%) | 132 (26.4%) | 128 (25.6%) | 240 (48%) |
| Schwarz | 0 (0%) | 0 (0%) | 2 (0.4%) | 9 [illegible] | 489 (97.8%) | 0 (0%) | 0 (0%) | 77 (15.4%) | 97 (19.4%) | 326 (65.2%) | 0 (0%) | 0 (0%) | 186 (37.2%) | 117 (23.4%) | 197 (39.4%) |
| ZS | 0 (0%) | 0 (0%) | 3 (0.6%) | 9 [illegible] | 488 (97.6%) | 0 (0%) | 0 (0%) | 101 (20.2%) | 96 (19.2%) | 303 (60.6%) | 0 (0%) | 0 (0%) | 228 (45.6%) | 99 (19.8%) | 173 (34.6%) |
| EIA | 0 (0%) | 0 (0%) | 2 (0.4%) | 9 [illegible] | 489 (97.8%) | 0 (0%) | 0 (0%) | 74 (14.8%) | 103 (20.6%) | 323 (64.6%) | 0 (0%) | 0 (0%) | 185 (37%) | 119 (23.8%) | 196 (39.2%) |
| | $\mu_2 = 2\mu_1$ | | | | | | | | | | | | | | |
| | $\sigma_1 = \sigma_2$ | | | | | $\sigma_2 = 2\sigma_1$ | | | | | $\sigma_2 = 3\sigma_1$ | | | | |
| | Very Strong | Strong | Positive | Weak | Negative | Very Strong | Strong | Positive | Weak | Negative | Very Strong | Strong | Positive | Weak | Negative |
| IP | 0 (0%) | 0 (0%) | 0 (0%) | 0 [illegible] | 500 (100%) | 0 (0%) | 0 (0%) | 11 (2.2%) | 13 (2.6%) | 476 (95.2%) | 12 (2.4%) | 52 (10.4%) | 109 (21.8%) | 53 (10.6%) | 274 (54.8%) |
| Robust | 0 (0%) | 0 (0%) | 0 (0%) | 0 [illegible] | 500 (100%) | 0 (0%) | 0 (0%) | 10 (2%) | 9 (1.8%) | 481 (96.2%) | 5 (1%) | 46 (9.2%) | 102 (20.4%) | 54 (10.8%) | 293 (58.6%) |
| TESS | 0 (0%) | 0 (0%) | 0 (0%) | 0 [illegible] | 500 (100%) | 0 (0%) | 0 (0%) | 5 (1%) | 12 (2.4%) | 483 (96.6%) | 5 (1%) | 38 (7.6%) | 90 (18%) | 53 (10.6%) | 314 (62.8%) |
| Conjugate | 0 (0%) | 0 (0%) | 0 (0%) | 0 [illegible] | 500 (100%) | 0 (0%) | 0 (0%) | 0 (0%) | 0 (0%) | 500 (100%) | 0 (0%) | 0 (0%) | 1 (0.2%) | 11 (2.2%) | 488 (97.6%) |
| Jeffrey | 0 (0%) | 0 (0%) | 0 (0%) | 0 [illegible] | 500 (100%) | 0 (0%) | 0 (0%) | 0 (0%) | 0 (0%) | 500 (100%) | 0 (0%) | 0 (0%) | 5 (1%) | 19 (3.8%) | 476 (95.2%) |
| Schwarz | 0 (0%) | 0 (0%) | 0 (0%) | 0 [illegible] | 500 (100%) | 0 (0%) | 0 (0%) | 0 (0%) | 0 (0%) | 500 (100%) | 0 (0%) | 0 (0%) | 13 (2.6%) | 21 (4.2%) | 466 (93.2%) |
| ZS | 0 (0%) | 0 (0%) | 0 (0%) | 0 [illegible] | 500 (100%) | 0 (0%) | 0 (0%) | 0 (0%) | 0 (0%) | 500 (100%) | 0 (0%) | 0 (0%) | 18 (3.6%) | 25 (5%) | 457 (91.4%) |
| EIA | 0 (0%) | 0 (0%) | 0 (0%) | 0 [illegible] | 500 (100%) | 0 (0%) | 0 (0%) | 0 (0%) | 0 (0%) | 500 (100%) | 0 (0%) | 0 (0%) | 13 (2.6%) | 21 (4.2%) | 466 (93.2%) |

**Table A3.** Frequency distribution for the balanced framework ($n_1 = n_2 = 50$) Student's $t$ random variables of the $2\log(B_{01})$ based on the scale proposed by [13]. Intrinsic priors (IP), Berger robust prior (Robust), BIC based on the effective sample size (TESS), conjugate, Jeffrey's, Schwarz, Zellner and Siow (ZS), and the expected arithmetic intrinsic prior of [24].

| | $\mu_1 = \mu_2$ | | | | | | | | | | | | | | |
|---|---|---|---|---|---|---|---|---|---|---|---|---|---|---|---|
| | $\sigma_1 = \sigma_2$ | | | | | $\sigma_2 = 2\sigma_1$ | | | | | $\sigma_2 = 3\sigma_1$ | | | | |
| | **Very Strong** | **Strong** | **Positive** | **Weak** | **Negative** | **Very Strong** | **Strong** | **Positive** | **Weak** | **Negative** | **Very Strong** | **Strong** | **Positive** | **Weak** | **Negative** |
| IP | 456 (91.2%) | 41 (8.2%) | 3 (0.6%) | 0 (0%) | 0 (0%) | 455 (91%) | 44 (8.8%) | 1 (0.2%) | 0 (0%) | 0 (0%) | 448 (89.6%) | 49 (9.8%) | 3 (0.6%) | 0 (0%) | 0 (0%) |
| Robust | 410 (82%) | 87 (17.4%) | 3 (0.6%) | 0 (0%) | 0 (0%) | 416 (83.2%) | 82 (16.4%) | 2 (0.4%) | 0 (0%) | 0 (0%) | 410 (82%) | 83 (16.6%) | 7 (1.4%) | 0 (0%) | 0 (0%) |
| TESS | 310 (62%) | 187 (37.4%) | 3 (0.6%) | 0 (0%) | 0 (0%) | 320 (64%) | 178 (35.6%) | 2 (0.4%) | 0 (0%) | 0 (0%) | 310 (62%) | 181 (36.2%) | 8 (1.6%) | 1 (0.2%) | 0 (0%) |
| Conjugate | 0 (0%) | 0 (0%) | 131 (26.2%) | 326 (65.2%) | 43 (8.6%) | 0 (0%) | 0 (0%) | 156 (31.2%) | 301 (60.2%) | 43 (8.6%) | 0 (0%) | 0 (0%) | 155 (31%) | 297 (59.4%) | 48 (9.6%) |
| Jeffrey | 0 (0%) | 0 (0%) | 404 (80.8%) | 85 (17%) | 11 (2.2%) | 0 (0%) | 0 (0%) | 412 (82.4%) | 74 (14.8%) | 14 (2.8%) | 0 (0%) | 0 (0%) | 396 (79.2%) | 86 (17.2%) | 18 (3.6%) |
| Schwarz | 0 (0%) | 0 (0%) | 459 (91.8%) | 37 (7.4%) | 4 (0.8%) | 0 (0%) | 0 (0%) | 457 (91.4%) | 39 (7.8%) | 4 (0.8%) | 0 (0%) | 0 (0%) | 454 (90.8%) | 36 (7.2%) | 10 (2%) |
| ZS | 0 (0%) | 0 (0%) | 479 (95.8%) | 18 (3.6%) | 3 (0.6%) | 0 (0%) | 0 (0%) | 474 (94.8%) | 24 (4.8%) | 2 (0.4%) | 0 (0%) | 0 (0%) | 474 (94.8%) | 17 (3.4%) | 9 (1.8%) |
| EIA | 0 (0%) | 0 (0%) | 457 (91.4%) | 39 (7.8%) | 4 (0.8%) | 0 (0%) | 0 (0%) | 457 (91.4%) | 39 (7.8%) | 4 (0.8%) | 0 (0%) | 0 (0%) | 454 (90.8%) | 36 (7.2%) | 10 (2%) |
| | $\mu_2 = 1.5\mu_1$ | | | | | | | | | | | | | | |
| | $\sigma_1 = \sigma_2$ | | | | | $\sigma_2 = 2\sigma_1$ | | | | | $\sigma_2 = 3\sigma_1$ | | | | |
| | Very Strong | Strong | Positive | Weak | Negative | Very Strong | Strong | Positive | Weak | Negative | Very Strong | Strong | Positive | Weak | Negative |
| IP | 378 (75.6%) | 92 (18.4%) | 22 (4.4%) | 5 (1%) | 3 (0.6%) | 395 (79%) | 88 (17.6%) | 14 (2.8%) | 1 (0.2%) | 2 (0.4%) | 421 (84.2%) | 69 (13.8%) | 10 (2%) | 0 (0%) | 0 (0%) |
| Robust | 327 (65.4%) | 132 (26.4%) | 31 (6.2%) | 5 (1%) | 5 (1%) | 347 (69.4%) | 129 (25.8%) | 19 (3.8%) | 3 (0.6%) | 2 (0.4%) | 375 (75%) | 111 (22.2%) | 14 (2.8%) | 0 (0%) | 0 (0%) |
| TESS | 259 (51.8%) | 187 (37.4%) | 39 (7.8%) | 9 (1.8%) | 6 (1.2%) | 271 (54.2%) | 199 (39.8%) | 23 (4.6%) | 4 (0.8%) | 3 (0.6%) | 284 (56.8%) | 191 (38.2%) | 24 (4.8%) | 1 (0.2%) | 0 (0%) |
| Conjugate | 0 (0%) | 0 (0%) | 125 (25%) | 259 (51.8%) | 116 (23.2%) | 0 (0%) | 0 (0%) | 109 (21.8%) | 289 (57.8%) | 102 (20.4%) | 0 (0%) | 0 (0%) | 139 (27.8%) | 283 (56.6%) | 78 (15.6%) |
| Jeffrey | 0 (0%) | 0 (0%) | 321 (64.2%) | 102 (20.4%) | 77 (15.4%) | 0 (0%) | 0 (0%) | 342 (68.4%) | 100 (20%) | 58 (11.6%) | 0 (0%) | 0 (0%) | 366 (73.2%) | 90 (18%) | 44 (8.8%) |
| Schwarz | 0 (0%) | 0 (0%) | 387 (77.4%) | 53 (10.6%) | 60 (12%) | 0 (0%) | 0 (0%) | 403 (80.6%) | 60 (12%) | 37 (7.4%) | 0 (0%) | 0 (0%) | 424 (84.8%) | 47 (9.4%) | 29 (5.8%) |
| ZS | 0 (0%) | 0 (0%) | 403 (80.6%) | 46 (9.2%) | 51 (10.2%) | 0 (0%) | 0 (0%) | 426 (85.2%) | 44 (8.8%) | 30 (6%) | 0 (0%) | 0 (0%) | 443 (88.6%) | 32 (6.4%) | 25 (5%) |
| EIA | 0 (0%) | 0 (0%) | 387 (77.4%) | 53 (10.6%) | 60 (12%) | 0 (0%) | 0 (0%) | 401 (80.2%) | 63 (12.6%) | 36 (7.2%) | 0 (0%) | 0 (0%) | 423 (84.6%) | 49 (9.8%) | 28 (5.6%) |
| | $\mu_2 = 2\mu_1$ | | | | | | | | | | | | | | |
| | $\sigma_1 = \sigma_2$ | | | | | $\sigma_2 = 2\sigma_1$ | | | | | $\sigma_2 = 3\sigma_1$ | | | | |
| | Very Strong | Strong | Positive | Weak | Negative | Very Strong | Strong | Positive | Weak | Negative | Very Strong | Strong | Positive | Weak | Negative |
| IP | 264 (52.8%) | 125 (25%) | 60 (12%) | 12 (2.4%) | 39 (7.8%) | 263 (52.6%) | 144 (28.8%) | 64 (12.8%) | 11 (2.2%) | 18 (3.6%) | 324 (64.8%) | 114 (22.8%) | 48 (9.6%) | 7 (1.4%) | 7 (1.4%) |
| Robust | 225 (45%) | 150 (30%) | 65 (13%) | 18 (3.6%) | 42 (8.4%) | 231 (46.2%) | 166 (33.2%) | 72 (14.4%) | 9 (1.8%) | 22 (4.4%) | 270 (54%) | 157 (31.4%) | 55 (11%) | 8 (1.6%) | 10 (2%) |
| TESS | 162 (32.4%) | 190 (38%) | 79 (15.8%) | 22 (4.4%) | 47 (9.4%) | 183 (36.6%) | 196 (39.2%) | 81 (16.2%) | 16 (3.2%) | 24 (4.8%) | 183 (36.6%) | 229 (45.8%) | 64 (12.8%) | 10 (2%) | 14 (2.8%) |
| Conjugate | 0 (0%) | 0 (0%) | 73 (14.6%) | 194 (38.8%) | 233 (46.6%) | 0 (0%) | 0 (0%) | 73 (14.6%) | 193 (38.6%) | 234 (46.8%) | 0 (0%) | 0 (0%) | 82 (16.4%) | 245 (49%) | 173 (34.6%) |
| Jeffrey | 0 (0%) | 0 (0%) | 224 (44.8%) | 87 (17.4%) | 189 (37.8%) | 0 (0%) | 0 (0%) | 229 (45.8%) | 102 (20.4%) | 169 (33.8%) | 0 (0%) | 0 (0%) | 261 (52.2%) | 110 (22%) | 129 (25.8%) |
| Schwarz | 0 (0%) | 0 (0%) | 268 (53.6%) | 77 (15.4%) | 155 (31%) | 0 (0%) | 0 (0%) | 269 (53.8%) | 98 (19.6%) | 133 (26.6%) | 0 (0%) | 0 (0%) | 330 (66%) | 75 (15%) | 95 (19%) |
| ZS | 0 (0%) | 0 (0%) | 287 (57.4%) | 72 (14.4%) | 141 (28.2%) | 0 (0%) | 0 (0%) | 298 (59.6%) | 82 (16.4%) | 120 (24%) | 0 (0%) | 0 (0%) | 349 (69.8%) | 64 (12.8%) | 87 (17.4%) |
| EIA | 0 (0%) | 0 (0%) | 268 (53.6%) | 78 (15.6%) | 154 (30.8%) | 0 (0%) | 0 (0%) | 268 (53.6%) | 100 (20%) | 132 (26.4%) | 0 (0%) | 0 (0%) | 330 (66%) | 77 (15.4%) | 93 (18.6%) |

**Table A4.** Frequency distribution for the balanced framework ($n_1 = n_2 = 50$) from the gamma random variables of the $2\log(B_{01})$ based on the scale proposed by [13]. Intrinsic priors (IP), Berger robust prior (Robust), BIC based on the effective sample size (TESS), conjugate, Jeffrey's, Schwarz, Zellner and Siow (ZS), and the expected arithmetic intrinsic prior of [24].

| | | | | | | | | $\mu_1 = \mu_2$ | | | | | | | |
|---|---|---|---|---|---|---|---|---|---|---|---|---|---|---|---|
| | | | $\sigma_1 = \sigma_2$ | | | | | $\sigma_2 = 2\sigma_1$ | | | | | $\sigma_2 = 3\sigma_1$ | | |
| | **Very Strong** | **Strong** | **Positive** | **Weak** | **Negative** | **Very Strong** | **Strong** | **Positive** | **Weak** | **Negative** | **Very Strong** | **Strong** | **Positive** | **Weak** | **Negative** |
| IP | 449 (89.8%) | 49 (9.8%) | 2 (0.4%) | 0 (0%) | 0 (0%) | 0 (0%) | 0 (0%) | 0 (0%) | 0 (0%) | 500 (100%) | 0 (0%) | 0 (0%) | 0 (0%) | 0 (0%) | 500 (100%) |
| Robust | 417 (83.4%) | 78 (15.6%) | 5 (1%) | 0 (0%) | 0 (0%) | 0 (0%) | 0 (0%) | 0 (0%) | 0 (0%) | 500 (100%) | 0 (0%) | 0 (0%) | 0 (0%) | 0 (0%) | 500 (100%) |
| TESS | 348 (69.6%) | 139 (27.8%) | 13 (2.6%) | 0 (0%) | 0 (0%) | 0 (0%) | 0 (0%) | 0 (0%) | 0 (0%) | 500 (100%) | 0 (0%) | 0 (0%) | 0 (0%) | 0 (0%) | 500 (100%) |
| Conjugate | 0 (0%) | 0 (0%) | 183 (36.6%) | 268 (53.6%) | 49 (9.8%) | 0 (0%) | 0 (0%) | 0 (0%) | 0 (0%) | 500 (100%) | 0 (0%) | 0 (0%) | 0 (0%) | 0 (0%) | 500 (100%) |
| Jeffrey | 0 (0%) | 0 (0%) | 412 (82.4%) | 62 (12.4%) | 26 (5.2%) | 0 (0%) | 0 (0%) | 0 (0%) | 0 (0%) | 500 (100%) | 0 (0%) | 0 (0%) | 0 (0%) | 0 (0%) | 500 (100%) |
| Schwarz | 0 (0%) | 0 (0%) | 452 (90.4%) | 31 (6.2%) | 17 (3.4%) | 0 (0%) | 0 (0%) | 0 (0%) | 0 (0%) | 500 (100%) | 0 (0%) | 0 (0%) | 0 (0%) | 0 (0%) | 500 (100%) |
| ZS | 0 (0%) | 0 (0%) | 465 (93%) | 25 (5%) | 10 (2%) | 0 (0%) | 0 (0%) | 0 (0%) | 0 (0%) | 500 (100%) | 0 (0%) | 0 (0%) | 0 (0%) | 0 (0%) | 500 (100%) |
| EIA | 0 (0%) | 0 (0%) | 451 (90.2%) | 32 (6.4%) | 17 (3.4%) | 0 (0%) | 0 (0%) | 0 (0%) | 0 (0%) | 500 (100%) | 0 (0%) | 0 (0%) | 0 (0%) | 0 (0%) | 500 (100%) |
| | | | | | | | | $\mu_2 = 1.5\mu_1$ | | | | | | | |
| | | | $\sigma_1 = \sigma_2$ | | | | | $\sigma_2 = 2\sigma_1$ | | | | | $\sigma_2 = 3\sigma_1$ | | |
| | Very Strong | Strong | Positive | Weak | Negative | Very Strong | Strong | Positive | Weak | Negative | Very Strong | Strong | Positive | Weak | Negative |
| IP | 30 (6%) | 141 (28.2%) | 186 (37.2%) | 63 (12.6%) | 80 (16%) | 0 (0%) | 3 (0.6%) | 33 (6.6%) | 35 (7%) | 429 (85.8%) | 0 (0%) | 0 (0%) | 0 (0%) | 0 (0%) | 500 (100%) |
| Robust | 21 (4.2%) | 119 (23.8%) | 191 (38.2%) | 68 (13.6%) | 101 (20.2%) | 0 (0%) | 0 (0%) | 22 (4.4%) | 39 (7.8%) | 439 (87.8%) | 0 (0%) | 0 (0%) | 0 (0%) | 0 (0%) | 500 (100%) |
| TESS | 8 (1.6%) | 109 (21.8%) | 186 (37.2%) | 72 (14.4%) | 125 (25%) | 0 (0%) | 0 (0%) | 16 (3.2%) | 33 (6.6%) | 451 (90.2%) | 0 (0%) | 0 (0%) | 0 (0%) | 0 (0%) | 500 (100%) |
| Conjugate | 0 (0%) | 0 (0%) | 2 (0.4%) | 32 (6.4%) | 466 (93.2%) | 0 (0%) | 0 (0%) | 0 (0%) | 0 (0%) | 500 (100%) | 0 (0%) | 0 (0%) | 0 (0%) | 0 (0%) | 500 (100%) |
| Jeffrey | 0 (0%) | 0 (0%) | 19 (3.8%) | 49 (9.8%) | 432 (86.4%) | 0 (0%) | 0 (0%) | 0 (0%) | 0 (0%) | 500 (100%) | 0 (0%) | 0 (0%) | 0 (0%) | 0 (0%) | 500 (100%) |
| Schwarz | 0 (0%) | 0 (0%) | 36 (7.2%) | 63 (12.6%) | 401 (80.2%) | 0 (0%) | 0 (0%) | 0 (0%) | 0 (0%) | 500 (100%) | 0 (0%) | 0 (0%) | 0 (0%) | 0 (0%) | 500 (100%) |
| ZS | 0 (0%) | 0 (0%) | 50 (10%) | 73 (14.6%) | 377 (75.4%) | 0 (0%) | 0 (0%) | 0 (0%) | 0 (0%) | 500 (100%) | 0 (0%) | 0 (0%) | 0 (0%) | 0 (0%) | 500 (100%) |
| EIA | 0 (0%) | 0 (0%) | 35 (7%) | 64 (12.8%) | 401 (80.2%) | 0 (0%) | 0 (0%) | 0 (0%) | 0 (0%) | 500 (100%) | 0 (0%) | 0 (0%) | 0 (0%) | 0 (0%) | 500 (100%) |
| | | | | | | | | $\mu_2 = 2\mu_1$ | | | | | | | |
| | | | $\sigma_1 = \sigma_2$ | | | | | $\sigma_2 = 2\sigma_1$ | | | | | $\sigma_2 = 3\sigma_1$ | | |
| | Very Strong | Strong | Positive | Weak | Negative | Very Strong | Strong | Positive | Weak | Negative | Very Strong | Strong | Positive | Weak | Negative |
| IP | 0 (0%) | 19 (3.8%) | 103 (20.6%) | 86 (17.2%) | 292 (58.4%) | 148 (29.6%) | 218 (43.6%) | 103 (20.6%) | 17 (3.4%) | 14 (2.8%) | 0 (0%) | 0 (0%) | 0 (0%) | 0 (0%) | 500 (100%) |
| Robust | 0 (0%) | 13 (2.6%) | 87 (17.4%) | 73 (14.6%) | 327 (65.4%) | 111 (22.2%) | 229 (45.8%) | 122 (24.4%) | 16 (3.2%) | 22 (4.4%) | 0 (0%) | 0 (0%) | 0 (0%) | 0 (0%) | 500 (100%) |
| TESS | 0 (0%) | 6 (1.2%) | 71 (14.2%) | 66 (13.2%) | 357 (71.4%) | 73 (14.6%) | 239 (47.8%) | 140 (28%) | 21 (4.2%) | 27 (5.4%) | 0 (0%) | 0 (0%) | 0 (0%) | 0 (0%) | 500 (100%) |
| Conjugate | 0 (0%) | 0 (0%) | 0 (0%) | 0 (0%) | 500 (100%) | 0 (0%) | 0 (0%) | 28 (5.6%) | 124 (24.8%) | 348 (69.6%) | 0 (0%) | 0 (0%) | 0 (0%) | 0 (0%) | 500 (100%) |
| Jeffrey | 0 (0%) | 0 (0%) | 0 (0%) | 2 (0.4%) | 498 (99.6%) | 0 (0%) | 0 (0%) | 107 (21.4%) | 130 (26%) | 263 (52.6%) | 0 (0%) | 0 (0%) | 0 (0%) | 0 (0%) | 500 (100%) |
| Schwarz | 0 (0%) | 0 (0%) | 0 (0%) | 5 (1%) | 495 (99%) | 0 (0%) | 0 (0%) | 157 (31.4%) | 139 (27.8%) | 204 (40.8%) | 0 (0%) | 0 (0%) | 0 (0%) | 0 (0%) | 500 (100%) |
| ZS | 0 (0%) | 0 (0%) | 0 (0%) | 7 (1.4%) | 493 (98.6%) | 0 (0%) | 0 (0%) | 200 (40%) | 115 (23%) | 185 (37%) | 0 (0%) | 0 (0%) | 0 (0%) | 0 (0%) | 500 (100%) |
| EIA | 0 (0%) | 0 (0%) | 0 (0%) | 5 (1%) | 495 (99%) | 0 (0%) | 0 (0%) | 154 (30.8%) | 143 (28.6%) | 203 (40.6%) | 0 (0%) | 0 (0%) | 0 (0%) | 0 (0%) | 500 (100%) |

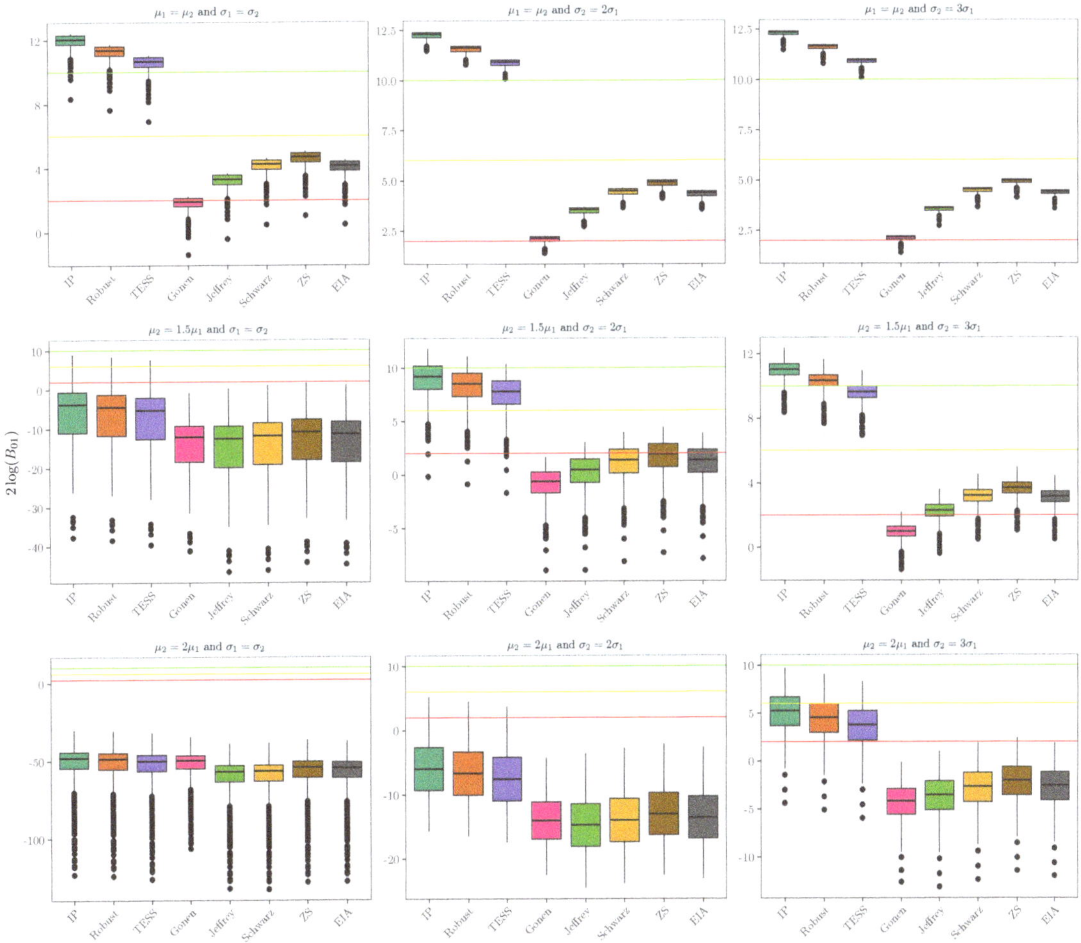


**Figure A1.** Evidence in the $2\log(B_{01})$ scale when comparing the population means of two samples that arise from normal distributions with several means and variances with equal sizes $n_1 = 50$ and $n_2 = 500$. Intrinsic priors (IP), Berger robust prior (Robust), BIC based on the effective sample size (TESS), conjugate, Jeffrey's, Schwarz, Zellner and Siow (ZS), and the expected arithmetic intrinsic prior of [24].

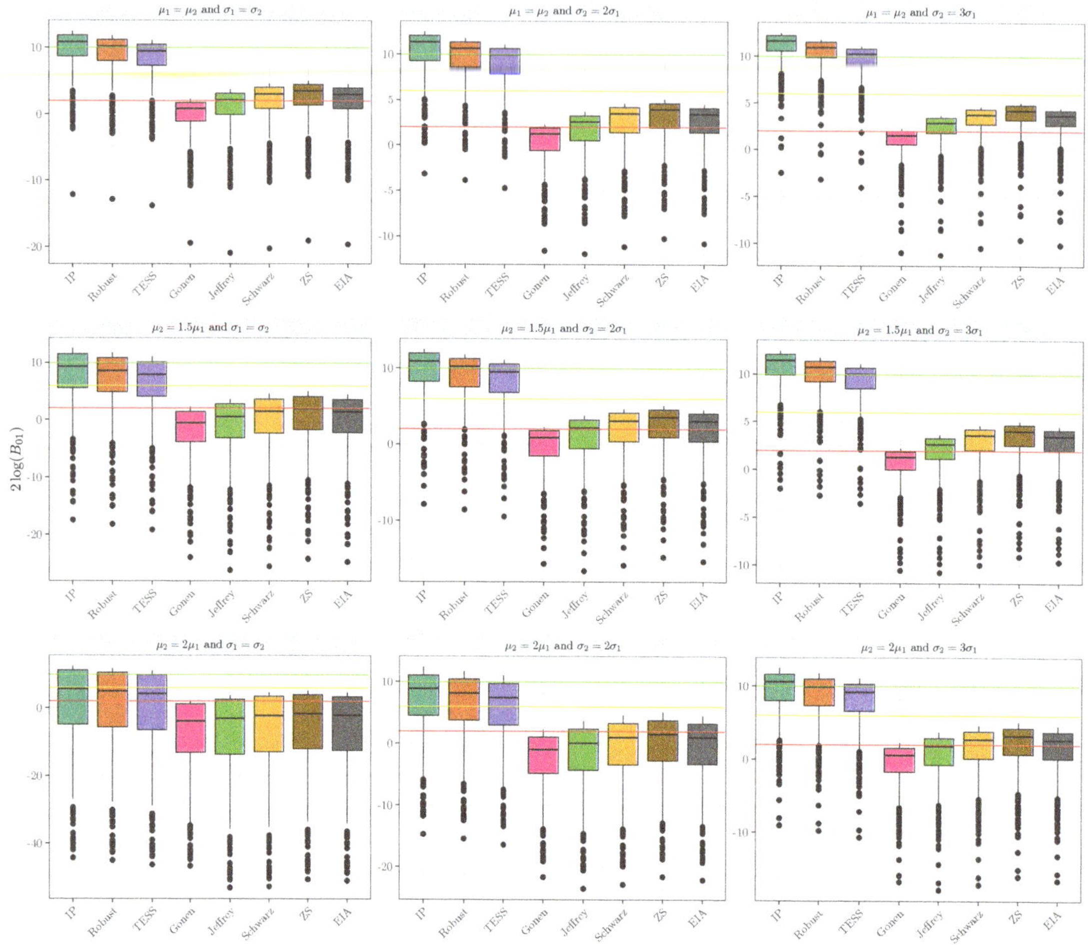


**Figure A2.** Evidence in the $2\log(B_{01})$ scale when comparing the population means of two samples that arise from a Student's *t* distributions with several means and variances with equal sizes $n_1 = 50$ and $n_2 = 500$. Intrinsic priors (IP), Berger robust prior (Robust), BIC based on the effective sample size (TESS), conjugate, Jeffrey's, Schwarz, Zellner and Siow (ZS), and the expected arithmetic intrinsic prior of [24].

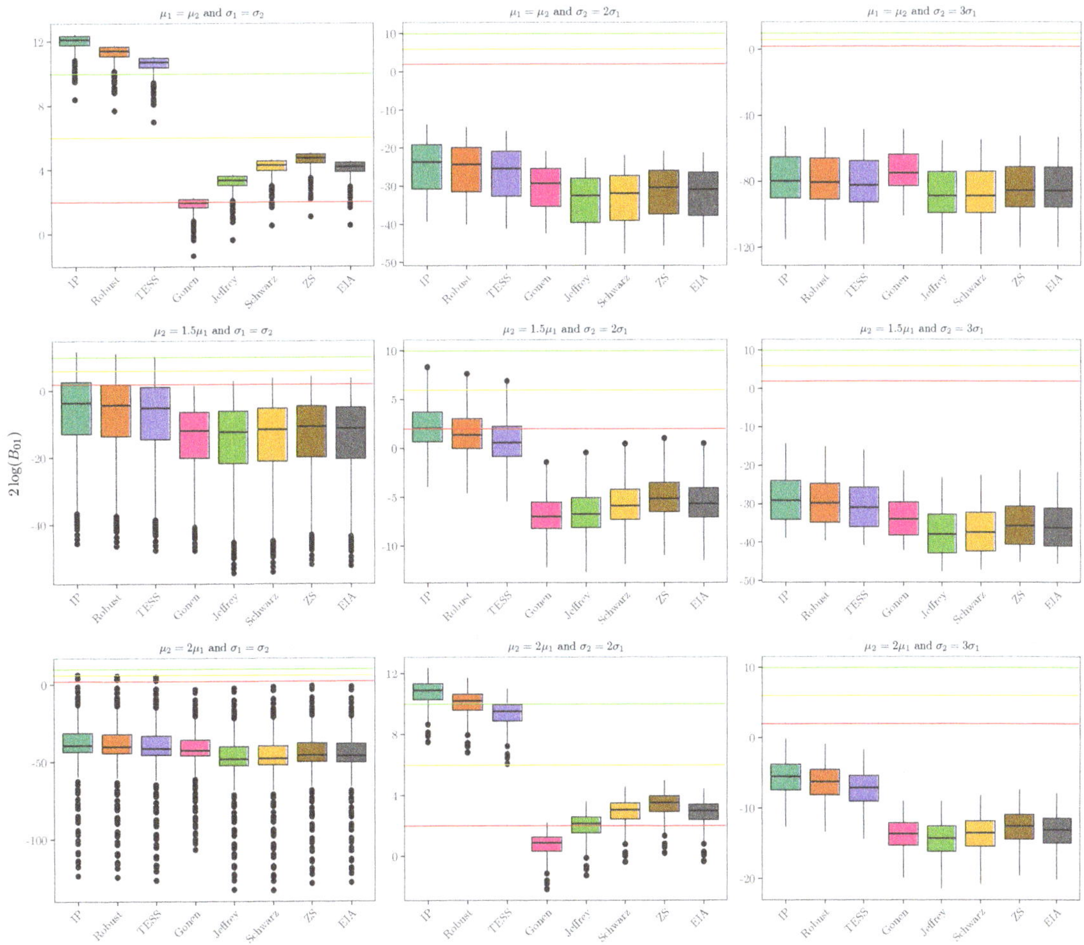


**Figure A3.** Evidence in the $2\log(B_{01})$ scale when comparing the population means of two samples that arise from gamma random samples with several means and variances with equal sizes $n_1 = 50$ and $n_2 = 500$. Intrinsic priors (IP), Berger robust prior (Robust), BIC based on the effective sample size (TESS), conjugate, Jeffrey's, Schwarz, Zellner and Siow (ZS), and the expected arithmetic intrinsic prior of [24].

## References

1. Student. The probable error of a mean. *Biometrika* **1908**, *6*, 1–25. [CrossRef]
2. Greenland, S.; Senn, S.J.; Rothman, K.J.; Carlin, J.B.; Poole, C.; Goodman, S.N.; Altman, D.G. Statistical tests, *p* values, confidence intervals, and power: A guide to misinterpretations. *Eur. J. Epidemiol.* **2016**, *31*, 337–350. [CrossRef] [PubMed]
3. Wasserstein, R.L.; Lazar, N.A. The ASA statement on *p*-values: Context, process, and purpose. *Am. Stat.* **2016**, *70*, 129–133. [CrossRef]
4. Vidgen, B.; Yasseri, T. *p*-values: Misunderstood and misused. *Front. Physics* **2016**, *4*, 6. [CrossRef]
5. Held, L.; Ott, M. On *p*-values and Bayes factors. *Annu. Rev. Stat. Its Appl.* **2018**, *5*, 393–419. [CrossRef]
6. Dienes, Z. How Bayes factors change scientific practice. *J. Math. Psychol.* **2016**, *72*, 78–89. [CrossRef]
7. Marden, J.I. Hypothesis testing: From *p* values to Bayes factors. *J. Am. Stat. Assoc.* **2000**, *95*, 1316–1320. [CrossRef]
8. Page, R.; Satake, E. Beyond *p* Values and Hypothesis Testing: Using the Minimum Bayes Factor to Teach Statistical Inference in Undergraduate Introductory Statistics Courses. *J. Educ. Learn.* **2017**, *6*, 254–266. [CrossRef]
9. Lavine, M.; Schervish, M.J. Bayes factors: What they are and what they are not. *Am. Stat.* **1999**, *53*, 119–122.

10. Berger, J.O.; Mortera, J. Default Bayes factors for nonnested hypothesis testing. *J. Am. Stat. Assoc.* **1999**, *94*, 542–554. [CrossRef]
11. Berger, J.; Pericchi, L. Bayes factors. In *Wiley StatsRef: Statistics Reference Online*; John Wiley & Sons: Hoboken, NJ, USA, 2014; pp. 1–14.
12. Jeffreys, H. *The Theory of Probability*; OUP Oxford: Oxford, UK, 1998.
13. Kass, R.E.; Raftery, A.E. Bayes factors. *J. Am. Stat. Assoc.* **1995**, *90*, 773–795. [CrossRef]
14. Gönen, M.; Johnson, W.O.; Lu, Y.; Westfall, P.H. The Bayesian two-sample t test. *Am. Stat.* **2005**, *59*, 252–257. [CrossRef]
15. Berger, J.O.; Pericchi, L.R.; Ghosh, J.; Samanta, T.; De Santis, F.; Berger, J.; Pericchi, L. *Objective Bayesian Methods for Model Selection: Introduction and Comparison*; Lecture Notes-Monograph Series; Institute of Mathematical Statistics: Beachwood, OH, USA, 2001; pp. 135–207.
16. Berger, J.O.; Pericchi, L.R. The intrinsic Bayes factor for linear models. *Bayesian Stat.* **1996**, *5*, 25–44.
17. Berger, J.O.; Pericchi, L.R. The intrinsic Bayes factor for model selection and prediction. *J. Am. Stat. Assoc.* **1996**, *91*, 109–122. [CrossRef]
18. Berger, J.O. Robust Bayesian analysis: Sensitivity to the prior. *J. Stat. Plan. Inference* **1990**, *25*, 303–328. [CrossRef]
19. Moreno, E. *Bayes Factors for Intrinsic and Fractional Priors in Nested Models. Bayesian Robustness*; Lecture Notes-Monograph Series; Institute of Mathematical Statistics: Beachwood, OH, USA, 1997; pp. 257–270.
20. Berger, J.O.; Berger, J. *Bayesian Analysis*; Springer: Berlin/Heidelberg, Germany, 1985.
21. Berger, J.; Bayarri, M.; Pericchi, L. The effective sample size. *Econom. Rev.* **2014**, *33*, 197–217. [CrossRef]
22. Schwarz, G. Estimating the dimension of a model. *Ann. Stat.* **1978**, *6*, 461–464. [CrossRef]
23. Zellner, A.; Siow, A. Posterior odds ratios for selected regression hypotheses. *Trab. Estad. Investig. Oper.* **1980**, *31*, 585–603. [CrossRef]
24. Kim, D.H.; Kang, S.G.; Lee, W.D. Intrinsic priors for testing two normal means with intrinsic bayes factors. *Commun. Stat. Methods* **2006**, *35*, 63–81. [CrossRef]
25. Cushny, A.R.; Peebles, A.R. The action of optical isomers: II. Hyoscines. *J. Physiol.* **1905**, *32*, 501. [CrossRef]
26. Senn, S.; Richardson, W. The first t-test. *Stat. Med.* **1994**, *13*, 785–803. [CrossRef]
27. Senn, S. A century of t-tests. *Significance* **2008**, *5*, 37–39. [CrossRef]
28. Falk, J.L.; Tang, M.; Forman, S. Schedule-induced chronic hypertension. *Psychosom. Med.* **1977**, *39*, 252–263. [CrossRef]

entropy

MDPI

*Article*

# On the Nuisance Parameter Elimination Principle in Hypothesis Testing

**Andrés Felipe Flórez Rivera *, Luis Gustavo Esteves, Victor Fossaluza and Carlos Alberto de Bragança Pereira**

Institute of Mathematics and Statistics, University of São Paulo, São Paulo 05508-090, Brazil; lesteves@ime.usp.br (L.G.E.); victorf@ime.usp.br (V.F.); cpereira@ime.usp.br (C.A.d.B.P.)
* Correspondence: afflorezr@gmail.com

**Abstract:** The Non-Informative Nuisance Parameter Principle concerns the problem of how inferences about a parameter of interest should be made in the presence of nuisance parameters. The principle is examined in the context of the hypothesis testing problem. We prove that the mixed test obeys the principle for discrete sample spaces. We also show how adherence of the mixed test to the principle can make performance of the test much easier. These findings are illustrated with new solutions to well-known problems of testing hypotheses for count data.

**Keywords:** $p$-values; Bayes factor; likelihood function; hypothesis testing

## 1. Introduction

Principles of Statistical Inference (or Data Reduction) constitute important guidelines on how to draw conclusions from data, especially when performing standard inferential procedures for unknown parameters of interest, like estimation and hypothesis testing. For instance, the Sufficiency Principle (SP) states that any sufficient statistic retains all relevant information about the unknown parameters that should be used to make inferences about them. It precisely recommends that if $T$ is a sufficient statistic for the statistical model under consideration and $x_1$ and $x_2$ are sample points such that $T(x_1) = T(x_2)$, then the observation of any of these points should lead to the same conclusions regarding the parameters of interest.

Besides the place of sufficiency in Statistical Inference, these recommendations cover several issues such as the contrast between post-experimental and pre-experimental reasoning and the roles of non-informative stopping rules, censoring mechanisms and nuisance parameters in data analysis. Among the main principles, the Sufficiency Principle is generally recognized as a cornerstone of Statistical Inference. On the other hand, the Likelihood Principle (LP) and its profound consequences are still subjects of intense debate. The reader will find a detailed discussion of the Likelihood Principle in [1–6].

In this work, we examine the Non-Informative Nuisance Parameter Principle (NNPP) introduced by Berger and Wolpert in 1988 in their remarkable book that concerns the problem of the way inferences about a parameter of interest should be made in the presence of nuisance parameters. Nuisance parameters usually affect inferences about the parameter of interest, like in the estimation of the mean of a normal distribution with unknown variance, in the estimation of the parameters of a linear regression model in the presence of unknown variance, and in the determination of $p$-values for specific hypotheses in the analysis of $2 \times 2$ contingency tables ([7]). In a few words, the NNPP states that under suitable conditions, it is irrelevant whether the value of a non informative nuisance parameter is known or not in order to draw conclusions about the parameter of interest. Despite the importance of the problem for eliminating nuisance parameters in data analysis, the authors have not explored this principle and its consequences in some depth as far as we have reviewed the literature. For this reason, we revisit the NNPP by formally stating it for the problem of hypothesis testing, present decision rules that meet the principle and show how the performance of a particular test in line with the NNPP can then be simplified.

This work is organized as follows: in Section 2, the NNPP for hypothesis testing is stated, discussed and illustrated under a Bayesian perspective. In Section 3, the Bayesian test procedure based on the concept of adaptive significance level and on an alternative $p$-value introduced by Pericchi and Pereira in [8], henceforth named the mixed test, is reviewed and is proven to satisfy the NNPP for discrete sample data when the (marginal) null hypothesis regarding the parameter of interest is a singleton (as a matter of fact, the result also holds when such a null hypothesis is specified by a hyperplane). In that section, we also define conditional versions of the adaptive significance level and $p$-value based on suitable statistics and prove that under those conditions, the performance of the mixed test is then simply the comparison between these new conditional quantities. These results are of great importance to make it easier to use the mixed test in various situations. In Section 4, we exemplify the main results by presenting new solutions by using the mixed test for well-known problems of test of hypotheses for count data under suitable reparametrizations of the corresponding models: we revisit the problems of comparison of Poisson population means and of testing the hypotheses of independence and symmetry in contingency tables. We make our final comments in Section 5. The proofs of the theorems and the calculations for one example in Section 4 are found in the Appendix A.

## 2. The Non-Informative Nuisance Parameter Principle for Hypothesis Testing

The problem of the elimination of nuisance parameters in statistical inference has a long history and remains a major issue. Proposals to deal with it include the marginalization of the likelihood function by integrating out the nuisance parameter ([9–11]), the construction of partial likelihood functions ([12–14], among others) and the consideration of conditional likelihood functions based on different notions of non-informativeness, sufficiency and ancillarity. Elimination of nuisance parameters and different notions of non-information have also been studied in more detail in [15–18], where, based on suitable statistics, the concepts of B, S and G non-information are presented. The generalized Sufficiency and Conditionality Principles are also discussed in [17]. On the other hand, Bayesian methods for eliminating nuisance parameters based on a suitable statistic $T$ involve different definitions of sufficiency: for instance, K-Sufficiency, Q-Sufficiency and L-Sufficiency (see for example [17] and references therein).

In this section, the Non-Informative Nuisance Parameter Principle (NNPP) by Berger and Wolpert is discussed and formally defined for the problem of hypothesis testing. As we will see, on the one hand, the NNPP seems to be fair under both the partial and the conditional non-Bayesian approaches mentioned in the previous paragraph; on the other hand, it sounds really reasonable under the Bayesian standpoint. Despite the relevance of the problem of the elimination of nuisance parameters in data analysis, Berger and Wolpert [1] presented the NNPP but has not explored the principle in-depth as far as we have examined in the literature.

Some notation is needed to continue. We denote by $\theta$ the unknown parameter and by $X$ the sample to be observed. $\Theta$ and $\mathfrak{X}$ represent the parameter and the sample spaces, respectively. The family of discrete probability distributions for $X$ is denoted by $\mathcal{P} = \{\mathbb{P}(\cdot|\theta) : \theta \in \Theta\}$. In addition, for $x \in \mathfrak{X}$, $L_x(\cdot)$ denotes the likelihood function for $\theta$ generated by the sample point $x$. By an experiment $\mathcal{E}$, we mean, as in [1] , a triplet $\mathcal{E} = (X, \theta, \mathcal{P})$, with $X$, $\theta$ and $\mathcal{P}$ as defined earlier. Finally, for a subset $\Theta_0$ of $\Theta$, we formulate the null hypothesis $H : \theta \in \Theta_0$ and the alternative one $A : \theta \notin \Theta_0$. We recall that a test function (procedure) for the hypotheses $H$ versus $A$ is a function $\varphi : \mathfrak{X} \to \{0, 1\}$ that takes the value 1 ($\varphi(x) = 1$) if $H$ is rejected when $x \in \mathfrak{X}$ is observed and takes the value 0 ($\varphi(x) = 0$) if $H$ is not rejected when $x$ is observed. Under the Bayesian perspective, we also consider a continuous prior density function $\pi(\cdot)$ for $\theta$ that induces, when combined with the likelihood function $L_x(\cdot)$, a continuous posterior density function for $\theta$ given $x$, $\pi(\cdot|x)$.

In [1], Berger and Wolpert presented the following principle on how to make inferences about an unknown parameter of interest $\theta_1$ in the presence of a nuisance parameter $\theta_2$: when a sample observation, say $x_0$, separates information concerning $\theta_1$ from information on $\theta_2$, it is irrelevant whether the value of $\theta_2$ is known or unknown in order to make inferences about $\theta_1$ based on the observation of $x_0$. In other terms, if the conclusions on $\theta_1$ were to be the same for every possible value of the nuisance parameter, were $\theta_2$ known, then the same conclusions on $\theta_1$ should be reached even if $\theta_2$ is unknown. These authors then consider the following mathematical setup to formalize these ideas.

Let $\theta = (\theta_1, \theta_2)$, with $\theta_1$ and $\theta_2$ defined as in the previous paragraph. Consider $\Theta = \Theta_1 \times \Theta_2$; that is, the parameter space is variation independent, where $\Theta_i \subseteq \mathbb{R}^{n_i}$ is the set of values for $\theta_i$, $n_i \in \mathbb{N}^*$, $i = 1, 2$. Suppose the experiment $\mathcal{E} = (X, \theta, \mathcal{P})$ is carried out to learn about $\theta$. Let $\bar{\mathcal{E}} = ((X, \theta_2), \theta_1, \bar{\mathcal{P}})$ be the "thought" experiment in which the pair $(X, \theta_2)$ is to be observed (instead of observing only $X$), where $\bar{\mathcal{P}}$ is the family of distributions for $(X, \theta_2)$ indexed by $\theta_1$. Suppose also that under experiment $\mathcal{E}$, the likelihood function generated by a specific $x_0 \in \mathfrak{X}$ for $\theta$ has the following factored form:

$$L_{x_0}(\theta_1, \theta_2) = L^1_{x_0}(\theta_1) L^2_{x_0}(\theta_2) \tag{1}$$

where $L^i_{x_0} : \Theta_i \to \mathbb{R}_+$, $i = 1, 2$; that is, $L^i_{x_0}$ depends on $\theta$ only through $\theta_i$.

Berger and Wolpert then states the **Non-Informative Nuisance Parameter Principle (NNPP):** *if $\mathcal{E}$ and $x_0 \in \mathfrak{X}$ are such that (1) holds, and if the inference about $\theta_1$ from the observation of $(x_0, \theta_2)$ when $\bar{\mathcal{E}}$ is performed does not depend on $\theta_2$, then the inferential statements made for $\theta_1$ from $\mathcal{E}$ and $x_0$ should be the same as (should coincide with) the inferential statements made from $\bar{\mathcal{E}}$ and $(x_0, \theta_2)$ for every $\theta_2 \in \Theta_2$.*

The authors named such a parameter $\theta_2$ a **Non-Informative Nuisance Parameter (NNP)**, as the conclusions or decisions regarding $\theta_1$ from $\bar{\mathcal{E}}$ and $(x_0, \theta_2)$ do not depend on $\theta_2$.

A likelihood function that satisfies (1) is named a likelihood function with separable parameters ([19]). The factored form of the likelihood function in (1) seems to capture the notion of "absence of information about a parameter, say $\theta_1$, from the other, $\theta_2$, and vice versa" under both Bayesian and non-Bayesian reasoning. Indeed, under the Bayesian paradigm, posterior independence between $\theta_1$ and $\theta_2$ (say, given $x_0$) reflects the fact that one´s opinion about the parameter $\theta_1$ after observing $x_0$ is not altered by any information about $\theta_2$, and consequently, decisions regarding $\theta_1$ should not depend on $\theta_2$. Since posterior independence between $\theta_1$ and $\theta_2$ given $x_0$ is equivalent to the factored form of the likelihood function generated by $x_0$ under prior independence, condition (1) sounds really reasonable as a mathematical description of separate information about the parameters. Thus, if a Bayesian statistician should make inferences regarding a parameter $\theta_1$ in the presence of a nuisance parameter $\theta_2$, it would be ideal that these parameters are independent a posteriori; that is, the factored form of the likelihood function holds. This last equivalence is proven in the theorem below.

**Theorem 1.** *Let $\mathcal{E} = (X, \theta, \mathcal{P})$ be an experiment and $\pi(\cdot)$ be the prior probability density function for $\theta = (\theta_1, \theta_2)$. Suppose $\theta_1$ is independent of $\theta_2$ ($\theta_1 \perp\!\!\!\perp \theta_2$) a priori. Then, for each $x \in \mathfrak{X}$,*

$$\theta_1 \perp\!\!\!\perp \theta_2 \mid X = x \iff \exists L^i_x : \Theta_i \to \mathbb{R}_+ \,,\; i = 1, 2, \tag{2}$$

*such that $L_x(\theta_1, \theta_2) = L^1_x(\theta_1) L^2_x(\theta_2)$.*

On the other hand, the condition (1) seems to also be a fair representation of non-informativeness of one parameter on another under a non-Bayesian perspective. In fact, such a factored form of the likelihood function arises, for instance, when the sample $X$ is conditioned on particular types of statistics that are simple to interpret under non-Bayesian paradigms. Note that for any statistic $T$, one can write

$$L_x(\theta_1,\theta_2) = P(X = x|\theta_1,\theta_2) = P(X = x|T(X) = T(x),\theta_1,\theta_2)P(T(X) = T(x)|\theta_1,\theta_2)\,.$$

If, in addition, $T$ is a statistic such that its distribution given $\theta$ depends only on $\theta_1$ and the conditional distribution of $X$ given $T(X) = T(x)$, and $\theta$ depends only on $\theta_2$, the factored form in (1) is easily obtained (such a statistic was named p-sufficient for $\theta_1$ by Basu ([17]). In this situation, all the relevant information on $\theta_1$ is summarized in $T$, and one can fully make inferences on $\theta_1$ taking into account only the conditional distribution of $T$ given $\theta$, which does not involve $\theta_2$. Similarly, if $T$ is a statistic such that its distribution given $\theta$ depends only on $\theta_2$ and the conditional distribution of $X$ given $T(X) = T(x)$ and $\theta$ depends only on $\theta_1$, the factored form in (1) holds. Such a statistic was named s-ancillary for $\theta_1$ by Basu ([17]), and it is somewhat evident that in this case, conclusions on $\theta_1$ should be drawn exclusively from the distribution of $X$ given $T(X)$ and $\theta$, which does not depend on $\theta_2$. Such a conditional approach to the problem of elimination of nuisance parameters had already been proposed by Basu ([17]) and in a sense is closely related to the NNPP by Berger and Wolpert. The next theorem formally presents such results.

**Theorem 2.** *Let $\mathcal{E} = (X,\theta,\mathcal{P})$ be an experiment in which $\theta = (\theta_1,\theta_2)$ and $\Theta$ is variation independent. Then, if $\exists\, T : \mathfrak{X} \to \mathcal{T}$ such that $T$ is either p-sufficient or s-ancillary for $\theta_1$, then for each $x \in \mathfrak{X}$, the likelihood function generated by $x$, $L_x(\cdot)$ can be factored as (1).*

In summary, it seems reasonable that inferences about $\theta_1$ and $\theta_2$ can be performed independently under condition (1). Thus, if only $\theta_1$ is of interest, then it seems sensible under (1) that we reach the same conclusions on $\theta_1$ when $x$ is observed either by using the whole likelihood function $L_x$ or only the factor $L_x^1$. That is, it makes sense to disregard the information contained in $L_x^2$ and focus on $L_x^1$. As mentioned by [19], examples of likelihood functions with separable parameters like (1) are rare, but if (1) holds, it would be a useful property for Bayesian and non-Bayesian statisticians to analyze statistical data, especially in the presence of nuisance parameters. This fact will be illustrated in Sections 3 and 4.

We end this section by formally adapting the general NNPP to the special problem of hypothesis testing, in which inference about an unknown parameter consists of deciding whether a statement about the parameter (a statistical hypothesis) should be rejected or accepted by using the observable quantity $X$.

As before, let $\mathcal{E} = (X,\theta,\mathcal{P})$ be an experiment, with $\Theta = \Theta_1 \times \Theta_2$. Let $\bar{\mathcal{E}} = ((X,\theta_2),\theta_1,\bar{\mathcal{P}})$ be the "thought" experiment in which, in addition to $X$, $\theta_2$ is observed. Then, consider the following definition.

**Definition 1.** ***Non-Informative Nuisance Parameter (NNP)**: Let $B \subseteq \Theta_1$ and $\bar{\varphi} : \mathfrak{X} \times \Theta_2 \to \{0,1\}$ be a test for the hypotheses*

$$\begin{aligned} \bar{H}:&\quad \theta_1 \in B \\ \bar{A}:&\quad \theta_1 \notin B \end{aligned} \tag{0}$$

*Then, we say that $\theta_2$ is a Non-Informative Nuisance Parameter (NNP) for testing $\bar{H}$ versus $\bar{A}$ by using $\bar{\varphi}$ if, for every $x \in \mathfrak{X}$ such that (1) holds, $\bar{\varphi}(x,\theta_2)$ does not depend on $\theta_2$; that is, it depends only on $x$.*

In a nutshell, Definition 1 tells us something that appears intuitive: if the decision between $H$ and $A$ does not depend on $\theta_2$, then $\theta_2$ does not provide any information about $\theta_1$. In the following example, we illustrate this idea.

**Example 1.** *Consider that $\Theta_1 = \Theta_2 = \mathbb{R}$ and the experiment $\bar{\mathcal{E}} = ((X, \theta_2), \theta_1, \mathcal{P})$. Let $B \subset \mathbb{R}$ and $\bar{\varphi} : \mathfrak{X} \times \Theta_2 \to \{0, 1\}$ be the test for the hypotheses*

$$\begin{aligned} \bar{H}: &\quad \theta_1 \in B \\ \bar{A}: &\quad \theta_1 \notin B, \end{aligned} \tag{4}$$

*such that the null hypothesis is rejected when the conditional probability of B given x and $\theta_2$ is small; that is,*

$$\bar{\varphi}(x, \theta_2) = 1 \Leftrightarrow P(\theta_1 \in B \,|\, x, \theta_2) < \delta, \tag{5}$$

*where $\delta \in (0, 1)$. Suppose, in addition, that $\theta_1$ and $\theta_2$ are independent a priori. Let us verify that $\theta_2$ is an NNP for testing these hypotheses by means of $\bar{\varphi}$. Let $x_0 \in \mathfrak{X}$ be such that $L_{x_0}(\theta_1, \theta_2) = L^1_{x_0}(\theta_1) L^2_{x_0}(\theta_2)$ for specific functions $L^1_{x_0}$ and $L^2_{x_0}$. Then,*

$$\begin{aligned} P(\theta_1 \in B \,|\, x_0, \theta_2) &= \int_B \pi(\theta_1 \,|\, x_0, \theta_2) d\theta_1 = \\ &= \int_B \Big[\frac{P(X = x_0|\theta_1, \theta_2)\pi(\theta_2|\theta_1)\pi_1(\theta_1)}{\int_{\Theta_1} P(X = x_0|\theta_1', \theta_2)\pi(\theta_2|\theta_1')\pi_1(\theta_1') d\theta_1'}\Big] d\theta_1 = \\ &= \frac{\int_B L_{x_0}(\theta_1, \theta_2)\pi_2(\theta_2)\pi_1(\theta_1) d\theta_1}{\int_{\Theta_1} L_{x_0}(\theta_1, \theta_2)\pi_2(\theta_2)\pi_1(\theta_1) d\theta_1} = \\ &= \frac{\int_B L^1_{x_0}(\theta_1) L^2_{x_0}(\theta_2)\pi_2(\theta_2)\pi_1(\theta_1) d\theta_1}{\int_{\Theta_1} L^1_{x_0}(\theta_1) L^2_{x_0}(\theta_2)\pi_2(\theta_2)\pi_1(\theta_1) d\theta_1} \Rightarrow \\ \Rightarrow P(\theta_1 \in B \,|\, x_0, \theta_2) &= \frac{\int_B L^1_{x_0}(\theta_1)\pi_1(\theta_1) d\theta_1}{\int_{\Theta_1} L^1_{x_0}(\theta_1)\pi_1(\theta_1) d\theta_1}, \end{aligned} \tag{6}$$

*where $\pi_i$ is the prior of $\theta_i$, $i = 1, 2$. Thus, we have that*

$$\bar{\varphi}(x_0, \theta_2) = 1 \Leftrightarrow \frac{\int_B L^1_{x_0}(\theta_1)\pi_1(\theta_1) d\theta_1}{\int_{\Theta_1} L^1_{x_0}(\theta_1)\pi_1(\theta_1) d\theta_1} < \delta. \tag{7}$$

*Note from Equation (7) that $\bar{\varphi}(x_0, \theta_2)$ does not depend on $\theta_2$. Thus, $\theta_2$ is an NNP for testing $\bar{H}$ versus $\bar{A}$ by using $\bar{\varphi}$.*

After defining an NNP, we formally state the Non-Informative Nuisance Parameter Principle (NNPP) for hypothesis testing.

**Definition 2.** ***Non-Informative Nuisance Parameter Principle (NNPP):*** *Let the parameter space be variation independent; that is, $\Theta = \Theta_1 \times \Theta_2$. Consider the experiments $\mathcal{E} = (X, \theta, \mathcal{P})$ and $\bar{\mathcal{E}} = ((X, \theta_2), \theta_1, \bar{\mathcal{P}})$. Let $B \subseteq \Theta_1$ be the subset of $\Theta_1$ of interest. In addition, let $\varphi : \mathfrak{X} \to \{0, 1\}$ and $\bar{\varphi} : \mathfrak{X} \times \Theta_2 \to \{0, 1\}$ be tests for the hypotheses*

$$\begin{aligned} H: &\quad \theta \in B \times \Theta_2 \\ A: &\quad \theta \notin B \times \Theta_2, \end{aligned} \qquad \text{and} \qquad \begin{aligned} \bar{H}: &\quad \theta_1 \in B \\ \bar{A}: &\quad \theta_1 \notin B, \end{aligned} \tag{8}$$

*respectively.*

*If $\theta_2$ is an NNP for testing $\bar{H}$ versus $\bar{A}$ by using $\bar{\varphi}$ and $x_0 \in \mathfrak{X}$ such that condition (1) holds, then*

$$\varphi(x_0) = 1 \Leftrightarrow \bar{\varphi}(x_0, \theta_2) = 1\,. \tag{9}$$

The NNPP for statistical hypothesis testing says that if one intends to test a hypothesis regarding only the parameter $\theta_1$, it is irrelevant whether $\theta_2$ is known or unknown if it is non-informative for such a decision-making problem. More formally, if one wants to test a hypothesis concerning only $\theta_1$ and he observes a sample point $x_0 \in \mathfrak{X}$ that separates information on $\theta_1$ from information on $\theta_2$—that is, (1) holds—then the performances of the tests $\varphi$ under the original experiment $\mathcal{E}$ and $\bar{\varphi}$ under the "thought" experiment $\bar{\mathcal{E}}$ should yield the same decision on the hypothesis $\theta_1 \in B$ if $\theta_2$ is non-informative for that purpose.

We should mention that the NNPP can be adapted to any other inferential procedure. However, in this work, we focus on the principle for the problem of hypothesis testing. We conclude this section by proving that tests based on the posterior probabilities of the hypotheses satisfy the NNPP under prior independence.

**Example 2** (continuation of Example 1)**.** *Consider the conditions of Example 1. Consider $\mathcal{E} = (X, \theta, \mathcal{P})$ and let $\varphi : \mathfrak{X} \to \{0,1\}$ be the test for the hypotheses*

$$\begin{aligned} H:&\quad \theta \in B \times \Theta_2 \\ A:&\quad \theta \notin B \times \Theta_2 \end{aligned} \tag{10}$$

*that rejects the null hypothesis $H$ if its posterior probability is small; that is,*

$$\varphi(x) = 1 \Leftrightarrow P(\theta \in B \times \Theta_2 \,|\, x) < \delta. \tag{11}$$

*Let $x_0 \in \mathfrak{X}$ be such that $L_{x_0}(\theta_1, \theta_2) = L^1_{x_0}(\theta_1) L^2_{x_0}(\theta_2)$. We can write the posterior probability on the right-hand side of (11) as*

$$\begin{aligned} P(\theta \in B \times \Theta_2 \,|\, x_0) &= \int_{B\times\Theta_2} \pi(\theta \,|\, x_0) d\theta = \frac{\int_{B\times\Theta_2} L_{x_0}(\theta)\pi(\theta) d\theta}{\int_{\Theta} L_{x_0}(\theta)\pi(\theta) d\theta} = \\ &= \frac{\int_{B\times\Theta_2} L^1_{x_0}(\theta_1) L^2_{x_0}(\theta_2) \pi_1(\theta_1)\pi_2(\theta_2) d\theta}{\int_{\Theta_1\times\Theta_2} L^1_{x_0}(\theta_1) L^2_{x_0}(\theta_2) \pi_1(\theta_1)\pi_2(\theta_2) d\theta} = \frac{\int_B L^1_{x_0}(\theta_1)\pi_1(\theta_1) d\theta_1}{\int_{\Theta_1} L^1_{x_0}(\theta_1)\pi_1(\theta_1) d\theta_1}, \end{aligned} \tag{12}$$

*where the last equality follows from Fubini's Theorem. Hence,*

$$\varphi(x) = 1 \Leftrightarrow \frac{\int_B L^1_{x_0}(\theta_1)\pi_1(\theta_1) d\theta_1}{\int_{\Theta_1} L^1_{x_0}(\theta_1)\pi_1(\theta_1) d\theta_1} < \delta. \tag{13}$$

*From Equations (7) and (13), we have that $\varphi(x) = 1 \Leftrightarrow \bar{\varphi}(x, \theta_2) = 1$. Thus, the NNP Principle is met by tests based on posterior probabilities, as in Example 1. This result also holds when $\Theta_i \subseteq \mathbb{R}^{n_i}$, $n_i \in \mathbb{N}^*$, $i = 1, 2$.*

In the next section, we examine a second test procedure that is in line with the NNPP. We review the mixed test introduced by Pericchi and Pereira ([8]) and prove that such a test meets the NNPP for simple hypotheses concerning the parameter of interest. We also show how the adherence of the mixed test to the NNPP can then simplify its use.

## 3. The Mixed Test Procedure

The mixed test formally introduced in ([8]) is a test procedure that combines elements from both Bayesian and frequentist views. On the one hand, it considers an (intrinsically Bayesian) prior distribution for the parameter from which predictive distributions for the data under the competing hypotheses and Bayes factors are derived. On the other hand, the performance of the test depends on ordering the sample space by the Bayes factor and on the integration of these predictive distributions over specific subsets of the sample space in a frequentist-like manner. The mixed test is an optimal procedure in the sense that it minimizes linear combinations of averaged (weighted) probabilities of errors of decision. It also meets a few logical requirements for multiple-hypothesis testing and obeys the Likelihood Principle for discrete sample spaces despite the integration over the sample space it involves. In addition, the test overcomes several of the drawbacks fixed-level tests have. However, a difficulty with the mixed test procedure is the need to evaluate the Bayes factor for every sample point to order the sample space, which may involve intensive calculations. Properties of the mixed test and examples of application are examined in detail in [8,20–25].

Next, we review the general procedure for the performance of the mixed test and then show the test satisfies the NNPP when the hypothesis regarding the parameter of interest is a singleton.

First, we determine the predictive distributions for $X$ under the competing hypotheses $H$ and $A$, $f_H$ and $f_A$, respectively. For the null hypothesis $H : \theta \in \Theta_0$, $\Theta_0 \subset \Theta$, $f_H$ is determined as follows: for each $x \in \mathfrak{X}$,

$$f_H(x) = \int_{\Theta_0} L_x(\theta) dP_H(\theta) , \tag{14}$$

where $P_H$ denotes the conditional distribution of $\theta$ given $\theta \in \Theta_0$. That is, for each $x \in \mathfrak{X}$, $f_H(x)$ is the expected value of the likelihood function generated by $x$ against $P_H$. Similarly, for the alternative hypothesis $A$: $\theta \in \Theta_0^c$ we define

$$f_A(x) = \int_{\Theta_0^c} L_x(\theta) dP_A(\theta) , \tag{15}$$

where $P_A$ denotes the conditional distribution of $\theta$ given $\theta \in \Theta_0^c$. From (14) and (15), we obtain the Bayes factor of $x \in \mathfrak{X}$ for the hypothesis $H$ over $A$ as

$$BF(x) = \frac{f_H(x)}{f_A(x)} . \tag{16}$$

Finally, the mixed test $\varphi^*$: $\mathfrak{X} \to \{0, 1\}$ for the hypotheses $H$ versus $A$ consists in rejecting $H$ when $x \in \mathfrak{X}$ is observed if and only if the Bayes factor $BF(x)$ is small. That is, for each $x \in \mathfrak{X}$,

$$\varphi^*(x) = 1 \Leftrightarrow BF(x) \leq b/a , \tag{17}$$

where the positive constants $a$ and $b$ reflect the decision maker's evaluation of the impact of the errors of the two types or, equivalently, his prior preferences for the competing hypotheses. A detailed discussion on the specification of such constants is found in [8,20–25].

The mixed test can also be defined as a function of a new significance index. That is, (17) can be rewritten as a comparison between such a significance index and a specific cut-off value. These quantities are defined below.

For the mixed test defined in (17), the $p$-value of the observation $x_0 \in \mathfrak{X}$ is the significance index given by

$$p\text{-}value(x_0) = \sum_{x \in \mathfrak{D}(x_0)} f_H(x) , \tag{18}$$

where $\mathfrak{D}(x_0) = \{x \in \mathfrak{X} : BF(x) \leq BF(x_0)\}$. Also, we define the adaptive type I error probability of $\varphi^*$ as

$$\alpha^* = \sum_{x \in \mathfrak{D}} f_H(x), \tag{19}$$

where $\mathfrak{D} = \{x \in \mathfrak{X} : BF(x) \leq b/a\}$. Alternatively, $\alpha^*$ is also known as the adaptive significance level of $\varphi^*$.

Pereira et al. [21] proved that the mixed test $\varphi^*$ for the hypotheses

$$\begin{array}{ll} H: & \theta \in \Theta_0 \\ A: & \theta \in \Theta_0^c \end{array} \tag{20}$$

can be written as

$$\varphi^*(x) = 1 \Leftrightarrow BF(x) \leq b/a \Leftrightarrow p\text{-}value(x) \leq \alpha^* . \tag{21}$$

Note that $\varphi^*$ consists of comparing the *p-value* with the cut-off $\alpha^*$, which depends on the specific statistical model under consideration and on the sample size, as opposed to a standard test with a fixed significance level that does not depend on the sample size.

The former does not have a few of the disadvantages of the latter, such as inconsistency ([8,26]) lack of correspondence between practical significance and statistical significance ([8,27]) and absence of logical coherence under multiple-hypothesis testing. We continue with the main results of the manuscript.

*The Mixed Test Obeys the NNPP*

In this subsection, we prove that the mixed test meets the NNPP when the hypothesis about the parameter of interest is simple. Next, we examine further the case in which there is a statistic s-ancillary for the parameter of interest and show how the introduction of the concepts of a conditional *p-value* and a conditional adaptive significance level can make performance of the mixed test much easier.

**Theorem 3.** *Let $\theta = (\theta_1, \theta_2)$ and $\Theta = \Theta_1 \times \Theta_2$ (that is, $\Theta$ is variation independent). Let $\mathcal{E} = (X, \theta, \mathcal{P})$ and $\bar{\mathcal{E}} = ((X, \theta_2), \theta_1, \bar{\mathcal{P}})$ be two experiments as defined in Section 2. Let $\theta_0 \in \Theta_1$. In addition, let $\varphi^* : \mathfrak{X} \to \{0,1\}$ and $\bar{\varphi}^* : \mathfrak{X} \times \Theta_2 \to \{0,1\}$ be the mixed tests for the hypotheses*

$$\begin{array}{ll} H: & \theta \in \{\theta_0\} \times \Theta_2 \\ A: & \theta \notin \{\theta_0\} \times \Theta_2 \end{array} \quad \text{and} \quad \begin{array}{ll} \bar{H}: & \theta_1 = \theta_0 \\ \bar{A}: & \theta_1 \neq \theta_0, \end{array} \tag{22}$$

*respectively. Assume $\theta = (\theta_1, \theta_2)$ is absolutely continuous with prior density function $\pi$, with $\theta_1 \perp\!\!\!\perp \theta_2$. Then, $\theta_2$ is a Non-Informative Nuisance Parameter for testing $\bar{H}$ versus $\bar{A}$ by using $\bar{\varphi}^*$, and for every $x \in \mathfrak{X}$ such that (1) holds,*

$$\varphi^*(x) = 1 \Leftrightarrow \bar{\varphi}^*(x, \theta_2) = 1 \tag{23}$$

Theorem 3 tells us that when the likelihood function may be factored as (1), the mixed test obeys the NNPP. That is to say, if one aims to test a simple hypothesis about the parameter of interest $\theta_1$ in the presence of a non-informative nuisance parameter $\theta_2$ by means of the mixed test, then he can disregard $\theta_2$ in the analysis. Under a purely mathematical viewpoint, when $x \in \mathfrak{X}$ satisfying (1) is observed, the decision between rejecting and accepting the null hypothesis regarding $\theta_1$ depends on $L_x$ only through the factor $L_x^1$, which is not a function of $\theta_2$, as we can see from Equation (A16) in Appendix A. It should be emphasized that Theorem 3 holds for null hypotheses more general than only simple ones. For instance, the Theorem is still valid when the null hypothesis $H$ is of the form $H : \theta \in \Theta_0 \times \Theta_2$, where $\Theta_0 \subset \Theta_1$ is a hyperplane of $\Theta_1$. The proof of this result is quite similar to the proof of Theorem 3 in Appendix A and for this reason is omitted.

The adherence to the NNPP is indeed an advantage of the mixed test. It may bring a considerable reduction in the calculations involved along the procedure of the mixed test, especially under statistical models for which a statistic s-ancillary for the parameter of interest can be found. Such cases are examined after Corollary 1, which follows straightforwardly from Theorems 2 and 3.

**Corollary 1.** *Assume the same conditions of Theorem 3 and suppose that* $\exists\, T : \mathfrak{X} \to \mathcal{T}$ *such that* $T$ *is p-sufficient for* $\theta_2$ *and s-ancillary for* $\theta_1$*. Then, for all* $x \in \mathfrak{X}$, $\varphi^*(x) = 1 \Leftrightarrow \bar{\varphi}^*(x, \theta_2) = 1$.

Now, let us suppose that under experiment $\mathcal{E} = (X, \theta, \mathcal{P})$, there is a statistic $T : \mathfrak{X} \to \mathcal{T}$ such that $T$ is s-ancillary for $\theta_1$. Let $H : \theta \in \{\theta_0\} \times \Theta_2$ be the hypothesis of interest. From the predictive distribution $f_H$ for $X$, we can define for each value $t \in T(\mathfrak{X}) = \{T(x) : x \in \mathfrak{X}\}$ the conditional probability function for $X$ given $T(X) = t$, $f_{H,t}$ by

$$f_{H,t}(x) \;=\; \frac{f_H(x)}{\sum\limits_{y \in \mathfrak{X}:T(y)=t} f_H(y)} \tag{24}$$

if $T(x) = t$, and $f_{H,t}(x) = 0$, otherwise.

Finally, from the conditional distribution in (24), we define two conditional statistics: the conditional *p-value* and the conditional adaptive significance level. Such quantities will be of great importance for the performance of the mixed test, as we will see in the next section.

**Definition 3.** ***Conditional p-value:*** *Let* $\mathcal{E} = (X, \theta, \mathcal{P})$ *be an experiment for which the statistic* $T : \mathfrak{X} \to \mathcal{T}$ *is s-ancillary for* $\theta_1$*. Let* $H : \theta \in \{\theta_0\} \times \Theta_2$ *be the hypothesis of interest, and* $f_{H,t}$*,* $t \in T(\mathfrak{X})$*, as in (24). We define the p-value conditional on T,* $p_T$*-value* $: \mathfrak{X} \to [0,1]$ *for each* $x_0 \in \mathfrak{X}$ *by*

$$p_T\text{-}value(x_0) \;=\; \sum_{x \,\in\, \mathfrak{D}(x_0)} f_{H,T(x_0)}(x) \;=\; \frac{\sum\limits_{x \,\in\, \mathfrak{D}^*_T(x_0)} f_H(x)}{\sum\limits_{x \,\in\, \mathfrak{D}_T(x_0)} f_H(x)}\,, \tag{25}$$

*where* $\mathfrak{D}^*_T(x_0) = \{x \in \mathfrak{X} : BF(x) \le BF(x_0), T(x) = T(x_0)\}$ *and* $\mathfrak{D}_T(x_0) = \{x \in \mathfrak{X} : T(x) = T(x_0)\}$*. From Equation (A14), the* $P_T - value$ *may be rewritten as*

$$p_T\text{-}value(x_0) \;=\; \frac{\sum\limits_{x \,\in\, \mathfrak{D}^*_T(x_0)} \left[L^1_x(\theta_0) \int_{\Theta_2} L^2_x(\theta_2)\pi_2(\theta_2)d\theta_2\right]}{\sum\limits_{x \,\in\, \mathfrak{D}_T(x_0)} \left[L^1_x(\theta_0) \int_{\Theta_2} L^2_x(\theta_2)\pi_2(\theta_2)d\theta_2\right]}\,, \tag{26}$$

*where* $L^1_x(\theta_0) = P(X = x|\, T(X) = T(x), \theta_0)$ *and* $L^2_x(\theta_2) = P(T(X) = T(x)|\, \theta_2)$ *since* $T$ *is s-ancillary for* $\theta_1$*. It follows that*

$$\begin{aligned}
p_T\text{-}value(x_0) \;&=\; \frac{\sum\limits_{x \,\in\, \mathfrak{D}^*_T(x_0)} \left[P(X = x|\, T(X) = T(x), \theta_0) \int_{\Theta_2} P(T(X) = T(x)|\, \theta_2)\pi_2(\theta_2)d\theta_2\right]}{\sum\limits_{x \,\in\, \mathfrak{D}_T(x_0)} \left[P(X = x|\, T(X) = T(x), \theta_0) \int_{\Theta_2} P(T(X) = T(x)|\, \theta_2)\pi_2(\theta_2)d\theta_2\right]} \\
&=\; \frac{\sum\limits_{x \,\in\, \mathfrak{D}^*_T(x_0)} \left[P(X = x|\, T(X) = T(x_0), \theta_0) \int_{\Theta_2} P(T(X) = T(x_0)|\, \theta_2)\pi_2(\theta_2)d\theta_2\right]}{\sum\limits_{x \,\in\, \mathfrak{D}_T(x_0)} \left[P(X = x|\, T(X) = T(x_0), \theta_0) \int_{\Theta_2} P(T(X) = T(x_0)|\, \theta_2)\pi_2(\theta_2)d\theta_2\right]} \;= \\
&=\; \frac{\sum\limits_{x \,\in\, \mathfrak{D}^*_T(x_0)} P(X = x|\, T(X) = T(x_0), \theta_0)}{\sum\limits_{x \,\in\, \mathfrak{D}_T(x_0)} P(X = x|\, T(X) = T(x_0), \theta_0)}\,;
\end{aligned}$$

*that is,*

$$p_T\text{-}value(x_0) \;=\; \sum_{x \,\in\, \mathfrak{D}^*_T(x_0)} P(X = x|\, T(X) = T(x_0), \theta_0)\,. \tag{27}$$

**Definition 4.** ***Conditional adaptive significance level:*** *Let $\mathcal{E} = (X, \theta, \mathcal{P})$ be an experiment for which the statistic $T : \mathfrak{X} \to \mathcal{T}$ is s-ancillary for $\theta_1$. Let $H : \theta \in \{\theta_0\} \times \Theta_2$ be the hypothesis of interest and $f_{H,t}$, $t \in T(\mathfrak{X})$ be as in (24). We define the conditional adaptive significance level given $T$, $\alpha_T^* : \mathfrak{X} \to [0,1]$, for each $x_0 \in \mathfrak{X}$ by*

$$\alpha_T^*(x_0) \;=\; \sum_{x \,\in\, \mathfrak{D}} f_{H,T(x_0)}(x) \;=\; \frac{\sum\limits_{x \,\in\, \mathfrak{D} \cap \mathfrak{D}_T(x_0)} f_H(x)}{\sum\limits_{x \,\in\, \mathfrak{D}_T(x_0)} f_H(x)} \,. \tag{28}$$

The conditional adaptive significance level $\alpha_T^*$ may be rewritten as

$$\alpha_T^*(x_0) \;=\; \sum_{x \,\in\, \mathfrak{D} \cap \mathfrak{D}_T(x_0)} P(X = x |\, T(X) = T(x_0), \theta_0) \,. \tag{29}$$

Definitions 3 and 4 are conditional versions of Definitions in (18) and (19), respectively. While calculation of the unconditional quantities involves the evaluation of the Bayes factor for every $x \in \mathfrak{X}$, the determination of the conditional statistics at a specific sample point $x_0 \in \mathfrak{X}$ depends only on the values of the Bayes factor for the sample points $x$ such that $T(x) = T(x_0)$, which may be much easier to accomplish. Note also that the $p_T$-value and $\alpha_T^*$ can be seen, respectively, as an alternative (conditional) measure of evidence in favor of the null hypothesis $H$ and an alternative threshold value for testing the competing hypotheses. As a matter of fact, one can substitute the *p-value* and the adaptive significance level with their conditional versions in order to perform the mixed test. This is exactly what the next theorem states.

**Theorem 4.** *Assume the same conditions as in Corollary 1 and Theorem 3. Then, for all $x_0 \in \mathfrak{X}$,*

$$\varphi^*(x_0) \;=\; 1 \;\Leftrightarrow\; p_T\text{-}value(x_0) \leqslant \alpha_T^*(x_0) \,.$$

The results of Theorems 3 and 4 and Corollary 1 suggest a way the mixed test may be used without doing so many calculations: when an ancillary statistic for the parameter of interest, $T$, is available, one can perform the test by comparing the conditional statistics $p_T$-value and $\alpha_T^*$ instead of comparing the unconditional ones in Definitions (18) and (19). This possibility is illustrated in the next section.

## 4. Examples

We now revisit three well-known problems of hypothesis testing for count data and present new solutions to them by means of the mixed test. In each problem, we consider a suitable reparametrization of the standard model in order to ensure that

1. There exists a statistic $T$ that is ancillary to the new parameter of interest;
2. The hypothesis about the new parameter of interest under the reparametrization is a singleton (or a hyperplane);
3. The new parameter of interest is independent of the new nuisance parameter a priori;
4. The distribution of the data $X$ given any value of the statistic $T$ is simple enough to render the calculations of the conditional *p-value* and the conditional adaptive significance level easy.

### 4.1. Comparison of Poisson Means

Suppose we are interested in testing the equality between two Poisson means: say $\theta_1$ and $\theta_2$. Let $\theta = (\theta_1, \theta_2)$. For this purpose, let $X = (X_1, X_2)$ be a random vector to be observed such that given $\theta$, $X_1$ and $X_2$ are independent Poisson random variables with parameters $n\theta_1$ and $n\theta_2$, respectively, where $n \in \mathbb{N}^* = \{1,2,3,\ldots\}$ is a known integer. The hypotheses to be tested are

$$\begin{aligned} H &: \theta \in \Theta_0 \\ A &: \theta \in \Theta_0^c, \end{aligned} \tag{30}$$

where $\Theta_0 = \{(\theta_1, \theta_2) \in \mathbb{R}_+^2 : \theta_1 = \theta_2\}$. The likelihood function for $\theta \in \mathbb{R}_+^2$ generated by $x = (x_1, x_2) \in \mathbb{N}^2$ is

$$L_x(\theta) = \frac{(n\theta_1)^{x_1}}{x_1!}\frac{(n\theta_2)^{x_2}}{x_2!}e^{-\theta_1 n}e^{-\theta_2 n}. \tag{31}$$

Suppose also that $\theta_1$ and $\theta_2$ are independent a priori and that $\theta_i$ is distributed as a Gamma random variable with parameters $a_i > 0$ and $c > 0$, $i = 1,2$. That is, the prior density function of $\theta$ is

$$\pi(\theta) = \frac{c^{a_1}}{\Gamma(a_1)}\theta_1^{a_1-1}e^{-c\theta_1}\mathbb{I}_{(0,\infty)}(\theta_1)\frac{c^{a_2}}{\Gamma(a_2)}\theta_2^{a_2-1}e^{-c\theta_2}\mathbb{I}_{(0,\infty)}(\theta_2). \tag{32}$$

Although one can determine an exact expression for the Bayes factor in this case (as a matter of fact, in [25], the authors first presented a solution to the problem of testing the equality of Poisson means by using weighted likelihoods in the context of a production process monitoring procedure), the use of the mixed test under the above parametrization may be computationally disadvantageous, as the sample space is $\mathbb{N}^2$ and one should determine infinitely many Bayes factors to perform the test. To overcome this difficulty, we next consider the following reparametrization of the model: let $\lambda = (\lambda_1, \lambda_2)$ be the new parameter, where

$$\lambda_1 = \frac{\theta_1}{\theta_1 + \theta_2} \quad \text{and} \quad \lambda_2 = \theta_1 + \theta_2. \tag{33}$$

The new parameter space is then $\Lambda = (0,1) \times \mathbb{R}_+$. Now, the hypotheses (30) can be rewritten as

$$\begin{aligned} \tilde{H} &: \lambda \in \Lambda_0 \\ \tilde{A} &: \lambda \in \Lambda_0^c, \end{aligned} \tag{34}$$

with $\Lambda_0 = \{\frac{1}{2}\} \times \mathbb{R}_+$. Note that the likelihood function (31) can be rewritten by conditioning on the statistic $T(X) = X_1 + X_2$ as follows:

$$\begin{aligned} L_x(\theta) = P(X_1 = x_1, X_2 = x_2 \,|\, \theta) &= P(X_1 = x_1, X_2 = x_2 \,|\, X_1 + X_2 = x_1 + x_2, \theta)P(X_1 + X_2 = x_1 + x_2 \,|\, \theta) \\ &= \binom{x_1 + x_2}{x_1}\left(\frac{\theta_1}{\theta_1 + \theta_2}\right)^{x_1}\left(\frac{\theta_2}{\theta_1 + \theta_2}\right)^{x_2}\frac{e^{-n(\theta_1+\theta_2)}[n(\theta_1 + \theta_2)]^{x_1+x_2}}{(x_1 + x_2)!}. \end{aligned} \tag{35}$$

Hence, the induced likelihood function for $\lambda$ generated by $(x_1, x_2)$ may be factored as

$$\tilde{L}_x(\lambda) = \left[\binom{x_1 + x_2}{x_1}\lambda_1^{x_1}(1 - \lambda_1)^{x_2}\right]\left[\frac{(n\lambda_2)^{x_1+x_2}}{(x_1 + x_2)!}e^{-\lambda_2 n}\right] \tag{36}$$

Note that $T$ is an ancillary statistic for $\lambda_1$, as it is distributed as a Poisson random variable with mean $n\lambda_2$, and the conditional distribution of $X$, given $T(X) = t$, $t \in \mathbb{N}$, depends on $\lambda$ only through $\lambda_1$. The prior distribution for $\lambda$ is given by

$$\tilde{\pi}(\lambda) = \frac{\Gamma(a_1 + a_2)}{\Gamma(a_1)\Gamma(a_2)}\lambda_1^{a_1-1}(1 - \lambda_1)^{a_2-1}\mathbb{I}_{(0,1)}(\lambda_1)\frac{c^{a_1+a_2}}{\Gamma(a_1 + a_2)}\lambda_2^{a_1+a_2-1}e^{-c\lambda_2}\mathbb{I}_{(0,\infty)}(\lambda_2). \tag{37}$$

Now, as (34), (36) and (37) hold, it follows from Theorem 3 that $\lambda_2$ is an NNP and that the performance of the mixed test for the hypothesis $\tilde{H} : \lambda \in \{\frac{1}{2}\} \times \mathbb{R}_+$ against $\tilde{A}$ based on $\tilde{L}_x$ and the prior $\tilde{\pi}$ is equivalent to the performance of the mixed test for the simple hypothesis $\lambda_1 = \frac{1}{2}$ against $\lambda_1 \neq \frac{1}{2}$ based on the binomial-like factor of $\tilde{L}_x$ that depends only on $\theta_1$ and the marginal Beta prior density for $\lambda_1$ ignoring the NNP $\lambda_2$. In addition, Theorem 4 implies that the test for $\tilde{H}$ versus $\tilde{A}$ reduces to the comparison of the statistics $p_T$-*value* and $\alpha_T^*$ at the observed sample point, say $x_0 = (x_{01}, x_{02})$. Note that in this case, one does not need to evaluate the Bayes factor for every point of $\mathbb{N}^2$ but only for those $x_{01} + x_{02} + 1$ of them for which the sum of the components is $x_{01} + x_{02}$. That is, one needs to evaluate the Bayes factor only for the elements of $\{(u,v) \in \mathbb{N}^2 : T(u,v) = T(x_0) = x_{01} + x_{02}\}$ when $x_0 = (x_{01}, x_{02})$ is observed.

From Equations (A14) and (A15), one gets the following predictive functions under $\tilde{H}$ and under $\tilde{A}$ for $X$:

$$f_{\tilde{H}}(\boldsymbol{x}) = (1/2)^{x_1+x_2}\binom{x_1+x_2}{x_1} \times K \tag{38}$$

and

$$f_{\tilde{A}}(\boldsymbol{x}) = \binom{x_1+x_2}{x_1}\left[\frac{\Gamma(x_1+a_1)\Gamma(x_2+a_2)}{\Gamma(x_1+x_2+a_1+a_2)}\right]\left[\frac{\Gamma(a_1+a_2)}{\Gamma(a_1)\Gamma(a_2)}\right] \times K\,, \tag{39}$$

where $K = \int_0^{\infty}\left[\frac{(n\lambda_2)^{x_1+x_2}}{(x_1+x_2)!}e^{-\lambda_2 n}\right]\frac{c^{a_1+a_2}}{\Gamma(a_1+a_2)}\lambda_2^{a_1+a_2-1}e^{-c\lambda_2}d\lambda_2$. Consequently, the Bayes factor $BF(x)$ is

$$BF(\boldsymbol{x}) = (1/2)^{x_1+x_2}\frac{\Gamma(a_1)\Gamma(a_2)}{\Gamma(a_1+a_2)}\frac{\Gamma(x_1+x_2+a_1+a_2)}{\Gamma(x_1+a_1)\Gamma(x_2+a_2)}. \tag{40}$$

Finally, it follows from (28) and (30) that for $x_0 = (x_{01}, x_{02}) \in \mathbb{N}^2$,

$$\begin{aligned} p_T\text{-value}(x_0) &= \sum_{(x_1,x_2)\,\in\,\mathfrak{D}_T^*(x_0)}\binom{x_1+x_2}{x_1}(1/2)^{x_1+x_2} \\ &= \sum_{x_1=0}^{T(x_0)}\binom{T(x_0)}{x_1}(1/2)^{T(x_0)}\mathbb{I}_{\mathfrak{D}(x_0)}(x_1, T(x_0)-x_1) \end{aligned} \tag{41}$$

and

$$\begin{aligned} \alpha_T^*(x_0) &= \sum_{(x_1,x_2)\,\in\,\mathfrak{D}\cap\mathfrak{D}_T(x_0)}\binom{x_1+x_2}{x_1}(1/2)^{x_1+x_2} \\ &= \sum_{x_1=0}^{T(x_0)}\binom{T(x_0)}{x_1}(1/2)^{T(x_0)}\mathbb{I}_{\mathfrak{D}}(x_1, T(x_0)-x_1)\,. \end{aligned} \tag{42}$$

Note that in this case, the conditional $p_T$*-value* resembles the frequentist *p-value* for the simple hypothesis $\theta = \frac{1}{2}$ under simple random sampling from the Bernoulli model with parameter $\theta$ (however, for the calculation of the $p_T$*-value*, the sample space is ordered by the Bayes factor instead of the likelihood ratio).

**Example 3 (Comparison of Poisson means).** *In [25], the authors consider that a methodology to detect a shift in a production process is to compare the quality index of the current rating period P, $\theta_2$, with the quality index of the previous rating period, $\theta_1$. Suppose that we want to test if a process is under control; that is, if $\theta_1 = \theta_2$. For this purpose, two audit samples of size $n = 10$ are collected at rating periods $P-1$ and P, respectively. Let $X_1$ represent the number of defects found in the first sample and $X_2$ represent the number of defects found in the second sample. Also suppose that $X_1$ and $X_2$ are Poisson random variables with parameters $n\theta_1$ and $n\theta_2$, respectively. Let $X = (X_1, X_2)$. For simplicity, we consider the hyperparameters in (32) as $a_1 = a_2 = c = 1$. Hence, the predictive functions under the competing hypothesis are given by:*

$$f_H(\boldsymbol{x}) = (1/2)^{x_1+x_2}\left[(x_1+x_2+1)\binom{x_1+x_2}{x_1}\right]\left[\left(\frac{n}{n+1}\right)^{x_1+x_2}\left(\frac{1}{n+1}\right)^2\right], \tag{43}$$

*and*

$$f_A(\boldsymbol{x}) = \left(\frac{n}{n+1}\right)^{x_1+x_2}\left(\frac{1}{n+1}\right)^2. \tag{44}$$

*Consequently, the Bayes factor at $x = (x_1, x_2) \in \mathbb{N}^2$ can be expressed by*

$$BF(\boldsymbol{x}) = (1/2)^{x_1+x_2}(x_1+x_2+1)\binom{x_1+x_2}{x_1}. \tag{45}$$

*Now, suppose that two defects are found at rating period $P-1$ and nine defects are found at period P. That is, suppose that $X = (2,9)$ is observed. In this case, one gets $BF(2,9) = 0.322$.*

*Considering* $\frac{b}{a} = 1$, *the conditional adaptive significance level and the conditional* $p_T$*-value at* $(2,9)$ *are, respectively,*

$$\alpha_T^*((2,9)) = \sum_{x_1 \in \{0,1,2,3,8,9,10,11\}} \binom{2+9}{x_1} (1/2)^{2+9} = 0.227 \quad and$$

$$P_T\text{-}value((2,9)) = \sum_{x_1 \in \{0,1,2,9,10,11\}} \binom{11}{x_1} (1/2)^{11} = 0.065\,.$$

*Since* $P_T$*-value*$((2,9)) < \alpha_T^*((2,9))$, *the decision is to reject the null hypothesis (34), where* $\lambda = (\frac{\theta_1}{\theta_1+\theta_2}, \theta_1 + \theta_2)$.

*Note that although the sample size is small, the null hypothesis can be rejected with a conditional* $P_T - value$ *of 0.065. Such a value is not compared with standard (fixed) cut-off values such as 0.01 or 0.05 but rather with the conditional adaptive significance level of 0.227 for* $X = (2,9)$. *Note also that performance of the mixed test by means of the conditional statistics* $p_T$*-value and* $\alpha_T^*$ *when* $X = (2,9)$ *is observed requires the calculation of only finitely many Bayes factors (twelve, precisely) even though the sample space is infinite.*

### 4.2. Test of Symmetry

Suppose we want to test the hypothesis of symmetry in an $r \times r$ two-way contingency table. Several methods have been proposed for testing diagonal symmetry: see, for example, [28–33] and references therein. Here we propose a solution to this problem by using the mixed test and its properties. We present the simplest case $r = 2$. The reader will find the general case $r > 2$ in Appendix A for the sake of readability.

Suppose each element (individual) of a sample of size $n$ is classified into four mutually exclusive combinations of the two-valued variables $X_1$ and $X_2$. Let Table 1 represent the observed frequencies of the cross-classifications, where $X_{ij}$ is the number of individuals classified into the $i-th$ category of $X_1$ and the $j-th$ category of $X_2$, $i,j = 1,2$. Let $\theta = (\theta_{11}, \theta_{12}, \theta_{21})$, with $\theta_{ij} \geq 0$ and $\theta_{11} + \theta_{12} + \theta_{21} \leq 1$, where $\theta_{ij}$ denotes the probability of classification into the $i-th$ category of $X_1$ and the $j-th$ category of $X_2$, $i,j = 1,2$.

**Table 1.** Observed frequencies of $(X_1, X_2)$ in the $2 \times 2$ case.

| | | **$X_2$** | |
|---|---|---|---|
| | $x_{11}$ | $x_{12}$ | $n_{1.}$ |
| $X_1$ | $x_{21}$ | $x_{22}$ | $n_{2.}$ |
| | $n_{.1}$ | $n_{.2}$ | $n$ |

The hypotheses for testing diagonal symmetry are

$$\begin{aligned} H &: \theta_{12} = \theta_{21} \\ A &: \theta_{12} \neq \theta_{21} \end{aligned} \tag{46}$$

We assume that the vector $X = (X_{11}, X_{12}, X_{21})$ is, given $\theta$, a multinomial random vector with parameters $n$ and $\theta$. The likelihood function generated by $x = (x_{11}, x_{12}, x_{21})$ is then given by

$$L_x(\theta) = \frac{n!}{x_{11}!x_{12}!x_{21}!x_{22}!} \theta_{11}^{x_{11}} \theta_{12}^{x_{12}} \theta_{21}^{x_{21}} \theta_{22}^{x_{22}}, \tag{47}$$

where $x_{22} = n - x_{11} - x_{12} - x_{21}$ and $\theta_{22} = 1 - \theta_{11} - \theta_{12} - \theta_{21}$. Assume also a prior Dirichlet distribution with parameter vector $\alpha = (\alpha_{11}, \alpha_{12}, \alpha_{21}; \alpha_{22})$, $\alpha_{ij} > 0$ for $\theta$. That is,

$$\pi(\theta) = \frac{\Gamma(\alpha_{11} + \alpha_{12} + \alpha_{21} + \alpha_{22})}{\Gamma(\alpha_{11})\Gamma(\alpha_{12})\Gamma(\alpha_{21})\Gamma(\alpha_{22})} \theta_{11}^{\alpha_{11}-1} \theta_{12}^{\alpha_{12}-1} \theta_{21}^{\alpha_{21}-1} \theta_{22}^{\alpha_{22}-1} \mathbb{I}_{\Theta}(\theta), \tag{48}$$

where $\Theta = \{(u_1, u_2, u_3) \in \mathbb{R}^3_+ : u_1 + u_2 + u_3 \leq 1\}$.

We should note that the determination of the predictive functions is much easier under the following reparametrization of the model: let us define

$$\lambda_{11} = \theta_{11} \quad \lambda_{21} = \theta_{12} + \theta_{21} \quad \text{and} \quad \lambda_{12} = \frac{\theta_{12}}{\theta_{12} + \theta_{21}}.$$

Let $\lambda = (\lambda_{12}, (\lambda_{11}, \lambda_{21}))$. Thus, the new parameter space is $\Lambda = (0,1) \times S_2$ , where $S_2 = \{(u, v) \in \mathbb{R}^2_+ : u + v \leq 1\}$.

Then, we can reformulate the hypotheses (46) as

$$\begin{array}{ll} \tilde{H}: & \boldsymbol{\lambda} \in \Lambda_0 \\ \tilde{A}: & \boldsymbol{\lambda} \in \Lambda_0^c, \end{array} \tag{49}$$

where $\Lambda_0 = \{\frac{1}{2}\} \times S_2$. Note that the likelihood function for $\theta$ generated by $x = (x_{11}, x_{12}, x_{21}) \in \{(a, b, c) \in \mathbb{N}^3 : a + b + c \leq n\}$ can be rewritten by conditioning on the statistic $T(X) = (X_{11}, X_{12} + X_{21})$ as

$$\begin{aligned} L_x(\theta) &= P(X = (x_{11}, x_{12}, x_{21}) \,|\, T(X) = (x_{11}, x_{12} + x_{21}) \,,\, \theta) P(T(X) = (x_{11}, x_{12} + x_{21}) \,|\, \theta) \\ &= \binom{x_{12} + x_{21}}{x_{12}} \left(\frac{\theta_{12}}{\theta_{12} + \theta_{21}}\right)^{x_{12}} \left(\frac{\theta_{21}}{\theta_{12} + \theta_{21}}\right)^{x_{21}} \frac{n!}{x_{11}!(x_{12} + x_{21})!x_{22}!} \theta_{11}^{x_{11}} (\theta_{12} + \theta_{21})^{x_{12} + x_{21}} \theta_{22}^{x_{22}}. \end{aligned} \tag{50}$$

Hence, the induced likelihood function for $\lambda$ generated by $x = (x_{11}, x_{12}, x_{21})$ may be factored as

$$\tilde{L}_x(\lambda) = \left[\binom{x_{12} + x_{21}}{x_{12}} \lambda_{12}^{x_{12}} (1 - \lambda_{12})^{x_{21}}\right] \left[\frac{n!}{x_{11}!(x_{12} + x_{21})!x_{22}!} \lambda_{11}^{x_{11}} \lambda_{21}^{x_{12} + x_{21}} (1 - \lambda_{11} - \lambda_{21})^{x_{22}}\right] \tag{51}$$

Note that $T$ is an ancillary statistic for $\lambda_{12}$ as it is a multinomial random vector with parameters $n$ and $(\lambda_{11}, \lambda_{21})$, and the conditional distribution of $X$ given $T(X) = t$, $t \in \{(u, v) \in \mathbb{N}^2 : u + v \leq n\}$ depends on $\lambda$ only through $\lambda_{12}$. The prior distribution for $\lambda$ is given by

$$\tilde{\pi}(\lambda) = \frac{\Gamma(\alpha_{12} + \alpha_{21})}{\Gamma(\alpha_{12})\Gamma(\alpha_{21})} \lambda_{12}^{\alpha_{12} - 1} (1 - \lambda_{12})^{\alpha_{21} - 1} \mathbb{I}_{(0,1)}(\lambda_{12})\, \tilde{\pi}_{(\lambda_{11}, \lambda_{21})}(\lambda_{11}, \lambda_{21}), \tag{52}$$

where $\tilde{\pi}_{(\lambda_{11}, \lambda_{21})}$ is the prior Dirichlet distribution for $(\lambda_{11}, \lambda_{21})$ with parameter vector $(\alpha_{11}, \alpha_{12} + \alpha_{21}, \alpha_{22})$.

As in the example of the previous subsection, the results from Section 3 imply that $(\lambda_{11}, \lambda_{21})$ is an NNP for testing the hypotheses $\tilde{H}$ versus $\tilde{A}$ in (50) by using the mixed test. In addition, we only need to compare the conditional $p_T$-$value$ with the conditional adaptive significance level to decide between the hypotheses.

From Equations (A14) and (A15), one gets the following predictive functions under $\tilde{H}$ and under $\tilde{A}$ for $X$:

$$f_{\tilde{H}}(x_{11}, x_{12}, x_{21}) = (1/2)^{x_{12} + x_{21}} \binom{x_{12} + x_{21}}{x_{12}} \times K \tag{53}$$

and

$$f_{\tilde{A}}(x) = \binom{x_{12} + x_{21}}{x_{12}} \left[\frac{\Gamma(x_{12} + \alpha_{12})\Gamma(x_{21} + \alpha_{21})}{\Gamma(x_{12} + x_{21} + \alpha_{12} + \alpha_{21})}\right] \left[\frac{\Gamma(\alpha_{12} + \alpha_{21})}{\Gamma(\alpha_{12})\Gamma(\alpha_{21})}\right] \times K, \tag{54}$$

where

$$K = \int_{S_2} \left[\frac{n!}{x_{11}!(x_{12} + x_{21})!x_{22}!} \lambda_{11}^{x_{11}} \lambda_{21}^{x_{12} + x_{21}} (1 - \lambda_{11} - \lambda_{21})^{x_{22}}\right] \tilde{\pi}_{(\lambda_{11}, \lambda_{21})}(\lambda_{11}, \lambda_{21}) d\lambda_{11} d\lambda_{21}.$$

Consequently, the Bayes factor $BF(x)$ is

$$BF(x) = (1/2)^{x_{12}+x_{21}} \frac{\Gamma(\alpha_{12})\Gamma(\alpha_{21})}{\Gamma(\alpha_{12}+\alpha_{21})} \frac{\Gamma(x_{12}+x_{21}+\alpha_{12}+\alpha_{21})}{\Gamma(x_{12}+\alpha_{12})\Gamma(x_{21}+\alpha_{21})}. \quad (55)$$

Finally, it follows from (28) and (30) that for $x = (x_{11}, x_{12}, x_{21})$,

$$\begin{aligned} p_T\text{-}value(x) &= \sum_{(y_{11},y_{12},y_{21}) \in \mathfrak{D}^*_T(x)} \binom{y_{12}+y_{21}}{y_{12}} (1/2)^{y_{12}+y_{21}} \\ &= \sum_{y_{12}=0}^{x_{12}+x_{21}} \binom{x_{12}+x_{21}}{y_{12}} (1/2)^{x_{12}+x_{21}} \mathbb{I}_{\mathfrak{D}(x)}(x_{11}, y_{12}, x_{12}+x_{21}-y_{12}) \end{aligned} \quad (56)$$

and

$$\begin{aligned} \alpha^*_T(x) &= \sum_{(y_{11},y_{12},y_{21}) \in \mathfrak{D}\cap\mathfrak{D}_T(x)} \binom{y_{12}+y_{21}}{y_{12}} (1/2)^{y_{12}+y_{21}} \\ &= \sum_{y_{12}=0}^{x_{12}+x_{21}} \binom{x_{12}+x_{21}}{y_{12}} (1/2)^{x_{12}+x_{21}} \mathbb{I}_{\mathfrak{D}}(x_{11}, y_{12}, x_{12}+x_{21}-y_{12}) \end{aligned} \quad (57)$$

In this example (as in the previous subsection), the conditional $p_T$*-value* looks like the frequentist $p$-value for the simple hypothesis $\theta = \frac{1}{2}$ regarding an unknown proportion. We should emphasize that for calculation of the $p_T$*-value*, the sample space is ordered by the Bayes factor in place of the likelihood ratio. Note also that the evaluation of this conditional statistic involves ordering at most $n+1$ points of the sample space (exactly those for which the statistic $T$ takes the value $T(x_0)$ when $x_0$ is the effectively observed sample point). On the other hand, if one performs the mixed test without using these conditional quantities, he shall order all $\binom{n+3}{3} = \frac{(n+3)(n+2)(n+1)}{6}$ elements of the sample space.

**Example 4 (Analysis of opinion swing).** *Suppose it is of interest to evaluate whether the proportion of individuals that did not support the US President before the State of the Union Address remained unchanged after his address. For this purpose, $n = 100$ individuals are surveyed with regard to their support for the President before and after his annual message. The survey results are displayed in the following $2 \times 2$ contingency Table 2:*

**Table 2.** Survey results.

| | | After | | |
|---|---|---|---|---|
| | | No | Yes | |
| Before | No | 20 | 17 | 37 |
| | Yes | 10 | 53 | 63 |
| | | 30 | 70 | 100 |

*Let $X_1$ ($X_2$) be the support—"No" or "Yes"—for the President before (after) the State of the Union Address. Let $\theta_{ij}$ be the probability that an individual is classified into the i-th category of $X_1$ and j-th category of $X_2$ (for instance, $\theta_{11}$ is the probability that an individual does not support the President both before and after his address). The hypothesis that the support for the President remains unchanged is $\theta_{21} + \theta_{22} = \theta_{12} + \theta_{22}$. This is equivalent to the hypothesis that the proportion of swings from "Yes" to "No" is equal to the proportion of swings from "No" to "Yes"; that is, this is equivalent to the symmetry hypothesis $\theta_{12} = \theta_{21}$. Thus, we can test such a hypothesis by means of the mixed test considering the mathematical setup of this subsection. Suppose $\alpha = (1,1,1,1)$. Then, the Bayes factor is given by*

$$BF(x_{11}, x_{12}, x_{21}) = (1/2)^{x_{12}+x_{21}} (x_{12}+x_{21}+1) \binom{x_{12}+x_{21}}{x_{12}}. \quad (58)$$

*For the observed data $x = (20, 17, 10)$, we obtain the Bayes factor $BF((20, 17, 10)) = 1.76$. Considering $a = b$ (that is $b/a = 1$), we do not reject the null hypothesis since $BF((20, 17, 10)) > 1$. In this case, the conditional adaptive significance level and the conditional $P_T$-value at the point $((20, 17, 10))$ are*

$$\alpha^*_T((20,17,10)) = \sum_{y_{12}\in\{0,\ldots,9\}\cup\{18,\ldots,27\}} \binom{17+10}{y_{12}} (1/2)^{17+10} = 0.122 \quad \textit{and}$$

$$P_T\text{-}value((20,17,10)) = \sum_{y_{12}\in\{0,\ldots,10\}\cup\{17,\ldots,27\}} \binom{27}{y_{12}} (1/2)^{27} = 0.248\,.$$

*Note that $p_T$-value$((20, 17, 10)) > \alpha^*_T((20, 17, 10))$, as it was expected. Note also that we ordered only 28 elements of the sample space by the Bayes factor to determine the above conditional quantities. To calculate the unconditional ones, we should have ordered all 176,851 points in the sample space.*

### 4.3. Test of Independence

Consider the same statistical model as in the previous subsection. However, now we want to evaluate whether there exists (or not) association between the variables $X_1$ and $X_2$. For this purpose, we may test the independence hypothesis between these variables. Consider the joint distribution for $(X_1, X_2)$ in Table 3 below:

**Table 3.** Joint distribution of $X_1$ and $X_2$ given $\theta$.

| | $X_2$ | | |
|---|---|---|---|
| $X_1$ | $\theta_{11}$<br>$\theta_{21}$ | $\theta_{12}$<br>$\theta_{22}$ | $\theta_{1.}$<br>$\theta_{2.}$ |
| | $\theta_{.1}$ | $\theta_{.2}$ | 1 |

The hypotheses to be tested are

$$\begin{aligned} H: \theta_{11} &= (\theta_{11}+\theta_{12})(\theta_{11}+\theta_{21}) \\ A: \theta_{11} &\neq (\theta_{11}+\theta_{12})(\theta_{11}+\theta_{21}) \end{aligned} \tag{59}$$

It is easy to check that hypotheses $H$ and $A$ can be rewritten as

$$\begin{aligned} H: \frac{\theta_{11}}{\theta_{11}+\theta_{12}} &= \frac{\theta_{21}}{1-(\theta_{11}+\theta_{12})} \\ A: \frac{\theta_{11}}{\theta_{11}+\theta_{12}} &\neq \frac{\theta_{21}}{1-(\theta_{11}+\theta_{12})} \end{aligned} \tag{60}$$

Let us define

$$\lambda_{11} = \frac{\theta_{11}}{\theta_{11}+\theta_{12}} \quad \lambda_{21} = \frac{\theta_{21}}{1-(\theta_{11}+\theta_{12})} \quad \text{and } \lambda_{12} = \theta_{11}+\theta_{12}$$

and consider the new parameter $\lambda = ((\lambda_{11}, \lambda_{21}), \lambda_{12})$, which takes value in $\Lambda = (0,1)^2 \times (0,1)$. Let $T(X) = T(X_{11}, X_{12}, X_{21}) = X_{11} + X_{12}$. Proceeding as in the previous subsections, we obtain the following induced likelihood function for $\lambda$ generated by $x = (X_{11}, x_{12}, x_{21})$

$$\tilde{L}_x(\lambda) = \left[\binom{x_{11}+x_{12}}{x_{11}} \lambda_{11}^{x_{11}} (1-\lambda_{11})^{x_{12}} \binom{x_{21}+x_{22}}{x_{21}} \lambda_{21}^{x_{21}} (1-\lambda_{21})^{x_{22}}\right] \left[\binom{n}{x_{11}+x_{12}} \lambda_{12}^{x_{11}+x_{12}} (1-\lambda_{12})^{x_{21}+x_{22}}\right] \tag{61}$$

Note that $T$ is an ancillary statistic for $(\lambda_{11}, \lambda_{21})$, as it is a binomial random variable with parameters $n$ and $\lambda_{12}$. In addition, for each possible value $t$ of the statistic $T$, the conditional distribution of $X$ given $T(X) = t$ depends on $\lambda$ only through $(\lambda_{11}, \lambda_{21})$.

The prior distribution for $\lambda$ is such that $\lambda_{11}$, $\lambda_{21}$ and $\lambda_{12}$ are independent Beta random variables with respective parameters $\alpha_{11}$ and $\alpha_{12}$, $\alpha_{21}$ and $\alpha_{22}$, and $\alpha_{11} + \alpha_{12}$ and $\alpha_{21} + \alpha_{22}$.

Finally, note that under the new parametrization, the independence hypothesis is

$$\begin{aligned} \tilde{H}: &\quad \lambda \in \Lambda_0 \\ \tilde{A}: &\quad \lambda \notin \Lambda_0 , \end{aligned} \tag{62}$$

where $\Lambda_0 = \{(u,v) \in (0,1)^2 : u = v\} \times (0,1)$.

From the results from Section 3, it follows that $\lambda_{12}$ is an NNP for testing the hypotheses $\tilde{H}$ versus $\tilde{A}$ above by using the mixed test. In addition, we only need to compare the conditional $P_T - value$ with the conditional adaptive significance level to decide between these hypotheses. In a sense, the test for the hypothesis of independence between $X_1$ and $X_2$ by using the conditional statistics resembles the test for the hypothesis of homogeneity were the marginal counts $X_{11} + X_{12}$ and $n - X_{11} - X_{12}$ fixed beforehand.

Considering as in the previous section $\alpha = (1,1,1,1)$, we obtain the following expression for the Bayes factor:

$$BF(x_{11}, x_{12}, x_{21}) = \frac{36\,(x_{11} + x_{21} + 1)!\,(n + 1 - x_{11} - x_{21})!}{x_{11}!\,x_{12}!\,x_{21}!\,x_{22}!\,(n+3)\binom{n+2}{x_{11}+x_{21}+1}} .$$

The conditional predictive probability function for $X$ given $T(X) = X_{11} + X_{12} = t$, $t = 0, \ldots, n$ is given by

$$f_{H,t}(x_{11}, x_{12}, x_{21}) = \frac{6\binom{t}{x_{11}}\binom{n-t}{x_{21}}}{(n+3)\binom{n+2}{x_{11}+x_{21}+1}}\,\mathbb{I}_{T^{-1}(t)}(x_{11}, x_{12}, x_{21}) , \tag{63}$$

where $T^{-1}(t) = \{(y_{11}, y_{12}, y_{21}) \in \mathfrak{X} : T(y_{11}, y_{12}, y_{21}) = y_{11} + y_{12} = t\}$.

From the above distribution, one may obtain the conditional $P_T - value$ and the conditional adaptive significance level $\alpha_T^*$ at each point in the sample space.

**Example 5 (Market's directional change).** *In [34] it is argued that the directional change of the stock market in January signals the directional change of the market for the remainder of the year. Suppose the following Table 4 summarizes the directional changes of the prices of a few stocks in both periods.*

**Table 4.** Survey results.

| | | After January | | |
|---|---|---|---|---|
| | | Up | Down | |
| January change | up | 5 | 0 | 5 |
| | down | 2 | 8 | 10 |
| | | 7 | 8 | 15 |

*In this case, the Bayes factor is given by*

$$BF(x_{11}, x_{12}, x_{21}) = \frac{36\,(x_{11} + x_{21} + 1)!\,(16 - x_{11} - x_{21})!}{x_{11}!\,x_{12}!\,x_{21}!\,x_{22}!\,18\binom{17}{x_{11}+x_{21}+1}} . \tag{64}$$

*For the observed data $x = (5,0,2)$, we obtain the Bayes factor $BF((5,0,2)) = 0.244$. Considering $a = b$ (that is $b/a = 1$), we reject the null hypothesis by using the mixed test since $BF((5,0,2)) < 1$. That is, the data from only a few stocks reveal that the directional change for* *the remainder of the year depends on the directional change in January. Note that although the sample size is small ($n = 15$) and a cell count is equal to zero, the mixed test can be fully performed, as opposed to standard tests for the hypothesis of independence that rely on asymptotic results. In this case, the conditional adaptive significance level and the conditional $p_T$-value at the point $((5,0,2))$ are*

$$\alpha_T^*((5,0,2)) \;=\; 0.0109 \quad and \quad P_T\text{-}value((5,0,2)) \;=\; 0.0022\,.$$

## 5. Discussion

Statistical hypothesis testing is an important quantitative method that may help the daily activity of scientists from different areas of knowledge. However, with recent computational advances, the misuse of standard tests have come to light. Thus, problems with tests of significance and fixed-level tests have brought a growing need for alternative approaches to hypothesis testing that do not have such drawbacks. Among these alternatives, we revisit in this manuscript the mixed test by Pericchi and Pereira, which combines aspects from two opposing viewpoints: the frequentist and the Bayesian. The mixed test satisfies various reasonable properties one desires when performing a test of hypotheses. Here we prove that the mixed test also meets the Non-Informative Nuisance Parameter Principle (NNPP) for simple hypotheses regarding the parameter of interest. The NNPP concerns the question of how to make inferences about a parameter in the presence of Non-Informative Nuisance Parameters: it states that it is irrelevant whether a Non-Informative Nuisance Parameter is known or unknown in order to draw conclusions about a quantity of interest from data. This principle, though important, has not been explored in some depth, and for this reason, we studied it further in hypothesis testing problems. Nuisance parameters typically affect inferences about a parameter of interest: when the variance is unknown, estimation of the mean of a normal distribution and estimation of the parameters of a linear regression model are examples of this.

Adherence of the mixed test to the NNPP allowed for much easier performance of the test, as the calculations involved were significantly reduced. Indeed, decision making between the competing statistical hypotheses was simplified in the three examples we examined: in each situation, conditioning on a suitable statistic and considering conditional versions of the $p$-value and the adaptive significance level were revealed to be an advantageous course of action to use the mixed test. The extent to which the adherence of the mixed test to the NNPP is valid and the use of the mixed test can then be made easier remains unanswered in this work. This issue is the goal of future investigation.

**Author Contributions:** All authors have contributed to the conceptualization, formal analysis and writing of the manuscript. All authors have read and agreed to the published version of the manuscript.

**Funding:** This work was partially supported by *Conselho Nacional de Desenvolvimento Científico e Tecnológico* [grant 141161/2018-3].

**Data Availability Statement:** No new data were created or analyzed in this study. Data sharing is not applicable to this article.

**Conflicts of Interest:** The authors declare no conflicts of interest.

## Appendix A

**Proof of Theorem 2.** Suppose there exists a statistic $T : \mathcal{X} \to \mathcal{T}$ such that it is p-sufficient for $\theta_1$ and s-ancillary for $\theta_2$. Then,

$$\begin{aligned} P(X = x|\,\theta) =& P(X = x, T(X) = T(x)\,|\,\theta) \\ =& P(X = x|T(X) = T(x), \theta_1, \theta_2) P(T(X) = T(x)\,|\,\theta_1, \theta_2) \end{aligned} \tag{A1}$$

The result is immediate: as the conditional distribution of $X$ given $T(X) = T(x)$ and $\theta$ depends only on $\theta_2$, and the marginal distribution of $T$ given $\theta$ depends only on $\theta_1$, one can write for each $x \in \mathfrak{X}$, $P(T(X) = T(x) \,|\, \theta_1, \theta_2) = L_x^1(\theta_1)$ and $P(X = x | T(X) = T(x) \,|\, \theta_1, \theta_2) = L_x^2(\theta_2)$. The proof when $T$ is p-sufficient for $\theta_2$ and s-ancillary for $\theta_1$ is analogous. □

**Proof of Theorem 1.** We first prove the ($\Rightarrow$) part of the theorem. Suppose that $x \in \mathfrak{X}$ is such that $\theta_1 \perp\!\!\!\perp \theta_2 \,|\, X = x$; that is, the posterior distribution of $\theta$ given $X = x$ can be factored as $\pi(\theta|\, x) = \pi_1(\theta_1|\, x)\pi_2(\theta_2|\, x)$. Then,

$$\pi(\theta|x) \;=\; \pi_1(\theta_1|x)\pi_2(\theta_2|x) \;\Rightarrow\; \frac{L_x(\theta)\pi(\theta)}{\int_\Theta L_x(\theta)\pi(\theta)d\theta} = \frac{\int_{\Theta_2} L_x(\theta)\pi(\theta)d\theta_2}{\int_\Theta L_x(\theta)\pi(\theta)d\theta}\frac{\int_{\Theta_1} L_x(\theta)\pi(\theta)d\theta_1}{\int_\Theta L_x(\theta)\pi(\theta)d\theta}. \tag{A2}$$

Due to the fact that $\theta_1 \perp\!\!\!\perp \theta_2$, it follows from the last equality in (A2) that

$$L_x(\theta)\pi_1(\theta_1)\pi_2(\theta_2) = \pi_1(\theta_1)\int_{\Theta_2} L_x(\theta)\pi_2(\theta_2)d\theta_2 \,\frac{\pi_2(\theta_2)\int_{\Theta_1} L_x(\theta)\pi_1(\theta_1)d\theta_1}{\int_\Theta L_x(\theta)\pi(\theta)d\theta}. \tag{A3}$$

The result follows considering, for instance,

$$L_x^1(\theta_1) = \int_{\Theta_2} L_x(\theta)\pi_2(\theta_2)d\theta_2 \quad \text{and} \quad L_x^2(\theta_2) = \frac{\int_{\Theta_1} L_x(\theta)\pi(\theta_1)d\theta_1}{\int_\Theta L_x(\theta)\pi(\theta)d\theta}. \tag{A4}$$

□

Next, we prove the converse. Suppose that the likelihood can be factored as $L_x(\theta) = L_x^1(\theta_1)L_x^2(\theta_2)$. Then,

$$\pi(\theta|x) = \frac{L_x(\theta)\pi(\theta)}{\int_\Theta L_x(\theta)\pi(\theta)d\theta} = \frac{L_x^1(\theta_1)L_x^2(\theta_2)\pi_1(\theta_1)\pi_2(\theta_2)}{\int_{\Theta_1\times\Theta_2} L_x^1(\theta_1)L_x^2(\theta_2)\pi_1(\theta_1)\pi_2(\theta_2)d\theta}. \tag{A5}$$

The posterior marginal density of $\theta_i$ is obtained from (A5) by integrating out the other component. Thus,

$$\pi_i(\theta_i|x) \;=\; \frac{L_x^i(\theta_i)\pi_i(\theta_i)}{\int_{\Theta_i} L_x^i(\theta_i)\pi_i(\theta_i)d\theta_i}\,,\; i = 1,2, \tag{A6}$$

and therefore, $\pi(\theta_1, \theta_2|x) = \pi_1(\theta_1|x)\pi_2(\theta_2|x)$; that is, $\theta_1 \perp\!\!\!\perp \theta_2 | X = x$. □

**Proof of Theorem 3.** We first verify that $\theta_2$ is an NNP for testing $\bar{H}$ versus $\bar{A}$ by means of $\bar{\varphi}^*$. Recall that

$$\bar{\varphi}^*(x, \theta_2) = 1 \Leftrightarrow \frac{\bar{f}_{\bar{H}}(x,\theta_2)}{\bar{f}_{\bar{A}}(x,\theta_2)} < \frac{b}{a}, \tag{A7}$$

where $\bar{f}_H$ ($\bar{f}_A$) is the predictive distribution for $(X, \theta_2)$ obtained under $\bar{H}$ ($\bar{A}$). In this case, the likelihood function generated by $(x_0, \theta_2)$ for $\theta_1$ with $x_0 \in \mathfrak{X}$ such that (1) holds and $\theta_2 \in \Theta_2$ is

$$\begin{aligned} \bar{L}_{(x_0,\theta_2)}(\theta_1) &= P(X = x_0 \,|\, \theta_1, \theta_2)\pi_2(\theta_2 \,|\, \theta_1) \;=\; L_{x_0}(\theta_1, \theta_2)\pi_2(\theta_2) \\ &= L_{x_0}^1(\theta_1)L_{x_0}^2(\theta_2)\pi_2(\theta_2) \end{aligned} \tag{A8}$$

Then, the predictive function under the null hypothesis $\bar{H}$ can be calculated as

$$\bar{f}_{\bar{H}}(x_0, \theta_2) \;=\; \int_{\{\theta_0\}} \bar{L}_{(x_0,\theta_2)}(\theta_1)dP_{\bar{H}}(\theta_1)\,, \tag{A9}$$

where $P_{\bar{H}}$ is degenerate at $\theta_0$ conditional distribution of $\theta_1|\theta_1 = \theta_0$. Thus,

$$\bar{f}_{\bar{H}}(x_0,\theta_2) = L^1_{x_0}(\theta_0)L^2_{x_0}(\theta_2)\pi_2(\theta_2). \tag{A10}$$

In addition, the predictive function under the alternative hypothesis $\bar{A}$ is given by

$$\begin{aligned} \bar{f}_{\bar{A}}(x_0,\theta_2) &= \int_{\Theta_1} L^1_{x_0}(\theta_1)L^2_{x_0}(\theta_2)\pi_2(\theta_2)dP_{\bar{H}_1}(\theta_1) \\ &= \int_{\Theta_1} L^1_{x_0}(\theta_1)L^2_{x_0}(\theta_2)\pi_2(\theta_2)\pi_1(\theta_1)d\theta_1 \\ &= L^2_{x_0}(\theta_2)\pi_2(\theta_2)\int_{\Theta_1} L^1_{x_0}(\theta_1)\pi_1(\theta_1)d\theta_1. \end{aligned} \tag{A11}$$

Thus, the Bayes factor can be expressed by

$$\begin{aligned} \frac{\bar{f}_{\bar{H}}(x_0,\theta_2)}{\bar{f}_{\bar{A}}(x_0,\theta_2)} &= \frac{L^1_{x_0}(\theta_0)L^2_{x_0}(\theta_2)\pi_2(\theta_2)}{L^2_{x_0}(\theta_2)\pi_2(\theta_2)\int_{\Theta_1} L^1_{x_0}(\theta_1)\pi_1(\theta_1)d\theta_1} \\ &= \frac{L^1_{x_0}(\theta_0)}{\int_{\Theta_1} L^1_{x_0}(\theta_1)\pi_1(\theta_1)d\theta_1}. \end{aligned} \tag{A12}$$

Note that Equation (A12) does not depend on $\theta_2$. As a result, the test in (A7) does not depend on $\theta_2$, and consequently, $\theta_2$ is an NNP for testing $\bar{H}$ versus $\bar{A}$ by means of $\bar{\varphi}^*$. Now, we shall determine the test $\varphi^*$ for $H$ versus $A$. The predictive distribution for $X$ at $x_0$ under the null hypothesis is

$$f_H(x_0) = \int_{\Theta_1\times\Theta_2} L_{x_0}(\theta_1,\theta_2)d\mathbb{P}_H(\theta_1,\theta_2). \tag{A13}$$

It is not difficult to verify that for fixed $\theta_0 \in \Theta_1$, the conditional distribution of $\theta$ given $\theta_1 = \theta_0$ is such that $\theta_1$ is degenerate at $\theta_0$, and $\theta_2$ is independent of $\theta_1$ with density $\pi_2$.

Then,

$$\begin{aligned} f_H(x_0) &= \int_{\Theta_1\times\Theta_2} L_{x_0}(\theta_1,\theta_2)dP_H(\theta_1,\theta_2) \\ &= \int_{\Theta_2} L^1_{x_0}(\theta_0)L^2_{x_0}(\theta_2)\pi_2(\theta_2)d\theta_2 \\ &= L^1_{x_0}(\theta_0)\int_{\Theta_2} L^2_{x_0}(\theta_2)\pi_2(\theta_2)d\theta_2. \end{aligned} \tag{A14}$$

For the alternative hypothesis, we have that

$$\begin{aligned} f_A(x_0) &= \int_{\Theta_1\times\Theta_2} L^1_{x_0}(\theta_1)L^2_{x_0}(\theta_2)dP_A(\theta_1,\theta_2) \\ &= \int_{\Theta_1\times\Theta_2} L^1_{x_0}(\theta_1)L^2_{x_0}(\theta_2)dP(\theta_1,\theta_2) \\ &= \int_{\Theta_1}\int_{\Theta_2} L^1_{x_0}(\theta_1)L^2_{x_0}(\theta_2)\pi_1(\theta_1)\pi_2(\theta_2)d\theta_1 d\theta_2 \\ &= \int_{\Theta_1} L^1_{x_0}(\theta_1)\pi_1(\theta_1)d\theta_1\int_{\Theta_2} L^2_{x_0}(\theta_2)\pi_2(\theta_2)d\theta_2. \end{aligned} \tag{A15}$$

Finally,

$$\begin{aligned} \frac{f_H(x_0)}{f_A(x_0)} &= \frac{L^1_{x_0}(\theta_0)\int_{\Theta_2} L^2_{x_0}(\theta_2)\pi_2(\theta_2)d\theta_2}{\int_{\Theta_1} L^1_{x_0}(\theta_1)\pi_1(\theta_1)d\theta_1\int_{\Theta_2} L^2_{x_0}(\theta_2)\pi_2(\theta_2)d\theta_2} \\ &= \frac{L^1_{x_0}(\theta_0)}{\int_{\Theta_1} L^1_{x_0}(\theta_1)\pi_1(\theta_1)d_{\theta_1}} = \frac{\bar{f}_{\bar{H}}(x_0,\theta_2)}{\bar{f}_{\bar{A}}(x_0,\theta_2)}. \end{aligned} \tag{A16}$$

Hence,

$$\frac{f_{H_0}(x_0)}{f_{H_1}(x_0)} < \frac{a}{b} \Leftrightarrow \frac{\bar{f}_{\bar{H}_0}(x_0, \theta_2)}{\bar{f}_{\bar{H}_1}(x_0, \theta_2)} < \frac{a}{b}, \tag{A17}$$

and consequently,

$$\varphi^*(x_0) = 1 \Leftrightarrow \bar{\varphi}^*(x_0, \theta_2) = 1. \tag{A18}$$

□

**Proof of Corollary 1.** The corollary follows directly from Theorems 2 and 3. □

**Proof of Theorem 4.** From Theorem 3 and Corollary 1, we have that for each $x_0 \in \mathfrak{X}$,

$$\varphi^*(x_0) \; = \; 1 \Leftrightarrow \; BF(x_0) \; \leqslant \frac{b}{a} \, . \tag{A19}$$

Then,

$$\varphi^*(x_0) \; = \; 1 \Rightarrow \; BF(x_0) \; \leqslant \; \frac{b}{a} \; \Rightarrow \mathfrak{D}(x_0) \; \subseteq \; \mathfrak{D} \; \Rightarrow$$

$$\Rightarrow \sum_{x \,\in\, \mathfrak{D}(x_0)} f_{H,T(x_0)}(x) \; \leq \; \sum_{x \,\in\, \mathfrak{D}} f_{H,T(x_0)}(x) \; \Rightarrow \; p_T\text{-value}(x_0) \; \leq \; \alpha^*_T(x_0) \, .$$

Thus,

$$\varphi^*(x_0) \; = \; 1 \Rightarrow \; P_T\text{-value}(x_0) \; \leq \; \alpha^*_T(x_0) \, . \tag{A20}$$

The converse is proven by the contrapositive.

$$\varphi^*(x_0) \; = \; 0 \Rightarrow \; \frac{b}{a} \; < \; BF(x_0) \; \Rightarrow \; \mathfrak{D} \, \cup \, \{x_0\} \; \subseteq \; \mathfrak{D}(x_0) \, .$$

As $x_0 \notin \mathfrak{D}$ if $BF(x_0) > \frac{b}{a}$, we obtain that

$$\varphi^*(x_0) \; = \; 0 \; \Rightarrow \; \sum_{x \,\in\, \mathfrak{D}} f_{H,T(x_0)}(x) \; + \; f_{H,T(x_0)}(x_0) \; \leq \; \sum_{x \,\in\, \mathfrak{D}(x_0)} f_{H,T(x_0)}(x) \, .$$

Since $x_0 \in \mathfrak{D}_T(x_0)$ and $BF(x_0) > \frac{b}{a} > 0$, it follows that $f_{H,T(x_0)}(x_0) > 0$. Thus,

$$\varphi^*(x_0) \; = \; 0 \; \Rightarrow \; \alpha^*_T(x_0) \; < \; P_T\text{-value}(x_0) \, , \tag{A21}$$

and consequently,

$$p_T\text{-value}(x_0) \; \leq \; \alpha^*_T(x_0) \; \Rightarrow \; \varphi^*(x_0) \; = \; 1 \, . \tag{A22}$$

From (A20) and (A22), the result follows. □

**Mixed test for symmetry hypothesis for $r \times r$ contingency tables**

In this case, Table A1 represents the observed frequencies of the cross-classification of $n$ units by the variables $X_1$ and $X_2$.

**Table A1.** Observed frequencies of $X_1$ and $X_2$ in the $3 \times 3$ case.

| | | $X_2$ | | |
|---|---|---|---|---|
| $X_1$ | $x_{11}$ | $x_{12}$ | $x_{13}$ | $n_{1.}$ |
| | $x_{21}$ | $x_{22}$ | $x_{23}$ | $n_{2.}$ |
| | $x_{31}$ | $x_{32}$ | $x_{33}$ | $n_{3.}$ |
| | $n_{.1}$ | $n_{.2}$ | $n_{.3}$ | $n$ |

Let $X = (X_{ij})$ be the $(r^2 - 1)$-dimensional vector of cell counts and $\theta = (\theta_{ij})$ be the $(r^2 - 1)$-dimensional vector of cell probabilities, where $X_{ij}$ and $\theta_{ij}$ are self explanatory.

Suppose that $X$ is a multinomial random vector with parameters $n$ and $\theta$. The likelihood function generated by $x \in \mathfrak{X}$ for $\theta$ is given by

$$L_x(\theta) = \frac{n!}{x_{11}! \ldots x_{rr}!} \theta_{11}^{x_{11}} \ldots \theta_{rr}^{x_{rr}}. \tag{A23}$$

The hypotheses for testing diagonal symmetry are

$$\begin{aligned} H &: \theta_{ij} = \theta_{ji} \quad \forall i \neq j. \\ A &: \theta_{ij} \neq \theta_{ji} \quad \text{for at least one } i \neq j. \end{aligned} \tag{A24}$$

We also assume a prior Dirichlet distribution with parameter $\alpha = (\alpha_{ij})$ for $\theta$. That is,

$$\pi(\theta) = \frac{\Gamma(\alpha_{11} + \ldots + \alpha_{rr})}{\Gamma(\alpha_{11}) \ldots \Gamma(\alpha_{rr})} \theta_{11}^{\alpha_{11}-1} \ldots \theta_{rr}^{\alpha_{rr}-1}. \tag{A25}$$

To perform the mixed test for the symmetry hypothesis, we consider the following reparametrization of the model: we define

$$\begin{aligned} \lambda_{ij} &= \frac{\theta_{ij}}{\theta_{ij}+\theta_{ji}} && \text{for} \quad i < j \\ \lambda_{ij} &= \theta_{ij} + \theta_{ji} && \text{for} \quad i > j \\ \lambda_{ij} &= \theta_{ij} && \text{for} \quad i = j. \end{aligned} \tag{A26}$$

Let $\lambda = (\lambda_1, \lambda_2)$, where $\lambda_1$ is the $(\frac{r^2-r}{2})$-dimensional vector for which the components are $\lambda_{ij}$'s such that $i < j$, and $\lambda_2$ is the $(\frac{r^2-r}{2} + r - 1)$-dimensional vector for which the components are $\lambda_{ij}$'s such that $i \geq j$. The new parameter space is then $\Lambda = (0,1)^{\frac{r^2-r}{2}} \times S_{\frac{r^2-r}{2}+r-1}$.

Then, we can rewrite the hypotheses (A24) as

$$\begin{aligned} \tilde{H} &: \lambda \in \Lambda_0 \\ \tilde{A} &: \lambda \in \Lambda_0^c. \end{aligned} \tag{A27}$$

where $\Lambda_0 = B \times S_{\frac{r^2-r}{2}+r-1}$, and $B$ is the singleton $B = \{(\frac{1}{2}, \ldots, \frac{1}{2})\}$.

As in previous sections, we consider a statistic $T$ that is s-ancillary for $\lambda_1$: $T$ is the $(\frac{r^2-r}{2} + r - 1)$-dimensional vector for which the components are the sums $X_{ij} + X_{ji}$ for $i < j$ and $X_{ii}$ for $i = 1, \ldots, r-1$. The induced likelihood function for $\lambda$ generated by $x$ is

$$\tilde{L}_x(\lambda) = \left[\prod_{i<j} \binom{x_{ij} + x_{ji}}{x_{ij}} \lambda_{ij}^{x_{ij}} (1 - \lambda_{ij})^{x_{ji}}\right] \left[\frac{n!}{\prod_i x_{ii}! \prod_{i>j} (x_{ij} + x_{ji})!} \prod_i \lambda_{ii}^{x_{ii}} \prod_{i>j} \lambda_{ij}^{x_{ij}+x_{ji}}\right]. \tag{A28}$$

We can easily see that the likelihood function in (A28) can be factored as $\tilde{L}_x(\lambda_1, \lambda_2) = \tilde{L}_x^1(\lambda_1)\tilde{L}_x^2(\lambda_2)$. In addition, the prior distribution for $\lambda$ is such that $\lambda_1$ and $\lambda_2$ are independent: $\lambda_2$ being a Dirichlet random vector and $\lambda_1$ a vector of independent Beta random variables. That is,

$$\tilde{\pi}(\lambda) = \tilde{\pi}_1(\lambda_1)\tilde{\pi}_2(\lambda_2) = \prod_{i<j} \frac{\Gamma(\alpha_{ij} + \alpha_{ji})}{\Gamma(\alpha_{ij})\Gamma(\alpha_{ji})} \lambda_{ij}^{\alpha_{ij}-1} (1 - \lambda_{ij})^{\alpha_{ij}-1} \mathbb{I}_{(0,1)}(\lambda_{ij}) \; \tilde{\pi}_2(\lambda_2) \tag{A29}$$

From Theorem 3, we have that $\lambda_2$ is an NNP for testing $\tilde{H}$ versus $\tilde{A}$ by means of the mixed test. In addition, the mixed test for $\tilde{H}$ reduces to the mixed test for the simple hypothesis $\lambda_1 = (\frac{1}{2}, \ldots, \frac{1}{2})$ were $\lambda_2$ known. From Theorem 4, it follows that we only need to compare the conditional $P_T - value$ with the conditional adaptive significance level to test $\tilde{H}$ against $\tilde{A}$. From (28), (30) and (A28), we obtain for $x = (x_{ij}) \in \mathfrak{X}$:

$$p_T\text{-value}(x) = \sum_{y \in \mathfrak{D}_T^*(x)} \prod_{i<j} \binom{y_{ij}+y_{ji}}{y_{ij}} (\frac{1}{2})^{y_{ij}+y_{ji}} = \sum_{y \in \mathfrak{D}_T^*(x)} \prod_{i<j} \binom{x_{ij}+x_{ji}}{y_{ij}} (\frac{1}{2})^{x_{ij}+x_{ji}} \tag{A30}$$

and

$$\alpha_T^*(x) = \sum_{y \in \mathfrak{D}\cap\mathfrak{D}_T(x)} \prod_{i<j} \binom{y_{ij}+y_{ji}}{y_{ij}} (\frac{1}{2})^{y_{ij}+y_{ji}} = \sum_{y \in \mathfrak{D}\cap\mathfrak{D}_T(x)} \prod_{i<j} \binom{x_{ij}+x_{ji}}{y_{ij}} (\frac{1}{2})^{x_{ij}+x_{ji}}. \tag{A31}$$

In this case, these conditional quantities are simply determined by the products of binomial-type probabilities.

## References

1. Berger, J.; Wolper, R. *The Likelihood Principle*; Institute of Mathematical Statistics: Hayward, CA, USA, 1988.
2. Mayo, D. On the Birnbaum Argument for the Strong Likelihood Principle. *Stat. Sci.* **2014**, *29*, 227–239. [CrossRef]
3. Dawid, A. Discussion of "On the Birnbaum Argument for the Strong Likelihood Principle". *Stat. Sci.* **2014**, *29*, 240–241. [CrossRef]
4. Evans, M. Discussion of "On the Birnbaum Argument for the Strong Likelihood Principle". *Stat. Sci.* **2014**, *29*, 242–246. [CrossRef]
5. Hannig, J. Discussion of "On the Birnbaum Argument for the Strong Likelihood Principle". *Stat. Sci.* **2014**, *29*, 254–258. [CrossRef]
6. Bjørnstad, J. Discussion of "On the Birnbaum Argument for the Strong Likelihood Principle". *Stat. Sci.* **2014**, *29*, 259–260. [CrossRef]
7. Shan, G. *Exact Statistical Inference for Categorical Data*; Academic Press: Cambridge, MA, USA, 2016.
8. Pericchi, L.; Pereira, C. Adaptive significance levels using optimal decision rules: Balancing by weighting the error probabilities. *Braz. J. Probab. Stat.* **2016**, *30*, 70–90. [CrossRef]
9. Butler, R.W. Predictive Likelihood Inference with Applications. *J. R. Stat. Soc. Ser. B* **1986**, *48*, 1–38. [CrossRef]
10. Severini, T. Integrated likelihoods for functions of a parameter. *Stat* **2018**, *7*, e212. [CrossRef]
11. Berger, J.; Liseo, B.; Wolpert, R. Integrated Likelihood Methods for Eliminating Nuisance Parameters. *Stat. Sci.* **1999**, *14*, 1–28. [CrossRef]
12. Cox, D.R. Partial likelihood. *Biometrika* **1975**, *62*, 269–276. [CrossRef]
13. Dawid, A.P. On the concepts of sufficiency and ancillarity in the presence of nuisance parameters. *J. R. Stat. Soc. Ser. B* **1975**, *37*, 248–258. [CrossRef]
14. Sprott, D.A. Marginal and conditional sufficiency. *Biometrika* **1975**, *62*, 599–605. [CrossRef]
15. Barndorff-Nielsen, O. Nonformation. *Biometrika* **1976**, *63*, 567–571. [CrossRef]
16. Barndorff-Nielsen, O. *Information and Exponential Families: In Statistical Theory*; Wiley: Chichester, UK, 1978.
17. Basu, D. On the Elimination of Nuisance Parameters. *J. Am. Stat. Assoc.* **1977**, *72*, 355–366. [CrossRef]
18. Jørgensen, B. The rules of conditional inference: Is there a universal definition of nonformation? *J. Ital. Stat. Soc.* **1994**, *3*, 355. [CrossRef]
19. Pace, L.; Salvan, A. *Principles of Statistical Inference: From a Neo-Fisherian Perspective*; World Scientific Publishing Company Pte Limited: Singapore, 1997.
20. Gannon, M.; Pereira, C.; Polpo, A. Blending Bayesian and Classical Tools to Define Optimal Sample-Size-Dependent Significance Levels. *Am. Stat.* **2019**, *73*, 213–222. [CrossRef]
21. Pereira, C.; Nakano, E.; Fossaluza, V.; Esteves, L.; Gannon, M.; Polpo, A. Hypothesis Tests for Bernoulli Experiments: Ordering the Sample Space by Bayes Factors and Using Adaptive Significance Levels for Decisions. *Entropy* **2017**, *19*, 696. [CrossRef]
22. Olivera, M. Definição do nivel de significancia em função do tamanho amostral. Master's Thesis, IME, Universidade de São Paulo, São Paulo, Brazil, 2014.
23. Pereira, B.; Pereira, C. A Likelihood approach to diagnostic test in clinical medicine. *Stat. J.* **2005**, *3*, 77–98.
24. Montoya, D.; Irony, T.; Pereira, C.; Whittle, M. An unconditional exact test for the Hardy-Weinberg equilibrium law: Sample space ordering using the Bayes factor. *Genet. Soc. Am.* **2001**, *158*, 875–883.
25. Irony, T.; Pereira, C. Bayesian hypothesis test: Using surface integrals to distribute prior information among the hypotheses. *Resenhas IME-USP* **1995**, *2*, 27–46.
26. DeGroot, M. *Probability and Statistics*; Adson Wesley: Boston, MA, USA, 1986.
27. Freeman, P. The role of $p$-values in analysing trial resultss. *Stat. Med.* **1993**, *12*, 15–16. [CrossRef]
28. Bowker, A. A Test for Symmetry in Contingency Tables. *J. Am. Stat. Assoc.* **1948**, *43*, 572–574. [CrossRef]
29. Ireland, C.; Ku, H.; Kullback, S. Symmetry and marginal homogeneity of an r $\times$ r contingency table. *J. Am. Stat. Assoc.* **1969**, *64*, 1323–1341. [CrossRef]
30. Kullback, S. Marginal Homogeneity of Multidimensional Contingency Tables. *Ann. Math. Stat.* **1971**, *42*, 594–606. [CrossRef]
31. Bernardo, G.; Lauretto, M.; Stern, J. The full Bayesian significance test for symmetry in contingency tables. *AIP Conf. Proc.* **2012**, *1443*, 198–205.
32. Agresti, A. *Categorical Data Analysis*, 3rd ed.; John Wiley & Sons: Hoboken, NJ, USA, 2013.

33. Tahata, K.; Tomizawa, S. Symmetry and asymmetry models and decompositions of models for contingency tables. *SUT J. Math.* **2014**, *50*, 131–165. [CrossRef]
34. McClave, J.T.; Benson, P.G.; Sincich, T.T. *Statistics for Business and Economics*; Number 519.5; Pearson: London, UK, 2001.

**Disclaimer/Publisher's Note:** The statements, opinions and data contained in all publications are solely those of the individual author(s) and contributor(s) and not of MDPI and/or the editor(s). MDPI and/or the editor(s) disclaim responsibility for any injury to people or property resulting from any ideas, methods, instructions or products referred to in the content.

entropy

MDPI

Article

# Stochastic Volatility Models with Skewness Selection

**Igor Martins * and Hedibert Freitas Lopes**

Insper Institute of Education and Research, Rua Quatá 300, São Paulo 04546-042, Brazil; hedibertfl@insper.edu.br
* Correspondence: igorfbm@al.insper.edu.br

**Abstract:** This paper expands traditional stochastic volatility models by allowing for time-varying skewness without imposing it. While dynamic asymmetry may capture the likely direction of future asset returns, it comes at the risk of leading to overparameterization. Our proposed approach mitigates this concern by leveraging sparsity-inducing priors to automatically select the skewness parameter as dynamic, static or zero in a data-driven framework. We consider two empirical applications. First, in a bond yield application, dynamic skewness captures interest rate cycles of monetary easing and tightening and is partially explained by central banks' mandates. In a currency modeling framework, our model indicates no skewness in the carry factor after accounting for stochastic volatility. This supports the idea of carry crashes resulting from volatility surges instead of dynamic skewness.

**Keywords:** stochastic volatility; sparsity; skewness

## 1. Introduction

Accurate representation of asset returns is one of the key topics in finance. Based on the theoretical results from [1,2], standard approaches to asset pricing have largely focused on the first and second moments. Stochastic volatility (SV) models, discussed, for example, by [3], are among the cornerstone models in modern financial econometrics. In their simplest form, SV models represent asset returns via normal distribution with persistent volatility and a mean that is either constant or a linear function of explanatory variables. Such models capture the first two moments of asset returns in a simple and elegant manner, being supported empirically and theoretically, as discussed in [4].

While we acknowledge the importance of the first two moments in asset pricing, we also recognize the potential benefits of including skewness when modeling returns. Due to its ability to capture the likely direction of returns, models with time-varying skewness may be more suitable for forecasting periods with a higher concentration of same sign returns, leading to better detection of both overperformance and underperformance periods. Ref. [5] is one key example of the empirical benefits of adding such feature for modeling cross-sectional stock momentum. While the momentum factor is known for delivering good mean–variance compensation, it is also subject to a long period of negative performance. By capturing such prolonged periods of likely negative returns via dynamic skewness, ref. [5] improves the performance of the stock momentum factor compared to traditional approaches that neglect skewness.

However, including dynamic skewness in traditional financial econometric models can be costly. While allowing for asymmetry may lead to a better representation of some financial time series, it may not be a vital feature, and its inclusion risks overparameterization. Therefore, we wish to include dynamic skewness only when required by the data and remove such a feature if it is not necessary.

This paper expands stochastic volatility models by allowing dynamic skewness without having to impose it. We replace the traditional hypothesis of Gaussian errors with a skew-normal distribution. Such a change preserves the usual features for the first two moments of SV models but allows for dynamic skewness. Since the inclusion of time-varying asymmetry may not always be necessary, we consider a sparsity-inducing scheme for its parameters. In particular, we consider a random-walk evolution for the asymmetry. When the standard deviation of the dynamic process is shrunk to zero, our model results in an SV model with constant skewness. Additionally, if the level of skewness is shrunk to zero, we recover a traditional SV model. By combining prior information with the likelihood of the model, our proposed approach automatically chooses between dynamic, static, or no skewness.

We consider two empirical applications. In our first application, we model Brazil and US bonds, obtaining three main results. First, our proposed model indicates that bond yield changes for both countries, better represented by including time-varying skewness, resulting in out-of-sample improvements for forecasting the direction of future yields when compared to generalized autoregressive score (GAS) models. Second, the recovered skewness is associated with interest rate cycles of monetary easing and tightening. Third, inflation and unemployment partially explain the recovered skewness, linking it to central banks' mandates. In a second application, we model the carry factor for currency returns. Our model indicates not only the lack of dynamics, but also no skewness at all for it after accounting for volatility. Therefore, similar to the crash mitigation via volatility scaling proposed in [6], the carry factor also experiences reduced crashes once dynamic volatility is considered, without requiring the inclusion of skewness.

This paper intersects and contributes to multiple areas. First, it contributes to the stochastic volatility literature by expanding the static skewness model of [7] to the dynamic case while also extending the sparsity-inducing scheme of [8] by allowing for dynamic skewness to shrink towards the static case. Second, it contributes to the toolbox of methods for recovering dynamic skewness. Ref. [9] relies on option data, while [10] uses rolling windows. Both approaches have limitations. While theoretically sound, option-based approaches require tradeable options with a large collection of strikes, high liquidity, and continuous expiration dates. Such requirements are hard to meet in many applications, especially for emerging markets such as in our Brazilian bond applications. Rolling window-based approaches artificially introduce dynamics into skewness by changing the sample period continually. Such changes come at the cost of outliers playing a large role in estimation, in addition to a trade-off based on window size, which affects the precision of the estimate and the speed at which the dynamics change. Third, it contributes to the interest rate literature by showing that inflation and unemployment partially explain skewness, linking it to central banks' mandates, and expanding the traditional mean and variance analysis of papers such as [11,12]. Fourth, it contributes to the debate of whether the carry factor presents dynamic skewness after accounting for heteroskedasticity, as discussed in [13,14], by claiming that skewness is unlikely to be dynamic and, in fact, is more likely to be zero after accounting for SV effects.

The paper is organized as follows. It starts by describing traditional SV models and moves on to our proposal with time-varying skewness in Section 2. Section 3 discusses the sparsity-inducing framework. Section 4 shows our Hmailtonian Monte Carlo (HMC) approach to simulate from the joint posterior. Section 5 presents the bond yield forecasting application while Section 6 shows the carry factor application. Section 7 concludes.

## 2. SV Model with Time-Varying Skewness

A traditional stochastic volatility model is defined in Equations (1)–(5). Equation (1) represents asset returns with a mean of zero and dynamic volatility of $exp(h_t/2)$. Equation (2) indicates persistent log-volatility with level $\mu$ and persistence $\phi$, having initial values given by the stationary distribution shown in Equation (3). In its simplest form, both measure and state equations have Gaussian errors as represented in Equations (4) and (5).

$$y_t = exp\left(\frac{h_t}{2}\right)\varepsilon_t, \tag{1}$$

$$h_t = \mu_h + \phi_h(h_{t-1} - \mu_h) + \sigma_h\eta_t, \tag{2}$$

$$h_0 \sim N\left(\mu_h, \frac{\sigma_h^2}{1-\phi_h^2}\right), \tag{3}$$

$$\varepsilon_t \sim N(0,1), \tag{4}$$

$$\eta_t \sim N(0,1). \tag{5}$$

In order to introduce asymmetry into the model, we replace the normal variable, $\varepsilon_t$ in Equation (4) with a skew-normal random variable, $z_t$. We utilize the skew-normal density representation described in [15,16] as shown in Equation (6), where $\phi(\cdot)$ and $\Phi(\cdot)$ represent standard normal density and distribution function, respectively. $\lambda$ controls the degree of asymmetry in the distribution, as depicted in Figure 1. Specifically, for $\lambda = 0$, the skew-normal reduces to standard normal distribution. Additionally, we can introduce location ($\xi$) and scale ($\omega$) parameters to the skew-normal, denoting $X = \xi + \omega z$ as $X \sim SN(\xi, \omega, \lambda)$, with its density presented in Equation (7). Appendix A describes the relationships between $\xi$, $\lambda$, and $\omega$ in terms of mean, variance, and skewness.

$$\text{If } Z \sim SN(\lambda), \text{ then } p(z;\lambda) = 2\phi(z)\Phi(\lambda z); \tag{6}$$

$$\text{If } X \sim SN(\xi,\omega,\lambda), \text{ then } p(x;\xi,\omega,\lambda) = 2\frac{1}{\omega}\phi\Big(\frac{x-\xi}{\omega}\Big)\Phi\Big(\lambda\frac{x-\xi}{\omega}\Big). \tag{7}$$

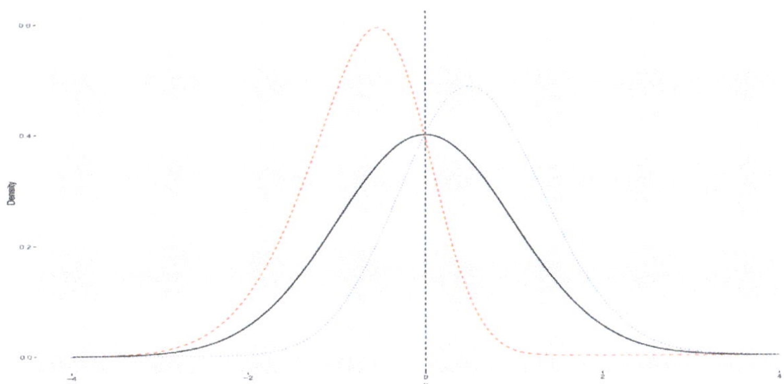

**Figure 1.** Skew-normal densities with $\xi = 0$ and $\omega = 1$ and $\lambda$ equal to $-2$, 0, and 1 for the dashed red, solid black and dotted blue lines, respectively. If $\lambda < 0$, the distribution is skewed to the left. If $\lambda = 0$, SN(0) reduces to the standard Gaussian distribution. Finally, if $\lambda > 0$, the distribution is skewed to the right.

We allow for the possibility of dynamic skewness by replacing static $\lambda$ with $\lambda_t$, which evolves according to a random walk starting at $\lambda_0$ as represented by Equations (8) and (9). Therefore, we modify our observation equation by enabling both volatility and skewness to vary with time, changing the observation equation to Equation (11). While Equation (1) implies that $y_t$ follows a symmetric distribution, Equation (11) indicates that $y_t$ comes from a potentially skewed distribution. Therefore, our model can be viewed as an extension of the stochastic volatility models with static skewness proposed in [7,8,17].

$$z_t \sim SN(\lambda_t), \tag{8}$$

$$\lambda_t = \lambda_{t-1} + \sigma_\lambda \eta_{\lambda,t} \text{ with } \eta_{\lambda,t} \sim N(0,1), \tag{9}$$

$$\lambda_0 = \alpha_0, \tag{10}$$

$$y_t = exp\left(\frac{h_t}{2}\right) z_t. \tag{11}$$

Since $\varepsilon_t \sim N(0,1)$, Equation (1) implies that $y_t$ follows a normal distribution with a location of zero and a scale of $exp(h_t/2)$. By replacing $\varepsilon_t$ with $z_t \sim SN(\lambda_t)$, Equation (11) implies that $y_t$ follows a skew-normal distribution with a location of zero, a scale of $exp(h_t/2)$, and skewness parameter $\lambda_t$.

We are not the first to consider models with dynamic skewness. For instance, refs. [18,19] introduced GAS models which induce time-varying skewness through the score of conditional density. More recently, refs. [5,20] used GAS models to model Bitcoin returns and manage momentum-based portfolios. However, unlike our proposal, GAS models are suitable for including time-varying higher moments within a GARCH-like framework, while our proposal is designed for SV models.

## 3. Sparsity-Inducing Approach

The inclusion of asymmetry may improve the representation of time series by capturing periods with a higher concentration of returns exhibiting the same sign, as demonstrated, for instance, in [5,16,21]. However, it may not always be necessary as it involves estimating additional parameters. To mitigate the risk of overparametrization, our aim is to incorporate time-varying skewness only when required by the data. One possible approach involves estimating multiple models with different skewness specifications and then selecting a model using the Bayes factor. Ref. [22] provides a comprehensive review of using Bayes factors for model selection. However, recovering Bayes factors can be a challenging problem, as highlighted in [23]. We propose a sparsity-inducing method that conveniently performs model selection without the need to estimate multiple models and entirely avoids the use of Bayes factors.

In the non-Bayesian literature, shrinkage is based on maximizing the likelihood of a model subject to a penalty function with the LASSO of [24] being the most commonly employed approach. From a Bayesian perspective, shrinkage problems can be framed as a penalization of the log-likelihood through a log-prior. In fact, the posterior mode of a linear model with Double Exponential prior having a location of zero and a scale of $2/\psi$ equals the point estimate of the LASSO with penalty $\psi$, as shown in [25]. Therefore, to shrink both $\sigma_\lambda$ and $\lambda_0$ towards zero, we utilize Double Exponential priors for both parameters, as illustrated in Equations (12) and (13).

Our proposal is consistent with the concept of sparsity in dynamic models, a principle also utilized in [26–29]. Our approach is considered sparsity-inducing in the sense that both the random walk variance and initial state for the skewness parameter are shrunk towards zero. Equation (9) governs the dynamics of the asymmetry parameter. When $\sigma_\lambda$ approaches zero, $\lambda_t$ becomes static and assumes the value of its initial point, $\lambda_0$. Furthermore, if the initial point is also zero, the model reduces to the vanilla SV model. Hence, by inducing sparsity for both $\sigma_\lambda$ and $\lambda_0$, we can encompass all three cases of interest.

$$\sigma_\lambda \sim \text{DoubleExponential}(0, 1/\kappa_{\sigma_\lambda}) \text{ with } \kappa_{\sigma_\lambda} \sim Gamma(a,b), \tag{12}$$

$$\alpha_\lambda \sim \text{DoubleExponential}(0, 1/\kappa_\alpha) \text{ with } \kappa_\alpha \sim Gamma(c,d). \tag{13}$$

To the best of our knowledge, we are the first to introduce sparsity in the dynamic skewness framework. The closest paper to ours is [8], which uses the spike and slab prior of [30] to estimate the posterior probability of inclusion of static skewness.

## 4. Remaining Priors and Posterior Inference

Our modeling approach involves the following unknown quantities: $\Theta = \mu_h, \phi_h, \sigma_h, \alpha_0, \sigma_\lambda, h_t, \lambda_t$. Our goal is to estimate the joint posterior distribution $p(\Theta|y)$, which, according to Bayes' rule, can be calculated as

$$p(\Theta|y) = \frac{p(y|\Theta)p(\Theta)}{\int p(y|\Theta)p(\Theta)d\Theta}.$$

$p(y|\Theta)$ is the likelihood component being characterized by our proposed sampling model. We consider independent components for each member of $p(\Theta)$. $p(\mu_h)$ and $p(\phi_h)$ follow Gaussian distributions, $p(\sigma_h^2)$ has inverse gamma distribution while $p(\alpha_0)$ and $p(\sigma_\lambda)$ have double exponential distribution, as discussed previously. The exact values for the prior parameters are described in Appendices B and C.

After defining $p(y|\Theta)$ and $p(\Theta)$, we must recover $p(\Theta|y)$. However, $\int p(y|\Theta)p(\Theta)d\Theta$ does not have an analytical solution. Moreover, due to the high dimensionality of $\Theta$, grid-based integration methods are computationally infeasible. Thus, we employ to Markov Chain Monte Carlo (MCMC) methods to sample from $p(\Theta|y)$. In this paper, we use a particular MCMC method, known as HMC, instead of the more traditional Random–Walk Metropolis Hastings (RWMH).

Both HMC and RWMH are MCMC methods. Thus, both methods generate a proposed value for unknown quantities $\Theta^{(i)}$ on each Markov chain iteration i in order to approximate $p(\Theta|y)$. We denote the sequence of $\Theta^{(i)}$ by $\{\Theta^{(i)}\}_{i=1}^{I}$. In our applications, we run our HMC scheme for 30,000 iterations with the first 15000 being used as burn-in draws. HMC and RWMH differ in their approach to generating $\Theta^{(i)}$ from $\Theta^{(i-1)}$. RWMH generates $\Theta^{(i)}$ as a random walk from the previously sampled $\Theta^{i-1}$. In contrast, HMC enhances the process by using guided proposals based on the gradient of the log posterior. This guidance helps direct the Markov chain toward regions of higher posterior density while also sampling tail areas properly, as discussed in [31,32]. Specifically, HMC generates proposals by solving the following Hamiltonian equations:

$$\frac{dq}{dt} = -\frac{\partial H(\Theta,q)}{\partial\Theta} = \nabla_\Theta logp(\Theta|y),$$
$$\frac{d\Theta}{dt} = \frac{\partial H(\Theta,q)}{\partial q} = \frac{\partial K(q)}{\partial q} = M^{-1}q,$$

where $H(\Theta,q)$ represents the Hamilton function. In the context of this paper, $H(\Theta,q) = -logp(\Theta|y) + \frac{1}{2}q^T M^{-1} p$. Additionally, $\nabla_\Theta logp(\Theta|y)$ is the gradient of the log posterior density. Due to $\nabla_\Theta logp(\Theta|y)$, ref. [31] claims that HMC generates guided proposals. We refer readers to [31,32] for a thorough review of HMC methods.

We choose HMC over RWMH for two main reasons. First, due to its more refined method to generate $\Theta^{(i)}$, HMC requires several iterations less than RWMH. This difference becomes even bigger if $\Theta$ is high-dimensional which is the case in this paper. Second, the software Stan verison 1.2, introduced in [33], offers convenient implementation of HMC. In our study, we utilize Stan in conjunction with R through the rStan package introduced in [34] (The codes and data for this project are available on the first author's GitHub page, github.com/igorfbmartins, shortly after publication).

## 5. Empirical Application: Bond Yields

The bond market is one of the largest in the world being key for investors and policy-makers. Most papers focus on the first two moments, e.g., refs. [11,12,35,36]. Our paper focuses on the much less explored third moment. Skewness captures the likely direction of returns allowing for an interest rate investor to improve their forecast about the sign of future yields. Such feature is explored in the literature in at least three ways. First, ref. [5] highlights the role of skewness in forecasting crashes in momentum portfolios. Second, works [37,38] highlight that even monetary 'surprises,' such as the differences between actual policy rates announced by the Federal Open Market Committee (FOMC) and expectations from professional forecasters, can be partially predicted by the option-implied skewness of the 10-year US bond. Third, ref. [17] demonstrates that allowing for skewness improves value-at-risk evaluation for multiple assets.

In our first application, we model the monthly yield changes in fixed 1-year maturity for both American and Brazilian bonds. We sample from the joint posterior via the HMC scheme presented in Section 3 by combining the likelihood implied by our proposed model in Section 2 and the priors described in Appendix B. In both cases, skewness is likely to be time-varying. It is associated with cycles of monetary easing and tightening. It is partially explained by the central bank's mandate and provides valuable information regarding the future direction of yield changes.

The sample of US bonds comes from the updated dataset of [39] made available by the Federal Reserve Board starting on July 1981 and lasting until August 2023. The sample of Brazilian bonds is based on the DI interest rate contracts available on the Brazilian stock and future exchange B3. The DI contracts are interpolated to form 1-year fixed maturity bonds using the same Nelson–Siegel procedure described in [39] resulting in a sample starting in February 2004 and ending in August 2023. Figure 2 plots both time series of monthly yield changes. Notably, both series fluctuate around zero with volatility clusters. Both series hint at the possibility of skewness. For example, the US series presents a persistent and negative yield change period in early 1990 and early 2000. In the Brazilian series, the negative and persistent yield changes are even clearer, with the period from August 2016 to March 2018 being one example.

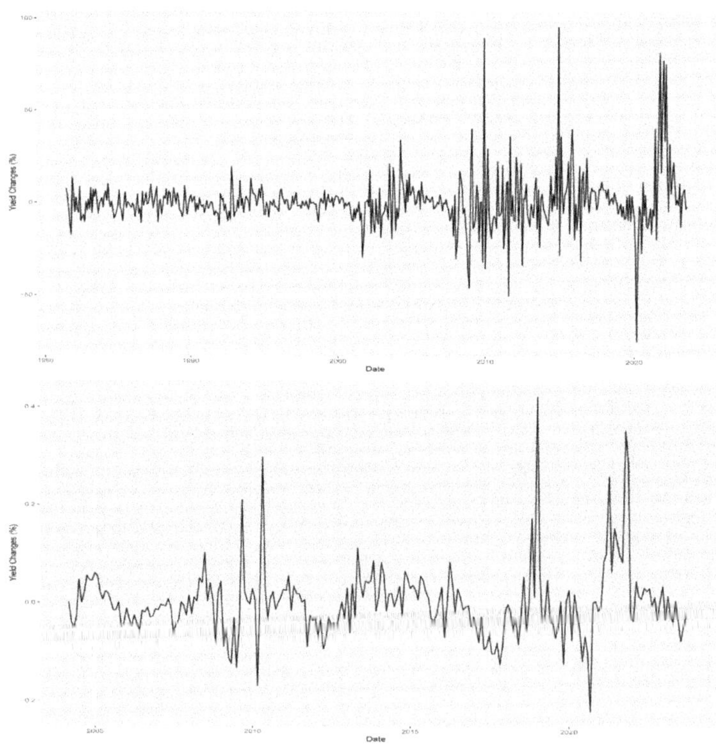

**Figure 2.** Change in yields from fixed 1-year maturity bonds from the US and Brazil. The top panel presents monthly changes in yields from 1-year bonds from the US government starting in July 1981 and lasting up to August 2023. Similarly, the bottom panel shows monthly changes in 1-year Brazilian bonds from February 2004 up to August 2023.

Some might express concern that the guidance provided by central banks regarding future rates entirely dictates yield changes. However, such concerns are unlikely to be substantial for several reasons. First, if central bank communication were the sole determinant of yields for 1-year fixed maturity bonds, yields would instantly adjust to incorporate the information from newly announced paths and persist at that level until subsequent announcements, in line with the efficient market hypothesis. Second, current yields not only reflect the anticipated average future short rate over a bond's lifespan, but also encompass a term premium component. As demonstrated, for instance, in [40,41], this term premium component is likely to be time-varying. Consequently, yields are expected to fluctuate over time even after accounting for the expected future short rate. Third, while central bank communication indeed aids in forecasting future yields, it is by no means the sole source of information, as exemplified in [42].

We apply our proposed model to both US and Brazilian bonds with the priors presented in Appendix B. To account for the Brazilian time series being shorter than the American, the estimation sample comes closer to the present than the American. Precisely, we consider an estimation period which lasts up to December 2018 for the US and up to December 2019 to the Brazilian case. Table 1 presents the posterior summaries for the parameters of both time series. The values of $\phi_h$ indicate high persistence in the log-scale which is reflected in Figure 3 that plots posterior summaries of $\{h_t\}$. In both cases, our approach captures the surges in volatility indicated in Figure 2. For instance, in the US series, our model captures spikes in volatility during the early 2000s and the financial crisis of 2008. Similarly, the Brazilian time series shows a volatility spike in 2008, which our model also captures. Additionally, both series are likely to have a dynamic skewness as shown by the posterior summaries of $\sigma_\lambda$ with the Brazilian bonds having a bigger range of variation for $\lambda_t$ than bonds from the US. This evidence is supported by the posterior summaries of $\{\lambda_t\}$ in Figure 4 as well.

Figure 5 plots the posterior mean of $\{\lambda_t\}$ alongside monetary easing–tightening cycles. The green shaded areas represent periods of monetary easing characterized by interest rate cuts implemented by the countries' central banks. Conversely, the red shaded areas represent periods of monetary tightening marked by interest rate hikes. Our approach identifies negative skewness in yield changes during easing periods and large positive skewness when a central bank is hiking interest rates. The monetary policy cycles for the US are based on the FED effective fund rate, while for the Brazilian case, they are derived from the target rate policy decisions of each meeting (Brazilian target policy rate is available at https://www.bcb.gov.br/controleinflacao/historicotaxasjuros (accessed on 28 November 2023)).

**Table 1.** Posterior summaries of the parameters from our proposed model. $\mu_h$, $\phi_h$ and $\sigma_h$ represent the log-scale level, persistence and standard deviation, respectively. $\sigma_\lambda$ captures the dynamic of the skewness component and $\alpha_0$ is the initial level of the skewness. Both series are likely to have a dynamic skewness as shown by the posterior summaries of $\sigma_\lambda$ with the Brazilian bonds having a bigger range of skewness variation than bonds from the US.

| | $\mu_h$ | $\phi_h$ | $\sigma_h$ | $\sigma_\lambda$ | $\alpha_0$ |
|---|---|---|---|---|---|
| US q05 | 2.94 | 0.92 | 0.32 | 0.09 | −0.62 |
| US Mean | 3.88 | 0.96 | 0.42 | 0.17 | −0.06 |
| US q95 | 4.84 | 0.99 | 0.55 | 0.27 | 0.42 |
| BR q05 | 2.59 | 0.59 | 0.38 | 0.63 | −2.67 |
| BR Mean | 3.08 | 0.79 | 0.63 | 1.09 | −0.46 |
| BR q95 | 3.59 | 0.94 | 0.91 | 1.75 | 0.79 |

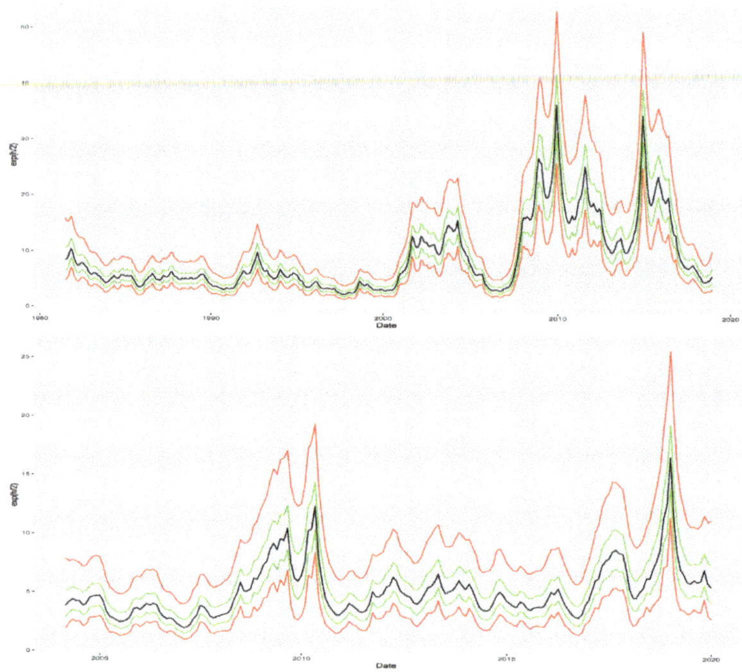


**Figure 3.** Scale recovered for the US and Brazilian bonds during the estimation period which lasts up to December 2018 for the US and up to December 2019 for the Brazilian case. Green lines represent quantiles 0.25 and 0.75 while solid red lines represent quantiles 0.05 and 0.95. For both series, time-varying volatility is plausible. Top panel indicates rises in yield change volatility during the early 2000s and around the global financial crisis for the US, while the bottom panel indicate peaks of volatility for Brazilian yield changes between 2009 to 2010 with a second spike in late 2018 and early 2019.

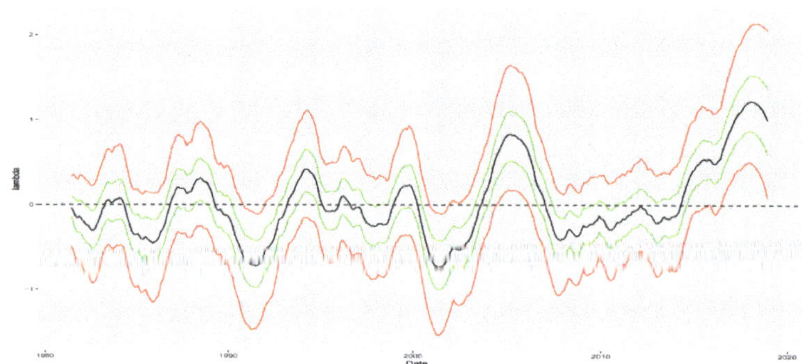


**Figure 4.** *Cont.*

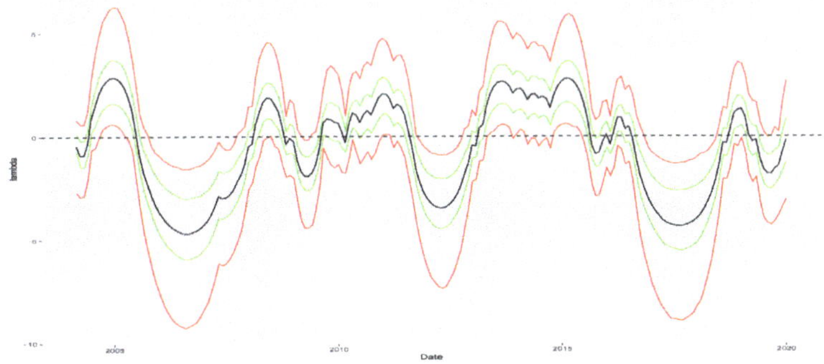


**Figure 4.** $\{\lambda_t\}$ recovered for the US and Brazilian bonds during the estimation period which lasts up to December 2018 for the US and up to December 2019 for the Brazilian case. While $\lambda$ is not the skewness itself, it can be transformed by using the formula in Appendix A. Green lines represent quantiles 0.25 and 0.75 while solid red lines represent quantiles 0.05 and 0.95. Time-varying skewness is likely in both cases. We obtain stronger evidence of dynamic skewness for Brazil in the bottom panel than for the US in the top one.

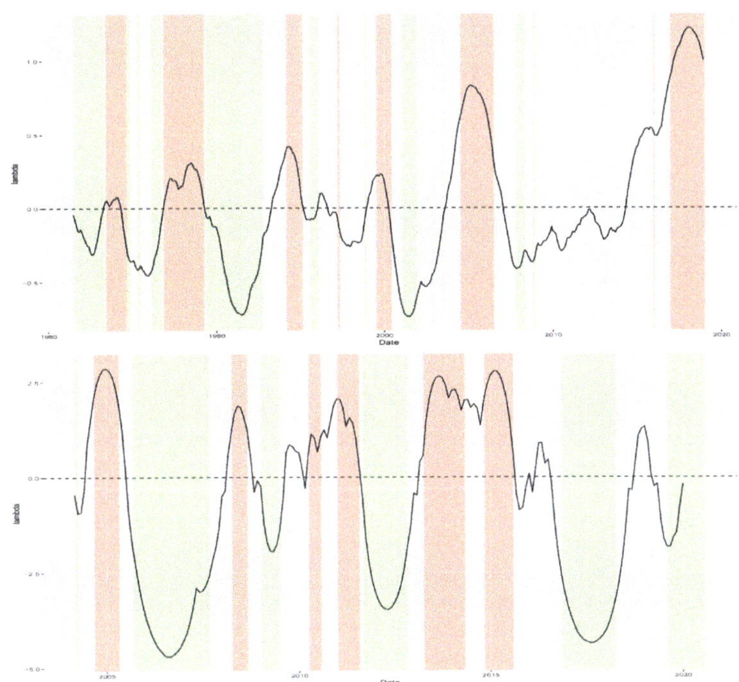


**Figure 5.** $\{\lambda_t\}$ recovered for the US, top panel, and Brazilian bonds, bottom panel, during the estimation period which lasts up to December 2018 for the US and up to December 2019 for the Brazilian case. Green shaded area indicate monetary easing periods while red ones indicate monetary tightening. In both cases, $\lambda_t$ seems able to capture the monetary cycles and reflect future direction of yield change. US monetary police cycles are based on the FED effective fund rate, while for the Brazilian case they are recovered from the target rate policy rate decision of each meeting.

If the asymmetry of yield changes is connected to interest rate cycles, then drivers of the monetary policy should help explain skewness. We test this hypothesis by regressing the posterior mean of $\{\lambda_t\}$, denoted $\hat{\lambda}$, into inflation and unemployment as represented by

Equation (14). Both variables are reasonable ex-ante since central banks have mandates of price stability and full employment.

$$\hat{\lambda}_t \sim N(X\beta, \sigma^2) \text{ with } X = [1, Inflation_t, Unemployment_t]. \tag{14}$$

Table 2 indicates that unemployment levels partially explain the asymmetry in yield changes for both countries. The negative sign of $\beta_{unemployment}$ is reasonable since central banks typically address high unemployment levels by implementing interest rate cuts to encourage consumption, and, as shown in Figure 5, easing cycles are associated with negative skewness on yield changes. Moreover, in the case of Brazil, inflation is likely to also influence this asymmetry. The positive sign of $\beta_{inflation}$ aligns with central banks' tendency to counter inflation surges by raising interest rates. As illustrated in Figure 5, this is associated with higher values of skewness. Regarding the US, although inflation posed challenges in the late 1970s and early 1980s, for most of our estimation sample, the American economy did not face significant inflationary pressures. Consequently, yields did not react substantially to inflation. Therefore, the nearly zero effect of $\beta_\lambda$ is justifiable.

**Table 2.** Linear regression of the posterior mean of $\{\lambda_t\}$ into inflation and unemployment during the estimation sample. For both countries, unemployment partially explains the skewness in yield changes, while the asymmetry in the Brazilian case is also partially explained by inflation.

| | Intercept | $\beta_{Inflation}$ | $\beta_{Unemployment}$ |
|---|---|---|---|
| US q05 | 0.39 | −0.01 | −0.11 |
| US mean | 0.58 | 0.00 | −0.09 |
| US q95 | 0.73 | 0.01 | −0.06 |
| BR q05 | −0.72 | 1.16 | −0.35 |
| BR mean | 0.39 | 2.47 | −0.23 |
| BR q95 | 1.57 | 3.52 | −0.09 |

We also evaluate the out-of-sample performance of our proposed model. If skewness is informative about the likely direction of changes in bond yields, then $sign(E_t\hat{\lambda}_{t+1})$ should agree with $sign(y_{t+1})$. We verify this claim within an increasing window framework, where the initial window corresponds to the estimation sample. For each window, we execute our HMC procedure and obtain $sign(E_t\hat{\lambda}_{t+1})$. Table 3 presents our findings. For US bonds, we observe that $sign(y_{t+1})$ matches $sign(E_t\lambda_{t+1})$ in 66.1% of cases, with an average change of 20.6% when correctly forecasted and only 8.7% when incorrect. Similarly, in the case of Brazilian bonds, $sign(y_{t+1})$ aligns with $sign(E_t[\lambda_{t+1}])$ in 72.7% of instances. Moreover, the average magnitude of correctly predicted yield changes is 8.2%, while it is only 2.4% when the prediction is incorrect. Therefore, out-of-sample analysis supports our assertion that dynamic skewness in bond yield changes serves as a predictive variable for future yield changes. Furthermore, we compare our results with skewness-based forecasts using GAS models via the implementation of [43] (check https://cran.r-project.org/web/packages/GAS/ (accessed on 20 November 2023)). While our proposal demonstrates similar performance to those of GAS models in the US case, it outperforms GAS in the Brazilian case. Thus, for our dataset, our proposed model not only predicts the future direction of yield changes, but also shows improvements over GAS models.

**Table 3.** If bond yield skewness captures the likely direction of yield changes, then we should expected yield increases when $E_t[\lambda_{t+1}] > 0$ and, otherwise, decreases. Our model provides evidence supporting such claims. In both cases, our model correctly predicts the correct yield change direction in at least 66.1% of times.

| | Proposal US (%) | GAS US (%) | Proposal Brazil (%) | GAS Brazil (%) |
|---|---|---|---|---|
| Hit Ratio | 66.1 | 64.3 | 72.7 | 54.5 |
| Avg when right | 20.6 | 20.7 | 8.2 | 7.8 |
| Avg when wrong | 8.7 | 8.8 | 2.4 | 5.2 |

## 6. Empirical Application: Carry Factor

In addition to the bond yield application detailed in Section 5, we explore application in the currency market. According to [44], two factors—dollar factor and carry—account for the cross-section of currency returns. Our focus is on the latter factor, which captures interest rate differentials between countries. It involves taking long positions on countries with high interest rate differentials relative to the US and short positions on countries with the smallest differentials. While our emphasis is on the FX markets, ref. [45] argues that carry-based factors can effectively explain the cross-section of various asset classes, including commodities and equities. For this analysis, we consider and update a sample of the carry factor described in [44] (readers can check out Lustig's carry factor on gsb-faculty.stanford.edu/hanno-lustig/files/2022/05/CurrencyPortfolios.xls), presented in Figure 6, which starts on November 1983 and lasts up to May 2021.

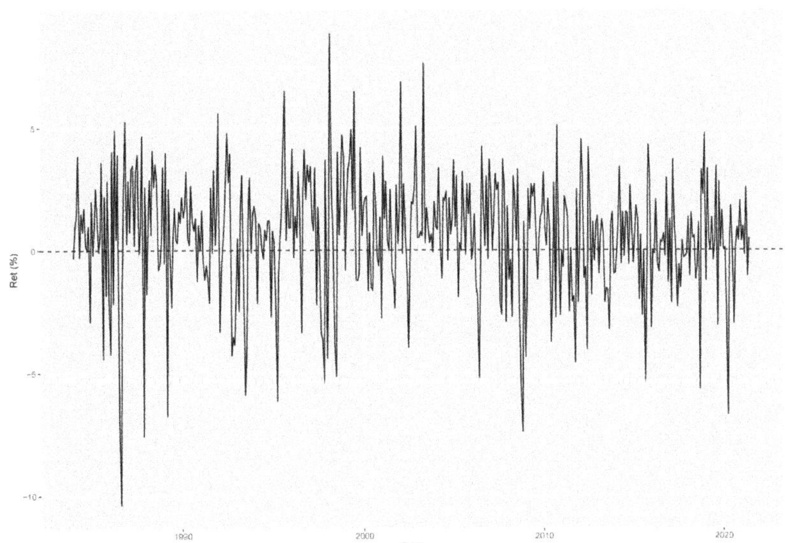


**Figure 6.** Updated version of the time series for the Carry factor introduced in [44]. Our sample lasts from November 1983 to May 2021.

We are not the first to study the skewness of carry returns. For example, refs. [10,13] identify a time-varying crash risk on the carry factor. This risk materializes in some occasions leading to large negative returns to the carry factor and skewing its distribution to the left. Conversely, ref. [14] uses out-of-the-money currency options hedging against large crashes and shows that carry remains profitable, indicating a small role for tail risk on currency returns. Additionally, ref. [14] presents evidence in favor of time varying volatility for carry returns and that the largest negative return of its sample, October 2008, occurs in a period of high volatility. Our model is well suited to evaluate such claims. Ref. [14] is not an isolated case. Ref. [6] provides another example of tail risk mitigation in tradeable factors after accounting for volatility without skewness playing a major role.

We consider the prior specification shown in Appendix C and sample from the posterior using the HMC scheme described in Section 4. Figure 7 plots the posterior mean (black), interquartile range (green) and q05-q95 interval (red) for both $\{exp\left(\frac{h_t}{2}\right)\}$ and $\{\lambda_t\}$ which are shown at the top and bottom panel, respectively. The top panel corroborates the evidence of time-varying volatility with a surge in volatility around October 2008 similarly to the description in [14]. The bottom panel indicates that it is likely that there is no skewness at all after accounting for stochastic volatility.

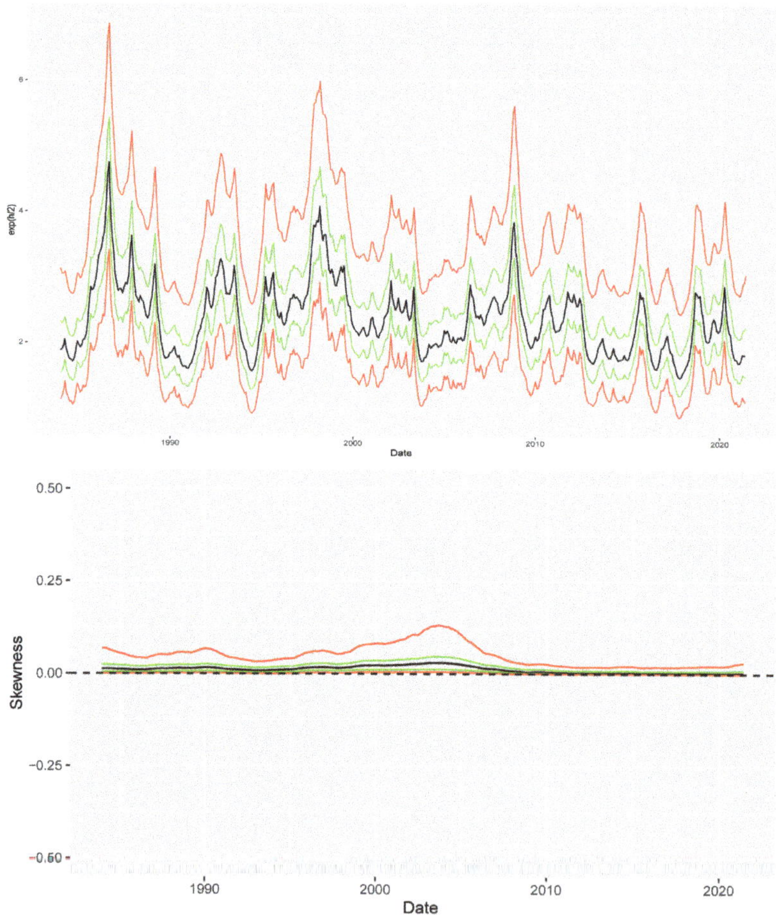


**Figure 7.** Skewness recovered from the carry factor. Green lines represent quantiles 0.25 and 0.75 while solid red lines represent quantiles 0.05 and 0.95. After controlling for volatility, we find no evidence of skewness in the carry factor.

Additionally, we assess the performance of the carry factor during periods of high volatility compared to low volatility. We say that volatility is high if it is above the average volatility recovered for the full sample and we say it is low otherwise. Table 4 reports the results of our analysis. The average return for the carry factor is the same in both environments. However, crash indicators such as the return on the fifth percentile and minimum return exhibit significant improvements. Therefore, in combination with the results shown in Figure 7, our results indicate that after accounting for volatility, it is unlikely that skewness plays a large role in affecting the returns of the carry factor.

**Table 4.** Summary statistics of the carry factor in high- and low-volatility environments for the sample starting in November 1983 and lasting up to December 2021. While the average return for the carry factor in both environments is the same, crash indicators such as the return on the 5th percentile and minimum return are severely improved.

| | High Vol | Low Vol |
|---|---|---|
| Mean | 0.58 | 0.57 |
| Sd | 3.34 | 1.41 |
| Q05 | −5.38 | −2.07 |
| Min | −10.38 | −3.21 |

## 7. Conclusions

This paper expands stochastic volatility models by allowing for time-varying skewness without having to impose it. By considering a LASSO-type regularization for both the standard deviation and the starting level of the skewness dynamics, our model selects among dynamic, static, and no skewness in a data-driven approach. In our bond yield application, we highlight the benefits of dynamic skewness by demonstrating its connection to monetary easing/tightening cycles and central banks' mandates. Additionally, we show that asymmetry provides information about the likely direction of future bond yield changes. In the second application, we shed light on the debate of carry average returns reflecting time-varying skewness versus no skewness but time-varying volatility. Our model indicates no skewness after accounting for stochastic volatility.

**Author Contributions:** Author Contributions: Conceptualization, I.M. and H.F.L.; Methodology, I.M. and H.F.L.; Software, I.M. All authors have read and agreed to the published version of the manuscript.

**Funding:** Hedibert F. Lopes receives support from FAPESP (Fundação de Amparo à Pesquisa do Estado de São Paulo) through Grant 2023/02538-0.

**Data Availability Statement:** Data used in this project is available at the first author's GitHub page: github.com/igorfbmartins.

**Conflicts of Interest:** The authors declare no conflict of interest.

## Appendix A. Moments of a Skew Normal Distribution

Following [15,46], $\xi$, $\omega$ and $\lambda$ relate to mean, variance and skewness by the following expressions:

If $Z \sim SN(\xi, \omega, \lambda)$, then

$$E[Z] = \xi + \sqrt{\omega}\delta\sqrt{\frac{2}{\pi}},$$

$$Var[Z] = \omega\left(1 - \frac{2}{\pi}\delta^2\right),$$

$$\gamma = \sqrt{\frac{2}{\pi}}\left(\frac{4}{\pi} - 1\right)\left(\frac{\lambda}{\sqrt{1+\lambda^2}}\right)^3\left(1 - \frac{2}{\pi}\frac{\lambda^2}{1+\lambda^2}\right)^{3/2},$$

where $\delta = \frac{\lambda}{\sqrt{1+\lambda^2}}$ and $\gamma$ is the skewness index. We note that $\gamma$ depends only on $\lambda$.

## Appendix B. Priors and Additional Results for the Bond Applications

We consider the following structure for bond yield applications:

$$\mu_h \sim N(4, 10^2),$$
$$\phi_h \sim N(0.95, 0.5^2),$$
$$\sigma \sim IG(0.1, 0.1),$$
$$\alpha_0 \sim DoubleExp(0, 1/\kappa_\alpha),$$
$$\sigma_\lambda \sim DoubleExp(0, 1/\kappa_{\sigma_\lambda}),$$
$$\kappa_\alpha \sim Gamma(0.1, 0.1),$$
$$\kappa_{\sigma_\lambda} \sim Gamma(0.1, 0.1).$$

This prior scheme reflects vague beliefs. $\mu_h \sim N(4, 10^2)$ implies an expected volatility level of $exp(4/2) =\approx$ 7.4%; however, the large standard deviation implies a vague belief for this parameter. $\phi_h$ with an expected value of 0.95 indicates a high persistence in volatility which is common in the SV literature. $\sigma$ following an IG reflects the restriction of the variance being non-negative. $\alpha_0$ and $\sigma_\lambda$ following Double exponential reflect our sparsity-inducing approach to the random walk variance and initial state for the skewness parameter. Gamma priors for $\kappa_\alpha$ and $\kappa_{\sigma_\lambda}$ impose non-negative values for the scale of the double exponential.

Also, Figure A1 plots the skewness itself using green and red shades to indicate easing and tightening periods in addition to the posterior for $\{\lambda_t\}$. While conclusions are the same, the version with skewness may help the reader to make a better assessment of the magnitude of skewness in each period.

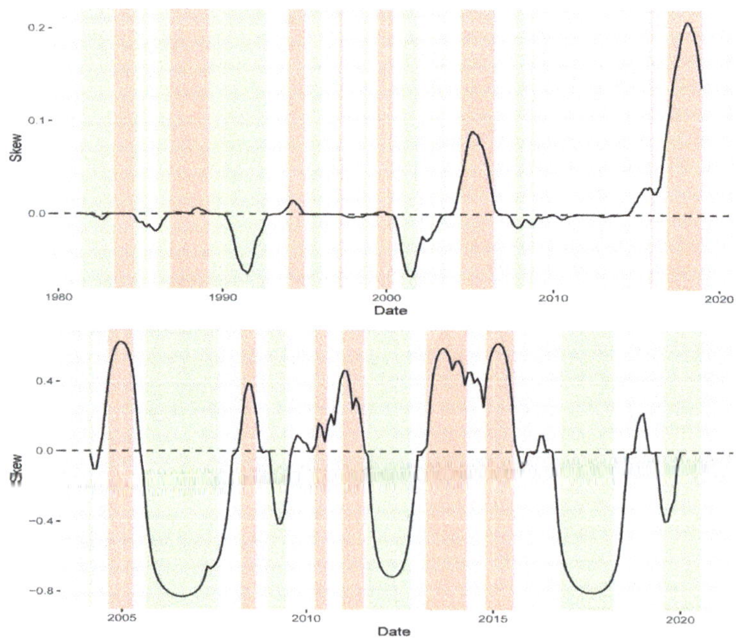


**Figure A1.** Skewness recovered based on the posterior median of $\{\lambda_t\}$ for the US, top panel, and Brazilian bonds, bottom panel, during the estimation period which lasts up to December 2018 for the

US and up to December 2019 for the Brazilian case. Green shaded areas indicate monetary easing periods while red ones indicate monetary tightening. US monetary police cycles are based on the FED fund effective rate changes, while for the Brazilian case they are recovered from the target rate policy rate decision of each meeting. In both countries, positive skewness is associated with tight monetary policy periods, while negative skewness is connected to easing cycles.

## Appendix C. Priors for the FX Application

We consider the following structure for the fx applications:

$$\mu_h \sim N(4, 10^2),$$
$$\phi_h \sim N(0.95, 0.5^2),$$
$$\sigma_h \sim IG(2, 2),$$
$$\alpha_0 \sim DoubleExp(0, 1/\kappa_\alpha),$$
$$\sigma_\lambda \sim DoubleExp(0, 1/\kappa_{\sigma_\lambda}),$$
$$\kappa_\alpha \sim Gamma(0.1, 0.1),$$
$$\kappa_{\sigma_\lambda} \sim Gamma(0.1, 0.1).$$

We note that our apporach for FX application reflects vague priors similarly to the bond yield case. Again, $\mu_h \sim N(4, 10^2)$ implies an expected volatility level of $exp(4/2) =\approx 7.4\%$; however, the large standard deviation implies a vague belief for this parameter. $\phi_h$ with an expected value of 0.95 indicates a high persistence in volatility, which is common in SV literature. $\sigma$ following an IG reflects the restriction of the variance being non-negative. $\alpha_0$ and $\sigma_\lambda$ following Double exponential reflect our sparsity-inducing approach to the random walk variance and initial state for the skewness parameter. Gamma priors for $\kappa_\alpha$ and $\kappa_{\sigma_\lambda}$ impose non-negative values for the scale of the double exponential.

## References


1. Markowitz, H. Portfolio selection. *J. Financ.* **1952**, *7*, 77–91.
2. Hansen, L.P.; Richard, S.F. The role of conditioning information in deducing testable restrictions implied by dynamic asset pricing models. *Econom. J. Econom. Soc.* **1987**, *55*, 587–613. [CrossRef]
3. Jacquier, E.; Polson, N.G.; Rossi, P.E. Bayesian analysis of stochastic volatility models. *J. Bus. Econ. Stat.* **2002**, *20*, 69–87. [CrossRef]
4. Shephard, N. *Stochastic Volatility: Selected Readings*; OUP: Oxford, UK, 2005.
5. Bianchi, D.; De Polis, A.; Petrella, I. Taming Momentum Crashes. Available online: https://ssrn.com/abstract=4182040 (accessed on 14 January 2023).
6. Barroso, P.; Santa-Clara, P. Momentum has its moments. *J. Financ. Econ.* **2015**, *116*, 111–120. [CrossRef]
7. Nakajima, J.; Omori, Y. Stochastic volatility model with leverage and asymmetrically heavy-tailed error using GH skew Student's t-distribution. *Comput. Stat. Data Anal.* **2012**, *56*, 3690–3704. [CrossRef]
8. Nakajima, J. Skew selection for factor stochastic volatility models. *J. Appl. Stat.* **2020**, *47*, 582–601. [CrossRef]
9. Trolle, A.B.; Schwartz, E.S. The swaption cube. *Rev. Financ. Stud.* **2014**, *27*, 2307–2353. [CrossRef]
10. Rafferty, B. Currency returns, skewness and crash risk. *SSRN Electron. J.* **2012**. [CrossRef]
11. Litterman, R.B.; Scheinkman, J. Common factors affecting bond returns. *J. Fixed Income* **1991**, *1*, 54–61. [CrossRef]
12. Joslin, S. Can unspanned stochastic volatility models explain the cross section of bond volatilities? *Manag. Sci.* **2018**, *64*, 1707–1726. [CrossRef]
13. Burnside, C.; Eichenbaum, M.; Kleshchelski, I.; Rebelo, S. Do peso problems explain the returns to the carry trade? *Rev. Financ. Stud.* **2011**, *24*, 853–891. [CrossRef]
14. Jurek, J.W. Crash-neutral currency carry trades. *J. Financ. Econ.* **2014**, *113*, 325–347. [CrossRef]
15. Azzalini, A. A class of distributions which includes the normal ones. *Scand. J. Stat.* **1985**, *12*, 171–178.
16. Azzalini, A. *The Skew-Normal and Related Families*; Cambridge University Press: Cambridge, UK, 2013; Volume 3.
17. Li, M.; Scharth, M. Leverage, asymmetry and heavy tails in the high-dimensional factor stochastic volatility model. *J. Bus. Econ. Stat.* **2020**, *40*, 281–301. [CrossRef]
18. Creal, D.; Koopman, S.J.; Lucas, A. Generalized autoregressive score models with applications. *J. Appl. Econom.* **2013**, *28*, 777–795. [CrossRef]

19. Harvey, A.C. *Dynamic Models for Volatility and Heavy Tails: With Applications to Financial and Economic Time Series*; Cambridge University Press: Cambridge, UK, 2013; Volume 52.
20. Vieira, L.I.; Laurini, M.P. Time-varying higher moments in Bitcoin. *Digit. Financ.* **2023**, *5*, 231–260. [CrossRef]
21. Rachev, S.T.; Menn, C.; Fabozzi, F.J. *Fat-Tailed and Skewed Asset Return Distributions: Implications for Risk Management, Portfolio Selection, and Option Pricing*; John Wiley & Sons: Hoboken, NJ, USA, 2005.
22. Turkman, M.A.A.; Paulino, C.D.; Müller, P. *Computational Bayesian statistics: An introduction*; Cambridge University Press: Cambridge, UK, 2019; Volume 11.
23. Lopes, H.F. A Tutorial on the Computation of Bayes Factor. 2014. Available online: http://repositorio.insper.edu.br/handle/11224/5960 (accessed on 14 January 2024).
24. Tibshirani, R. Regression shrinkage and selection via the lasso. *J. R. Stat. Soc. Ser. B (Methodol.)* **1996**, *58*, 267–288. [CrossRef]
25. Park, T.; Casella, G. The bayesian lasso. *J. Am. Stat. Assoc.* **2008**, *103*, 681–686. [CrossRef]
26. Frühwirth-Schnatter, S.; Wagner, H. Stochastic model specification search for Gaussian and partial non-Gaussian state space models. *J. Econom.* **2010**, *154*, 85–100. [CrossRef]
27. Belmonte, M.A.; Koop, G.; Korobilis, D. Hierarchical shrinkage in time-varying parameter models. *J. Forecast.* **2014**, *33*, 80–94. [CrossRef]
28. Bitto, A.; Frühwirth-Schnatter, S. Achieving shrinkage in a time-varying parameter model framework. *J. Econom.* **2019**, *210*, 75–97. [CrossRef]
29. Lopes, H.F.; McCulloch, R.E.; Tsay, R.S. Parsimony inducing priors for large scale state–space models. *J. Econom.* **2022**, *230*, 39–61. [CrossRef]
30. George, E.I.; McCulloch, R.E. Variable selection via Gibbs sampling. *J. Am. Stat. Assoc.* **1993**, *88*, 881–889. [CrossRef]
31. Betancourt, M. A conceptual introduction to Hamiltonian Monte Carlo. *arXiv* **2017**, arXiv:1701.02434.
32. Thomas, S.; Tu, W. Learning hamiltonian monte carlo in r. *Am. Stat.* **2021**, *75*, 403–413. [CrossRef]
33. Carpenter, B.; Gelman, A.; Hoffman, M.D.; Lee, D.; Goodrich, B.; Betancourt, M.; Brubaker, M.A.; Guo, J.; Li, P.; Riddell, A. Stan: A probabilistic programming language. *J. Stat. Softw.* **2017**, *76*, 1. [CrossRef]
34. Guo, J.; Gabry, J.; Goodrich, B.; Weber, S. Package 'rstan'. 2020. Available online: https://cran.râĂŢproject.org/web/packages/rstan/ (accessed on 28 November 2023).
35. Collin-Dufresne, P.; Goldstein, R.S. Do bonds span the fixed income markets? Theory and evidence for unspanned stochastic volatility. *J. Financ.* **2002**, *57*, 1685–1730. [CrossRef]
36. Cochrane, J.H.; Piazzesi, M. Bond risk premia. *Am. Econ. Rev.* **2005**, *95*, 138–160. [CrossRef]
37. Bauer, M.D.; Swanson, E.T. A reassessment of monetary policy surprises and high-frequency identification. *NBER Macroecon. Annu.* **2023**, *37*, 87–155. [CrossRef]
38. Cieslak, A.; McMahon, M. Tough Talk: The Fed and the Risk Premium. 2023. Avaliable online: https://ssrn.com/abstract=4560220 (accessed on 14 January 2024).
39. Gürkaynak, R.S.; Sack, B.; Wright, J.H. The US Treasury yield curve: 1961 to the present. *J. Monet. Econ.* **2007**, *54*, 2291–2304. [CrossRef]
40. Cieslak, A.; Povala, P. Expected returns in Treasury bonds. *Rev. Financ. Stud.* **2015**, *28*, 2859–2901. [CrossRef]
41. Adrian, T.; Crump, R.K.; Moench, E. Pricing the term structure with linear regressions. *J. Financ. Econ.* **2013**, *110*, 110–138. [CrossRef]
42. de Andrade Alves, C.R.; Joseph Abraham, K.; Poletti Laurini, M. Can Brazilian Central Bank Communication help to predict the yield curve? *J. Forecast.* **2023**, *42*, 1429–1444. [CrossRef]
43. Ardia, D.; Boudt, K.; Catania, L. Generalized Autoregressive Score Models in R: The GAS Package. *J. Stat. Softw.* **2019**, *88*, 1–28. [CrossRef]
44. Lustig, H.; Roussanov, N.; Verdelhan, A. Common risk factors in currency markets. *Rev. Financ. Stud.* **2011**, *24*, 3731–3777. [CrossRef]
45. Koijen, R.S.; Moskowitz, T.J.; Pedersen, L.H.; Vrugt, E.B. Carry. *J. Financ. Econ.* **2018**, *127*, 197–225. [CrossRef]
46. Bayes, C.L.; Branco, M.D. Bayesian inference for the skewness parameter of the scalar skew normal distribution. *Braz. J. Probab. Stat.* **2007**, *21*, 141–163.

*entropy*

MDPI

*Article*

# Bayesian Non-Parametric Inference for Multivariate Peaks-over-Threshold Models

**Peter Trubey * and Bruno Sansó**

Department of Statistics, University of California, Santa Cruz, CA 95064, USA; bsanso@ucsc.edu
* Correspondence: ptrubey@ucsc.edu

**Abstract:** We consider a constructive definition of the multivariate Pareto that factorizes the random vector into a radial component and an independent angular component. The former follows a univariate Pareto distribution, and the latter is defined on the surface of the positive orthant of the infinity norm unit hypercube. We propose a method for inferring the distribution of the angular component by identifying its support as the limit of the positive orthant of the unit $p$-norm spheres and introduce a projected gamma family of distributions defined through the normalization of a vector of independent random gammas to the space. This serves to construct a flexible family of distributions obtained as a Dirichlet process mixture of projected gammas. For model assessment, we discuss scoring methods appropriate to distributions on the unit hypercube. In particular, working with the energy score criterion, we develop a kernel metric that produces a proper scoring rule and presents a simulation study to compare different modeling choices using the proposed metric. Using our approach, we describe the dependence structure of extreme values in the integrated vapor transport (IVT), data describing the flow of atmospheric moisture along the coast of California. We find clear but heterogeneous geographical dependence.

**Keywords:** multivariate extremes; peak over threshold models; bayesian non-parametric models; dirichlet process mixtures

## 1. Introduction

The statistical analysis of extreme values focuses on inferences for rare events that correspond to the tails of probability distributions. As such, it is a key ingredient in the risk assessment of phenomena that can have strong societal impacts like floods, heat waves, high concentration of pollutants, crashes in the financial markets, among others. The fundamental challenge of extreme value theory (EVT) is to use information, collected over limited periods of time, to extrapolate to long time horizons. This sets EVT apart from most of statistical inference, where the focus is on the bulk of the distribution. Extrapolation to the tails of the distributions is possible thanks to theoretical results that give asymptotic descriptions of the probability distributions of extreme values.

Inferential methods for the extreme values of univariate observations are well established, and software is widely available; see, for example, [1]. For variables in one dimension, the application of EVT methods considers the asymptotic distribution of either the maxima calculated for regular blocks of data, or the values that exceed a certain threshold. The former leads to a generalized extreme value (GEV) distribution that depends on three parameters. The latter leads to a generalized Pareto (GP) distribution, which depends on a shape and a scale parameter. Likelihood-based approaches to inference can be readily implemented in both cases. In the multivariate case, the GEV theory is well developed; see, for example, [2], but the inferential problem is complicated by the fact that there is no parametric representation of the GEV. This problem is inherited by the peaks over threshold (PoT) approach and compounded by the fact that there is no unique definition of an exceedance of a multivariate threshold, as there is an obvious dependence on the norm that is used to measure the size of a vector.

During the last decade or so, much work has been done in the exploration of the definition and properties of an appropriate generalization of the univariate GP distribution to a multivariate setting. To mention some of the papers on the topic, the work of [3] defines the generalized Pareto distribution, with further analysis of these classes of distributions presented in [4,5]. A recent review of the state of the art in multivariate peaks over threshold modeling using generalized Pareto is provided in [6] while [7] provides insight on the theoretical properties of possible parametrizations. These are used in [8] for likelihood-based models for PoT estimation. A frequently used method for describing dependence in multivariate distributions is to use a copula. Refs. [9,10] provide successful examples of this approach in an EVT framework.

Ref. [11] presents a constructive definition of the Pareto process, which generalizes the GP to an infinite-dimensional setting. It consists of decomposing the process into independent radial and angular components. Such an approach can be used in the finite-dimensional case, where the angular component contains information pertaining to the dependence structure of the random vector. Based on this definition, we present a novel approach for modeling the angular component with families of distributions that provide flexibility and can be applied in a moderately large dimensional setting. Our focus on the angular measure is similar to that in [12–14], which consider Bayesian non-parametric approaches. Yet, our approach differs in that it is established in the peaks-over-threshold regime and uses a constructive definition of the multivariate GP based on the infinity norm. The approach proposed in this paper adds to the growing literature on Bayesian models for multivariate extreme value analysis (see, for example, [12–15]), providing a model that has strong computational advantages due its structural simplicitly, achieves flexibility using a mixture model, and scales well to moderately large dimensions.

The remainder of this paper is outlined as follows. Section 2 comprises a brief review of multivariate PoT, detailing the separation of the radial measure from the angular measure. Section 3 details our approach for estimating the angular measure, based on transforming an arbitrary distribution supported in $\mathbb{R}^d_+$ onto unit hyper-spheres defined by $p$-norms. Section 4 develops criteria for model selection in the support of the angular measure. Section 5 explores the efficacy of the proposed approach on a set of simulated data, and, acknowledging the relevance of extreme value theory to climatological events [16–18], estimates the extremal dependence structure for a measure of water vapor flow in the atmosphere, used for identifying atmospheric rivers. Finally, Section 6 presents our conclusions and discussion.

Throughout the paper, we adopt the operators $\wedge$ to denote minima and the $\vee$ to denote maxima. Thus $\wedge_i s_i = \min_i s_i$, and $\vee_i s_i = \max_i s_i$. These operators can also be applied component-wise between vectors such as $\boldsymbol{a} \wedge \boldsymbol{b} = (a_1 \wedge b_1, a_2 \wedge b_2, \ldots)$. Similarly, we apply inequality and arithmetic operators operators to vectors. For example, $\boldsymbol{a} \leq \boldsymbol{b}$, and interpret them component-wise. We use uppercase to indicate random variables, lowercase to indicate points, and bold-face to indicate vectors or matrices thereof.

## 2. A Multivariate PoT Model

To develop a multivariate PoT model for extreme values, consider a $d$-dimensional random vector $\boldsymbol{W} = (W_1, \ldots, W_d)$ with cumulative distribution $F$. A common assumption on $\boldsymbol{W}$ is that it is in the so-called domain of attraction of a multivariate max-stable distribution, $G$. Thus, following [7], assume that there exists sequences of vectors $\boldsymbol{a}_n$ and $\boldsymbol{b}_n$, such that $\lim_{n\to\infty} F^n(\boldsymbol{a}_n \boldsymbol{w} + \boldsymbol{b}_n) = G(\boldsymbol{w})$. $G$ is a $d$-variate generalized extreme value distribution. Notice that, even though the univariate marginals are obtained from a three-parameter family, there is no parametric form to represent $G$. Taking logarithms and expanding, we have that

$$\lim_{n\to\infty} n(1 - F(\boldsymbol{a}_n \boldsymbol{w} + \boldsymbol{b}_n)) = -\log G(\boldsymbol{w}),$$

$\forall \boldsymbol{w} \in \mathbb{R}^d$ such that $G(\boldsymbol{w}) > 0$. It follows that

$$\lim_{n\to\infty} \Pr\left[\boldsymbol{a}_n^{-1}(\boldsymbol{W} - \boldsymbol{b}_n) \le \boldsymbol{w} \mid \boldsymbol{W} \not\le \boldsymbol{b}_n)\right] = \frac{\log G(\boldsymbol{w}\wedge \boldsymbol{0}) - \log G(\boldsymbol{w})}{\log G(\boldsymbol{0})} = H(\boldsymbol{w}),$$

where $\boldsymbol{a}_n^{-1}$ indicates element-wise inversion, and $\{\boldsymbol{W} \not\le \boldsymbol{b}_n\}$ denotes the set where at least one coordinate is above the corresponding component of $\boldsymbol{b}_n$. $H$ is a multivariate Pareto distribution. It corresponds to a joint distribution conditional on exceeding a multivariate threshold. $H$ is defined by a non-parametric function governing the multivariate dependence and two $d$-dimensional vectors of parameters that control the shapes and scales of the marginals. We denote these as $\boldsymbol{\xi}$ for the shapes and $\boldsymbol{\sigma}$ for the scales. Ref. [7] provides a number of stochastic representations for $H$. In this paper, we focus on a particular one that is proposed in [11]. To this end, we denote as $Z$ a random variable with distribution $H$ where $\boldsymbol{\xi} = 1$ and $\boldsymbol{\sigma} = 0$. Then, $\boldsymbol{Z} = R\boldsymbol{V}$ where $R$ and $\boldsymbol{V}$ are independent. $R = \|\boldsymbol{Z}\|_\infty = \vee_{i=1}^d Z_i$ is distributed as a standard Pareto random variable, and $\boldsymbol{V} = \boldsymbol{Z}/\|\boldsymbol{Z}\|_\infty$ is a random vector in $\mathbb{S}_\infty^{d-1}$, the positive orthant of the unit sphere under $\mathcal{L}_\infty$ norm, with distribution $\Phi$. This representation is central to the methods proposed in this paper. $R$ and $\boldsymbol{V}$ are referred to, respectively, as the *radial* and *angular* components of $H$. The angular measure controls the dependence structure of $\boldsymbol{Z}$ in the tails. In view of this, to obtain a PoT model, we seek a flexible model for the distribution of $\boldsymbol{V} \in \mathbb{S}_\infty^{d-1}$, based on a Bayesian non-parametric model.

The approach considered in [6] focuses on the limiting conditional distribution $H$. An alternative approach to obtaining a limiting PoT distribution consists of assuming that regular variation (see, for example, [19]) holds for the limiting distribution of $\boldsymbol{W}$, implying that

$$\lim_{n\to\infty} n\Pr\left[n^{-1}\boldsymbol{W} \in A\right] = \mu(A),$$

for some measure $\mu$ that is referred to as the exponent measure. $\mu$ has the homogeneity property $\mu(tA) = t^{-1}\mu(A)$. Letting $\rho = \|W\|_p, p > 0$ and $\boldsymbol{\theta} = \boldsymbol{W}/\rho$, define $\Psi(B) = \mu(\{\boldsymbol{w} : \rho > 1, \boldsymbol{\theta} \in B\})$, which is referred to as the angular measure. After some manipulations, we obtain that

$$\lim_{r\to\infty} \Pr[\boldsymbol{\theta} \in A|\rho > r] = \frac{\Psi(A)}{\Psi(\mathbb{S}_p^{d-1})}. \tag{1}$$

Thus, a model for the exponent measure induces a model for the limiting distribution conditional on the observations being above a threshold defined with respect to their $p$-norm. The constraint that all marginals of $\mu$ correspond to a standard Pareto distribution leads to the so-called moment constraints on $\Psi$, consisting of

$$\int_{\mathbb{S}_p^{d-1}} w_i \, d\Psi(\boldsymbol{w}) = \frac{1}{d}, \quad i = 1,\ldots,d.$$

Inference for the limiting distribution of the exceedances needs to account for the normalizing constant in Equation (1) as well as the moment constraints. Because of these issues, in this paper, we prefer to follow the limiting conditional distribution approach. An example of the application of the regular variation approach using $p = 1$ is developed in [13].

## 3. Estimation of the Angular Measure

To infer the PoT distribution, we consider two steps: First we estimate the shape and scale parameters for the multivariate Pareto distribution, using the univariate marginals; then we focus on the dependence structure in extreme regions by proposing a flexible model for the distribution of $\boldsymbol{V}$. Consider $\boldsymbol{w}_i$, $i = 1,\ldots,n$ a collection of realizations of $\boldsymbol{W}$. We start by setting a large threshold $b_{t,\ell}$ for the $\ell$-th marginal, $\ell = 1,\ldots,d$. Then, the distribution of $W_\ell$, conditional on exceeding the threshold, can be approximated with a generalized univariate Pareto. Thus,

$$\Pr[W_\ell > w_{i\ell} \mid W_\ell > b_{t,\ell}] = \left(1 + \xi_\ell \frac{w_{i\ell} - b_{t,\ell}}{\sigma_\ell}\right)_+^{-1/\xi_\ell}$$

where $(\cdot)_+$ indicates the positive part function. We set $b_{t,l} = \hat{F}_\ell^{-1}(1 - 1/t)$, the empirical $(1 - 1/t)$-quantile. We then estimate $\xi_\ell$ and $\sigma_\ell$, for each $\ell$, using likelihood-based methods. To estimate the angular distribution, we standardize each of the marginals. The standardization yields

$$z_{i\ell} = \left(1 + \xi_\ell \frac{w_{i\ell} - b_{t,\ell}}{\sigma_\ell}\right)_+^{1/\xi_\ell}. \tag{2}$$

Note that $z_{i\ell} > 1$ implies that $w_{i\ell} > b_{t,\ell}$, meaning that the observation $\boldsymbol{w}_i$ is extreme in the $\ell$-th dimension. Thus, $r_i = \|z_i\|_\infty > 1$ implies that at least one dimension has an extreme observation and corresponds to a very extreme observation when $t$ is large. We focus on the observations that are such that $r_i > 1$. These provide a sub-sample of the standardized original sample. We define $\boldsymbol{v}_i = z_i/r_i \in \mathbb{S}_\infty^{d-1}$. These vectors are used for the estimation of $\Phi$.

### 3.1. Projected Gamma Family

At the core of our PoT method is the development of a distribution on $\mathbb{S}_p^{d-1} = \{\boldsymbol{s} : \boldsymbol{s} \in \mathbb{R}_+^d, \|\boldsymbol{s}\|_p = 1\}$, where, for $p > 0$, $\|\cdot\|_p$ is the $\mathcal{L}_p$-norm of a vector $\boldsymbol{x} \in \mathbb{R}^d$, defined as

$$\|\boldsymbol{x}\|_p = \left(\Sigma_{\ell=1}^d |x_\ell|^p\right)^{\frac{1}{p}}.$$

The absolute and Euclidean norms are obtained for $p = 1$ and $p = 2$ respectively, and the $\mathcal{L}_\infty$ norm can be obtained as a limit:

$$\|\boldsymbol{x}\|_\infty = \lim_{p\to\infty} \|\boldsymbol{x}\| = \bigvee_{\ell=1}^d x_\ell.$$

To obtain a distribution on $\mathbb{S}_p^{d-1}$, we start with a vector in $\boldsymbol{x} \in \mathbb{R}_+^d$ and normalize it to obtain $\boldsymbol{y} = \boldsymbol{x}/\|\boldsymbol{x}\|_p \in \mathbb{S}_p^{d-1}$. Figure 1a shows the progression of $\mathbb{S}_p^1$ asymptotically towards $\mathbb{S}_\infty^1$ as $p$ increases; Figure 1b shows the relative positions of data points normalized to $\mathbb{S}_p^1$ for selected $p$. A natural distribution to consider in $\mathbb{R}_+^d$ is given by a product of independent univariate Gamma distributions. Let $\boldsymbol{X} \sim \prod_{\ell=1}^d \text{Ga}(X_\ell \mid \alpha_\ell, \beta_\ell)$. $\alpha_\ell$ and $\beta_\ell$ are the shape and scale parameters, respectively. For any finite $p > 0$, letting $y_d = (1 - \Sigma_{\ell=1}^{d-1} y_\ell^p)^{1/p}$, the transformation

$$T(x_1, \ldots, x_d) = \left(\|\boldsymbol{x}\|_p, \frac{x_1}{\|\boldsymbol{x}\|_p}, \ldots, \frac{x_{d-1}}{\|\boldsymbol{x}\|_p}\right) = (r, y_1, \ldots, y_{d-1}) \tag{3}$$

is invertible with

$$T^{-1}(r, y_1, \ldots, y_{d-1}) = \left(ry_1, \ldots, ry_{d-1}, r\left(1 - \Sigma_{\ell=1}^{d-1} y_\ell^p\right)^{\frac{1}{p}}\right). \tag{4}$$

The Jacobian of the transformation takes the form

$$r^{d-1}\left[\left(1 - \Sigma_{\ell=1}^{d-1} y_\ell^p\right)^{\frac{1}{p}} + \Sigma_{\ell=1}^{d-1} y_\ell^p \left(1 - \Sigma_{l=1}^{d-1} y_\ell^p\right)^{\frac{1}{p}-1}\right]. \tag{5}$$

The normalization provided by $T$ maps a vector in $\mathbb{R}_+^d$ onto $\mathbb{S}_p^{d-1}$. With a slight abuse of terminology, we refer to it as a projection. Using Equations (3)–(5), we have the joint density

$$f(r, \boldsymbol{y}) = \prod_{\ell=1}^d \left[\frac{\beta_\ell^{\alpha_\ell}}{\Gamma(\alpha_\ell)} (ry_\ell)^{\alpha_\ell - 1} \exp\{-\beta_\ell r y_\ell\}\right] \times r^{d-1}\left[y_d + \Sigma_{\ell=1}^{d-1} y_\ell^p y_d^{1-p}\right]. \tag{6}$$

Integrating out $r$ yields the resulting *Projected Gamma* density

$$\mathrm{PG}(\boldsymbol{y} \mid \boldsymbol{\alpha}, \boldsymbol{\beta}) = \prod_{\ell=1}^{d} \left[ \frac{\beta_\ell^{\alpha_\ell}}{\Gamma(\alpha_\ell)} y_\ell^{\alpha_\ell - 1} \right] \times \left[ y_d + \sum_{\ell=1}^{d-1} y_\ell^p y_d^{1-p} \right] \times \frac{\Gamma(\sum_{\ell=1}^d \alpha_\ell)}{\left( \sum_{\ell=1}^d \beta_\ell y_\ell \right)^{\sum_{\ell=1}^d \alpha_\ell}}, \tag{7}$$

defined for $\boldsymbol{y} \in \mathbb{S}_p^{d-1}$ and for any finite $p > 0$. To avoid identifiability problems when estimating the shape and scale parameters, we set $\beta_1 = 1$. Ref. [20] obtain the density in Equation (7) for $p = 2$ as a multivariate distribution for directional data using spherical coordinates. For $\boldsymbol{y} \in \mathbb{S}_1^{d-1}$ and $\beta_\ell = \beta$ for all $\ell$, the density in Equation (7) corresponds to that of a Dirichlet distribution.

The projected gamma family is simple to specify and has very tractable computational properties. Thus, we use it as a building block for the angular measure $\Phi$ models. To build a flexible family of distributions in $\mathbb{S}_p^{d-1}$, we consider mixtures of projected gamma densities defined as

$$f(\boldsymbol{y}) = \int_\Theta \mathcal{PG}(\boldsymbol{y} \mid \boldsymbol{\theta}) dG(\boldsymbol{\theta}), \tag{8}$$

where $\boldsymbol{\theta} = (\boldsymbol{\alpha}, \boldsymbol{\beta})$. Following a Bayesian non-parametric approach [21–23], we assume that $G$ is drawn from a random measure. In particular, assuming a Dirichlet process prior for $G$, we have a hierarchical formulation of the mixture model that, for a vector of observations $\boldsymbol{y}_i$, is given by

$$\boldsymbol{y}_i \sim \mathrm{PG}(\boldsymbol{y}_i \mid \boldsymbol{\theta}_i) \quad \boldsymbol{\theta}_i \sim G \quad G \sim \mathcal{DP}(\eta, G_0) \tag{9}$$

where $\mathcal{DP}$ denotes a Dirichlet process, $\eta$ is the precision parameter, and $G_0$ is the centering distribution.

Unfortunately, in the limit when $p \to \infty$, the normalizing transformation is not differentiable. Thus, a closed-form expression like Equation (7) for the projected gamma density on $\mathbb{S}_\infty^{d-1}$ is not available. Instead, we observe that for a sufficiently large $p$, $\mathbb{S}_p^{d-1}$ will approach $\mathbb{S}_\infty^{d-1}$. With that in mind, our strategy consists of describing the angular distribution $\Phi$ using a sample-based approach with the following steps: (i) Apply the transformation in Equation (2) to the original data; (ii) Obtain the subsample of the standardized observations that satisfy $R > 1$; (iii) Take a finite $p$ and project the observations onto $\mathbb{S}_p^{d-1}$; (iv) Fit the model in Equation (8) to the resulting data and obtain samples from the fitted model; (v) project the resulting samples onto $\mathbb{S}_\infty^{d-1}$. For step (iv), we use a Bayesian approach that is implemented using a purposely developed Markov chain Monte Carlo sampler described in the next section.

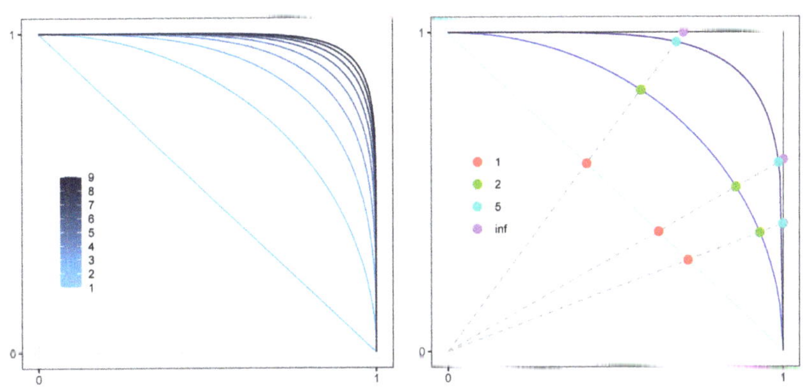


**(a)** $\mathbb{S}_p^1$ for $p = 1, \ldots, 10$ **(b)** Projection of data on $\mathbb{S}_\infty^1$ onto $\mathbb{S}_p^1$

**Figure 1.** The positive orthant of the $p$-norm sphere for $d = 2$.

### 3.2. Tail Probabilities for the PoT Model

A measure that is used to characterize the strength of the dependence in the tail for two random variables, $Z_1$ and $Z_2$, with marginal distributions $F_1$ and $F_2$ is given by [1]

$$\chi_{12} = \lim_{u \uparrow 1} \Pr[F_1(Z_1) > u \mid F_2(Z_2) > u].$$

$\chi_{12}$ provides information about the distribution of extremes for the variable $Z_1$ given that $Z_2$ is very large. When $\chi_{12} > 0$, $Z_1$ and $Z_2$ are said to be asymptotically dependent; otherwise, they are asymptotically independent. The following result provides the asymptotic dependence coefficient between two components of $\mathbf{Z}$ for our proposed PoT model.

**Proposition 1.** *Suppose that* $\mathbf{Z} = R\mathbf{V}$ *with* $R \sim Pa(1)$, $Pr[V_\ell > 0] = 1$ *and* $\mathrm{E}[V_\ell]$ *exists, for* $\ell = 1, \ldots, d$, *then*

$$\chi_{j\ell} = \mathrm{E}\left[\frac{V_j}{\mathrm{E}[V_j]} \wedge \frac{V_\ell}{\mathrm{E}[V_\ell]}\right] \tag{10}$$

**Proof.** Denote as $F_\ell$ the marginal distribution of $Z_\ell$. To obtain $\chi_{j\ell}$, we need $Pr(Z_j > z_j, Z_\ell > z_\ell)$, where $z_\ell = F_\ell^{-1}(u) = \mathrm{E}[V_\ell]/(1-u)$, $\ell = 1, \ldots, d$. Using the fact that $V_\ell > 0, \forall \ell$ almost surely, we have that the former is equal to

$$\Pr\left[R > \frac{z_j}{V_j} \vee \frac{z_\ell}{V_\ell}\right] = \mathrm{E}\left[1 \wedge \left(\frac{z_j}{V_j} \vee \frac{z_\ell}{V_\ell}\right)^{-1}\right] = \mathrm{E}\left[\frac{V_j}{z_j} \wedge \frac{V_\ell}{z_\ell}\right] = (1-u)\mathrm{E}\left[\frac{V_j}{\mathrm{E}[V_j]} \wedge \frac{V_\ell}{\mathrm{E}[V_\ell]}\right]$$

where the second identity is justified by the fact that $V_i$ is bounded and $z_i \to \infty$. The proof is completed by noting that $\Pr[F_i(Z_i) > u] = 1 - u$. □

Equation (10) implies that $\chi_{j\ell} > 0$, and so, no asymptotic independence is possible under our proposed model. For the analysis of extreme values, it is of interest to calculate the multivariate conditional survival function. The following result provides the relevant expression as a function of the angular measure.

**Proposition 2.** *Assume the same conditions as Proposition 1. Let* $\alpha \subset \{1, \ldots, d\}$ *be a collections of indexes. Then*

$$\Pr\left[\bigcap_{\ell \in \alpha} Z_\ell > z_\ell \mid \bigcap_{\ell \notin \alpha} Z_\ell > z_\ell\right] = \frac{\mathrm{E}\left[\bigwedge_{k=1}^{d} 1 \wedge \frac{V_k}{z_k}\right]}{\mathrm{E}\left[\bigwedge_{k \notin \alpha} 1 \wedge \frac{V_k}{z_k}\right]}. \tag{11}$$

The proof uses a similar approach to the proof of Proposition 1.

Equations (10) and (11) provide relevant tools for inference on the tail behavior of the joint distribution of the observations. The expressions can be readily calculated within a sample-based inferential approach like the one considered in the following section.

### Inference for the Projected Gamma Mixture Model

To perform inference for our proposed PoT model, we develop an iterative sample-based approach. We implement a Markov chain Monte Carlo method that, for a given iteration, groups observations into stochastically assigned clusters, where members of a cluster share distributional parameters [23,24]. Building out the methods of inference for Equation (9), let $n_j^{(-i)}$ be the number of observations in cluster $j$, not including observation $i$. Let $J^{(-i)}$ be the number of extant clusters, not including any singleton containing observation $i$. Under this model, the probability of cluster membership for a given observation is proportional to

$$\Pr[\delta_i = j \mid \ldots] \propto \begin{cases} n_j^{(-i)} \mathcal{PG}(y_i \mid \alpha_j, \beta_j) \\ \eta \int \mathcal{PG}(y_i \mid \alpha_j, \beta_j) dG_0(\alpha_j, \beta_j), \end{cases}$$

where the top case is iterating over extant clusters $j = 1, \ldots, J^{(-i)}$, and the bottom case is for a *new* cluster. If $G_0$ is not a conjugate prior for the kernel density, the integral in the above formula may not be available in closed form. We sidestep this using Algorithm 8 from [25]: by Monte Carlo integration, we draw $m$ candidate clusters, $\alpha_j, \beta_j$ for $j = J^{(-i)} + 1, \ldots, J^{(-i)} + m$ from $G_0$. Then, we sample the cluster indicator $\gamma_i$ from extant or candidate clusters, where the probability of cluster membership is proportional to

$$\Pr[\delta_i = j \mid \ldots] \propto \begin{cases} n_j^{(-i)} \mathcal{PG}(y_i \mid \alpha_j, \beta_j) \\ \frac{\eta}{m} \mathcal{PG}(y_i \mid \alpha_j, \beta_j). \end{cases} \tag{12}$$

Again, the top case is iterating over extant clusters, and now the bottom case is iterating over new *candidate* clusters. If a candidate cluster is selected, then $\gamma_i = J = J^{(-i)} + 1$, and the associated cluster parameters are saved.

A key feature of the the projected Gamma distribution is its computational properties. We augment $\mathcal{PG}(y_i \mid \alpha_i, \beta_i)$ by introducing a latent radial component $r_i$, for each observation. Using Equation (6) we observe that the full conditional of $r_i$ is easy to sample from, as it is given as

$$r_i \mid \alpha_i, \beta_i \sim \mathcal{G}\left(r_i \,\middle|\, \sum_{\ell=1}^d \alpha_{i\ell}, \sum_{\ell=1}^d \beta_\ell y_{i\ell}\right). \tag{13}$$

Moreover, the full conditional for $\alpha_j, \beta_j$ is then proportional to

$$f(\alpha_j, \beta_j \mid \mathbf{Y}, \mathbf{r}, \delta, \ldots) \propto \prod_{i:\gamma_i = j} \prod_{\ell=1}^d \mathcal{G}\left(r_i y_{i\ell} \mid \alpha_{j\ell}, \beta_{j\ell}\right) \times dG_0(\alpha_j, \beta_j). \tag{14}$$

Note that the ordering of the products can be reversed in Equation (14), indicating that with appropriate choice of centering distribution, the full conditionals for $\alpha_j, \beta_j$ can become separable by dimension, and thus inference on $\alpha_{j\ell}, \beta_{j\ell}$ can be done in parallel for all $j, \ell$. We first consider a centering distribution given by a product of independent Gammas:

$$G_0(\alpha_j, \beta_j \mid \xi, \tau, \zeta, \sigma) = \prod_{\ell=1}^d \mathcal{G}(\alpha_{j\ell} \mid \xi_\ell, \tau_\ell) \times \prod_{\ell=2}^d \mathcal{G}(\beta_{j\ell} \mid \zeta_\ell, \sigma_\ell). \tag{15}$$

This model is completed with independent Gamma priors on $\xi_\ell$, $\tau_\ell$, $\zeta_\ell$, and $\sigma_\ell$. We also assume a Gamma prior on $\eta$, which is updated via the procedure outlined in [26]. We refer to this model as the *projected gamma-gamma* (PG-G) model. An advantage of the PG-G model is that, thanks to conjugacy, the rate parameters $\beta_{j\ell}$ can easily be integrated out for inference on $\alpha_j$. Then, the full conditional for $\alpha_{j\ell}$ takes the form

$$\pi(\alpha_{j\ell} \mid \mathbf{r}, \mathbf{Y}, \gamma, \xi_\ell, \tau_\ell, \zeta_\ell, \sigma_\ell) \propto \frac{\left(\prod_{i:\gamma_i=j} r_i y_{i\ell}\right)^{\alpha_{j\ell}-1} \alpha_{j\ell}^{\xi_\ell - 1} e^{-\tau_\ell \alpha_{j\ell}}}{\Gamma^{n_j}(\alpha_{j\ell})} \times \frac{\Gamma\left(n_j \alpha_{j\ell} + \zeta_\ell\right)}{\left(\sum_{i:\gamma_i=j} r_i y_{i\ell} + \sigma_\ell\right)^{n_j \alpha_{j\ell} + \zeta_\ell}} \tag{16}$$

for $\ell = 2, \ldots, d$. For $\ell = 1$, as $\beta_1 := 1$, the full conditional takes the simpler form

$$\pi(\alpha_{j1} \mid \mathbf{r}, \mathbf{Y}, \gamma, \xi_1, \tau_1) \propto \frac{\left(\prod_{i:\gamma_i=j} r_i y_{i1}\right)^{\alpha_{j1}-1} \alpha_{j1}^{\xi_1 - 1} e^{-\tau_1 \alpha_{j1}}}{\Gamma^{n_j}(\alpha_{j1})}. \tag{17}$$

Samples of $\alpha_{j\ell}$ can thus be obtained using a Metropolis step. In our analysis, we first transform $\alpha_{j\ell}$ to the log scale and use a normal proposal density. The full conditional for $\beta$ is

$$\beta_{j\ell} \mid \boldsymbol{r}, \mathbf{Y}, \alpha, \zeta_\ell, \sigma_\ell \sim \mathcal{G}\left( \beta_{j\ell} \,\middle|\, n_j\alpha_{j\ell} + \zeta_\ell, \sum_{i:\gamma_i=j} r_i y_{i\ell} + \sigma_\ell \right), \tag{18}$$

for $\ell = 2, \ldots, d$. Updating $\beta_{j\ell}$ is done via a Gibbs step. The hyper-parameters $\xi_\ell, \tau_\ell, \zeta_\ell, \sigma_\ell$ follow similar gamma-gamma update relationships. We also explore a restricted form of this model, where $\beta_\ell = 1$ for all $\ell$. Under this model, we use the full conditional in Equation (17) for all $\ell$ and omit inference on $\boldsymbol{\zeta}, \boldsymbol{\sigma}$. We refer to this model as the *projected restricted gamma-gamma* (PRG-G) model.

The second form of centering distribution we explore is a multivariate log-normal distribution on the shape parameters $\boldsymbol{\alpha}_j$ with independent gamma $\beta_{j\ell}$ rate parameters.

$$G_0\left(\boldsymbol{\alpha}_j, \boldsymbol{\beta}_j \mid \boldsymbol{\mu}, \boldsymbol{\Sigma}, \zeta, \sigma\right) = \mathcal{LN}\left(\boldsymbol{\alpha}_j \mid \boldsymbol{\mu}, \boldsymbol{\Sigma}\right) \times \prod_{\ell=2}^{d} \mathcal{G}\left(\beta_{j\ell} \mid \zeta_\ell, \sigma_\ell\right). \tag{19}$$

This model is completed with a normal prior on $\boldsymbol{\mu}$, an inverse Wishart prior on $\boldsymbol{\Sigma}$, and Gamma priors on $\zeta_\ell$, $\sigma_\ell$, and $\eta$. This model is denoted as the *projected gamma-log-normal* (PG-LN) model. We also explore a restricted Gamma form of this model as above, where $\beta_\ell = 1$ for all $\ell$. This is denoted as the *projected restricted gamma-log-normal* (PRG-LN) model. Updates for $\boldsymbol{\alpha}$ can be accomplished using a joint Metropolis step, where $\beta_{j\ell}$ for $\ell = 2, \ldots, d$ have been integrated out of the log-density. That is,

$$\begin{aligned} \pi(\boldsymbol{\alpha}_j \mid \mathbf{Y}, \boldsymbol{r}, \boldsymbol{\delta}, \boldsymbol{\mu}, \boldsymbol{\Sigma}, \boldsymbol{\zeta}, \boldsymbol{\sigma}) \propto \exp\left\{ -\frac{1}{2}(\log \boldsymbol{\alpha}_j - \mu)^T \boldsymbol{\Sigma}^{-1} (\log \boldsymbol{\alpha}_j - \mu) \right\} \times \frac{1}{\prod_{\ell=1}^{d} \alpha_{j\ell}} \\ \times \frac{\left(\prod_{i:\gamma_i=j} r_i y_{i1}\right)^{\alpha_{j1}-1}}{\prod_{\ell=1}^{d} \Gamma^{n_j}(\alpha_{j\ell})} \times \prod_{\ell=2}^{d} \frac{\Gamma\left(n_j\alpha_{j\ell} + \zeta_\ell\right)}{\left(\sum_{i:\gamma_i=j} r_i y_{i\ell} + \sigma_\ell\right)^{n_j\alpha_{j\ell}+\zeta_\ell}} \end{aligned}$$

The inferential forms for $\beta_{j\ell}$ and its priors are the same as for PG-G. The normal prior for $\mu$ is conjugate for the log-normal $\boldsymbol{\alpha}_j$ and can be sampled via a Gibbs step. Finally, the inverse Wishart prior for $\Sigma$ is again conjugate to the log-normal $\boldsymbol{\alpha}_j$, implying that it can also be sampled via a Gibbs step.

To effectively explore the sample space with a joint Metropolis step, as well as to speed convergence, we implement a parallel tempering algorithm [27] for the log-normal models. This technique runs parallel MCMC chains at ascending temperatures. That is, for chain $s$, the posterior density is exponentiated by the reciprocal of temperature $t_s$. For the *cold* chain, $t_1 := 1$. Let $E_s$ be the log-posterior density under the current parameter state for chain $s$. Then states between chains $r, s$ are exchanged via a Metropolis step with probability

$$\alpha_{rs} = \min\left[1, \exp\left\{(t_r^{-1} - t_s^{-1})(E_r - E_s)\right\}\right].$$

Higher temperatures serve to *flatten* the posterior distribution, meaning hotter chains have a higher probability of making a given transition or will make larger transitions. As such, they will more quickly explore the parameter space and share information gained through state exchange.

## 4. Scoring Criteria for Distributions on the Infinity-Norm Sphere

In order to assess and compare the estimation of a distribution on $\mathbb{S}_\infty^{d-1}$, we consider the theory of proper scoring rules developed in [28]. As mentioned in Section 3.1, our approach does not provide a density on $\mathbb{S}_\infty^{d-1}$, restricting our ability to construct model selection criteria to sample-based approaches. To this end, we employ the *energy score* criterion introduced therein.

The energy score criterion, defined for a general probability distribution $P$ with a finite expectation, is developed as

$$S_{\text{ES}}(P, \boldsymbol{x}_i) = \text{E}_P[g(\boldsymbol{X}_i, \boldsymbol{x}_i)] - \frac{1}{2}\text{E}_P[g(\boldsymbol{X}_i, \boldsymbol{X}_i')], \tag{20}$$

where $g$ is a kernel function. The score defined in Equation (20) can be evaluated using samples from $P$ with the help of the law of large numbers. Moreover, Theorem 4 in [28] states that if $g(\cdot, \cdot)$ is a negative definite kernel, then $\text{S}(P, \boldsymbol{x})$ is a *proper* scoring rule. Recall that a real valued function $g$ is a negative definite kernel if it is symmetric in its arguments, and $\sum_{i=1}^{n}\sum_{j=1}^{n} a_i a_j g(x_i, x_j) \leq 0$ for all positive integers $n$ and any collection $a_1, \ldots, a_n \in \mathbb{R}$ such that $\sum_{i=1}^{n} a_i = 0$.

In a Euclidean space, these conditions are satisfied by the Euclidean distance [29]. However, for observations on different faces of $\mathbb{S}_{\infty}^{d-1}$, the Euclidean distance will underestimate the geodesic distance, the actual distance required to travel between the two points. Let

$$\mathbb{C}_{\ell}^{d-1} = \{\boldsymbol{x} : \boldsymbol{x} \in \mathbb{S}_{\infty}^{d-1}, x_{\ell} = 1\}$$

comprise the $\ell$th *face*. For points on the same face, the Euclidean distance corresponds to the length of the shortest possible path in $\mathbb{S}_{\infty}^{d-1}$. For points on different faces, the Euclidean distance is a lower bound for that length.

For a finite $p$, the shortest connecting path between two points in $\mathbb{S}_{p}^{d-1}$ is the minimum geodesic; its length satisfying the definition of a distance. Thus its length can be used as a negative definite kernel for the purpose of defining an energy score. Unfortunately, as $p \to \infty$, the resulting surface $\mathbb{S}_{\infty}^{d-1}$ is not differentiable, implying that routines to calculate geodesics are not readily available. However, as $\mathbb{S}_{\infty}^{d-1}$ is a portion of a $d$-cube, we can borrow a result from geometry [30] stating that the length of the shortest path between two points on a geometric figure corresponds to the length of a straight line drawn between the points on an appropriate unfolding, rotation, or *net* of the figure from a $d$-dimensional to a $d-1$-dimensional space. The optimal net will have the shortest straight line between the points, as long as that line is fully contained within such a net. As $\mathbb{S}_{\infty}^{d-1}$ has $d$ faces—each face pairwise adjacent, there are $d!$ possible nets. However, we are only interested in nets that begin and end on the source and destination faces, respectively, reducing the number of nets under consideration to $\sum_{k=0}^{d-2}\binom{d-2}{k}$. This is still computationally burdensome for a large number of dimensions. However, we can efficiently establish an upper bound on the geodesic length. We use this upper bound on geodesic distance as the kernel function for the energy score.

To calculate the energy score, we define the kernel

$$g(\boldsymbol{a}, \boldsymbol{b}) = \min_{c \in \mathbb{C}_{j}^{d-1} \cap \mathbb{C}_{\ell}^{d-1}} \{\|\boldsymbol{c} - \boldsymbol{a}\|_2 + \|\boldsymbol{b} - \boldsymbol{c}\|_2\}.$$

where $\boldsymbol{a} \in \mathbb{C}_{\ell}^{d-1}$, and $\boldsymbol{b} \in \mathbb{C}_{j}^{d-1}$ for $\ell, j \in \{1, \ldots, d\}$. Evaluating $g$ as described requires the solution of a $(d-2)$-dimensional optimization problem. The following proposition provides a straightforward approach.

**Proposition 3.** *Let $\boldsymbol{a} \in \mathbb{C}_{\ell}^{d-1}$, and $\boldsymbol{b} \in \mathbb{C}_{j}^{d-1}$, for $\ell, j \in \{1, \ldots, d\}$. For $\ell \neq j$, the transformation $P_{j\ell}(\cdot)$ required to rotate the $j$th face along the $\ell$th axis produces the vector $\boldsymbol{b}'$, where*

$$b_i' = P_{j\ell}(\boldsymbol{b}) = \begin{cases} b_i & \text{for } i \neq j, \ell \\ 1 & \text{for } i = \ell \\ 2 - b_{\ell} & \text{for } i = j \end{cases}, \tag{21}$$

*Then $g(\boldsymbol{a}, \boldsymbol{b}) = \|\boldsymbol{a} - \boldsymbol{b}'\|_2$.*

**Proof.** Notice that for $\boldsymbol{c} \in \mathbb{C}_j^{d-1} \cap \mathbb{C}_\ell^{d-1}$, $\|\boldsymbol{b} - \boldsymbol{c}\|_2 = \|\boldsymbol{b}' - \boldsymbol{c}\|_2$. We then have that

$$\begin{aligned} g(\boldsymbol{a}, \boldsymbol{b}) &= \min_{\boldsymbol{c} \in \mathbb{C}_j^{d-1} \cap \mathbb{C}_\ell^{d-1}} \{\|\boldsymbol{c} - \boldsymbol{a}\|_2 + \|\boldsymbol{b} - \boldsymbol{c}\|_2\} \\ &= \min_{\boldsymbol{c} \in \mathbb{C}_j^{d-1} \cap \mathbb{C}_\ell^{d-1}} \{\|\boldsymbol{c} - \boldsymbol{a}\|_2 + \|\boldsymbol{b}' - \boldsymbol{c}\|_2\} \\ &= \|\boldsymbol{a} - \boldsymbol{b}'\|_2. \end{aligned}$$

The last equality is due to the fact that $\boldsymbol{a}$ and $\boldsymbol{b}'$ belong to the same hyperplane. □

Using the rotation in Proposition 3, we obtain the following result.

**Proposition 4.** *$g$ is a negative definite kernel.*

**Proof.** For a given $n$, consider an arbitrary set of points $\boldsymbol{a}_1, \dots, \boldsymbol{a}_n \in \mathbb{S}_\infty^{d-1}$, and $\alpha_1, \dots, \alpha_n \in \mathbb{R}$, such that $\sum_{i=1}^n \alpha_i = 0$. Then

$$\sum_{i,j} \alpha_i \alpha_j g(\boldsymbol{a}_i, \boldsymbol{a}_j) = \sum_{i,j} \alpha_i \alpha_j \|\boldsymbol{a}_i - \boldsymbol{a}_j'\|_2 \leq 0,$$

where $\boldsymbol{a}_j'$ is defined as in Proposition 3. The last equality holds as $\|\boldsymbol{x} - \boldsymbol{x}'\|_2, \boldsymbol{x}, \boldsymbol{x}' \in \mathbb{R}^d$ is negative definite [28] □

Proposition 3 provides a computationally efficient way to evaluate the proper scoring rule $S_{\text{ES}}$ defined on $\mathbb{S}_\infty^{d-1}$ for each observation. For the purpose of model assessment and comparison, we report the average $S_{\text{ES}}$ taken across all observed data and notice that the smaller the score, the better.

## 5. Data Illustrations

We apply the aforementioned models to simulated angular data. We then consider the analysis of atmospheric data. To tackle the difficult problem of assessing the convergence an MCMC chain for a large-dimensional model, we monitor the log-posterior density. In all the examples considered, MCMC samples produced stable traces of the log-posterior in less than 40,000 iterations. We use that as a burn-in and thereafter sample 10,000 additional iterations. We then thin the chain by retaining one every ten samples, to obtain 1000 total samples. These are used to generate samples from the posterior predictive densities. We used two different strategies to implement the MCMC samplers. For the models whose DP prior is centered around a log-normal distribution, we used parallel tempering. This serves to overcome the very slow mixing that we observed in these cases. The temperature ladder was set as $t_s = 1.3^s$ for $s \in \{0, 1, \dots, 5\}$. This was set empirically in order to produce acceptable swap probabilities both for the simulated data and real data. Parallel tempering produces chains with good mixing properties but has a computational cost that grows linearly with the number of temperatures. Thus, for the gamma-centered models, we used a single chain. We leverage the fast speed of each iteration to obtain a large number of samples, which are appropriately thinned to deal with a mild autocorrelation. In summary, the strategy for log-normal centered models is based on a costly sampler with good mixing properties. The strategy for the gamma-centered models is based on a cheap sampler that can be run for a large number of iterations.

Our hyperprior parameters are set as follows: For the gamma-centered models (PG-G, PRG-G), the shape parameter for the centering distribution $\xi_\ell \sim \mathcal{G}(1,1)$, and rate parameter $\tau_\ell \sim \mathcal{G}(2,2)$. For the log-normal centered models (PG-LN, PRG-LN), the centering distribution's log-mean $\boldsymbol{\mu} \sim \mathcal{N}_d(0, \boldsymbol{I}_d)$, and covariance matrix $\Sigma \sim \mathcal{IW}(d+10, (d+10)\boldsymbol{I}_d)$. These values are intended such that draws from the prior for $\Sigma$ will weakly tend towards the identity matrix. For models learning rate parameters $\beta_{j\ell}$ (PG-G, PG-LN), the centering distribution's shape parameter $\zeta \sim \mathcal{G}(1,1)$ and rate parameter $\sigma \sim \mathcal{G}(2,2)$. The choice of the $\mathcal{G}(2,2)$ for rate parameters places little mass near 0 in order to draw estimates for the value away from 0 for numerical stability.

### 5.1. Simulation Study

The challenging problem in multivariate EVT is to capture the dependence structure of the limiting distribution. To this end, we focus our simulation study specifically on the angular component. To evaluate our proposed approach for angular measure estimation, we consider simulated datasets on $\mathbb{S}_\infty^{d-1}$ for values of $d$ ranging from 2 to 32. We generated each dataset as a mixture of multivariate log-normal distributions projected onto $\mathbb{S}_\infty^{d-1}$. The generation procedure is detailed in Algorithm 1. We produced ten replicates of each configuration. We consider two gamma-centered and two log-normal-centered DP mixture models, with and without restrictions in each case. To perform a comparative analysis, we fitted the pairwise betas model proposed in [31]. We chose this model for comparison, as it similarly works to capture a complex dependence structure on an $\mathbb{S}_p^{d-1}$ sphere, albeit with $p = 1$, and is implemented in the readily available package `BMAmevt` in R [32], which can provide samples from the posterior predictive distribution. These samples are needed for the calculation of the energy scores that are at the basis of our comparison. In addition, `BMAmevt` can be fitted to moderately large multivariate observations. For the DP mixture models, the data are projected onto $\mathbb{S}_{10}^{d-1}$. For the other two models, they are projected onto $\mathbb{S}_1^{d-1}$. We sampled each model for 50,000 iterations, dropping the first 40,000 as burn-in and thinning to keep every 10th iteration after. These settings were intended to provide a consistent sampling strategy that would work with every model, even if inefficient for some.

**Algorithm 1** Simulated Angular Dataset Generation Routine. $\mu_j$, $\Sigma_j$ are the parameters of the mixture component distribution; $\pi$ is the probability vector assigning weight mixture components; $\delta_i$ is the mixture component identifier for each simulated observation.

```
for n_iter in [1,...,10] do
    for n_mix in [1,2,4,8] do
        for j in 1,...,n_mix do
            Generate μ_j ~ N_32(0, I)
            Generate Σ_j ~ IW_32(70, 70I)
        end for
        Generate π ~ Dirichlet(10_{n_mix})
        for i in 1,...,1000 do
            Generate δ_i ~ Categorical(π)
            Generate X_i ~ LN(μ_[δ_i], Σ_[δ_i])
        end for
        for n_col in [2,4,8,16,24,32] do
            Project columns 1 to n_col of X onto S_∞^{n_col − 1} and save.
        end for
    end for
end for
```

Figure 2 shows the average rise over baseline in energy score, as calculated on $\mathbb{S}_\infty^{d-1}$ using the kernel metric described in Proposition 3, for models trained on simulated data. After training a model, a posterior predictive dataset is generated, and the energy score is calculated as a Monte Carlo approximation of Equation (20). In our analysis, after burn-in and thinning, we had 1000 replicates from the posterior distribution and generated 10 posterior predictive replicates per iteration. The *baseline* value is the energy score of a new dataset from the same generating distribution as the training dataset evaluated against the training dataset. For the simulated data, we observe that the projected gamma models dominate the other two options considered, regardless of the choice of centering distribution. The projected restricted gamma models with a multivariate log-normal centering distribution appear to be dominated by the models based on the alternative centering distributions. Moreover, the performance deteriorates with the increase in dimensionality. Additionally, models centered around the log-normal distribution incur the computational cost of multivariate normal evaluation and parallel tempering, taking approximately six times longer to sample relative to the gamma models. We also note that the computational cost of the pairwise betas model grows combinatorially, with a sample space of dimension $\binom{d}{2}+1$. By comparison, the sample space for PG-G and PRG-G are $2(J+1)d$ and $(J+1)d$, respectively, where $J$ is the number of extant clusters, with much of that inference able to be done in parallel. In our testing, for low-dimensional problems, `BMAmevt` was substantially faster than any of our proposed DP mixture models. However, for examples with high numbers of dimensions, the computational time for `BMAmevt` was greater than that for PG-G. We compare computing times in our data analysis in Table 1b.

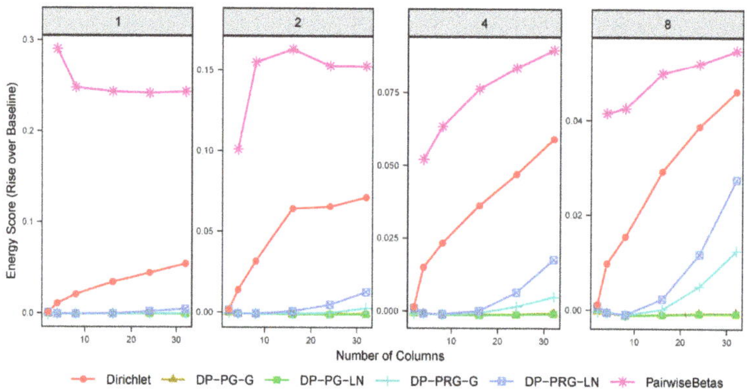


**Figure 2.** Average energy score rise over baseline (on $\mathbb{S}_{\infty}^{d-1}$) for various models fitted to simulated data, with ascending count of mixture components (indicated by plot heading) and number of dimensions (indicated by horizontal axis). Note that pairwise betas is a moment-restricted model.

**Table 1.** Model fit assessment and computation time on ERA-Interim and ERA5 data. (a) Energy score criterion from fitted models against the IVT data. Lower is better. (b) Time to sample (in minutes) 50,000 iterations for various models.

(a)

| Source | Pairwise Betas | PG-G | PG-LN | PRG-G | PRG-LN |
|---|---|---|---|---|---|
| ERA-Interim | 0.8620 | 0.8003 | 0.7986 | **0.7966** | 0.7970 |
| ERA5 | 2.0311 | 1.6404 | 1.5576 | **1.4349** | 1.5051 |

(b)

| Source | Pairwise Betas | PG-G | PG-LN | PRG-G | PRG-LN |
|---|---|---|---|---|---|
| ERA-Interim | 1.7 | 10.5 | 88.4 | 14.8 | 57.9 |
| ERA5 | 53.1 | 19.4 | 153.4 | 24.6 | 121.4 |

## 5.2. Integrated Vapor Transport

The *integrated vapor transport* (IVT) is a two-component vector that tracks the flow of the total water volume in a column of air over a given area [33]. IVT is increasingly used in the study of atmospheric rivers because of its direct relationship with orographically induced precipitation [34]. Atmospheric rivers (AR) are elongated areas of high local concentration of water vapor in the atmosphere that transport water from the tropics around the world. AR can cause extreme precipitation, something that is usually associated with very large values of the IVT magnitude over a whole geographical area. In spite of this, AR are fundamental for the water supply of areas like California. Thus, the importance of understanding the extreme behavior of IVT includes extreme tail dependence. We consider datasets that correspond to IVT estimated at two different spatial resolutions. The coarse-resolution dataset is obtained from the European Centre for Medium-Range Weather Forecasts (ECMWF) Interim reanalysis (ERA-Interim) [35,36]. The high-resolution dataset corresponds to the latest ECMWF observational product, ERA5 [37].

Our data correspond to daily average values for the IVT magnitude along the coast of California. The ERA-Interim data used cover the time period 1979 through 2014 (37 years), omitting leap days, and eight grid cells that correspond to the coast of California. The ERA5 data cover the time period 1979 through 2019 (42 years) with the same restriction and 47 grid cells for the coast of California. This gives us the opportunity to illustrate the performance of our method in multivariate settings of very different dimensions. Figure 3 provides a visual representation of the area these grid cells cover.

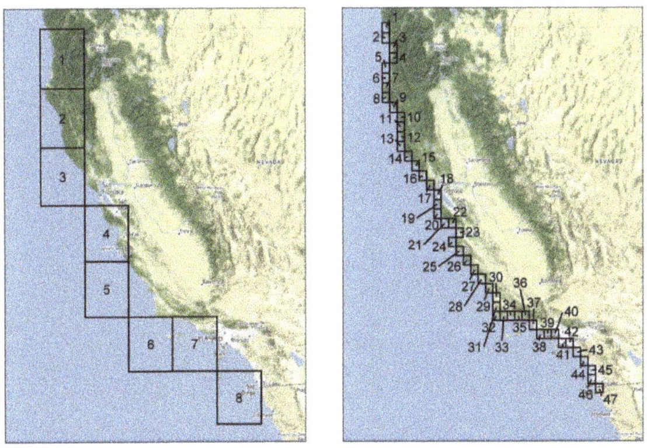

**Figure 3.** Grid cell locations for ERA-Interim (**left**) and ERA5 (**right**).

Fitting our models to the IVT data requires some pre-processing. First, we subset the data to the rainy season, which in California runs roughly from November to March. Following the approach described in Section 3, we estimate the shape and scale parameters of a univariate GP in each dimension, using maximum likelihood. We set the threshold in each dimension $\ell$ as $b_{t,\ell} = \hat{F}_\ell^{-1}(1 - t^{-1})$, where $\hat{F}$ is the empirical CDF and $t = 20$, which corresponds to the 95 percentile. We then use the transformation in Equation (2) to standardize the observations. Dividing each standardized observation by its $\mathcal{L}_\infty$ norm, we obtain a projection onto $\mathcal{S}_\infty^{d-1}$. As the data correspond to a daily time series, the observations are temporally correlated. For each group of consecutive standardized vectors $z_i$ such that $\|z_i\|_\infty > 1$, we retain only the vector with the largest $\mathcal{L}_\infty$ norm. The complete procedure is outlined in Algorithm 2.

After subsetting the ERA-Interim data to the rainy season, we have 5587 observations. After the processing and declustering described in Algorithm 2, this number reduces to 511 observations. A pairwise plot of the transformed data after processing and declustering is presented in Figure 4. From this, we note that the marginal densities display strong similarities, with a large spike near 0 and a small spike near 1. A value of 1 in a particular axis indicates that the standardized threshold exceedance was the largest in that dimension. The off-diagonal plots correspond to pairwise density plots. We observe that some site pairs, such as $(1,2)$, $(7,8)$, and especially $(4,5)$, have the bulk of their data concentrated in a small arc along the 45°; in other site combinations, such as $(3,6)$, $(2,7)$, or $(1,8)$, the data is split, favoring one side or the other of the 45° line. For the ERA5 data, after subsetting, we have 6342 observations, which reduces to 532 observations after processing and declustering. We fit the PG-G, PRG-G, PG-LN, and PRG-LN models to both datasets.

**Algorithm 2** Data preprocessing to isolate and transform data exhibiting extreme behavior. $r_i$ represents the radial component, and $v_i$ the angular component. The declustering portion is relevant for data correlated in time.

**for** $\ell = 1, \ldots, d$ **do**
  Set $b_{t,\ell} = \hat{F}_\ell^{-1}\left(1 - \frac{1}{t}\right)$.
  With $x_\ell > b_{t,\ell}$, fit $\sigma_\ell, \xi_\ell$ via MLE according to generalized Pareto likelihood.
**end for**
**for** $i = 1, \ldots, n$ **do**
  Define $z_{i,\ell} = \left(1 + \xi_\ell \frac{x_{i,\ell} - b_{t,\ell}}{\sigma_\ell}\right)_+^{1/\xi_\ell}$;  then $r_i = \|z_i\|_\infty$, $v_i = \frac{z_i}{\|z_i\|_\infty}$
**end for**
Subset $r, v$ such that $r_i \geq 1$
**if** declustering **then**
  **for** $i = 1, \ldots, n$ **do**
    If $r_i \geq 1$ and $r_{i-1} \geq 1$, drop the lesser (and associated $v_i$) from dataset.
  **end for**
**end if**

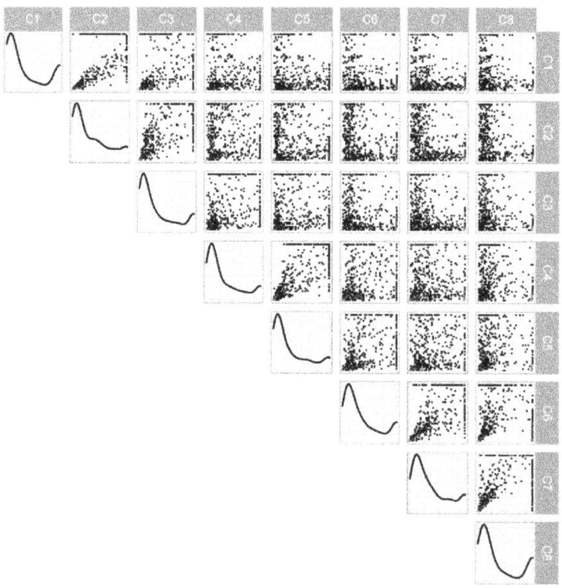


**Figure 4.** Pairwise plots from ERA-Interim data after transformation and projection to $\mathbb{S}_\infty^7$. Down the diagonal are marginal kernel densities with two-dimensional histograms on the off-diagonal. In those plots, red indicates a higher density. All data are between 0 and 1.

Table 1a shows the values of the estimated energy scores for the different models considered. We observe that, contrary to the results in the simulation study in Figure 2, the preferred model is the projected restricted gamma models, though for the lower-dimensional ERA-Interim data, all models perform comparably. Table 1b shows the computing times needed to fit the different models to the two datasets. We see the effect of dimensionality on the various models; for gamma-centered models, it grows linearly; for the log-normal centered model, it will grow superlinearly as matrix inversion becomes the most costly operation. For `BMAmevt`, its parameter space grows combinatorially with the number of dimensions, and thus so does computational complexity and sampling time.

We consider an exploration of the pairwise extremal dependence using Monte Carlo estimates of the coefficients in Equation (10). For this, we use samples obtained from the

PRG-G model. Figure 5 provides a graphical analysis of the results. The coefficients achieve values between 0.286 and 0.759 for the ERA-Interim data and between 0.181 and 0.840 for the ERA5 data. The greater range in dependence scores observed in the ERA5 data versus ERA-Interim speaks to the greater granularity of the ERA5 data, indicating that distance between locations is a strong contributor to the strength of the pairwise asymptotic dependence. The highest coefficients are 0.759 for locations 4 and 5 in the ERA-Interim data and 0.840 for locations 1 and 2 in the ERA5 data. Clearly, pairwise asymptotic dependence coefficients tell a limited story, as a particular dependence may include more than two locations. We can, however, glean some information from the patterns that emerge in two dimensions. For the ERA-Interim data, we observe a possible cluster between cells 5–8, indicating a strong dependence among these cells. Analogously, for the ERA5 data, we observe three possible groups of locations.

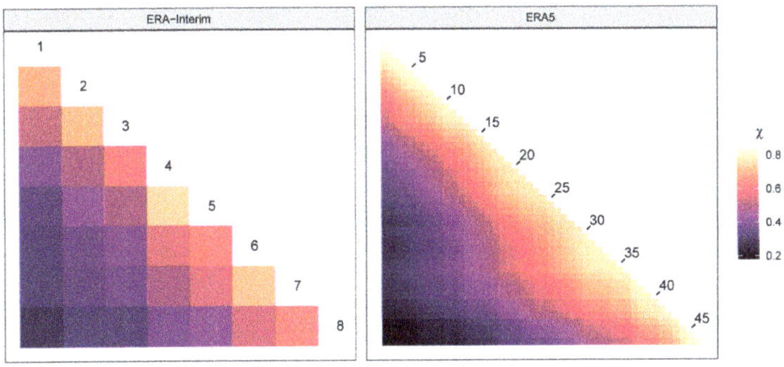


**Figure 5.** Pairwise extremal dependence coefficients for IVT data using the PRG-G model.

Figure 6 shows, for the ERA-Interim data under the PRG-G model, the conditional survival curve defined in Equation (11) for one dimension conditioned on all other dimensions being greater than their (fitted) 90th percentile. Figure 7 presents the bi-variate conditional survival function, conditioning on all other dimensions. These results illustrate quantitatively how extremal dependence affects the shape of the conditional survival curves. The two top panels represent the joint survival function between grid locations 4 and 5, which are shown in Figure 5 to exhibit strong extremal dependence. We observe that the joint survival surface is strongly convex. The bottom panels represent the joint survival surface between grid locations 1 and 5, which exhibited low extremal dependence. In this case, the shape of the contours tends to be concave, quite different from the shapes observed in the top panels.

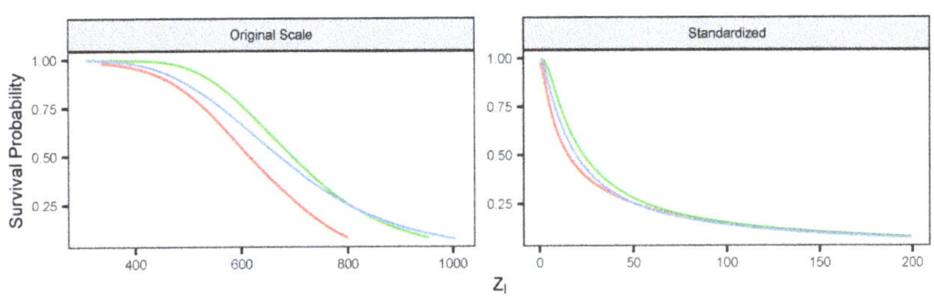


**Figure 6.** Conditional survival curves for selected locations using ERA-Interim and PRG-G model conditioning on all other dimensions at greater than 90th percentile (fitted). The left panel uses original units. Right panel uses standardized units.

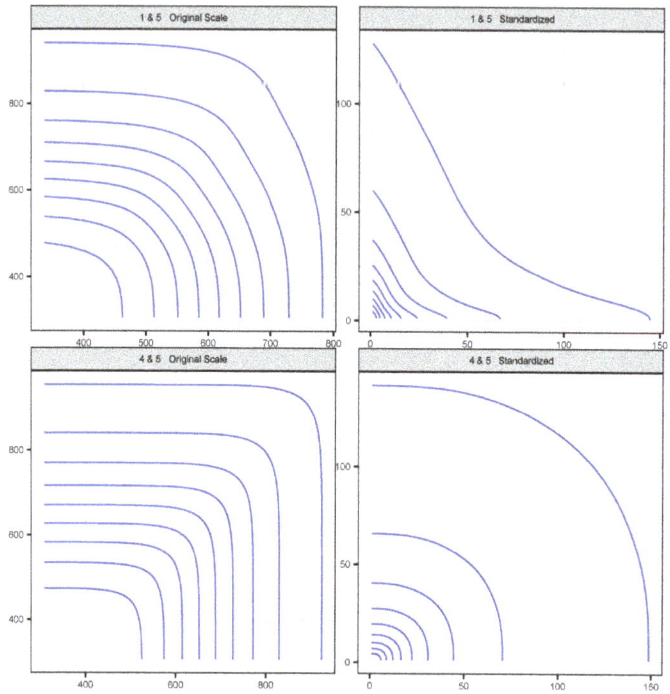


**Figure 7.** Pairwise conditional survival curves for selected locations, using ERA-Interim and PRG-G models, conditioning on all other dimensions at greater than the 90th percentile (fitted).

Using our proposed scoring criteria, we explored the effect of the choice of $p$ on the final results. Using the simulated data, generated from a mixture of projected gammas, we were unable to observe sizeable differences in the scores for $p$ ranging between 1 and 15. However, for the IVT data, we observed a drop in the energy score associated with higher $p$, with a diminishing effect as $p$ increased. We observed no significant differences in the performance of the model that uses $p = 10$, which corresponds to the analysis presented, relative to the one that uses $p = 15$.

## 6. Conclusions

In this paper, we have built upon the definition of the multivariate Pareto described in [11] to establish a useful representation of its dependence structure through the distribution of its angular component, which is supported on the positive orthant of the unit hypersphere under the $\mathcal{L}_\infty$ norm, $\mathbb{S}_\infty^{d-1}$. Due to the inherent difficulty of obtaining the likelihood of distributions with support on $\mathbb{S}_\infty^{d-1}$, our method transforms the data to $\mathbb{S}_p^{d-1}$, fits then using mixtures of products of independent gammas, then transforms the predictions back to $\mathbb{S}_\infty^{d-1}$. As $\mathbb{S}_p^{d-1}$ converges to $\mathbb{S}_\infty^{d-1}$ as $p \to \infty$, we expect the proposed resampling to be efficient for large enough $p$. In fact, our exploration of the simulated and real data indicates that the procedure is robust to the choice of moderately large values of $p$. Our method includes two inferential steps. The first consists of the estimation of the marginal Pareto distributions; the second consists of the estimation of the angular density. Parameter uncertainty incurred in the former is not propagated to the latter. Conceptually, an integrated approach that accounts for all the estimation uncertainty is conceivable. Unfortunately, this leads to posterior distributions with complex data-dependent restrictions that are very difficult to explore, especially in large dimensional settings. In fact, our attempts to fit a simple parametric model for the marginals and the angular measures jointly in several dimensions were not successful.

In this paper, we have focused on a particular representation of the multivariate Pareto distribution for PoT inference on extreme values. To this end, our model provides a computationally efficient and flexible approach. An interesting extension of the proposed model is to consider regressions of extreme value responses, due to extreme value inputs following the ideas in [38]. This will produce PoT-based Bayesian non-parametric extreme value regression models. More generally, models that allow for covariate-dependent extremal dependence [39] could be considered. In addition, we notice that our approach is based on flexibly modeling angular distributions for any $p$-norm. As such, it can be applied to other problems focused on high-dimensional directional statistics constrained to a cone of directions.

Developing an angular measure specifically in $\mathbb{S}_\infty^{d-1}$ provides two benefits over $\mathbb{S}_p^{d-1}$. First, the transformation to $\mathbb{S}_\infty^{d-1}$ is unique. Recall that Equation (4) gives $y_d$ as a function of $y_1, \ldots, y_{d-1}$. An analogous expression can be obtained for any $y_\ell$. This indicates that there are $d$ equivalent transformations, each yielding a different Jacobian and, for $p > 1$, potentially resulting in a different density. Second, the evaluation of geodesic distances on $\mathbb{S}_p^{d-1}$ is not straightforward. However, we have demonstrated a computationally efficient upper bound on geodesic distance on $\mathbb{S}_\infty^{d-1}$. Accepting these foibles, it would be interesting to explore the distribution of $\mathbb{S}_p^{d-1}$.

The computations in this paper were performed on a desktop computer with an AMD Ryzen 5000 series processor. The program is largely single-threaded, so computation time is not dependent on the available core count. In each case, we run the MCMC chain for 50,000 iterations, with a burn-in of 40,000 samples. Fitting the PG-G model on the ERA5 dataset took approximately 15 min. Work is in progress to optimize the code and explore parallelization where possible. We are also exploring alternative computational approaches that will make it feasible to tackle very high dimensional problems, such as variational Bayes. In fact, to elaborate on the study of IVT, there is a need to consider several hundreds, if not thousands, of grid cells over the Pacific Ocean in order to obtain a good description of atmospheric events responsible for large storm activity over California.

**Author Contributions:** Conceptualization, methodology, visualization, writing, P.T.; Supervision, editing, B.S. All authors have read and agreed to the published version of the manuscript.

**Funding:** This material is based on work supported by the National Science Foundation under Grant No. SES-2050012 and DMS-2153277.

**Institutional Review Board Statement:** Not applicable.

**Data Availability Statement:** The raw data supporting the conclusions of this article will be made available by the authors on request.

**Conflicts of Interest:** The authors declare no conflicts of interest.

## References

1. Coles, S.G. *An Introduction to Statistical Modelling of Extreme Values*; Springer: Berlin/Heidelberg, Germany, 2001. [CrossRef]
2. De Haan, L.; Ferreira, A. *Extreme Value Theory: An Introduction*; Springer: Berlin/Heidelberg, Germany, 2006; Volume 21. [CrossRef]
3. Rootzén, H.; Tajvidi, N. Multivariate generalized Pareto distributions. *Bernoulli* **2006**, *12*, 917–930. [CrossRef]
4. Falk, M.; Guillou, A. Peaks-over-Threshold stability of multivariate generalized Pareto distributions. *J. Multivar. Anal.* **2008**, *99*, 715–734. [CrossRef]
5. Michel, R. Some notes on multivariate generalized Pareto distributions. *J. Multivar. Anal.* **2008**, *99*, 1288–1301. [CrossRef]
6. Rootzén, H.; Segers, J.; Wadsworth, J.L. Multivariate peaks over thresholds models. *Extremes* **2018**, *21*, 115–145. [CrossRef]
7. Rootzén, H.; Segers, J.; Wadsworth, J.L. Multivariate generalized Pareto distributions: Parametrizations, representations, and properties. *J. Multivar. Anal.* **2018**, *165*, 117–131. [CrossRef]
8. Kiriliouk, A.; Rootzén, H.; Segers, J.; Wadsworth, J.L. Peaks Over Thresholds Modeling With Multivariate Generalized Pareto Distributions. *Technometrics* **2019**, *61*, 123–135. [CrossRef]

9. Renard, B.; Lang, M. Use of a Gaussian copula for multivariate extreme value analysis: Some case studies in hydrology. *Adv. Water Resour.* **2007**, *30*, 897–912. [CrossRef]
10. Falk, M.; Padoan, S.A.; Wisheckel, F. Generalized Pareto copulas: A key to multivariate extremes. *J. Multivar. Anal.* **2019**, *174*, 104538. [CrossRef]
11. Ferreira, A.; de Haan, L. The generalized Pareto process; with a view towards application and simulation. *Bernoulli* **2014**, *20*, 1717–1737. [CrossRef]
12. Boldi, M.O.; Davison, A.C. A mixture model for multivariate extremes. *J. R. Stat. Soc. Ser. Stat. Methodol.* **2007**, *69*, 217–229. [CrossRef]
13. Sabourin, A.; Naveau, P. Bayesian Drichlet mixture model for multivariate extremes: A re-parametrization. *Comput. Stat. Data Anal.* **2014**, *71*, 542–567. [CrossRef]
14. Hanson, T.E.; de Carvalho, M.; Chen, Y. Bernstein polynomial angular densities of multivariate extreme value distributions. *Stat. Probab. Lett.* **2017**, *128*, 60–66. [CrossRef]
15. Guillotte, S.; Perron, F.; Segers, J. Non-parametric Bayesian inference on bivariate extremes. *J. R. Stat. Soc. Ser. (Stat. Methodol.)* **2011**, *73*, 377–406. [CrossRef]
16. Jentsch, A.; Kreyling, J.; Beierkuhnlein, C. A new generation of climate-change experiments: Events, not trends. *Front. Ecol. Environ.* **2007**, *5*, 365–374. [CrossRef]
17. Vousdoukas, M.I.; Mentaschi, L.; Voukouvalas, E.; Verlaan, M.; Jevrejeva, S.; Jackson, L.P.; Feyen, L. Global probabilistic projections of extreme sea levels show intensification of coastal flood hazard. *Nat. Commun.* **2018**, *9*, 2360. [CrossRef]
18. Li, C.; Zwiers, F.; Zhang, X.; Chen, G.; Lu, J.; Li, G.; Norris, J.; Tan, Y.; Sun, Y.; Liu, M. Larger increases in more extreme local precipitation events as climate warms. *Geophys. Res. Lett.* **2019**, *46*, 6885–6891. [CrossRef]
19. Resnick, S. *Extreme Values, Regular Variation, and Point Processes*; Applied Probability; Springer: Berlin/Heidelberg, Germany, 2008.
20. Núñez-Antonio, G.; Geneyro, E. A multivariate projected Gamma model for directional data. *Commun. Stat.-Simul. Comput.* **2021**, *50*, 2721–2742. [CrossRef]
21. Ferguson, T.S. Prior Distributions on Spaces of Probability Measures. *Ann. Stat.* **1974**, *2*, 615–629. [CrossRef]
22. Antoniak, C.E. Mixtures of Dirichlet Processes with Applications to Bayesian Nonparametric Problems. *Ann. Stat.* **1974**, *2*, 1152–1174. [CrossRef]
23. Müller, P.; Quintana, F.A.; Jara, A.; Hanson, T. *Bayesian Nonparametric Data Analysis*; Springer: Berlin/Heidelberg, Germany, 2015; Volume 1.
24. Ascolani, F.; Lijoi, A.; Rebaudo, G.; Zanella, G. Clustering consistency with Dirichlet process mixtures. *Biometrika* **2022**, *110*, 551–558. [CrossRef]
25. Neal, R.M. Markov Chain Sampling Methods for Dirichlet Process Mixture Models. *J. Comput. Graph. Stat.* **2000**, *9*, 249–265. [CrossRef]
26. Escobar, M.D.; West, M. Bayesian density estimation and inference using mixtures. *J. Am. Stat. Assoc.* **1995**, *90*, 577–588. [CrossRef]
27. Earl, D.J.; Deem, M.W. Parallel tempering: Theory, applications, and new perspectives. *Phys. Chem. Chem. Phys.* **2005**, *7*, 3910–3916. [CrossRef]
28. Gneiting, T.; Raftery, A.E. Strictly Proper Scoring Rules, Prediction, and Estimation. *J. Am. Stat. Assoc.* **2007**, *102*, 359–378. [CrossRef]
29. Berg, C.; Christensen, J.P.R.; Ressel, P. *Harmonic Analysis on Semigroups: Theory of Positive Definite and Related Functions*; Springer: Berlin/Heidelberg, Germany, 1984; Volume 100.
30. Pappas, T. *The Joy of Mathematics: Discovering Mathematics All Around You*; Wide World Pub Tetra: Frederick, MD, USA, 1989.
31. Cooley, D.; Davis, R.A.; Naveau, P. The pairwise beta distribution: A flexible parametric multivariate model for extremes. *J. Multivar. Anal.* **2010**, *101*, 2103–2117. [CrossRef]
32. Sabourin, A. *BMAmevt: Multivariate Extremes: Bayesian Estimation of the Spectral Measure*, R Package Version 1.0.5; 2023. Available online: https://CRAN.R-project.org/package=BMAmevt (accessed on 10 April 2024).
33. Ralph, F.M.; Iacobellis, S.; Neiman, P.; Cordeira, J.; Spackman, J.; Waliser, D.; Wick, G.; White, A.; Fairall, C. Dropsonde observations of total integrated water vapor transport within North Pacific atmospheric rivers. *J. Hydrometeorol.* **2017**, *18*, 2577–2596. [CrossRef]
34. Neiman, P.J.; White, A.B.; Ralph, F.M.; Gottas, D.J.; Gutman, S.I. A water vapour flux tool for precipitation forecasting. In *Proceedings of the Institution of Civil Engineers-Water Management*; Thomas Telford Ltd.: London, UK, 2009; Volume 162, pp. 83–94. [CrossRef]
35. Berrisford, P.; Kållberg, P.; Kobayashi, S.; Dee, D.; Uppala, S.; Simmons, A.; Poli, P.; Sato, H. Atmospheric conservation properties in ERA-Interim. *Q. J. R. Meteorol. Soc.* **2011**, *137*, 1381–1399. [CrossRef]
36. Dee, D.P.; Uppala, S.; Simmons, A.; Berrisford, P.; Poli, P.; Kobayashi, S.; Andrae, U.; Balmaseda, M.; Balsamo, G.; Bauer, P.; et al. The ERA-Interim reanalysis: Configuration and performance of the data assimilation system. *Q. J. R. Meteorol. Soc.* **2011**, *137*, 553–597. [CrossRef]
37. Hersbach, H.; Bell, B.; Berrisford, P.; Hirahara, S.; Horányi, A.; Muñoz-Sabater, J.; Nicolas, J.; Peubey, C.; Radu, R.; Schepers, D.; et al. The ERA5 global reanalysis. *Q. J. R. Meteorol. Soc.* **2020**, *146*, 1999–2049. [CrossRef]

38. de Carvalho, M.; Kumukova, A.; Dos Reis, G. Regression-type analysis for multivariate extreme values. *Extremes* **2022**, 25, 595–622. [CrossRef]
39. Mhalla, L.; de Carvalho, M.; Chavez-Demoulin, V. Regression-type models for extremal dependence. *Scand. J. Stat.* **2019**, *46*, 1141–1167. [CrossRef]

entropy

MDPI

*Article*

# Bayesian Spatio-Temporal Modeling of the Dynamics of COVID-19 Deaths in Peru

**César Raúl Castro Galarza [1,†], Omar Nolberto Díaz Sánchez [1,†], Jonatha Sousa Pimentel [2,*,†], Rodrigo Bulhões [3], Javier Linkolk López-Gonzales [1] and Paulo Canas Rodrigues [3]**

[1] Escuela de Posgrado, Universidad Peruana Unión, Lima 15468, Peru; cesarcastrogalarza@gmail.com (C.R.C.G.); omarndisa@gmail.com (O.N.D.S.); javierlinkolk@gmail.com (J.L.L.-G.)
[2] Department of Statistics, Federal University of Pernambuco, Recife 50740-540, PE, Brazil
[3] Department of Statistics, Federal University of Bahia, Salvador 40170-110, BA, Brazil; rbulhoes@ufba.br (R.B.); paulocanas@gmail.com (P.C.R.)
* Correspondence: jsppimentel9@gmail.com
† These authors contributed equally to this work.

**Abstract:** Amid the COVID-19 pandemic, understanding the spatial and temporal dynamics of the disease is crucial for effective public health interventions. This study aims to analyze COVID-19 data in Peru using a Bayesian spatio-temporal generalized linear model to elucidate mortality patterns and assess the impact of vaccination efforts. Leveraging data from 194 provinces over 651 days, our analysis reveals heterogeneous spatial and temporal patterns in COVID-19 mortality rates. Higher vaccination coverage is associated with reduced mortality rates, emphasizing the importance of vaccination in mitigating the pandemic's impact. The findings underscore the value of spatio-temporal data analysis in understanding disease dynamics and guiding targeted public health interventions.

**Keywords:** COVID-19; spatio-temporal modeling; areal unit data; spatio-temporal generalized linear model; Bayesian statistics

## 1. Introduction

The emergence of Coronavirus Disease 2019 (COVID-19) in December 2019 marked the beginning of a global crisis, with the World Health Organization (WHO) declaring it a pandemic in March 2020 due to its alarming severity and rapid spread. COVID-19, caused by the SARS-CoV-2 virus, belongs to the family of coronaviruses and has since posed significant health, social, and economic challenges worldwide [1–3].

Peru has faced immense challenges in combating the COVID-19 pandemic, like many other countries. The first case of COVID-19 was confirmed on 6 March 2021, triggering a rapid escalation in cases and subsequent waves of infection. The pandemic has had significant impacts in Peru, including economic challenges, disruptions to education, and mental health concerns, leaving many children orphaned and highlighting vulnerabilities in healthcare systems [4,5]. Peru was one of the worst-affected countries in cases and deaths [6].

To combat the pandemic, scientific collaborations expedited the development and authorization of COVID-19 vaccines, which have become pivotal in preventing the spread of the disease and reducing mortality rates [7,8]. However, achieving widespread vaccination coverage remains challenging, particularly in regions with limited healthcare resources [9].

In this context, spatio-temporal data analysis plays a crucial role in understanding the dynamics of the pandemic, identifying high-risk areas, and informing public health interventions for similar future outbreaks. Despite its importance, few studies have been conducted to help understand the spatial and temporal trends of COVID-19 in Peru. An exception is the study of [10], which demonstrated the feasibility and value of implementing a decentralized SARS-CoV-2 RNA wastewater monitoring system to assess the spatio-temporal distribution of COVID-19 in three major cities in Peru. On the other hand, several studies have proposed using spatio-temporal approaches to model the number of deaths and the number of cases of COVID-19 data as outlined by a review that summarizes the contribution of spatio-temporal modeling methodologies in the field of COVID-19 [11]. For example, [12] proposed a spatio-temporal modeling approach of COVID-19 incident cases in Italy, ref. [13] used a model based on discrete latent variables, which are spatially associated and time-specific, for the analysis of incident cases in Italy, ref. [14] studied the association between COVID-19 spread and environmental conditions in Catalonia, Spain, ref. [15] studied the association between deaths and impact of key risk factors in England, ref. [16] studied risk clusters of COVID-19 transmission in northeastern Brazil, ref. [17] analyzed the behavior and forecast of the number of deaths in the 26 Brazilian states, the federal district, and Italy, and [18] presented a spatio-temporal modeling analysis of initial COVID-19 diffusion in China and in the United States.

Despite the wealth of spatio-temporal COVID data available, there remains a gap in the literature regarding applying advanced statistical spatio-temporal models to analyze and understand the dynamics of these datasets, particularly for Peru. This work aims to fill this gap in two ways. Firstly, it provides a descriptive and exploratory analysis of the spatial and temporal dynamics of COVID-19 data in Peru. Then, we employ a spatio-temporal generalized linear model tailored for areal unit data, with parameter inferences conducted within a Bayesian framework. By leveraging this model, we aim to elucidate the spatial and temporal patterns of COVID-19 deaths, investigate the impact of vaccination efforts, and provide valuable insights for guiding public health policies and interventions.

This paper is structured as follows. Section 2 describes the data sources and preprocessing steps and outlines the methodology, including the Bayesian spatio-temporal generalized linear model and Bayesian inference framework. Section 3 presents the results and discussion of the analysis, including the descriptive and exploratory analysis of the temporal and spatial dynamics of the data and the results of the statistical model. Finally, Section 4 concludes with a summary of key findings and suggestions for future research.

## 2. Materials and Methods

This section provides an overview of the data utilized in our analysis, including the collection, processing, and organization procedures of both the response variable and the covariates. We then detail the construction of the spatio-temporal generalized linear model tailored for areal unit data, whose parameter inferences are performed within a Bayesian framework.

### 2.1. The Data

This study examines data spanning two years, from 3 March 2020 to 13 December 2021. The data include information from three distinct sources:

(i) Records of COVID-19 deaths across Peru sourced from the Ministerio de Salud (MINSA) and accessible through the Plataforma Nacional De Datos Abiertos (www.datosabiertos.gob.pe/);
(ii) Records of COVID-19 cases across Peru sourced from the MINSA;
(iii) Vaccination records against COVID-19, also obtained from the MINSA.

Peru is geographically divided into three levels: 26 regions, 194 provinces, and 1838 districts. Furthermore, the shapefile includes Lake Titicaca because of its extension. It is located on the border between Peru and Bolivia in the Andes Mountains and is one of the largest lakes in South America. Therefore, this part of the territory will not be included in the analysis despite being represented in the figures. For the modeling phase, the data were aggregated at the province level to provide spatial coverage across the country. This division is illustrated in Figure 1. Temporally, the data were organized daily, resulting in a panel format dataset. Each column represents one of the 194 Peruvian provinces, and each row represents a date, resulting in 651 observations for each province. The cutoff date for the analysis was set as 13 December 2021, corresponding to the date of the last death recorded in the dataset of deceased individuals by COVID-19.

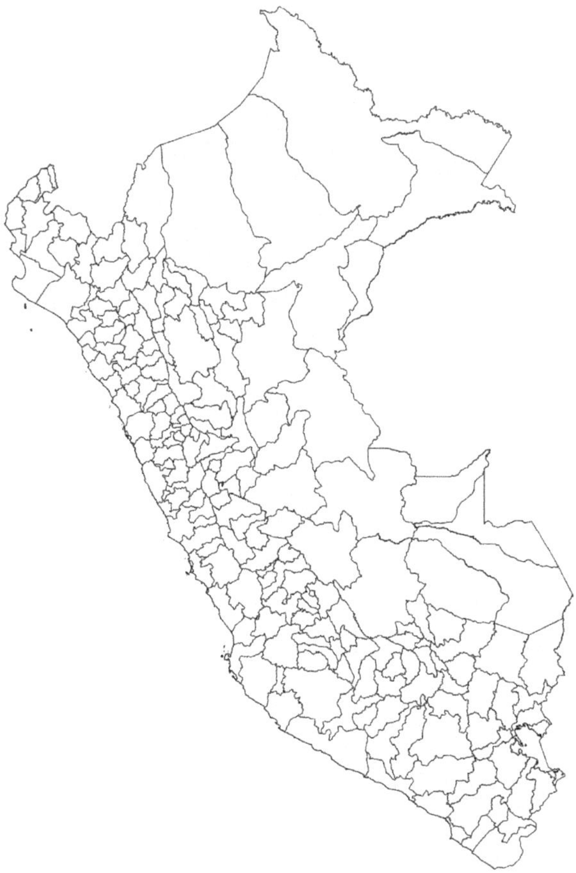

**Figure 1.** Map of Peru subdivided by its 194 provinces and Lake Titicaca.

Given the diverse formats for the datasets, several approaches were employed to transform them into the final format required for analysis. Detailed descriptions of data collection, processing, and organization are provided below to ensure transparency and facilitate reproducibility in scientific research.

The response variable, the number of deaths from COVID-19, initially resided in a single file encompassing all recorded deaths within Peruvian territory from 3 March 2020 to 13 December 2021. Over this period, slightly over 200,000 deaths from COVID-19 were documented, corresponding to the total number of entries in the dataset. Deaths were aggregated based on the date and province of occurrence to derive the final dataset, resulting in a structured dataset with 651 rows and 194 columns. Each row represents a day within the analysis period, while each column represents a Peruvian province. We assume that a zero value was assigned for days where no observations were recorded in a particular province, meaning the absence of reported deaths during that specific day in that location.

The variable total COVID-19 cases was initially consolidated into a single file containing all cases registered across the Peruvian territory between 6 March 2020 and 31 December 2023. However, due to the absence of response variable data for a period equivalent to the variables, the analysis period was restricted to 3 March 2020 to 13 December 2021. Thus, the three days of difference between the beginning of recording cases and deaths were assumed as zero cases. This raw file comprised over ten variables, including information about people, such as age, sex, geographic information, and district and province of case notification. Throughout this period, slightly over 4.5 million COVID-19 cases were documented in Peru, corresponding to the total number of entries in the database. Subsequently, reported cases were aggregated based on the notification date and province of residence for model development and application. This process yielded a dataset with dimensions of 651 rows and 194 columns, where each row represents a day within the analysis period and each column represents a Peruvian province. Similarly to the number of deaths, we assume that a zero value was assigned for days where no observations were recorded in a given province, meaning the absence of reported cases during that specific day in that location.

Due to its considerable size, the COVID-19 vaccination database posed significant challenges in reading and processing. The original dataset comprises a single file containing all records of COVID-19 vaccines administered in Peru from 27 April 2020 to 29 November 2023, totaling over 90 million doses administered nationwide, corresponding to the total number of rows in the database. Similarly to the previous variables, the data are limited between 3 March 2020 and 13 December 2021. The raw file contains 14 variables, including the vaccination location, the vaccinated individual's risk group (whether the person who was vaccinated belonged to a risk group for worsening the disease), gender, and vaccine manufacturer (i.e., the company responsible for the vaccine). The number of vaccines administered was aggregated based on the location and day of administration. Additionally, the data were segmented into four distinct subsets corresponding to the first four doses administered, each comprising 651 rows (representing the number of days) and 194 columns (representing provinces).

The dataset used for the analysis and modeling consists, for each Peruvian province, of the number of deaths from COVID-19, the response variable in this study, and the explanatory variables total number of COVID-19 cases and number of vaccine doses against COVID-19 administered, divided into four categories corresponding to the first four doses. The response variable and the five covariates were transformed into seven-day moving averages to correct for large weekly fluctuations. Furthermore, a difference of 14 days was adopted between the response variable number of deaths and the explanatory variables, which can be justified by the incubation time and presentation of symptoms that varied between 2 and 14 days [19–21].

All analyses were performed using the R programming language (version 4.3.2) [22] on a personal computer equipped with a 2.50 GHz Intel Core i5-10300H processor and 8 GB of RAM, running on the Windows 11 64-bit operating system.

### 2.2. Bayesian Spatio-Temporal Model

The conventional linear regression model typically assumes independent observations and overlooks temporal and spatial dependencies. However, considering the nature of our panel data, which varies across time and space, it becomes imperative to account for these dependencies. To address this challenge, we adopted a Bayesian spatio-temporal generalized linear model specifically tailored for areal unit data, which was proposed by [23] and whose main ideas were previously developed by [24,25]. This model is well suited for fitting areal unit data observed in discrete periods while including relevant explanatory variables. Next, we will briefly review the formulation of this model that we will apply to analyze our data.

Let $Y_{k,t}$ be the response variable in areal unit $k$ and time $t$, where $k \in \{1,\ldots,K\}$, $t \in \{1,\ldots,N\}$, $K$ is the total of areal units, and $N$ is the number of periods of time. Suppose that $Y_{k,t} \mid \mu_{k,t} \sim \text{Poisson}(E_{k,t}\mu_{k,t})$ and $\ln \mu_{k,t} = \mathbf{x}_{k,t}^{\mathsf{T}}\boldsymbol{\beta} + O_{k,t} + \psi_{k,t}$, where $\mu_{k,t}$ is the risk of death in areal unit $k$ and time $t$ relative to the expected counts $E_{k,t}$, $\mathbf{x}_{k,t}$ is a $p$-variate vector of known covariates for areal unit $k$ and time $t$, $\boldsymbol{\beta} = (\beta_1, \ldots, \beta_p)$ is a $p$-dimensional vector of covariate regression parameters, and $O_{k,t}$ is an offset for areal unit $k$ and time $t$. Including a random effects term $\psi_{k,t}$ for areal unit $k$ and time $t$ allows us to effectively capture the inherent dependencies of our dataset that vary over time and space. Other model specifications are given by

$$
\begin{aligned}
\boldsymbol{\beta} &\sim \text{Normal}(\boldsymbol{\mu}_{\beta}, \boldsymbol{\Sigma}_{\beta}) && (1)\\
\psi_{k,t} &= (\beta_1 + \phi_k) + (\alpha + \delta_k)\frac{t - \bar{t}}{N} && (2)\\
\phi_k \mid \boldsymbol{\phi}_{-k}, \mathbf{W} &\sim \text{Normal}\left(\mu_{\phi_k|\boldsymbol{\phi}_{-k},\mathbf{W}}, \sigma^2_{\phi_k|\boldsymbol{\phi}_{-k},\mathbf{W}}\right) && (3)\\
\delta_k \mid \delta_{-k}, \mathbf{W} &\sim \text{Normal}\left(\mu_{\delta_k|\delta_{-k},\mathbf{W}}, \sigma^2_{\delta_k|\delta_{-k},\mathbf{W}}\right) && (4)\\
\alpha &\sim \text{Normal}(\mu_{\alpha}, \sigma^2_{\alpha}), && (5)
\end{aligned}
$$

where

- $\bar{t} = \sum_{t=1}^{N} t/N$ is the average time;
- $\psi_{k,t}$ is a latent component for the province $k$ and day $t$ embracing one or more sets of spatio-temporally autocorrelated random effects, which are known as *correlated linear time trends* [26];
- $\mathbf{W} = [w_{k,j}]$ is a binary neighborhood matrix $K \times K$, with $w_{k,j} = 0$ if $k = j$ (diagonal elements equal to zero), $w_{k,j} = 1$ if the provinces $k$ and $j$ share a common border, and $w_{k,j} = 0$ if the provinces $k$ and $j$ do not share a common border;
- The random effects $\boldsymbol{\phi} = (\phi_1, \ldots, \phi_K)$ and $\boldsymbol{\delta} = (\delta_1, \ldots, \delta_K)$ are modeled as spatially autocorrelated by the CAR (conditional autoregressive) prior, satisfying $\sum_{k=1}^{K} \phi_k = \sum_{k=1}^{K} \delta_k = 0$ to avoid a lack of identifiability, with $\boldsymbol{\phi}_{-k}$ and $\delta_{-k}$ denoting the vectors $\boldsymbol{\phi}$ and $\boldsymbol{\delta}$ without their corresponding $k$th entries, respectively;
- The quantities $\mu_{\phi_k|\boldsymbol{\phi}_{-k},\mathbf{W}}$, $\sigma^2_{\phi_k|\boldsymbol{\phi}_{-k},\mathbf{W}}$, $\mu_{\delta_k|\delta_{-k},\mathbf{W}}$, and $\sigma^2_{\delta_k|\delta_{-k},\mathbf{W}}$ are given, respectively, by

$$
\mu_{\phi_k|\boldsymbol{\phi}_{-k},\mathbf{W}} = \frac{\rho_{int} \sum_{j=1}^{K} w_{k,j}\phi_j}{\rho_{int} \sum_{j=1}^{K} w_{k,j} + 1 - \rho_{int}}, \tag{6}
$$

$$
\sigma^2_{\phi_k|\boldsymbol{\phi}_{-k},\mathbf{W}} = \frac{\tau^2_{int}}{\rho_{int} \sum_{j=1}^{K} w_{k,j} + 1 - \rho_{int}}, \tag{7}
$$

$$
\mu_{\delta_k|\delta_{-k},\mathbf{W}} = \frac{\rho_{slo} \sum_{j=1}^{K} w_{k,j}\delta_j}{\rho_{slo} \sum_{j=1}^{K} w_{k,j} + 1 - \rho_{slo}}, \tag{8}
$$

and

$$
\sigma^2_{\delta_k|\delta_{-k},\mathbf{W}} = \frac{\tau^2_{slo}}{\rho_{slo} \sum_{j=1}^{K} w_{k,j} + 1 - \rho_{slo}}. \tag{9}
$$

The model captures the spatio-temporal pattern in the mean response by incorporating a spatially varying linear time trend. Each province (indexed by $k$) possesses its own individual linear time trend, characterized by a spatially varying intercept $\beta_1 + \phi_k$ and a spatially varying slope $\alpha + \delta_k$.

The parameters $\rho_{int}$ and $\rho_{slo}$ are spatial dependence parameters, with zero corresponding to independence and one corresponding to strong spatial smoothness. Each parameter follows a uniformly distributed prior distribution over the unit interval. The random effects variances are specified with the conjugate prior distributions $\tau^2_{int} \sim$ Inverse-Gamma$(a, b)$ and $\tau^2_{slo} \sim$ Inverse-Gamma$(a, b)$.

To have flat prior distributions for all model parameters, we specify the following hyperparameters: $\mu_\beta = \mathbf{0}_p$, $\mathbf{\Sigma}_\beta = 10^5 \cdot \mathbf{I}_p$, $a = 0$, $b = 0.01$, $\mu_\alpha = 0$, and $\sigma^2_\alpha = 1000$. This statistical model is implemented in the function *ST.CARlinear* of the R package `CARBayesST` [26], which estimates the model parameters using the MCMC (Markov chain Monte Carlo) algorithm.

The spatio-temporal modeling aims to characterize the total number of COVID-19 deaths in Peru over a specified period, aggregated by provinces and days. Our analysis incorporates explanatory variables such as the total number of COVID-19 cases and the cumulative count of the first four doses of the COVID-19 vaccine administered in the respective provinces.

## 3. Results and Discussion

### 3.1. Descriptive and Exploratory Analysis

Our study aims to compare the dynamics of COVID-19 deaths in Peru over a span of two years, examining the impacts of vaccination efforts and the spatial distribution of the disease on mortality. When analyzing the relationship between the number of COVID-19 cases and deaths during the study period spanning from 3 March 2020 to 13 December 2021, as depicted in Figure 2, we observed spikes in cases and deaths in periods of similar behavior between the two series. Specifically, increases in COVID-19 cases correspond to rises in deaths, indicating a consistent pattern across the two variables.

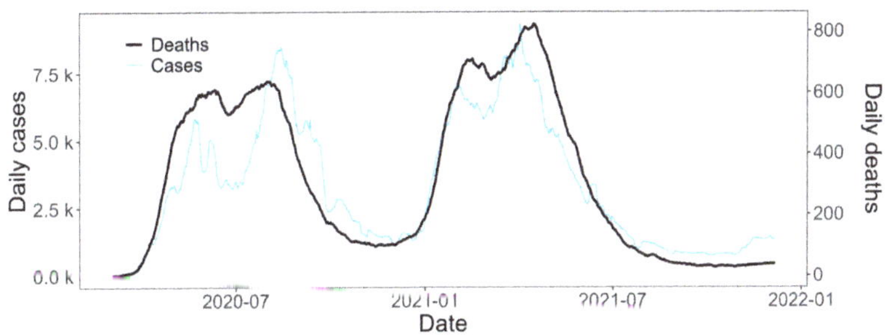


**Figure 2.** Seven-day moving average for the total COVID-19 cases and deaths in Peru between 3 March 2020 and 13 December 2021. The 14-day delay used in the modeling phase is not represented in this image.

The peaks in COVID-19 cases and deaths are also evident in Figures 3 and 4, which display the cumulative cases and deaths over six-month periods. Specifically, we observe a higher concentration of cases during the second half of 2020 and the first half of 2021, corresponding to the periods where the highest peaks occurred in the series (Figure 2). Similarly, the number of deaths also exhibits distinct periods, with notable variations across the three periods encompassing 2020 and the first half of 2021.

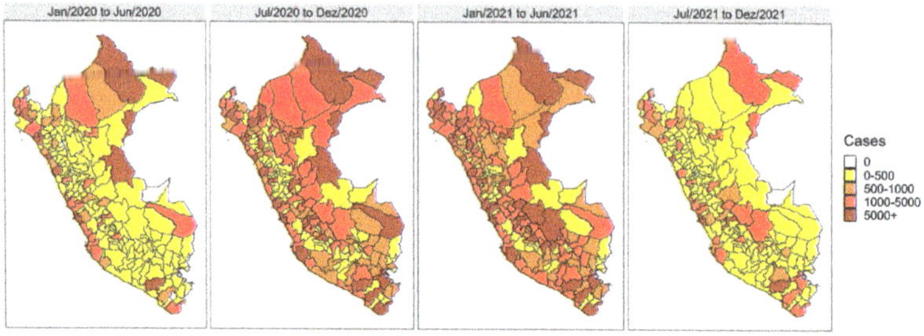


**Figure 3.** Heatmaps with the evolution in the total number of COVID-19 cases in Peru semiannually between 3 March 2020 and 13 December 2021.

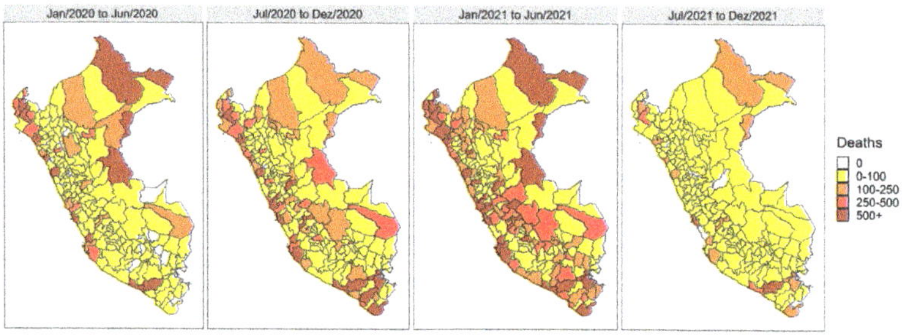


**Figure 4.** Heat maps with the evolution in the total number of COVID-19 deaths in Peru semiannually between 3 March 2020 and 13 December 2021.

Figures A1–A4 of Appendix A show the heat maps with the vaccine coverage of the first four COVID-19 doses, respectively, every three months during the COVID-19 pandemic across all 194 provinces of Peru and Lake Titicaca.

### 3.2. *Bayesian Spatio-Temporal Modeling*

After the initial descriptive and exploratory analysis, it became apparent that the (seven-day moving average) number of deaths exhibits spatial and temporal dependencies. Acknowledging this dependence, a spatio-temporal model was estimated for the entire period. In this context, we utilized the Bayesian spatio-temporal generalized linear model proposed by [23], chosen for its suitability in handling count data and enabling the incorporation of explanatory variables. The percentage of the population per province has been included as an offset for our model to account for the population difference between provinces.

We analyzed data from $K = 194$ provinces over a period of $N = 651$ days. We assessed the correlation strength between each candidate variable and the response variable in each model to select explanatory variables for each model, and we used different combinations of models with the available variables, selecting the one in which the variables were jointly statistically significant, in a backward manner. We ran the MCMC algorithm 20,000 times to estimate the model parameters, excluding the first 2000 iterations (warm-up period) and taking samples from the posterior distribution every 6th iteration to reduce autocorrelation in the chains (thinning).

During the estimation process, two models (with and without a 14-day lag between the number of cases and other variables) were compared based on the deviance information criterion (DIC), the log marginal predictive likelihood (LMPL), and the Watanabe–Akaike information criterion (WAIC). The model that considered a 14-day lag between the number of cases and other variables showed an improvement of about 10% in the evaluation metrics DIC, WAIC, and LMPL. Table 1 presents the most relevant coefficients of the model, including the degree of spatial dependence and the significance of the coefficients associated with the covariates.

Under the Bayesian framework employed in this study, we consider each component of $\beta$ to be statistically significant when the value of zero falls outside the credibility interval formed by the 2.5th and 97.5th percentiles of its corresponding posterior distribution. Among the covariates considered, it was observed that the (seven-day moving average) number of cases and the second and third doses of the COVID-19 vaccine were statistically significant and kept in the model. Moreover, based on the coefficients, it is evident that the (seven-day moving average) number of cases positively influences the number of deaths. At the same time, both doses of the vaccine exert a negative influence, with the third dose showing a more pronounced reduction effect.

**Table 1.** Posterior mean, 2.5th, and 97.5th percentiles of the posterior distribution of the model parameters. The acceptance percentage, effective sample size, and Geweke statistic for each model parameter are provided. The sample size of the posterior distribution of each parameter is equal to one thousand. DIC: 621,729; WAIC: 640,586; LMPL: −316,548.

| Parameter | Posterior Mean | 2.5th Perc. | 97.5th Perc. | % Accept. | Effective Samples | Geweke |
|---|---|---|---|---|---|---|
| Intercept | 0.0722 | 0.0657 | 0.0789 | 13 | 128 | −0.3 |
| $\beta_{Cases}$ | 0.0020 | 0.0020 | 0.0020 | 13 | 285 | 0.4 |
| $\beta_{Vaccine2}$ | −0.1354 | −0.1462 | −0.1243 | 13 | 105 | −0.1 |
| $\beta_{Vaccine3}$ | −0.4078 | −0.4334 | −0.3808 | 13 | 105 | −0.1 |
| $\alpha$ | −0.1337 | −0.1535 | −0.1148 | 38 | 2263 | −1.4 |
| $\tau^2_{int}$ | 0.0888 | 0.0675 | 0.1228 | 100 | 1610 | −0.2 |
| $\tau^2_{slo}$ | 0.1506 | 0.1124 | 0.2063 | 100 | 1907 | 0.1 |
| $\rho_{int}$ | 0.0335 | 0.0010 | 0.1171 | 41.6 | 1523 | 0.1 |
| $\rho_{slo}$ | 0.0287 | 0.0008 | 0.1003 | 43.2 | 1524 | −0.2 |

The term $\delta_k$ is known as the "differential trend of the $k$th areal unit", which is the interaction between the time effect and the area effect. An interpretation for the time effect is provided by [24] as follows: a value of $\delta_k < 0$ implies that the temporal trend of the areal unit $k$ is less steep than the mean trend $\alpha$, while a value of $\delta_k > 0$ implies that the temporal trend of areal unit $k$ is steeper than the mean trend $\alpha$.

Figure 5 depicts the posterior average of the parameter $\delta_k$, where $k$ denotes the $k$th province. The areal units whose trend is steeper than the average trend are further east and north. From this map, it is evident that a diverse array of behaviors and temporal trends are present. Provinces closer to the capital and along the coast exhibit negative temporal trends more frequently. Conversely, provinces located farther from the capital and in the country's northern regions display positive temporal trends, indicating an upward trend in the (seven-day moving average) number of deaths over the study period.

Based on Table 1, the MCMC algorithm achieves convergence. When the Geweke statistic takes high values, say, outside the interval $(-1.96, 1.96)$, it indicates convergence problems [27], which is not observed for any of the model parameters. Although acceptance rates for certain parameters were low, visual diagnosis based on trace plots (Figure A5 shows the trace plot related to $\beta_{Cases}$) also shows convergence.

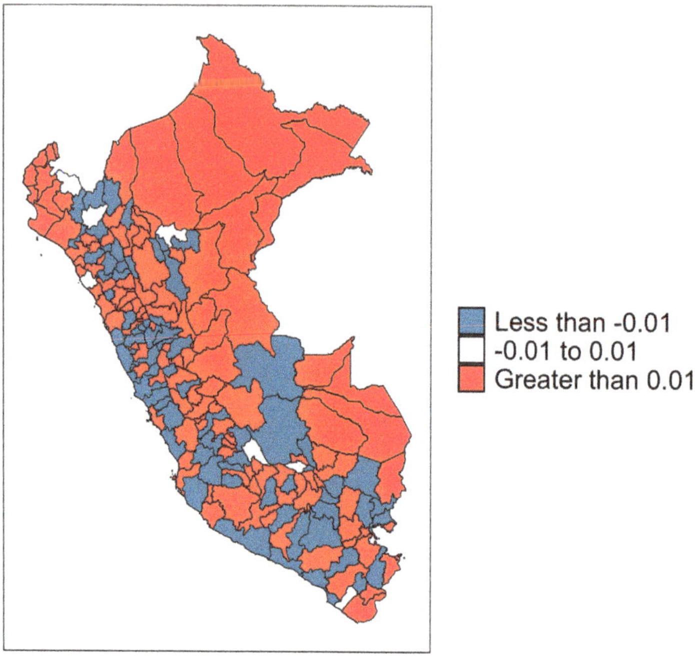


**Figure 5.** Heatmaps with the posterior mean of the parameter $\delta_k$ of the spatio-temporal model across all provinces of Peru, where $k$ indicates the $k$th province.

## 4. Concluding Remarks

In conclusion, our study sheds light on the complex spatial and temporal dynamics of COVID-19 in Peru and underscores the critical role of vaccination in mitigating mortality rates. The findings highlight the effectiveness of vaccination campaigns in reducing the impact of the pandemic and emphasize the importance of continued efforts to enhance vaccine coverage. Furthermore, our analysis underscores the value of spatio-temporal data analysis in guiding targeted public health interventions and the importance of effective case management and prevention strategies. Moving forward, policymakers and healthcare authorities should prioritize vaccination efforts and implement evidence-based interventions to control the spread of COVID-19 and minimize its impact on communities. By leveraging advanced statistical models and comprehensive data analysis, we can better understand disease dynamics and inform strategies to combat future outbreaks effectively. Overall, this study contributes valuable insights to the global effort to address the COVID-19 pandemic and provides a foundation for further research in this critical area of public health.

For future research, it is essential to continue monitoring the spatial and temporal dynamics of COVID-19, particularly in the context of emerging variants and changing vaccination strategies. Longitudinal studies are needed to assess the long-term effectiveness of vaccination campaigns and the persistence of immunity over time. Furthermore, research on the socio-economic and demographic determinants of COVID-19 mortality could provide valuable insights into disparities in disease burden and inform targeted interventions to address health inequities. Additionally, incorporating real-time data and advanced modeling techniques could enhance our ability to effectively predict and respond to future outbreaks. Moreover, exploring the application of spatio-temporal modeling techniques to other fields of study, such as infectious disease epidemiology [28], environmental health [29–31], natural disaster management [32], and climate change [33–35], could provide further insights into complex systems' dynamics and inform evidence-based decision making across various domains. Overall, continued research in this area is crucial for informing evidence-based strategies to control the spread of COVID-19 and other infectious diseases and minimize their impact on public health.

**Author Contributions:** Conceptualization, C.R.C.G., O.N.D.S. and P.C.R.; methodology, J.S.P. and R.B.; software, J.S.P. and R.B.; validation, J.S.P., R.B., J.L.L.-G. and P.C.R.; formal analysis, J.S.P., R.B. and P.C.R.; investigation, J.S.P., R.B. and P.C.R.; writing—original draft preparation, C.R.C.G., O.N.D.S. and J.S.P.; writing—review and editing, J.S.P., R.B., J.L.L.-G. and P.C.R.; visualization, J.S.P.; supervision, P.C.R. All authors have read and agreed to the published version of the manuscript.

**Funding:** This research received no external funding. The APC was funded by the Universidad Peruana Unión.

**Data Availability Statement:** The data used in this paper are available at https://github.com/SaLLy-laboratory/COVID19-Peru (accessed on 27 May 2024).

**Conflicts of Interest:** The authors declare no conflicts of interest.

## Appendix A. Supplementary Figures

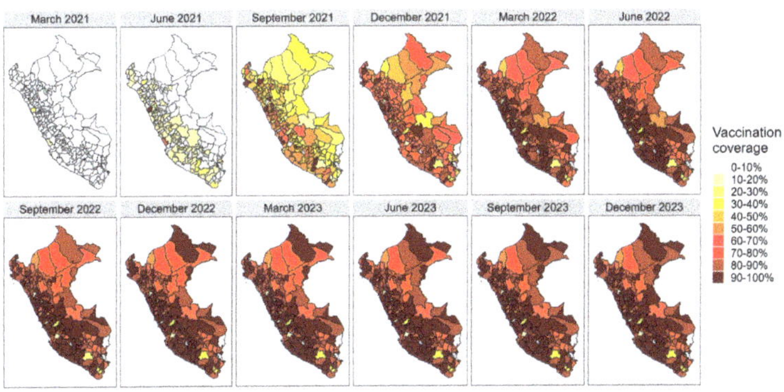


**Figure A1.** Heatmaps with the vaccine coverage of the first COVID-19 dose every three months during the COVID-19 pandemic across all 194 provinces of Peru and Lake Titicaca.

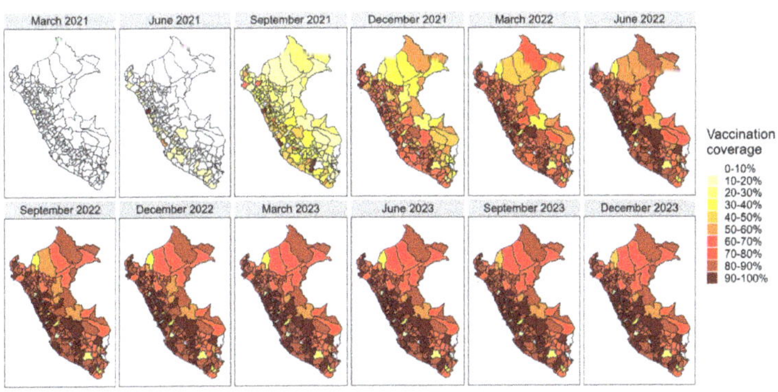


**Figure A2.** Heat maps with the vaccine coverage of the second COVID-19 dose every three months during the COVID-19 pandemic across all 194 provinces of Peru and Lake Titicaca.

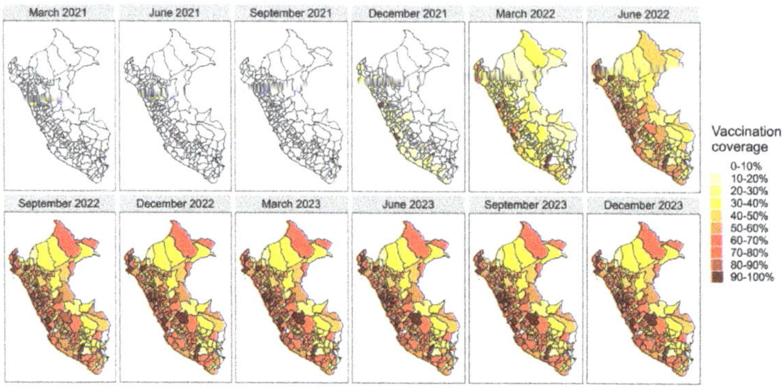


**Figure A3.** Heat maps with the vaccine coverage of the third COVID-19 dose every three months during the COVID-19 pandemic across all 194 provinces of Peru and Lake Titicaca.

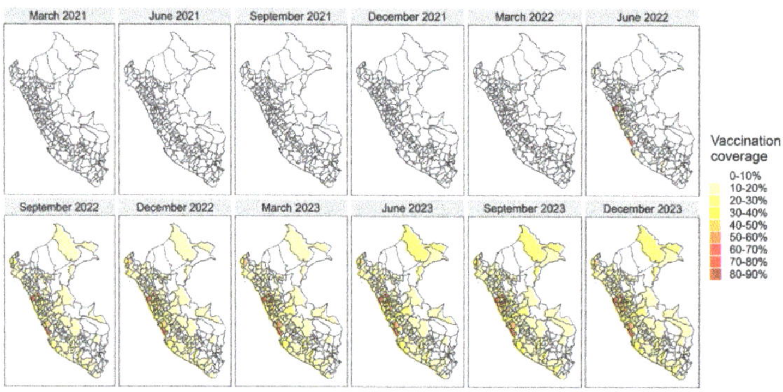


**Figure A4.** Heat maps with the vaccine coverage of the fourth COVID-19 dose every three months during the COVID-19 pandemic across all 194 provinces of Peru and Lake Titicaca.

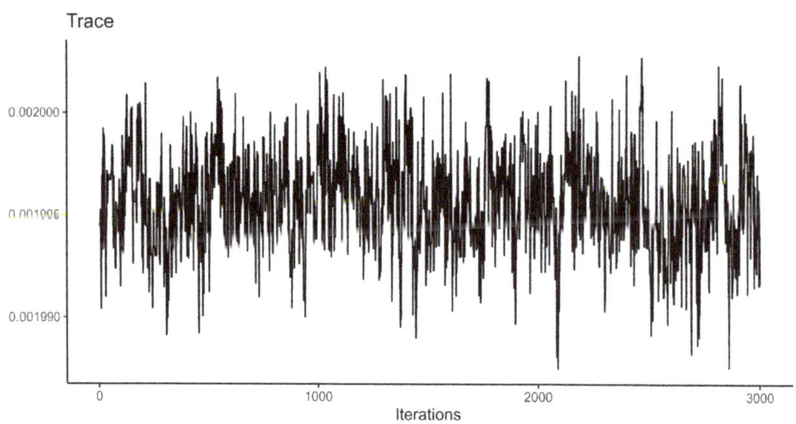


**Figure A5.** Trace plots for model parameter $\beta_{Cases}$.

## References


1. Baloch, S.; Baloch, M.A.; Zheng, T.; Pei, X. The coronavirus disease 2019 (COVID-19) pandemic. *Tohoku J. Exp. Med.* **2020**, *250*, 271–278. [CrossRef] [PubMed]
2. Ciotti, M.; Ciccozzi, M.; Terrinoni, A.; Jiang, W.C.; Wang, C.B.; Bernardini, S. The COVID-19 pandemic. *Crit. Rev. Clin. Lab. Sci.* **2020**, *57*, 365–388. [CrossRef] [PubMed]
3. Abenavoli, L.; Gentile, I. COVID-19: Where We Are and Where We Are Going. *Diseases* **2023**, *11*, 40. [CrossRef] [PubMed]
4. Alvarez-Risco, A.; Mejia, C.R.; Delgado-Zegarra, J.; Del-Aguila-Arcentales, S.; Arce-Esquivel, A.A.; Valladares-Garrido, M.J.; Del Portal, M.R.; Villegas, L.F.; Curioso, W.H.; Sekar, M.C.; et al. The Peru approach against the COVID-19 infodemic: Insights and strategies. *Am. J. Trop. Med. Hyg.* **2020**, *103*, 583–586. [CrossRef] [PubMed]
5. Schwalb, A.; Seas, C. The COVID-19 pandemic in Peru: What went wrong? *Am. J. Trop. Med. Hyg.* **2021**, *104*, 1176. [CrossRef] [PubMed]
6. Karlinsky, A.; Kobak, D. Tracking excess mortality across countries during the COVID-19 pandemic with the World Mortality Dataset. *eLife* **2021**, *10*, e69336. [CrossRef] [PubMed]
7. Ndwandwe, D.; Wiysonge, C.S. COVID-19 vaccines. *Curr. Opin. Immunol.* **2021**, *71*, 111–116. [CrossRef] [PubMed]
8. Lopez Bernal, J.; Andrews, N.; Gower, C.; Gallagher, E.; Simmons, R.; Thelwall, S.; Stowe, J.; Tessier, E.; Groves, N.; Dabrera, G.; et al. Effectiveness of COVID-19 vaccines against the B. 1.617. 2 (Delta) variant. *N. Engl. J. Med.* **2021**, *385*, 585–594. [CrossRef]
9. Calina, D.; Docea, A.O.; Petrakis, D.; Egorov, A.M.; Ishmukhametov, A.A.; Gabibov, A.G.; Shtilman, M.I.; Kostoff, R.; Carvalho, F.; Vinceti, M.; et al. Towards effective COVID-19 vaccines: Updates, perspectives and challenges. *Int. J. Mol. Med.* **2020**, *46*, 3–16. [CrossRef] [PubMed]
10. Pardo-Figueroa, B.; Mindreau-Ganoza, E.; Reyes-Calderon, A.; Yufra, S.P.; Solorzano-Ortiz, I.M.; Donayre-Torres, A.J.; Antonini, C.; Renom, J.M.; Quispe, A.M.; Mota, C.R.; et al. Spatiotemporal surveillance of SARS-CoV-2 in the sewage of three major urban areas in Peru: Generating valuable data where clinical testing is extremely limited. *Acs Es T Water* **2022**, *2*, 2144–2157. [CrossRef]
11. Wang, P.; Zheng, X.; Liu, H. Simulation and forecasting models of COVID-19 taking into account spatio-temporal dynamic characteristics: A review. *Front. Public Health* **2022**, *10*, 1033432. [CrossRef] [PubMed]
12. Mingione, M.; Di Loro, P.A.; Farcomeni, A.; Divino, F.; Lovison, G.; Maruotti, A.; Lasinio, G.J. Spatio-temporal modelling of COVID-19 incident cases using Richards' curve: An application to the Italian regions. *Spat. Stat.* **2022**, *49*, 100544. [CrossRef] [PubMed]
13. Bartolucci, F.; Farcomeni, A. A spatio-temporal model based on discrete latent variables for the analysis of COVID-19 incidence. *Spat. Stat.* **2022**, *49*, 100504. [CrossRef] [PubMed]
14. Briz-Redón, Á. The impact of modelling choices on modelling outcomes: A spatio-temporal study of the association between COVID-19 spread and environmental conditions in Catalonia (Spain). *Stoch. Environ. Res. Risk Assess.* **2021**, *35*, 1701–1713. [CrossRef] [PubMed]
15. Sartorius, B.; Lawson, A.; Pullan, R. Modelling and predicting the spatio-temporal spread of COVID-19, associated deaths and impact of key risk factors in England. *Sci. Rep.* **2021**, *11*, 5378. [CrossRef] [PubMed]
16. Gomes, D.S.; Andrade, L.A.; Ribeiro, C.J.N.; Peixoto, M.; Lima, S.; Duque, A.; Cirilo, T.M.; Góes, M.; Lima, A.; Santos, M.; et al. Risk clusters of COVID-19 transmission in northeastern Brazil: Prospective space–time modelling. *Epidemiol. Infect.* **2020**, *148*, e188. [CrossRef] [PubMed]
17. Pereira, C.A.d.B.; Nakamura, L.R.; Rodrigues, P.C. Naive statistical analyses for COVID-19: Application to data from Brazil and Italy. *Rev. Bras. Biom.* **2021**, *39*, 158–176. [CrossRef]
18. Griffith, D.; Li, B. Spatial-temporal modeling of initial COVID-19 diffusion: The cases of the Chinese Mainland and Conterminous United States. *Geo-Spat. Inf. Sci.* **2021**, *24*, 340–362. [CrossRef]
19. Lauer, S.A.; Grantz, K.H.; Bi, Q.; Jones, F.K.; Zheng, Q.; Meredith, H.R.; Azman, A.S.; Reich, N.G.; Lessler, J. The incubation period of coronavirus disease 2019 (COVID-19) from publicly reported confirmed cases: Estimation and application. *Ann. Intern. Med.* **2020**, *172*, 577–582. [CrossRef]
20. Ejima, K.; Kim, K.S.; Ludema, C.; Bento, A.I.; Iwanami, S.; Fujita, Y.; Ohashi, H.; Koizumi, Y.; Watashi, K.; Aihara, K.; et al. Estimation of the incubation period of COVID-19 using viral load data. *Epidemics* **2021**, *35*, 100454. [CrossRef]
21. Men, K.; Li, Y.; Wang, X.; Zhang, G.; Hu, J.; Gao, Y.; Han, A.; Liu, W.; Han, H. Estimate the incubation period of coronavirus 2019 (COVID-19). *Comput. Biol. Med.* **2023**, *158*, 106794. [CrossRef] [PubMed]
22. R Core Team. *R: A Language and Environment for Statistical Computing*; R Foundation for Statistical Computing: Vienna, Austria, 2023.
23. Lee, D.; Rushworth, A.; Napier, G. Spatio-temporal areal unit modeling in R with conditional autoregressive priors using the CARBayesST package. *J. Stat. Softw.* **2018**, *84*, 1–39. [CrossRef]
24. Bernardinelli, L.; Clayton, D.; Pascutto, C.; Montomoli, C.; Ghislandi, M.; Songini, M. Bayesian analysis of space—Time variation in disease risk. *Stat. Med.* **1995**, *14*, 2433–2443. [CrossRef] [PubMed]
25. Leroux, B.; Lei, X.; Breslow, N. Estimation of Disease Rates in Small Areas: A new Mixed Model for Spatial Dependence. In *Statistical Models in Epidemiology, the Environment, and Clinical Trials*; Bernado, J.M., Berger, J.O., Dawid, A.P., Smith, A.F.M., Eds.; Springer: Berlin/Heidelberg, Germany, 2000; pp. 179–191.
26. Lee, D. A tutorial on spatio-temporal disease risk modelling in R using Markov chain Monte Carlo simulation and the CARBayesST package. *Spat. Spatio-Temporal Epidemiol.* **2020**, *34*, 100353. [CrossRef] [PubMed]

27. Geweke, J. Evaluating the Accuracy of Sampling-Based Approaches to the Calculation of Posterior Moments. In *Bayesian Statistics*; Bernado, J.M., Berger, J.O., Dawid, A.P., Smith, A.F.M., Eds.; Oxford University Press: Oxford, UK, 1992; Volume 4.
28. Ganesan, S.; Subramani, D. Spatio-temporal predictive modeling framework for infectious disease spread. *Sci. Rep.* **2021**, *11*, 6741. [CrossRef] [PubMed]
29. López-Gonzales, J.L.; Gómez Lamus, A.M.; Torres, R.; Canas Rodrigues, P.; Salas, R. Self-Organizing Topological Multilayer Perceptron: A Hybrid Method to Improve the Forecasting of Extreme Pollution Values. *Stats* **2023**, *6*, 1241–1259. [CrossRef]
30. Solci, C.C.; Reisen, V.A.; Rodrigues, P.C. Robust local bootstrap for weakly stationary time series in the presence of additive outliers. *Stoch. Environ. Res. Risk Assess.* **2023**, *37*, 2977–2992. [CrossRef]
31. da Silva, K.L.S.; López-Gonzales, J.L.; Turpo-Chaparro, J.E.; Tocto-Cano, E.; Rodrigues, P.C. Spatio-temporal visualization and forecasting of PM 10 in the Brazilian state of Minas Gerais. *Sci. Rep.* **2023**, *13*, 3269. [CrossRef] [PubMed]
32. Aubrecht, C.; Fuchs, S.; Neuhold, C. Spatio-temporal aspects and dimensions in integrated disaster risk management. *Nat. Hazards* **2013**, *68*, 1205–1216. [CrossRef]
33. Awe, O.O.; Mahmoudvand, R.; Rodrigues, P.C. Non-negative time series reconstruction via singular spectrum analysis: A case study of precipitation dynamics in Nigeria. *Fluct. Noise Lett.* **2020**, *19*, 2050045. [CrossRef]
34. Oliveira Filho, F.M.; Guedes, E.F.; Rodrigues, P.C. Networks analysis of Brazilian climate data based on the DCCA cross-correlation coefficient. *PLoS ONE* **2023**, *18*, e0290838. [CrossRef] [PubMed]
35. Laurini, M.P. A spatio-temporal approach to estimate patterns of climate change. *Environmetrics* **2019**, *30*, e2542. [CrossRef]

entropy

MDPI

Article

# A Metric Based on the Efficient Determination Criterion

Jesús E. García, Verónica A. González-López * and Johsac I. Gomez Sanchez

Department of Statistics, University of Campinas, Campinas 13083-859, São Paulo, Brazil;
jg@ime.unicamp.br (J.E.G.); johsacgomez16@gmail.com or j216401@dac.unicamp.br (J.I.G.S.)
* Correspondence: veronica@ime.unicamp.br

**Abstract:** This paper extends the concept of metrics based on the Bayesian information criterion (BIC), to achieve strongly consistent estimation of partition Markov models (PMMs). We introduce a set of metrics drawn from the family of model selection criteria known as efficient determination criteria (EDC). This generalization extends the range of options available in BIC for penalizing the number of model parameters. We formally specify the relationship that determines how EDC works when selecting a model based on a threshold associated with the metric. Furthermore, we improve the penalty options within EDC, identifying the penalty $\ln(\ln(n))$ as a viable choice that maintains the strongly consistent estimation of a PMM. To demonstrate the utility of these new metrics, we apply them to the modeling of three DNA sequences of dengue virus type 3, endemic in Brazil in 2023.

**Keywords:** partition Markov models; Bayesian information criterion; entropy

## 1. Introduction

This article embarks on an exploration of the efficient determination criterion (EDC), as introduced in [1], with a particular emphasis on formulating an EDC-based metric. Our endeavor is bolstered by the presence of a Bayesian information criterion (BIC) metric proposed in [2], designed to provide consistent estimations of partition Markov models [2]. Our aim is to extend the scope of the BIC-based metric, thereby broadening the array of algorithms available for identifying partition Markov models.

To achieve our goal, we furnish a theoretical framework delineating the operational principles underlying the BIC/EDC, the BIC-based metric, and additionally, we conduct a brief survey of the current research landscape within this domain to provide context for our approach.

Let $(X_t)$ be a discrete-time order $o$ Markov chain on a finite and discrete alphabet $\Delta$, with $o < \infty$; let us call $\Omega = \Delta^o$ the state space. Denote the string $a_k a_{k+1} \dots a_m$ by $a_k^m$, where $a_i \in \Delta$, $k \le i \le m$. For each $a \in \Delta$ and $s \in \Omega$, the transition probability from the state $s$ to $a$ is

$$P(a|s) = \text{Prob}(X_t = a | X_{t-o}^{t-1} = s). \tag{1}$$

Let $\mathcal{P} = \{\Gamma_1, \Gamma_2, \dots, \Gamma_{|\mathcal{P}|}\}$ be a partition of $\Omega$, then for each pair of parts $\Gamma_i$ and $\Gamma_j$, $i \neq j$, $i, j \in \{1, \dots, |\mathcal{P}|\}$, $\Gamma_i \cap \Gamma_j = \emptyset$, and $\Omega = \cup_{i=1}^{|\mathcal{P}|} \Gamma_i$.

Note that a part $\Gamma$ of the partition is constituted by a collection of states coming from $\Omega$; we reformulate the notion introduced by Equation (1) as follows, for $a \in \Delta$, $\Gamma \in \mathcal{P}$:

$$\begin{aligned} P(\Gamma, a) &= \sum_{s \in \Gamma} \text{Prob}(X_{t-o}^{t-1} = s, X_t = a), \\ P(\Gamma) &= \sum_{s \in \Gamma} \text{Prob}(X_{t-o}^{t-1} = s), \\ P(a|\Gamma) &= \frac{P(\Gamma, a)}{P(\Gamma)} \quad \text{if} \quad P(\Gamma) > 0. \end{aligned} \tag{2}$$

Given the previous notation, we appeal to a model in $(X_t)$ which allows a more efficient estimation of the transition probabilities, introduced by Equation (1); see [2].

**Definition 1.** *Let $(X_t)$ be a discrete-time order $o$ Markov chain on a finite and discrete alphabet $\Delta, o < \infty$. Two states $s, r \in \Omega = \Delta^o$ are equivalent (denoted by $s \sim_p r$) if $P(a|s) = P(a|r)$ $\forall a \in \Delta$. For any $s \in \Omega$, the equivalence class of $s$ is given by the set of states $\{r \in \Omega : r \sim_p s\}$.*

The previous notion allows the definition of a Markov chain with minimal partition $\mathcal{P}$, that is, one which follows the equivalence relationship.

**Definition 2.** *Let $(X_t)$ be a discrete-time order $o$ Markov chain on a finite and discrete alphabet $\Delta, o < \infty$, and let $\mathcal{P} = \{\Gamma_1, \Gamma_2, \ldots, \Gamma_{|\mathcal{P}|}\}$ be a partition of $\Omega = \Delta^o$; $(X_t)$ is a Markov chain with minimal partition $\mathcal{P}$ if $\mathcal{P}$ is defined by the relationship $\sim_p$ introduced by Definition 1.*

As previously indicated, the objective of this model is to allow a more efficient estimation of the probabilities introduced by Equation (1), which occurs in the most efficient way possible by identifying the parts of the minimal partition (Definition 2), and thus, being able to use all the states inserted in each part to estimate a single probability per part. To identify the partition $\mathcal{P}$ introduced in Definition 2, a strategy must be implemented as shown below.

In a given sample $x_1^n$, of size $n$, coming from the stochastic process $(X_t)$ under the assumptions of Definition 2, given the state $s \in \Omega$ and the element of the alphabet $a \in \Delta$, we denote the number of occurrences of $s$ followed by $a$ in the sample $x_1^n$ by $N_n(s,a) = |\{t : o < t \leq n, x_{t-o}^{t-1} = s, x_t = a\}|$ and $N_n(s) = \sum_{a \in \Delta} N_n(s,a)$ is the number of occurrences of $s$ in the sample $x_1^n$. Also, given a partition $\mathcal{P}$ of $\Omega$, denote the number of occurrences of elements into $\Gamma$ (part of $\mathcal{P}$) followed by $a$ as

$$N_n(\Gamma, a) = \sum_{s \in \Gamma} N_n(s,a), \; a \in \Delta, \tag{3}$$

the accumulated number of values $N_n(s)$ for $s \in \Gamma$ is denoted by

$$N_n(\Gamma) = \sum_{s \in \Gamma} N_n(s). \tag{4}$$

Note that $N_n(\Gamma, a)$ and $N_n(\Gamma)$ can be computed for any partition $\mathcal{P}$ of $\Omega$, not only for the partition introduced by Definition 2.

The counts of occurrences, in this case $N_n(\Gamma, a)$ and $N_n(\Gamma)$, allow the estimation of probabilities (Equation (2)) subject to a modification of the likelihood function of the sample. The likelihood of the sample is

$$P(x_1^n) = P(x_1^o) \prod_{a \in \Delta, \Gamma \in \mathcal{P}} P(a|\Gamma)^{N_n(\Gamma,a)},$$

then, the maximum of the modified log likelihood is

$$\sum_{a \in \Delta, \Gamma \in \mathcal{P}} N_n(\Gamma, a) \ln\left(\frac{N_n(\Gamma,a)}{N_n(\Gamma)}\right), \text{ with } N_n(\Gamma) > 0, \forall \Gamma.$$

And,

$$\frac{N_n(\Gamma,a)}{N_n(\Gamma)}, \text{ with } N_n(\Gamma) > 0, \tag{5}$$

is the maximum likelihood estimator of $P(a|\Gamma)$ given in Equation (2).

As shown in [2], under the assumptions of Definition 2, the partition $\mathcal{P}$ can be consistently (strong consistency) retrieved using the Bayesian information criterion (BIC), defined as

$$\mathrm{BIC}(x_1^n, \mathcal{P}) = \sum_{a \in \Delta, \Gamma \in \mathcal{P}} N_n(\Gamma, a) \ln\left(\frac{N_n(\Gamma, a)}{N_n(\Gamma)}\right) - \frac{(|\Delta| - 1)|\mathcal{P}|}{\alpha} \ln(n), \tag{6}$$

with $\alpha > 0$, a constant value. Then, the BIC takes into consideration the maximum of the modified log-likelihood term penalized by $\frac{(|\Delta|-1)|\mathcal{P}|}{\alpha} \ln(n)$, where $(|\Delta| - 1)|\mathcal{P}|$ is the number of probabilities to be estimated.

In practice, candidates to be the partition according to Definition 2 are compared, and the partition with the higher BIC value is considered more suitable. Also, in [2] a metric is introduced based on the BIC criterion, along with clustering algorithms, which are used to obtain $\mathcal{P}$; the metric is defined below. To achieve consistent estimation, such a metric operates on partitions of the state space that follow certain rules. The metric is then able to refine partitions until it identifies the one cited by Definition 2. The partitions in which we will apply the metric, are made up of members (parts) formed by states sharing all the transition probabilities. The definition to follow formalizes the concept.

**Definition 3.** *Let $(X_t)$ be a Markov chain of order $o$, with finite and discrete alphabet $\Delta, o < \infty$, and state space $\Omega = \Delta^o$. Set a partition of $\Omega$, $\mathcal{P} = \{\Gamma_1, ..., \Gamma_{|\mathcal{P}|}\}$,*

*i. given a part $\Gamma$ of $\mathcal{P}$, $\Gamma$ is a good part if $\forall a, a \in \Delta$, $P(a|s) = P(a|r)$, $\forall r, s \in \Gamma, r \neq s$.*
*ii. $\mathcal{P}$ is a good partition of $\Omega$ if $\Gamma$ satisfies i. $\forall \Gamma \in \mathcal{P}$.*

Under the validity of Definition 3-i, the probabilities introduced by Equation (2) are

$$P(a|\Gamma) = \mathrm{Prob}(X_t = a | X_{t-o}^{t-1} = s) \;\; \forall a \in \Delta, \forall s \in \Gamma, \tag{7}$$

since all the elements of the good part $\Gamma$ of $\mathcal{P}$ share the transition probabilities. Note that the partition identified by Definition 2 verifies Definition 3-ii, but the reciprocal is naturally not valid. A straightforward example of a good partition is one composed of all the states being isolated.

The following introduces a notion used to estimate the minimal partition (Definition 2). This criterion operates on good parts (Definition 3-i).

**Definition 4.** *Let $(X_t)$ be a Markov chain of order $o$, with finite and discrete alphabet $\Delta, o < \infty$, and state space $\Omega = \Delta^o$; $x_1^n$ is a sample of the process and let $\mathcal{P} = \{\Gamma_1, ..., \Gamma_{|\mathcal{P}|}\}$ be a good partition of $\Omega$,*

$$d_{\mathcal{P}}(i,j) = \frac{\alpha}{(|\Delta| - 1)\ln(n)} \sum_{a \in \Delta} \left\{ \sum_{k \in \{i,j\}} N_n(\Gamma_k, a) \ln\left(\frac{N_n(\Gamma_k, a)}{N_n(\Gamma_k)}\right) - N_n(\Gamma_{ij}, a) \ln\left(\frac{N_n(\Gamma_{ij}, a)}{N_n(\Gamma_{ij})}\right) \right\}.$$

*where $\alpha$ is a constant and positive value, $N_n(\Gamma_{ij}) = N_n(\Gamma_i) + N_n(\Gamma_j)$, $N_n(\Gamma_{ij}, a) = N_n(\Gamma_i, a) + N_n(\Gamma_j, a)$, $\forall a \in \Delta$.*

In [2], it is proved that $d_{\mathcal{P}}$ of Definition 4 is a metric, meaning that, if $\Gamma_l \in \mathcal{P}, l \in \{i, j, k\}$,

i. $d_{\mathcal{P}}(i,j) > 0$, with equality, if and only if $\frac{N_n(\Gamma_i,a)}{N_n(\Gamma_i)} = \frac{N_n(\Gamma_j,a)}{N_n(\Gamma_j)}$ $\forall a \in \Delta$;
ii. $d_{\mathcal{P}}(i,j) = d_{\mathcal{P}}(j,i)$;
iii. $d_{\mathcal{P}}(i,k) \leq d_{\mathcal{P}}(i,j) + d_{\mathcal{P}}(j,k)$.

As a consequence of the property i of a metric, the ability of $d_{\mathcal{P}}$ to operate adequately depends on the accuracy of the maximum likelihood estimation of the transition probabilities $P(a|\Gamma_i)$ and $P(a|\Gamma_j)$, $\forall a \in \Delta$. That is, when the estimators of those probabilities

$\frac{N_n(\Gamma_i,a)}{N_n(\Gamma_i)}, \frac{N_n(\Gamma_j,a)}{N_n(\Gamma_j)}$ $\forall a \in \Delta$ are near and the sample size $n$ is large enough, we have evidence of proximity between $P(a|\Gamma_i)$ and $P(a|\Gamma_j), \forall a \in \Delta$. And, such a finding indicates that the elements of both parts must be together.

Partition Markov models, commonly referred to as those delineated by Definition 2, have found application in diverse realms. For instance, they have been employed in data compression in conjunction with Huffman coding, as exemplified in [3]. Across these investigations, the utilization of the BIC-based metric $d_{\mathcal{P}}$ has proven indispensable. Also, in [2], this metric has been pivotal for modeling the behavior of internet users. The partition Markov model allows identifying the chances of a user visiting a certain internet site in their next step, based on their history, and identifies equivalent histories in the sense introduced by Definition 2.

Since the support of $d_{\mathcal{P}}$ is the BIC criterion, the question arises whether there is a broader criterion than BIC that is capable of maintaining strong consistency in the estimation of $\mathcal{P}$. The next section shows that such a criterion exists (a generalization of BIC) and was proved by [4]. Then, the next question that we propose to answer is whether such a generalization of the BIC allows the creation of a metric that generalizes the one introduced in [2].

The next section (Section 2) addresses the problem by introducing the efficient determination criterion, and then, presenting how this criterion is linked to a metric, also introducing a cut-off point that enables the practical use of the metric based on the efficient determination criterion, for sufficiently large values of $n$. Section 3 shows an application in which different fits of model—Definition 2—are compared, inferred by variants of the efficient determination criterion, indicated as recommended in Section 2. This article ends with the Conclusions—Section 4—in which we highlight the main contributions, and the Bibliography section.

## 2. Efficient Determination Criterion

Ref. [1] proposes a criterion generalizing the BIC criterion, the efficient determination criterion (EDC). In that paper, the proposal is to introduce a sequence $\{w_n\}_{n\geq 1}$ in the place of $\{\ln(n)\}_{n\geq 1}$; see Equation (6). The generalization also offers more options in the penalty term of Equation (6), instead of the number of parameters a function $\gamma(\cdot)$ is introduced acting over the number of parameters; this function is strictly increasing in the number of parameters. Under the assumptions of Definition 2, the criterion is formulated as follows:

$$\mathrm{EDC}(x_1^n, \mathcal{P}) = \sum_{a\in\Delta, \Gamma\in\mathcal{P}} N_n(\Gamma, a) \ln\left(\frac{N_n(\Gamma, a)}{N_n(\Gamma)}\right) - \gamma\Big(\frac{(|\Delta|-1)|\mathcal{P}|}{\alpha}\Big) w_n. \tag{8}$$

With $\alpha > 0$ a constant value, $\gamma(\cdot)$ being a strictly increasing function, and $\{w_n\}$ a sequence of positive numbers depending on $n$. As well as BIC, candidates to be the partition according to Definition 2 are compared, and the higher the EDC, the more indicated the partition is. Note that if we choose $\gamma(\cdot)$ as being the identity function, $\gamma\big(\frac{(|\Delta|-1)|\mathcal{P}|}{\alpha}\big) = \frac{(|\Delta|-1)|\mathcal{P}|}{\alpha}$, and $w_n = \ln(n)$, then Equation (6) is recovered. Then, clearly the EDC criterion is a generalization of the BIC criterion.

Ref. [4] proves that the EDC criterion provides a strongly consistent way to estimate the partition $\mathcal{P}$ of Definition 2 if

$$\lim_{n\to\infty} \frac{w_n}{n} = 0 \quad \text{and} \quad \lim_{n\to\infty} \frac{w_n}{\ln(\ln(n))} = \infty. \tag{9}$$

Note that if we take $w_n = n^a$ for $a \in (0,1)$, the conditions given in Equation (9) are valid. Also, we can use $w_n = a\ln(n)$ for $a > 0$. Another option is to use $w_n = n^a \ln(n)$ for $a \in (0,1)$. Figure 1 shows penalty functions $w_n$ verifying Equation (9). We see in the figure that functions $w_n$ are positioned between the functions $n$ and $\ln(\ln(n))$. And between $n$ and $\ln(\ln(n))$ is also the $w_n$ related to the BIC criterion ($w_n = \ln(n)$).

Clearly, the penalty $\ln(\ln(n))$ does not verify the second statement of Equation (9), but according to [5] it is an optimal penalty term for estimating the order of a Markov chain. With such inspiration in mind, the following proposition guarantees that $\ln(\ln(n))$ can also be used to obtain a consistent estimate of $\mathcal{P}$. To state the proposition we introduce the notion of relative entropy.

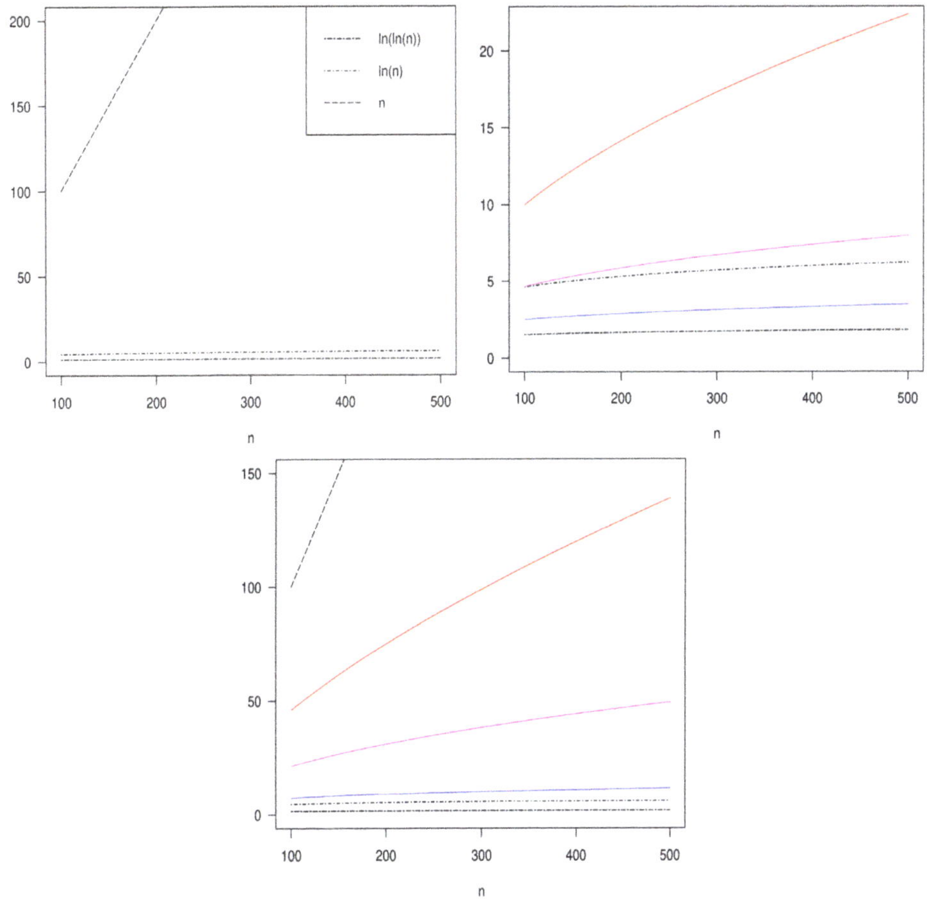


**Figure 1. Top left**: Double-dashed line, $\ln(\ln(n))$; dotted-dashed line, $\ln(n)$; long-dashed line, $n$. **Top right**: $w_n = n^{1/2}$ (in red); $w_n = n^{1/3}$ (in magenta); $w_n = n^{1/5}$ (in blue); double-dashed line, $\ln(\ln(n))$; dotted-dashed line, $\ln(n)$. **Bottom**: $w_n = n^{1/2}\ln(n)$ (in red); $w_n = n^{1/3}\ln(n)$ (in magenta); $w_n = n^{1/10}\ln(n)$ (in blue); double-dashed line, $\ln(\ln(n))$; dotted-dashed line $\ln(n)$; long-dashed line $n$.

**Definition 5.** *Let $P$ and $Q$ be probability distributions on $\Delta$. The relative entropy between $P$ and $Q$ is given by $D(P(\cdot)||Q(\cdot)) = \sum_{a\in\Delta} P(a)\ln\left(\frac{P(a)}{Q(a)}\right)$, with $Q(a) \neq 0, \forall a \in \Delta$.*

**Proposition 1.** *Let $(X_t)$ be a Markov chain of order $o$, with finite and discrete alphabet $\Delta, o < \infty$, and state space $\Omega = \Delta^o$; $x_1^n$ is a sample of the process and let $\mathcal{P} = \{\Gamma_1, ..., \Gamma_{|\mathcal{P}|}\}$ be a partition of $\Omega$, and $P(\cdot|\Gamma)$ be the probability given by Equation (2) related to a good part $\Gamma$ (Definition 3-i). To any $\delta > 0$ there exists $\kappa > 0$ (depending on $P(\cdot|\cdot)$) such that, eventually, almost surely as $n \to \infty$*

$$\left|\frac{N_n(\Gamma,a)}{N_n(\Gamma)} - P(a|\Gamma)\right| < \sqrt{\frac{\delta \ln(\ln(n))}{N_n(\Gamma)}},$$

*for all* $\Gamma$*, good part, with* $N_n(\Gamma) \geq 1$ *and* $o < \kappa \ln(\ln(n))$.

**Proof.** From the proof of Corollary 2 of [6] (on page 1621), we obtain that for any $\epsilon > 0$ there is $\kappa > 0$ (depending on $P(\cdot|\cdot)$) such that, eventually, almost surely as $n \to \infty$

$$\left|\frac{N_n(s,a)}{N_n(s)} - P(a|s)\right| < \sqrt{\frac{\epsilon \ln(\ln(n))}{N_n(s)}}, \tag{10}$$

for all $s \in \Omega$ with $N_n(s) \geq 1$ and $o < \kappa \ln(\ln(n))$.

Consider $\delta > 0$ and set $\epsilon = \frac{\delta}{|\Delta|^{2o}}$, in Equation (10), then

$$\begin{aligned}
\frac{N_n(s,a)}{N_n(s)} - P(a|s) &\leq \sqrt{\frac{\delta \ln(\ln(n))}{|\Delta|^{2o} N_n(s)}} \\
N_n(s,a) - N_n(s)P(a|s) &\leq \sqrt{\frac{\delta \ln(\ln(n))}{|\Delta|^{2o}} N_n(s)}.
\end{aligned}$$

Because $\Gamma$ is a good part of $\mathcal{P}$, $s \in \Gamma$, we obtain

$$\sum_{s\in\Gamma} N_n(s,a) - P(a|\Gamma) \sum_{s\in\Gamma} N_n(s) \leq \sum_{s\in\Gamma} \sqrt{\frac{\delta \ln(\ln(n))}{|\Delta|^{2o}} N_n(s)}.$$

Following Equations (3), (4) and (7), we have

$$N_n(\Gamma,a) - P(a|\Gamma)N_n(\Gamma) \leq \frac{\sqrt{\delta \ln(\ln(n))}}{|\Delta|^o} \sum_{s\in\Gamma} \sqrt{N_n(s)},$$

then,

$$\begin{aligned}
\frac{N_n(\Gamma,a)}{N_n(\Gamma)} - P(a|\Gamma) &\leq \frac{\sqrt{\delta \ln(\ln(n))}}{|\Delta|^o N_n(\Gamma)} |\Gamma| \sqrt{\max_{s\in\Gamma}(N_n(s))} \\
&\leq \frac{\sqrt{\delta \ln(\ln(n))}}{|\Delta|^o N_n(\Gamma)} |\Delta|^o \sqrt{\sum_{s\in\Gamma} N_n(s)} \\
&= \frac{\sqrt{\delta \ln(\ln(n))}}{N_n(\Gamma)} \sqrt{N_n(\Gamma)} \\
&= \sqrt{\frac{\delta \ln(\ln(n))}{N_n(\Gamma)}}.
\end{aligned}$$

□

The next results show that despite $\ln(\ln(n))$ violating the second condition imposed by Equation (9), the EDC (with $\ln(\ln(n))$) provides a consistent estimate of the minimal partition.

**Theorem 1.** *Let* $(X_t)$ *be a Markov chain of order* $o$*, with finite and discrete alphabet* $\Delta, o < \infty$*, and state space* $\Omega = \Delta^o$*;* $x_1^n$ *is a sample of the process and let* $\mathcal{P} = \{\Gamma_1, ..., \Gamma_{|\mathcal{P}|}\}$ *be a partition of* $\Omega$*, and suppose that* $i$ *and* $j$ *exist;* $i \neq j$ *such that* $\Gamma_i$ *and* $\Gamma_j$ *following Definition 3-i. Then,* $P(a|\Gamma_i) = P(a|\Gamma_j), \forall a \in \Delta$ *if, and only if, eventually, almost surely as* $n \to \infty$*,*

$$EDC(x_1^n, \mathcal{P}^{ij}) > EDC(x_1^n, \mathcal{P}).$$

*where $EDC(x_1^n, \mathcal{P})$ is defined by Equation (8), with $w_n = \ln(\ln(n))$ and $EDC(x_1^n, \mathcal{P}^{ij})$ is given by Equation (8) (with $w_n = \ln(\ln(n))$) over the partition $\mathcal{P}^{ij} = \Big\{\{\mathcal{P} \setminus \{\Gamma_i\}\} \setminus \{\Gamma_j\}\Big\} \cup \Gamma_{ij}$ and $\Gamma_{ij} = \{\Gamma_i \cup \Gamma_j\}$.*

**Proof.** The proof is a variant of the one presented in [2], theorem 1. $\Leftarrow$ is direct from that proof, just considering (i) $\frac{\ln(\ln(n))}{n} \to 0$ instead of $\frac{\ln(n)}{n} \to 0$, when $n \to \infty$ and considering (ii) that $\gamma(\cdot)$ is an increasing function. For $\Rightarrow$, we have that $P(a|\Gamma_i) = P(a|\Gamma_j), \forall a \in \Delta$, and we want to prove that $EDC(x_1^n, \mathcal{P}) - EDC(x_1^n, \mathcal{P}^{ij}) < 0$. Again, following the steps in such a proof, we obtain that $EDC(x_1^n, \mathcal{P}) - EDC(x_1^n, \mathcal{P}^{ij})$ is bounded above by

$$N_n(\Gamma_i) D\left(\frac{N_n(\Gamma_i,.)}{N_n(\Gamma_i)}\bigg|\bigg|P(.|\Gamma_i)\right) + N_n(\Gamma_j) D\left(\frac{N_n(\Gamma_j,.)}{N_n(\Gamma_j)}\bigg|\bigg|P(.|\Gamma_j)\right)$$
$$-\Big(\gamma\big(\frac{(|\Delta|-1)|\mathcal{P}|}{\alpha}\big) - \gamma\big(\frac{(|\Delta|-1)(|\mathcal{P}|-1)}{\alpha}\big)\Big)\ln(\ln(n)),$$

where $D(P(\cdot)||Q(\cdot))$ is the relative entropy, given by Definition 5.

For each $\Gamma \in \{\Gamma_i, \Gamma_j\}$, $\frac{N_n(\Gamma,.)}{N_n(\Gamma)}$ and $P(.|\Gamma)$ are probabilities on $\Delta$; then, Equation (11) follows from lemma 6.3 in [7]. On the other hand, since $\Gamma \in \{\Gamma_i, \Gamma_j\}$ is a good part, by hypothesis, from Proposition 1, for any $\delta > 0$ and large enough $n$, Equation (12) follows,

$$D\left(\frac{N_n(\Gamma,.)}{N_n(\Gamma)}\bigg|\bigg|P(.|\Gamma)\right) \leq \sum_{a\in\Delta} \frac{\left(\frac{N_n(\Gamma,a)}{N_n(\Gamma)} - P(a|\Gamma)\right)^2}{P(a|\Gamma)} \tag{11}$$

$$\leq \sum_{a\in\Delta} \frac{\frac{\delta\ln(\ln(n))}{N_n(\Gamma)}}{P(a|\Gamma)}. \tag{12}$$

Then, set $c_0 = \Big(\gamma\big(\frac{(|\Delta|-1)|\mathcal{P}|}{\alpha}\big) - \gamma\big(\frac{(|\Delta|-1)(|\mathcal{P}|-1)}{\alpha}\big)\Big)$, which is $>0$, since $\gamma(\cdot)$ in a strictly increasing function. For any $\delta > 0$ and large enough $n$,

$$\begin{aligned} EDC(x_1^n, \mathcal{P}) - EDC(x_1^n, \mathcal{P}^{ij}) &\leq \frac{2\delta|\Delta|}{p}\ln(\ln(n)) - c_0\ln(\ln(n)) \\ &= \ln(\ln(n))\left(\frac{2\delta|\Delta|}{p} - c_0\right) \end{aligned}$$

where $p = \min\{P(a|\Gamma) : a \in \Delta, \Gamma \in \{\Gamma_i, \Gamma_j\}\}$. In particular, taking $\delta < \frac{pc_0}{2|\Delta|}$, for a large enough $n$, $EDC(x_1^n, \mathcal{P}) - EDC(x_1^n, \mathcal{P}^{ij}) < 0$. □

As a result of the previous theorem, it turns out that it is possible to guarantee that the EDC with the penalty term $w_n = \ln(\ln(n))$ allows the consistent estimation of the minimal partition. As a consequence, we have:

**Corollary 1.** *Let $(X_t)$ be a Markov chain of order $o$, with finite and discrete alphabet $\Delta, o < \infty$, and state space $\Omega = \Delta^o$; $x_1^n$ is a sample of the process. Let $\Psi$ be the set of all the partitions of $\Omega$. Define*

$$\mathcal{P}_n^* = argmax_{\mathcal{P}\in\Psi}\{EDC(x_1^n, \mathcal{P})\}$$

*where $EDC(x_1^n, \mathcal{P})$ is defined by Equation (8), with $w_n = \ln(\ln(n))$. Then, eventually, almost surely as $n \to \infty$, $\mathcal{P}^* = \mathcal{P}_n^*$, where $\mathcal{P}^*$ is the partition of $\Omega$, following Definition 2.*

**Proof.** Following the same steps as the proof of Theorem 3 of [2]. It is enough to replace the BIC criterion with the EDC criterion (Equation (8)) with $w_n = \ln(\ln(n))$ and apply Theorem 1 instead of Theorem 1 and Corollary 1 of [2]. □

Corollary 1 complements the results of [4], showing that the minimal partition (Definition 2) is consistently recovered by the EDC (Equation (8)) when it is formulated by a strictly increasing function $\gamma$ and $w_n$ follows Equation (9), or when $w_n = \ln(\ln(n))$.

In order to generalize the BIC-based metric $d_{\mathcal{P}}$, given by Definition 4, the following notion is introduced.

**Definition 6.** *Let $(X_t)$ be a Markov chain of order $o$, with finite and discrete alphabet $\Delta, o < \infty$, and state space $\Omega = \Delta^o$; $x_1^n$ is a sample of the process, let $\mathcal{P} = \{\Gamma_1, ..., \Gamma_{|\mathcal{P}|}\}$ be a good partition of $\Omega$, and $1 \le i, j \le |\mathcal{P}|, i \neq j$:*

$$\delta_{\mathcal{P}}(i,j) = v_n \sum_{a \in \Delta} \left\{ \sum_{k \in \{i,j\}} N_n(\Gamma_k, a) \ln\left(\frac{N_n(\Gamma_k, a)}{N_n(\Gamma_k)}\right) - N_n(\Gamma_{ij}, a) \ln\left(\frac{N_n(\Gamma_{ij}, a)}{N_n(\Gamma_{ij})}\right) \right\},$$

*where $N_n(\Gamma_{ij}) = N_n(\Gamma_i) + N_n(\Gamma_j)$, $N_n(\Gamma_{ij}, a) = N_n(\Gamma_i, a) + N_n(\Gamma_j, a)$, $\forall a \in \Delta$. With $v_n^{-1} = w_n\left(\gamma(\frac{(|\Delta|-1)|\mathcal{P}|}{\alpha}) - \gamma(\frac{(|\Delta|-1)(|\mathcal{P}|-1)}{\alpha})\right)$, $\alpha$ a constant and positive value, $\gamma(\cdot)$ being a strictly increasing function, and $\{w_n\}$ a sequence of positive numbers depending on $n$.*

It is evident that if we take $\gamma(\frac{(|\Delta|-1)|\mathcal{P}|}{\alpha}) = \frac{(|\Delta|-1)|\mathcal{P}|}{\alpha}$ and $w_n = \ln(n)$, Definition 6 coincides with Definition 4.

The next result shows the relationship between the EDC criterion and the notion introduced in Definition 6.

**Theorem 2.** *Let $(X_t)$ be a Markov chain of order $o$, with finite and discrete alphabet $\Delta, o < \infty$, and $\Omega = \Delta^o$; $x_1^n$ is a sample of the process. Let $\mathcal{P} = \{\Gamma_1, ..., \Gamma_{|\mathcal{P}|}\}$ be a good partition of $\Omega$, and $1 \le i, j \le |\mathcal{P}|, i \neq j$, then,*

$$EDC(x_1^n, \mathcal{P}) < EDC(x_1^n, \mathcal{P}^{ij}) \Leftrightarrow \delta_{\mathcal{P}}(i,j) < 1.$$

*where $\delta_{\mathcal{P}}(i,j)$ is given by Definition 6, $EDC(x_1^n, \mathcal{P})$ is defined by Equation (8), and $EDC(x_1^n, \mathcal{P}^{ij})$ is given by Equation (8) over the partition $\mathcal{P}^{ij} = \left\{\{\mathcal{P} \setminus \{\Gamma_i\}\} \setminus \{\Gamma_j\}\right\} \cup \Gamma_{ij}$ and $\Gamma_{ij} = \{\Gamma_i \cup \Gamma_j\}$.*

**Proof.**

$$\begin{aligned} \mathrm{EDC}(x_1^n, \mathcal{P}) - \mathrm{EDC}(x_1^n, \mathcal{P}^{ij}) &= \sum_{a \in \Delta} \sum_{k \in \{i,j\}} N_n(\Gamma_k, a) \ln\left(\frac{N_n(\Gamma_k, a)}{N_n(\Gamma_k)}\right) - \\ &\quad \sum_{a \in \Delta} N_n(\Gamma_{ij}, a) \ln\left(\frac{N_n(\Gamma_{ij}, a)}{N_n(\Gamma_{ij'})}\right) - v_n^{-1} \end{aligned} \tag{13}$$

Note that $\mathrm{EDC}(x_1^n, \mathcal{P}) < \mathrm{EDC}(x_1^n, \mathcal{P}^{ij}) \Leftrightarrow \mathrm{EDC}(x_1^n, \mathcal{P}) - \mathrm{EDC}(x_1^n, \mathcal{P}^{ij}) < 0$, and $\mathrm{EDC}(x_1^n, \mathcal{P}) - \mathrm{EDC}(x_1^n, \mathcal{P}^{ij}) < 0 \Leftrightarrow \delta_{\mathcal{P}}(i,j) < 1$, applying Equation (13), since $v_n > 0$. □

**Remark 1.** *In order to guarantee the consistent estimation of the partition given by Definition 2, we note that Theorem 2 must be used for a large enough $n$ and with weights $w_n$ following Equation (9) or $w_n = \ln(\ln(n))$.*

The following theorem characterizes the notion given by Definition 6 as being a metric.

**Theorem 3.** *Let $(X_t)$ be a Markov chain of order $o$ over a finite and discrete alphabet $\Delta, o < \infty$, $\Omega = \Delta^o$ the state space, and $x_1^n$ a sample of the Markov process. If $\mathcal{P} = \{\Gamma_1, \ldots, \Gamma_{|\mathcal{P}|}\}$ is a good partition of $\Omega$, for each $n$, and for any $i, j, k \in \{1, 2, ..., |\mathcal{P}|\}$, given $\delta_{\mathcal{P}}$ as Definition 6,*

*i.* $\delta_{\mathcal{P}}(i,j) \ge 0$, *with equality, if and only if,* $\frac{N_n(\Gamma_i, a)}{N_n(\Gamma_i)} = \frac{N_n(\Gamma_j, a)}{N_n(\Gamma_j)}$ $\forall a \in \Delta$;

*ii.* $\delta_{\mathcal{P}}(i,j) = \delta_{\mathcal{P}}(j,i)$;

iii. $\delta_{\mathcal{P}}(i,k) \leq \delta_{\mathcal{P}}(i,j) + \delta_{\mathcal{P}}(j,k)$.

**Proof.** Here, we only prove iii. since item i. is straightforward from Theorem 2 [2] and ii. follows from definition. Consider the relative entropy between two probabilities $P$ and $Q$ on the alphabet $\Delta$, $D(P(\cdot)||Q(\cdot)) = \sum_{a\in\Delta} P(a)\ln(P(a)/Q(a))$. $D$ is non-negative, furthermore $D$ is zero if and only if $P(\cdot) = Q(\cdot)$. Returning to our goal, iii. occurs if and only if

$$0 \leq v_n^{-1}(\delta_{\mathcal{P}}(i,j) + \delta_{\mathcal{P}}(j,k) - \delta_{\mathcal{P}}(i,k)) = (*) \tag{14}$$

since $v_n > 0$. We inspect the right side of Equation (14),

$$\begin{aligned}
(*) \quad &= \sum_{s=i,k}\sum_{a\in\Delta} N_n(\Gamma_j,a)\Big(\ln\Big(\frac{N_n(\Gamma_j,a)}{N_n(\Gamma_j)}\Big) - \ln\Big(\frac{N_n(\Gamma_{js},a)}{N_n(\Gamma_{js})}\Big)\Big) + \\
&\quad \sum_{s=i,k}\sum_{a\in\Delta} N_n(\Gamma_s,a)\Big(\ln\Big(\frac{N_n(\Gamma_{ik},a)}{N_n(\Gamma_{ik})}\Big) - \ln\Big(\frac{N_n(\Gamma_{sj},a)}{N_n(\Gamma_{sj})}\Big)\Big) \\
&= \sum_{s=i,k} N_n(\Gamma_j)\sum_{a\in\Delta}\frac{N_n(\Gamma_j,a)}{N_n(\Gamma_j)}\ln\Big(\frac{N_n(\Gamma_j,a)}{N_n(\Gamma_j)}\Big/\frac{N_n(\Gamma_{js},a)}{N_n(\Gamma_{js})}\Big) + \\
&\quad \sum_{s=i,k}\sum_{a\in\Delta} N_n(\Gamma_s,a)\ln\Big(\frac{N_n(\Gamma_{ik},a)}{N_n(\Gamma_{ik})}\Big/\frac{N_n(\Gamma_{sj},a)}{N_n(\Gamma_{sj})}\Big) \\
&=^{(1)} N_n(\Gamma_j)\sum_{s=i,k} D\Big(\frac{N_n(\Gamma_j,\cdot)}{N_n(\Gamma_j)}\Big|\Big|\frac{N_n(\Gamma_{js},\cdot)}{N_n(\Gamma_{js})}\Big) + \\
&\quad \sum_{s=i,k}\sum_{a\in\Delta} N_n(\Gamma_s,a)\frac{N_n(\Gamma_{ik})}{N_n(\Gamma_{ik},a)}\frac{N_n(\Gamma_{ik},a)}{N_n(\Gamma_{ik})}\ln\Big(\frac{N_n(\Gamma_{ik},a)}{N_n(\Gamma_{ik})}\Big/\frac{N_n(\Gamma_{sj},a)}{N_n(\Gamma_{sj})}\Big) \\
&\geq^{(2)} N_n(\Gamma_j)\sum_{s=i,k} D\Big(\frac{N_n(\Gamma_j,\cdot)}{N_n(\Gamma_j)}\Big|\Big|\frac{N_n(\Gamma_{js},\cdot)}{N_n(\Gamma_{js})}\Big) + \sum_{s=i,k}\frac{1}{n}D\Big(\frac{N_n(\Gamma_{ik},\cdot)}{N_n(\Gamma_{ik})}\Big|\Big|\frac{N_n(\Gamma_{sj},\cdot)}{N_n(\Gamma_{sj})}\Big) \geq^{(3)} 0.
\end{aligned}$$

where (1) follows from the definition of the relative entropy $D$, between two empirical laws $\frac{N_n(\Gamma_j,\cdot)}{N_n(\Gamma_j)}$ and $\frac{N_n(\Gamma_{js},\cdot)}{N_n(\Gamma_{js})}$. (2) follows from $\frac{1}{N_n(\Gamma_{ik},a)} \geq \frac{1}{n}$ and $N_n(\Gamma_s,a)N_n(\Gamma_{ik}) \geq 1$, and using the relative entropy $D$ between the two empirical laws $\frac{N_n(\Gamma_{ik},\cdot)}{N_n(\Gamma_{ik})}$ and $\frac{N_n(\Gamma_{sj},\cdot)}{N_n(\Gamma_{sj})}$. The last inequality (3) is valid since $D$ is non-negative. Then, Equation (14) is valid. □

We saw by Theorem 2 that the improvement in the construction of the partition, when joining the parts $\Gamma_i$ and $\Gamma_j$ is detected by the metric $\delta_{\mathcal{P}}$ when it takes a value less than 1, a value that could be used as a reference. It is clear that this property should only be used for large enough values of $n$, and a penalization term following Equation (9), according to [4], or when $w_n = \ln(\ln(n))$ according to Theorem 1 and Corollary 1, which is when the EDC criterion is capable of consistently estimating the partition that follows Definition 2.

The following section shows an example of applying the metric—Definition 6—to real data. We seek to show how the model—Definition 2—varies by varying the penalty term $w_n$ for cases where the consistency of the estimate is guaranteed, when $n$ is large enough, that is, with terms $w_n$ following Remark 1.

In the application we consider genetic sequences of dengue virus in FASTA format. In [8], a variant of the model specified in Definition 2 is designed specifically to model the first DNA sequence (FASTA format) of SARS-CoV-2 virus, Genbank number MN908947 (accessible at: https://www.ncbi.nlm.nih.gov/nuccore/MN908947, accessed on 10 March 2024). Furthermore, partition Markov models have been instrumental in modeling the DNA of the SARS-CoV 2 virus, exposing the evolution of the various variants during the pandemic period (see, for example, [9]).

## 3. Application

We examine and model three DNA sequences sourced from dengue virus type 3 (DENV-3), originating from Brazil. These sequences were sequenced and made publicly available in early 2023 (https://www.ncbi.nlm.nih.gov/, accessed on 10 March 2024). We then proceed to compare the models derived from these sequences by applying the metric—Definition 6—and employing the agglomerative algorithm. Our analysis focuses on observing the variations in partition composition and probability magnitudes as we change the penalization term $w_n$.

According to [10], the genesis of the initial autochthonous case of DENV-3 (GIII-American-I lineage) in Brazil dates back to December 2000, specifically within Rio de Janeiro. Over the course of the 2000s multiple incursions of this lineage were documented from the Caribbean into Brazil. The northern and southeastern regions of Brazil swiftly emerged as the epicenters of dissemination. The advent of this lineage precipitated a significant dengue outbreak in Brazil, in Rio de Janeiro, in 2002, followed by subsequent outbreaks in diverse locales.

However, since 2010, publicly available data indicate a downward tendency in the prevalence of DENV-3; DENV-3 has represented a mere fraction (<1%) of the total dengue cases in Brazil, with scant confirmed instances reported. Consequently, the transmission of DENV-3 has not been substantiated in recent years, pointing out a potential extinction of the DENV-3 (GIII-American-I lineage) within Brazil. The resurgence of DENV-3 is a real challenge in Brazil, since it is expected that the population will not have immunity, given the time that this virus has not been found in the region.

Table 1 shows the GenBank numbers, collection date, and origins of three sequences, introduced by [10]. The records correspond to three complete genetic sequences in FASTA format (alphabet $\Delta = \{a,c,g,t\}$), of DENV-3, which is already native to Brazil.

**Table 1.** Three autochthonous sequences of DENV-3 in FASTA format, $\Delta = \{a,c,g,t\}$.

| Origin | Collection Date | GenBank | Sequence Nickname | Size |
|---|---|---|---|---|
| Roraima, Canta (Brazil) | 4 March 2023 | OQ706226 | *A* | 10,697 |
| Roraima, Boa Vista (Brazil) | 22 January 2023 | OQ706227 | *B* | 10,511 |
| Roraima, Boa Vista (Brazil) | 3 January 2023 | OQ706228 | *C* | 10,553 |

We assume that each of these sequences is a sample of a process that meets Definition 2. We proceed to fit the model—Definition 2—using the metric—Definition 6—and the agglomerative algorithm. For this, we take into account the alphabet $\Delta = \{a,c,g,t\}$, with cardinal $|\Delta| = 4$, where the sequences take their values. In Table 2, we show the frequencies for each element of the alphabet.

**Table 2.** Frequencies $N_n(a), a \in \Delta = \{a,c,g,t\}$.

| GenBank | Sequence Nickname | $N_n(a)$ | $N_n(c)$ | $N_n(g)$ | $N_n(t)$ |
|---|---|---|---|---|---|
| OQ706226 | *A* | 3435 | 2209 | 2782 | 2271 |
| OQ706227 | *B* | 3378 | 2164 | 2736 | 2233 |
| OQ706228 | *C* | 3395 | 2173 | 2743 | 2242 |

Considering that min{10,697, 10,511, 10,553} = 10,511 and $\log_{|\Delta|}(10{,}511) = 6.68$, with integer part equal to 6, we adopt $o = 3$, since $3 < 6$ and the elements of the genetic alphabet $\Delta$ are organized in multiples of 3.

We fit four scenarios for each of the three sequences OQ706226, OQ706227, and OQ706228, with each scenario governed by a different penalty $w_n$. All of them are considered in Definition 6, $\Delta = \{a,c,g,t\}, o = 3, \alpha = 2$ (see [11]), and the $\gamma$ function is the identity function. For each penalty, we identify, using the metric (Definition 6), the estimated partition of the partition given by Definition 2, and then, determine the transition probabilities of each part for each element of $\Delta$. We denote by $\Gamma_i^v$ the part $i$ estimated for the sequence $v$, where $v$ can be $A, B, C$, corresponding to OQ706226, OQ706227, and OQ706228, respectively. In Tables 3 and 4, we record the results for the three sequences with penalty $w_n = n^{1/2}$; Tables 5 and 6 report the results for the three sequences with penalty $w_n = n^{1/3}$. While Tables 7 and 8 show, for the three sequences, the results using the usual BIC penalty

($w_n = \ln(n)$). Finally, Tables 9–11 report the results with the penalty $w_n = \ln(\ln(n))$ (see Corollary 1): for the sequence OQ706226, Table 9; for the sequence OQ706227, Table 10; and for the sequence OQ706228, Table 11.

**Table 3.** Minimal partition—Definition 2—estimated by Definition 6. From top to bottom, for the sequences $A$ (GenBank OQ706226), $B$ (GenBank OQ706227), and $C$ (GenBank OQ706228). $\Delta = \{a,c,g,t\}, o = 3, w_n = n^{1/2}, \alpha = 2, \gamma$ function given by the identity.

| Sequence | Part | States |
|---|---|---|
| OQ706226 | $\Gamma_1^A$ | ccc, tgc, cgc, ggc, gac, gtc, acg, att, gct, gcc, atc, agc, ggt, gag, ata, tcc, agt, tct, ctc, ttc, cct, ctt, gtt, aaa, ttt, aag, ccg, gcg, tgg, gtg, tat, agg, ctg, gat, ttg, aat, tcg, cgg, cat, ggg, act, atg |
| | $\Gamma_2^A$ | cag, cac, taa, cgt, aga, gga, tta, tac, cga, acc, tag, gta, cca, tga, tca, cta, gca, aac, tgt, gaa, caa, aca |
| OQ706227 | $\Gamma_1^B$ | ccc, ggc, cgc, gac, gtc, acg, gct, tag, gcc, atc, agc, ggt, gag, ata, att, tcc, agt, tgc, tct, gtt, ctc, ttc, cct, ctt, aaa, ttt, aag, ccg, gcg, tgg, gtg, tat, agg, ctg, ttg, aat, gat, tcg, cgg, cat, act, ggg, atg |
| | $\Gamma_2^B$ | cag, cgt, aga, gga, tta, tac, cga, cac, acc, taa, tga, cta, cca, tca, gca, gta, aac, tgt, gaa, caa, aca |
| OQ706228 | $\Gamma_1^C$ | ccc, cgc, ggc, gac, tgc, gct, tcc, tct, agt, gtc, acg, att, tag, gcc, atc, agc, ggt, gag, ata, ctc, cct, ttc, aaa, ctt, gtt, ttt, aag, ccg, gcg, tgg, gtg, agg, ctg, ttg, aat, gat, tcg, cat, tat, cgg, ggg, atg, act |
| | $\Gamma_2^C$ | cag, cgt, tta, cac, aga, gga, cga, tac, acc, taa, tga, cta, gca, cca, tca, gta, aac, tgt, gaa, caa, aca |

**Table 4.** Transition probabilities—Equation (2)—estimated by Equation (5). From top to bottom, for the sequences $A$ (GenBank OQ706226), $B$ (GenBank OQ706227), and $C$ (GenBank OQ706228). $\Delta = \{a,c,g,t\}, w_n = n^{1/2}$; full estimated partitions displayed in Table 3. In bold, the highest probability per part.

| OQ706226 | $i$ | $P(a\|\Gamma_i^A)$ | $P(c\|\Gamma_i^A)$ | $P(g\|\Gamma_i^A)$ | $P(t\|\Gamma_i^A)$ |
|---|---|---|---|---|---|
| | 1 | **0.37032** | 0.21336 | 0.21256 | 0.20376 |
| | 2 | 0.20595 | 0.19061 | **0.37152** | 0.23192 |
| OQ706227 | $i$ | $P(a\|\Gamma_i^B)$ | $P(c\|\Gamma_i^B)$ | $P(g\|\Gamma_i^B)$ | $P(t\|\Gamma_i^B)$ |
| | 1 | **0.36846** | 0.21441 | 0.21374 | 0.20339 |
| | 2 | 0.20723 | 0.18508 | **0.37341** | 0.23428 |
| OQ706228 | $i$ | $P(a\|\Gamma_i^C)$ | $P(c\|\Gamma_i^C)$ | $P(g\|\Gamma_i^C)$ | $P(t\|\Gamma_i^C)$ |
| | 1 | **0.36871** | 0.21373 | 0.21387 | 0.20369 |
| | 2 | 0.20760 | 0.18681 | **0.37167** | 0.23392 |

**Table 5.** Minimal partition—Definition 2—estimated by Definition 6. From top to bottom, for the sequences $A$ (GenBank OQ706226), $B$ (GenBank OQ706227), and $C$ (GenBank OQ706228). $\Delta = \{a,c,g,t\}, o = 3, w_n = n^{1/3}, \alpha = 2, \gamma$ function given by the identity.

| Sequence | Part | States |
|---|---|---|
| OQ706226 | $\Gamma_1^A$ | ccc, tgc, cgc, ggc, gac, gtc, acg, att, gct, gcc, atc, agc, ggt, gag, ata |
| | $\Gamma_2^A$ | tcc, tct, agt, ctc, ttc, cct, ctt, gtt, aaa, ttt |
| | $\Gamma_3^A$ | aag, ccg, gcg, tgg, gtg, agg, ctg, gat, ttg, aat, tcg, cgg, cat, ggg, tat, act, atg |
| | $\Gamma_4^A$ | cag, cac, taa, cta, cgt, aga, gga, tta, tac, cga, acc, tag, gta, cca, tga, tca, aac, tgt, gaa, caa, aca, gca |
| OQ706227 | $\Gamma_1^B$ | ccc, tgc, tct, gtt, cgc, ggc, gac, gtc, gct, acg, att, tag, gcc, atc, agc, ggt, gag, ata |
| | $\Gamma_2^B$ | tcc, agt, ctc, ttc, cct, ctt, aaa, ttt |
| | $\Gamma_3^B$ | aag, ccg, gcg, tgg, gtg, agg, ctg, ttg, aat, gat, tcg, cgg, cat, tat, act, ggg, atg |
| | $\Gamma_4^B$ | cag, cgt, aga, gga, tta, tac, cga, cac, acc, tgt, gaa, caa, taa, tga, cta, cca, tca, aca, gca, gta, aac |
| OQ706228 | $\Gamma_1^C$ | ccc, cgc, ggc, gac, tcc, tct, agt, tgc, gct, gtc, acg, att, gcc, atc, agc, ggt, gag, ata |
| | $\Gamma_2^C$ | ctc, cct, ttc, aaa, ctt, gtt, ttt |
| | $\Gamma_3^C$ | aag, ccg, gcg, tat, tgg, gtg, agg, ctg, ttg, aat, gat, tcg, cat, cgg, act, ggg, atg |
| | $\Gamma_4^C$ | cag, taa, tta, cac, cgt, cga, tac, acc, aga, gga, tag, gta, cca, tca, tga, cta, gca, aac, tgt, gaa, caa, aca |

**Table 6.** Transition probabilities—Equation (2)—estimated by Equation (5). From top to bottom, for the sequences *A* (GenBank OQ706226), *B* (GenBank OQ706227), and *C* (GenBank OQ706228). $\Delta = \{a,c,g,t\}, w_n = n^{1/3}$; full estimated partitions displayed in Table 5. In bold, the highest probability per part.

| OQ706226 | $i$ | $P(a\|\Gamma_i^A)$ | $P(c\|\Gamma_i^A)$ | $P(g\|\Gamma_i^A)$ | $P(t\|\Gamma_i^A)$ |
|---|---|---|---|---|---|
| | 1 | **0.29882** | 0.22627 | 0.25608 | 0.21882 |
| | 2 | **0.40166** | 0.18760 | 0.25987 | 0.15087 |
| | 3 | **0.41291** | 0.22673 | 0.11709 | 0.24328 |
| | 4 | 0.20595 | 0.19061 | **0.37152** | 0.23192 |
| OQ706227 | $i$ | $P(a\|\Gamma_i^B)$ | $P(c\|\Gamma_i^B)$ | $P(g\|\Gamma_i^B)$ | $P(t\|\Gamma_i^B)$ |
| | 1 | **0.30233** | 0.22596 | 0.25963 | 0.21208 |
| | 2 | **0.40612** | 0.18593 | 0.25902 | 0.14893 |
| | 3 | **0.41410** | 0.22668 | 0.11608 | 0.24314 |
| | 4 | 0.20723 | 0.18508 | **0.37341** | 0.23428 |
| OQ706228 | $i$ | $P(a\|\Gamma_i^C)$ | $P(c\|\Gamma_i^C)$ | $P(g\|\Gamma_i^C)$ | $P(t\|\Gamma_i^C)$ |
| | 1 | **0.31038** | 0.22205 | 0.26436 | 0.20321 |
| | 2 | **0.42182** | 0.17773 | 0.24578 | 0.15467 |
| | 3 | **0.41362** | 0.22573 | 0.11644 | 0.24422 |
| | 4 | 0.20761 | 0.19017 | **0.37147** | 0.23075 |

**Table 7.** Minimal partition—Definition 2—estimated by Definition 6. From top to bottom, for the sequences *A* (GenBank OQ706226), *B* (GenBank OQ706227), and *C* (GenBank OQ706228). $\Delta = \{a,c,g,t\}, o = 3, w_n = \ln(n), \alpha = 2, \gamma$ function given by the identity.

| Sequence | Part | States |
|---|---|---|
| OQ706226 | $\Gamma_1^A$ | ccc, tgc, cgc, ggc, gac, gtc, acg, att, gct, gcc, atc, agc, ggt, gag, ata |
| | $\Gamma_2^A$ | tcc, agt, ctc, tct, ttc, cct, ctt, gtt, aaa, ttt |
| | $\Gamma_3^A$ | aag, ccg, gcg, tgg, gtg, act, agg, ctg, gat, ttg, aat, tcg, cgg, cat, ggg, tat, atg |
| | $\Gamma_4^A$ | cag, cac, taa, cgt, aga, gga, tta, tac, cga, acc, tag, gta, cca, tca, tga, cta, aac |
| | $\Gamma_5^A$ | tgt, gaa, caa, aca, gca |
| OQ706227 | $\Gamma_1^B$ | ccc, tgc, tct, gtt, cgc, ggc, gac, gtc, gct, acg, att, tag |
| | $\Gamma_2^B$ | gcc, atc, agc, ggt, gag, ata |
| | $\Gamma_3^B$ | tcc, agt, ctc, ttc, cct, ctt, aaa, ttt |
| | $\Gamma_4^B$ | aag, ccg, gcg, tgg, gtg, agg, ctg, ttg, aat, gat, tcg, cgg, cat, tat, act, ggg, atg |
| | $\Gamma_5^B$ | cag, cgt, aga, gga, tta, tac, cga, cac, acc |
| | $\Gamma_6^B$ | tgt, gaa, caa, taa, tga, cta, cca, tca, aca, gca, gta, aac |
| OQ706228 | $\Gamma_1^C$ | ccc, cgc, ggc, gac, tcc, tct, agt, tgc, gct, gtc, acg, att |
| | $\Gamma_2^C$ | gcc, atc, agc, ggt, gag, ata |
| | $\Gamma_3^C$ | ctc, cct, ttc, aaa, ctt, gtt, ttt |
| | $\Gamma_4^C$ | aag, ccg, gcg, tgg, gtg, agg, ctg, ttg, aat, gat, tcg, cgg, cat, tat, act, ggg, atg |
| | $\Gamma_5^C$ | cag, taa, tta, cac, cgt, cga, tac, acc, aga, gga |
| | $\Gamma_6^C$ | tag, gta, cca, tca, tga, cta, gca, aac, tgt, gaa, caa, aca |

We observe from Tables 3, 5, 7 and 9 (right)–11 (right) that as the penalty $w_n$ is reduced (that is, when $w_n$ approaches the lower limit $\ln(\ln(n))$), the model is allowed to acquire more parameters, in this case, more parts.

Given a penalization $w_n$, the three sequences, *A* (GenBank OQ706226), *B* (GenBank OQ706227), and *C* (GenBank OQ706228), show a similar number of parts. More specifically, for the penalty $w_n = n^{1/2}$ the behavior of the three sequences is represented by two parts (Table 3), for $w_n = n^{1/3}$ the behavior of the three sequences is described by four parts (Table 5). For $w_n = \ln(n)$, OQ706226 is modeled by five parts while the other two are modeled by six parts (see Table 7). For penalty $w_n = \ln(\ln(n))$, OQ706226 is modeled by a partition with 13 parts (see Table 9, right) while the other two sequences are modeled by 14 parts, see Tables 10 (right) and 11 (right).

**Table 8.** Transition probabilities—Equation (2)—estimated by Equation (5). From top to bottom, for the sequences $A$ (GenBank OQ706226), $B$ (GenBank OQ706227), and $C$ (GenBank OQ706228). $\Delta = \{a,c,g,t\}, w_n = \ln(n)$; full estimated partitions displayed in Table 7. In bold, the highest probability per part.

| OQ706226 | $i$ | $P(a\|\Gamma_i^A)$ | $P(c\|\Gamma_i^A)$ | $P(g\|\Gamma_i^A)$ | $P(t\|\Gamma_i^A)$ |
|---|---|---|---|---|---|
| | 1 | **0.29882** | 0.22627 | 0.25608 | 0.21882 |
| | 2 | **0.40166** | 0.18760 | 0.25987 | 0.15087 |
| | 3 | **0.41291** | 0.22673 | 0.11709 | 0.24328 |
| | 4 | 0.18351 | 0.20596 | **0.35967** | 0.25086 |
| | 5 | 0.26507 | 0.15017 | **0.40273** | 0.18203 |
| OQ706227 | $i$ | $P(a\|\Gamma_i^B)$ | $P(c\|\Gamma_i^B)$ | $P(g\|\Gamma_i^B)$ | $P(t\|\Gamma_i^B)$ |
| | 1 | **0.30945** | 0.21394 | 0.28167 | 0.19493 |
| | 2 | **0.28468** | 0.25573 | 0.20507 | 0.25452 |
| | 3 | **0.40612** | 0.18593 | 0.25902 | 0.14893 |
| | 4 | **0.41410** | 0.22668 | 0.11608 | 0.24314 |
| | 5 | 0.18868 | 0.20926 | **0.31990** | 0.28216 |
| | 6 | 0.21860 | 0.17026 | **0.40620** | 0.20494 |
| OQ706228 | $i$ | $P(a\|\Gamma_i^C)$ | $P(c\|\Gamma_i^C)$ | $P(g\|\Gamma_i^C)$ | $P(t\|\Gamma_i^C)$ |
| | 1 | **0.31933** | 0.21040 | 0.28482 | 0.18545 |
| | 2 | **0.28451** | 0.25570 | 0.20528 | 0.25450 |
| | 3 | **0.42182** | 0.17773 | 0.24578 | 0.15467 |
| | 4 | **0.41362** | 0.22573 | 0.11644 | 0.24422 |
| | 5 | 0.19202 | 0.20975 | **0.31905** | 0.27917 |
| | 6 | 0.21932 | 0.17546 | **0.41088** | 0.19434 |

**Table 9.** Sequence OQ706226. Right: Minimal partition—Definition 2—estimated by Definition 6. Left: Transition probabilities—Equation (2)—estimated by Equation (5); in bold, the highest probability per part. $\Delta = \{a,c,g,t\}, o = 3, \gamma$ function given by the identity, $w_n = \ln(\ln(n))$.

| $i$ | $P(a\|\Gamma_i^A)$ | $P(c\|\Gamma_i^A)$ | $P(g\|\Gamma_i^A)$ | $P(t\|\Gamma_i^A)$ | Part | States |
|---|---|---|---|---|---|---|
| 1 | **0.31140** | 0.19342 | 0.28411 | 0.21107 | $\Gamma_1^A$ | ccc, tgc, cgc, ggc, gac |
| 2 | **0.32218** | 0.25314 | 0.19456 | 0.23013 | $\Gamma_2^A$ | gcc, atc |
| 3 | **0.38732** | 0.19249 | 0.27934 | 0.14085 | $\Gamma_3^A$ | tcc, tct, agt, ctc, ttc, cct |
| 4 | 0.23757 | 0.25967 | 0.21823 | **0.28453** | $\Gamma_4^A$ | agc, ggt, gag, ata |
| 5 | **0.28879** | 0.26078 | 0.27371 | 0.17672 | $\Gamma_5^A$ | gtc, acg, att, gct |
| 6 | **0.40686** | 0.21316 | 0.14272 | 0.23726 | $\Gamma_6^A$ | aag, ccg, gcg, tgg, gtg, ttg, tat |
| 7 | 0.19113 | 0.20930 | **0.32195** | 0.27762 | $\Gamma_7^A$ | cag, cac, taa, cgt, aga, gga, tta, tac, cga, acc |
| 8 | 0.17164 | 0.29104 | **0.41791** | 0.11940 | $\Gamma_8^A$ | tag, gta |
| 9 | **0.46675** | 0.21455 | 0.08532 | 0.23337 | $\Gamma_9^A$ | tcg, cgg, cat, ggg, act, atg |
| 10 | **0.34566** | 0.27172 | 0.11275 | 0.26987 | $\Gamma_{10}^A$ | agg, ctg, gat, aat |
| 11 | 0.26507 | 0.15017 | **0.40273** | 0.18203 | $\Gamma_{11}^A$ | tgt, gaa, caa, aca, gca |
| 12 | **0.43116** | 0.17754 | 0.21981 | 0.17150 | $\Gamma_{12}^A$ | ctt, gtt, aaa, ttt |
| 13 | 0.17246 | 0.18610 | **0.41439** | 0.22705 | $\Gamma_{13}^A$ | cca, tca, tga, cta, aac |

The formal determination of whether the identified models, under each penalty, exhibit significant differences lies beyond the scope of this application. However, we acknowledge it as an open question worthy of further exploration.

The following observation applies to all three sequences. Observing the magnitudes of the transition probabilities, marked in bold, we note that, as reported in Tables 6, 8, and 9 (left)–11 (left), there is a predominant number of parts whose prevalence is the transition to element a of the alphabet $\{a,c,g,t\}$, and secondly, parts that indicate a prevalence for element g of the alphabet. As for Table 4, which reports the most penalized case ($w_n = n^{1/2}$), one part is recorded with prevalence for a and another with prevalence for g, which is natural, since the model only has two parts. As Tables 9–11 show, based on the penalty $w_n = \ln(\ln(n))$, the three sequences show the same part {agc,ggt,gag,ata} with a prevalence for the element t of the alphabet $\Delta$, of lower magnitude, than those previously mentioned.

**Table 10.** Sequence OQ706227. Right: Minimal partition—Definition 2—estimated by Definition 6. Left: Transition probabilities—Equation (2)—estimated by Equation (5); in bold, the highest probability per part. $\Delta = \{a,c,g,t\}, o = 3, \gamma$ function given by the identity, $w_n = \ln(\ln(n))$.

| $i$ | $P(a\|\Gamma_i^B)$ | $P(c\|\Gamma_i^B)$ | $P(g\|\Gamma_i^B)$ | $P(t\|\Gamma_i^B)$ | Part | States |
|---|---|---|---|---|---|---|
| 1 | **0.34479** | 0.19313 | 0.27725 | 0.18483 | $\Gamma_1^B$ | ccc, tgc, gtt, tct |
| 2 | **0.31992** | 0.25636 | 0.19280 | 0.23093 | $\Gamma_2^B$ | gcc, atc |
| 3 | **0.39127** | 0.19183 | 0.27978 | 0.13712 | $\Gamma_3^B$ | tcc, agt, ctc, ttc, cct |
| 4 | 0.23810 | 0.25490 | 0.22129 | **0.28571** | $\Gamma_4^B$ | agc, ggt, gag, ata |
| 5 | **0.29094** | 0.19737 | 0.28509 | 0.22661 | $\Gamma_5^B$ | cgc, ggc, gac |
| 6 | 0.27672 | 0.26908 | **0.28435** | 0.16985 | $\Gamma_6^B$ | gtc, gct, acg, att, tag |
| 7 | **0.40705** | 0.21628 | 0.14945 | 0.22722 | $\Gamma_7^B$ | aag, ccg, gcg, tgg, gtg |
| 8 | 0.18868 | 0.20926 | **0.31990** | 0.28216 | $\Gamma_8^B$ | cag, cgt, aga, gga, tta, tac, cga, cac, acc |
| 9 | **0.47018** | 0.20642 | 0.08601 | 0.23739 | $\Gamma_9^B$ | tcg, cgg, cat, tat, act, ggg, atg |
| 10 | **0.35015** | 0.26558 | 0.11424 | 0.27003 | $\Gamma_{10}^B$ | agg, ctg, ttg, aat, gat |
| 11 | 0.27992 | 0.13996 | **0.42191** | 0.15822 | $\Gamma_{11}^B$ | tgt, gaa, caa |
| 12 | **0.43490** | 0.17450 | 0.21880 | 0.17181 | $\Gamma_{12}^B$ | ctt, aaa, ttt |
| 13 | 0.21127 | 0.17647 | **0.39188** | 0.22038 | $\Gamma_{13}^B$ | taa, tga, cta, cca, tca, aca, gca |
| 14 | 0.11330 | 0.20690 | **0.45321** | 0.22660 | $\Gamma_{14}^B$ | gta, aac |

**Table 11.** Sequence OQ706228. Right: Minimal partition—Definition 2—estimated by Definition 6. Left: Transition probabilities—Equation (2)—estimated by Equation (5); in bold, the highest probability per part. $\Delta = \{a,c,g,t\}, o = 3, \gamma$ function given by the identity, $w_n = \ln(\ln(n))$.

| $i$ | $P(a\|\Gamma_i^C)$ | $P(c\|\Gamma_i^C)$ | $P(g\|\Gamma_i^C)$ | $P(t\|\Gamma_i^C)$ | Part | States |
|---|---|---|---|---|---|---|
| 1 | **0.30740** | 0.18975 | 0.28463 | 0.21822 | $\Gamma_1^C$ | ccc, cgc, ggc, gac |
| 2 | **0.31924** | 0.25581 | 0.19450 | 0.23044 | $\Gamma_2^C$ | gcc, atc |
| 3 | **0.35319** | 0.20914 | 0.29501 | 0.14266 | $\Gamma_3^C$ | tcc, tct, agt |
| 4 | 0.23889 | 0.25556 | 0.21944 | **0.28611** | $\Gamma_4^C$ | agc, ggt, gag, ata |
| 5 | **0.30048** | 0.24642 | 0.27345 | 0.17965 | $\Gamma_5^C$ | tgc, gct, gtc, acg, att |
| 6 | **0.41354** | 0.17708 | 0.26875 | 0.14063 | $\Gamma_6^C$ | ctc, ttc, cct |
| 7 | **0.41304** | 0.21196 | 0.14565 | 0.22935 | $\Gamma_7^C$ | aag, ccg, gcg, tat, tgg, gtg |
| 8 | 0.19202 | 0.20975 | **0.31905** | 0.27917 | $\Gamma_8^C$ | cag, taa, tta, cac, cgt, cga, tac, acc, aga, gga |
| 9 | 0.17778 | 0.28889 | **0.41481** | 0.11852 | $\Gamma_9^C$ | tag, gta |
| 10 | **0.47315** | 0.20716 | 0.08440 | 0.23529 | $\Gamma_{10}^C$ | tcg, cat, cgg, act, ggg, atg |
| 11 | **0.31564** | 0.26588 | [illegible] | 0.27474 | $\Gamma_{11}^C$ | agg, ctg, ttg, aat, gat |
| 12 | 0.27205 | 0.15097 | **0.41555** | 0.16144 | $\Gamma_{12}^C$ | tgt, gaa, caa, aca |
| 13 | **0.43154** | 0.17848 | 0.21883 | 0.17115 | $\Gamma_{13}^C$ | ctt, gtt, aaa, ttt |
| 14 | 0.18957 | 0.17653 | **0.40722** | 0.22668 | $\Gamma_{14}^C$ | cca, tca, tga, cta, gca, aac |

## 4. Conclusions

The main objective of this paper, developed in Section 2, is to introduce a new notion based on the Equation (8), as given in Definition 6. This concept is used to identify the minimal partition of a Markov chain—Definition 2. Theorem 3 proves that the concept in Definition 6 constitutes a metric. Furthermore, Theorem 2 establishes the relationship between this new metric and the operation of the EDC criterion, showing that in an iterative process, selecting a partition with a higher EDC value is equivalent to using the value 1 as a threshold in the metric. In this way, we achieve our main goal of proposing an EDC-based metric to estimate the minimal partition.

Our results add to those of [4], in the search to characterize penalty terms that can be used in the EDC criterion to obtain the consistent estimation of the minimal partition. Ref. [4] demonstrates that the EDC, under certain conditions on the term $w_n$ (Equation (9)), provides a strongly consistent estimate of the minimal partition, as defined in Definition 2. Building on the results from [5], we conjectured that using $w_n = \ln(\ln(n))$ might preserve strong consistency, even though this term does not satisfy the second condition imposed by Equation (9). We confirm in Theorem 1 and Corollary 1 that strong consistency is indeed achieved using the EDC with the penalization term $w_n = \ln(\ln(n))$.

We conclude the article with an application demonstrating the effect of the metric introduced in Definition 6 on estimating the minimal partition—Definition 2, using various penalty terms discussed in Remark 1. For this purpose, we analyze three Dengue virus type 3 sequences, native to Brazil and collected in 2023, in FASTA format. The application shows that relaxing the penalty results in higher cardinalities for the estimated partition. We identify which parts (collections of states) of the Dengue sequences have a greater or lesser preference for transitioning to the next element (a, c, g, or t) in the alphabet $\Delta = \{a, c, g, t\}$. As expected, the models identified for each sequence exhibit similar features when the penalty is applied, which is natural given that the sequences share the same collection date and region of origin.

**Author Contributions:** Conceptualization, J.E.G. and V.A.G.-L.; Methodology, J.E.G. and V.A.G.-L.; Software, J.E.G. and V.A.G.-L.; Validation, J.E.G., V.A.G.-L. and J.I.G.S.; Formal analysis, J.E.G. and V.A.G.-L.; Investigation, J.E.G., V.A.G.-L. and J.I.G.S.; Resources, J.E.G. and V.A.G.-L.; Data curation, J.E.G. and V.A.G.-L.; Writing—original draft, J.E.G. and V.A.G.-L.; Writing—review & editing, J.E.G. and V.A.G.-L.; Visualization, J.E.G. and V.A.G.-L.; Supervision, J.E.G. and V.A.G.-L.; Project administration, J.E.G. and V.A.G.-L.; Funding acquisition, J.E.G. and V.A.G.-L. All authors have read and agreed to the published version of the manuscript.

**Funding:** Johsac I. Gomez Sanchez gratefully acknowledge the financial support provided by CAPES with fellowships from the Master Graduate Program in Statistics—University of Campinas.

**Data Availability Statement:** The National Center for Biotechnology Information Advances Science and Health, https://www.ncbi.nlm.nih.gov/ (accessed on 10 March 2024).

**Acknowledgments:** The authors wish to express their gratitude to the three referees and the editors for their helpful comments on an earlier draft of this paper.

**Conflicts of Interest:** The authors declare no conflict of interest.

## References


1. Zhao, L.C.; Dorea, C.C.Y.; Gonçalves, C.R. On determination of the order of a Markov chain. *Stat. Inference Stoch. Process.* **2001**, *4*, 273–282. [CrossRef]
2. García Jesús, E.; González-López, V.A. Consistent Estimation of Partition Markov Models. *Entropy* **2017**, *19*, 160. [CrossRef]
3. García, J.E.; González-López, V.A.; Tasca, G.H.; Yaginuma, K.Y. An Efficient Coding Technique for Stochastic Processes. *Entropy* **2022**, *24*, 65. [CrossRef]
4. Pereira, D.F.S. Critério de Determinação Eficiente Para Estimação de Cadeias de Markov de Partição Mínima. Master's Thesis, University of Brasilia, Brasilia, Federal District, Brazil, 2021. Available online: http://repositorio2.unb.br/jspui/handle/10482/42891 (accessed on 10 March 2024).
5. Dorea, C.C.Y. Optimal penalty term for EDC Markov chain order estimator. *Ann. de l'ISUP* **2008**, *52*, 15–25. Available online: https://hal.science/hal-03633210 (accessed on 10 March 2024).
6. Csiszár, I. Large-scale typicality of Markov sample paths and consistency of MDL order estimators. *IEEE Trans. Inf. Theory* **2002**, *48*, 1616–1628. [CrossRef]
7. Csiszár, I.; Talata, Z. Context tree estimation for not necessarily finite memory processes, via BIC and MDL. *IEEE Trans. Inf. Theory* **2006**, 52, 1007–1016. [CrossRef]
8. García, J.E.; González-López, V.A.; Tasca, G.H. Partition Markov Model for COVID-19 Virus. *4open* **2020**, *3*, 13. [CrossRef]
9. García, J.E.; González-López, V.A.; Tasca, G.H. Multiple partition Markov model for B.1.1.7, B.1.351, B.1.617.2, and P.1 variants of SARS-CoV 2 virus. *Comput. Stat.* **2022**. [CrossRef]

10. Naveca, F.G.; Santiago, G.A.; Maito, R.M.; Meneses, C.A.R.; do Nascimento, V.A.; de Souza, V.C.; do Nascimento, F.O.; Silva, D.; Mejía, M.; Gonçalves, L.; et al. Reemergence of dengue virus serotype 3, Brazil, 2023. *Emerg. Infect. Dis.* **2023**, *29*, 1482–1484. [CrossRef]
11. Schwarz, G. Estimating the dimension of a model. *Ann. Stat.* **1978**, *6*, 461–464. [CrossRef]

entropy

MDPI

*Article*

# Likelihood Inference for Factor Copula Models with Asymmetric Tail Dependence

**Harry Joe * and Xiaoting Li**

Department of Statistics, University of British Columbia, Vancouver, BC V6T 1Z4, Canada; xiaoting.li@stat.ubc.ca
* Correspondence: harry.joe@ubc.ca

**Abstract:** For multivariate non-Gaussian involving copulas, likelihood inference is dominated by the data in the middle, and fitted models might not be very good for joint tail inference, such as assessing the strength of tail dependence. When preliminary data and likelihood analysis suggest asymmetric tail dependence, a method is proposed to improve extreme value inferences based on the joint lower and upper tails. A prior that uses previous information on tail dependence can be used in combination with the likelihood. With the combination of the prior and the likelihood (which in practice has some degree of misspecification) to obtain a tilted log-likelihood, inferences with suitably transformed parameters can be based on Bayesian computing methods or with numerical optimization of the tilted log-likelihood to obtain the posterior mode and Hessian at this mode.

**Keywords:** copula; latent variable; likelihood; prior; Bayesian computing; numerical optimization

## 1. Introduction

Dependence models with multivariate copulas have had many applications in the past two decades to handle non-Gaussian dependence; in particular, for applications such as risk analysis where variables can have more dependence in the joint tails than with Gaussian dependence with the same strength of central dependence.

When pairwise scatterplots of variables suggest lower and upper tail dependence, possibly asymmetric in the strength in the joint lower tails (extreme of lower quadrant) versus the strength in the joint upper tails (extreme of upper quadrant), several different parametric copula families with tail dependence are among the best based on information criteria such as the Akaike information criterion (AIC). However model-based bivariate lower and upper tail dependence measures can be quite different for these different parametric copulas, and the comparisons of lower and upper tail dependence measures might not match the visual comparisons on the pairwise scatterplots. This is because likelihood methods are influenced a lot by data in the middle (rather than extremes), and all simple parametric models have some degree of misspecification.

For univariate distributions, it is well known that inferences involving large quantiles should not be based on a fitted parametric distribution because extrapolation is not reliable when the data values in the middle have the most influence in the parameter estimates. There are two approaches for univariate inferences involving extremes: (a) from univariate extreme value theory with the assumption of a well-behaved tail density, the peaks-over-threshold method based on generalized Pareto distribution [1] can be used, or (b) splicing models [2] can be used with different flexible densities for the body and tail, if inferences are also needed for non-extremes. For the joint tail region, there is a multivariate Pareto approach such as that in [3], but there is no convenient way to combine with a density for the body.

The goal in this article is to propose a method that incorporates "prior" information on the relations of bivariate lower/upper tail dependence pairs, thereby placing more weight on joint extreme observations when estimating the dependence parameters of the multivariate copula; the splicing of densities for the body and the joint tails is avoided. This approach should lead to parameter estimates of copula dependence parameters with more reliable inference for tail dependence and other tail-based quantities.

How different parametric copula models lead to quite different tail inferences is illustrated with some financial returns data over a few consecutive years. Consider the financial returns for different market indexes or stocks in the same sector of a market; for dependence analysis, commonly, a copula-GARCH model (see [4]) is applied to GARCH-filtered returns. Pairwise normal scores plots after rank transform to $N(0,1)$ show tail dependence with the clouds of points being sharper than the elliptical shape in the extreme lower and upper quadrants. Often, there appears to be a stronger dependence in the joint lower tail than in the joint upper tail.

When different flexible parametric multivariate copula families, such as vine and factor copula models, are fit to multivariate GARCH-filtered returns, the best-fitting models based on AIC imply lower and upper tail dependence for any pair of returns. This is based on the results of [5,6], which imply that if bivariate copulas, for pairs of variables in the first tree of the vine or with a variable linked to a latent variable, have lower and upper tail dependence, then the bivariate copulas of all pairs of variables have lower and upper tail dependence. Note that factor copulas are vine copulas that include latent variables.

However, if model-based tail dependence parameters are computed based on the best few fitted models, they can be quite different among the models and sometimes may not match what is seen in the normal score plots. For example, (a) sometimes, a model-based lower tail dependence parameter may be closer to 0 than expected based on the plot, or (b) the model-based lower tail dependence parameter may be smaller than the model-based upper tail dependence parameter, in contrast to the the visual inspection of the plot.

With the non-parametric method for empirical tail dependence measures in [7], it is possible to compare empirical and model-based lower and upper tail dependence to show quantitatively that model-based measures might not be reliable for all bivariate margins. This is because the fit of parametric multivariate models based on likelihood tends to be dominated by the data in the middle of the distribution. Inference concerning the middle (e.g., medians and non-extreme marginal orthant probabilities) can be reliable but not necessarily inference concerning the extremes (e.g., extreme marginal orthant probabilities or multivariate quantiles of the form defined in [8]).

This article shows the use of a tilted likelihood to estimate parameters of the 1-factor copula so that inferences in the joint tails are improved.The 1-factor copula for $d$ variables has a vector parameter $\boldsymbol{\vartheta}_j$ for the bivariate linking copula of the $j$th variable and the latent variable (the latter explains the joint dependence of the observed variables). The tilting depends on the nature of the variables. For $d$ GARCH-filtered stock returns for stocks in the same sector, the dependence parameters $\{\boldsymbol{\vartheta}_j : 1 \le j \le d\}$ can be considered a sample from a super-population so that it is reasonable to assume a common prior distribution for the $\boldsymbol{\vartheta}_j$. The tilted log-likelihood is based on the sum of the 1-factor copula log-likelihood and the logarithm of this prior density that is based on tail dependence summaries from some "previous data".

There is a numerical data example in Section 2 for preliminaries to show explicitly why likelihood inference can be inadequate for tail inference; tail dependence parameters are defined, and examples of normal score plots are given in this section. Sections 3 and 4 contain the theory and numerical methods to develop a "prior" to help with tail inference for the 1-factor copula model with asymmetric tail-dependent copulas linking to the latent variable. Section 5 illustrates the theory for a data example with GARCH-filtered stock returns from stocks in a S&P sector to show improved tail inference. Section 6 has some simulation results to compare with the data example. Section 7 concludes with a discussion on the generality of the approach proposed for the 1-factor model; the basis is a "super-population" assumption for some bivariate margins with lower and upper tail dependence.

The background results for tail dependence, copulas, and factor models are given in Appendix A.

## 2. Numerical Data Example to Illustrate Discrepancy for Tail Inference

In this section, a numerical low-dimensional data example is used to clarify what is meant by the possible poor joint tail inference following maximum likelihood.

Definitions of bivariate tail dependence and the copula as summaries of dependence are presented to explain concepts of dependence in joint tails.

Let $F_{1:d}$ be an absolutely continuous $d$-variate distribution with univariate margins $F_1, \ldots, F_d$ and copula $C_{1:d}$ such that $F_{1:d} = C_{1:d}(F_1, \ldots, F_d)$. Let $\mathbf{Y} = (Y_1, \ldots, Y_d) \sim F_{1:d}$.

For the bivariate margin $F_{jk} = C_{jk}(F_j, F_k)$ with $j \neq k$, the probabilistic version of the lower and upper tail dependence parameters is:

$$\begin{aligned}
\lambda_{jk,L} &= \lim_{u \to 0^+} \Pr(Y_j \le F_j^{-1}(u) | Y_k \le F_k^{-1}(u)) \\
&= \lim_{u \to 0^+} u^{-1} \Pr(Y_j \le F_j^{-1}(u), Y_k \le F_k^{-1}(u)) = \lim_{u \to 0^+} C_{jk}(u,u)/u, \\
\lambda_{jk,U} &= \lim_{u \to 0^+} \Pr(Y_j \ge F_j^{-1}(1-u) | Y_k \ge F_k^{-1}(1-u)) \\
&= \lim_{u \to 0^+} u^{-1} \Pr(Y_j \ge F_j^{-1}(1-u), Y_k \ge F_k^{-1}(1-u)) \\
&= \lim_{u \to 0^+} \overline{C}_{jk}(1-u, 1-u)/u,
\end{aligned}$$

where $\overline{C}_{jk}(u_j, u_k) = 1 - u_j - u_k + C_{jk}(u_j, u_k)$ for $0 \le u_j, u_k \le 1$.

Consider a random sample from $F_{1:d}$ with $\boldsymbol{y}_i = (y_{i1}, \ldots, y_{id})$ for $i = 1, \ldots, n$. Because $\lambda_{jk,L}$ and $\lambda_{jk,U}$ are limiting quantities (as $u \to 0^+$), there are no direct empirical (data) versions. For the numerical examples in this section and later sections, the sample version comes from a limit of tail-weighted dependence measures.

A general reference for concepts (in the above and in later sections) with copulas and dependence is [9], and the estimator of tail dependence from a limit of tail-weighted dependence measures is given in [7]. For the probabilistic version, the tail-weighted dependence measures are indexed by a parameter $\alpha > 1$ and the limit, as $\alpha \to \infty$ is the tail dependence parameter. After computing the empirical tail-weighted dependence measure for a grid of $\alpha$ values, typically in the interval $[10, 20]$, a regression model is fit for the empirical measure versus a power of $\alpha^{-1}$, and then the tail dependence parameter is estimated as the extrapolation with $\alpha^{-1} \to 0$.

The data example involves GARCH-filtered stock returns with all stocks in the same sector. Appendix A.1 has some background for GARCH time series and copula-GARCH models.

The S&P 500 data set of GARCH-filtered stock returns (January 2013 to December 2015, good economic conditions) used for illustration is analyzed in [10]. The sample consists of $n = 754$ days. For the finance sector, some initial descriptive statistics analyses based on 10 stocks were chosen from 64; the ticker symbols of the 10 stocks are COF, RJF, SCHW, FRC, GL, FD, TROW, GS, BLK, and ICE. Normal score plots of GARCH-filtered returns for a few pairs amongst these 10 stocks are given in Figure 1 (see Appendix A.3 for the mathematical definition of the transform). They show tail dependence, with the clouds of the points being sharper than the elliptical shape and having a stronger correlation in the lower quadrant than in the upper quadrant.

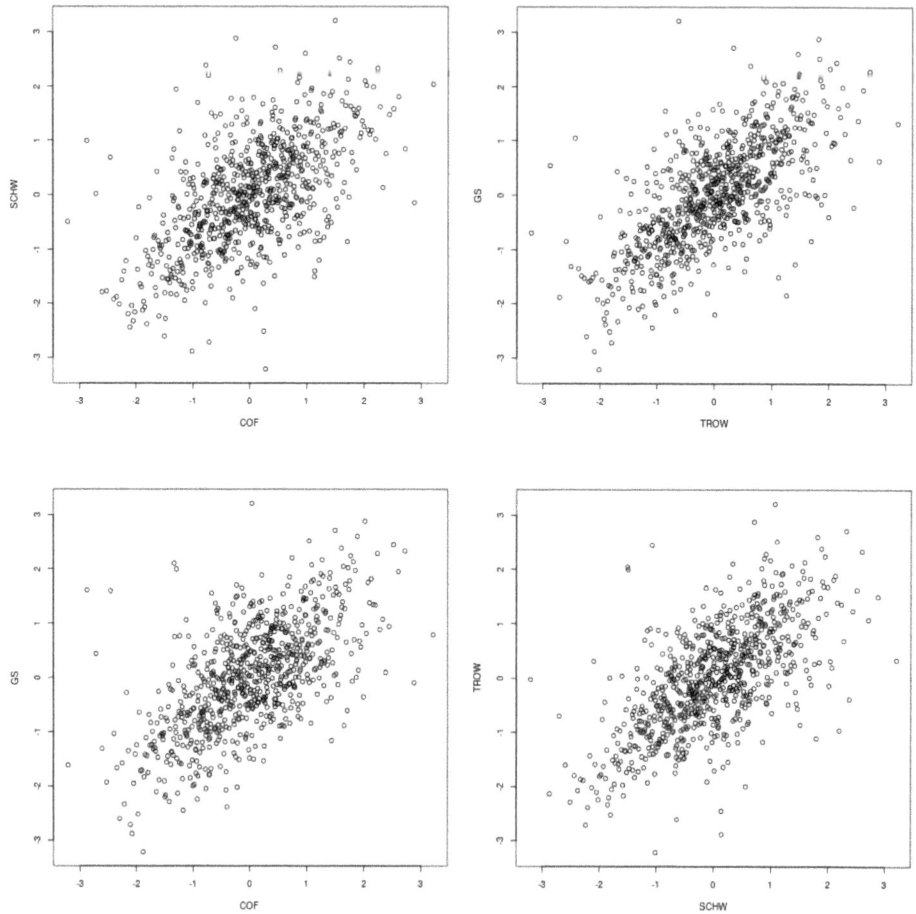


**Figure 1.** Normal score plots for some pairs of GARCH-filtered stock returns. Lower and upper semi-correlations, as used in Section 2.4 of [9], show more dependence in the lower quadrant than in the upper quadrant and suggest asymmetric tail dependence.

These few stocks are used to demonstrate (in small tables) a typical situation of differences in empirical and model-based tail quantities. To check that a 1-factor dependence structure is reasonable, the non-parametric transform to normal scores is applied to GARCH-filtered returns, and factor analysis (see [11]) is applied to the resulting correlation matrix. The loadings are, respectively, 0.741, 0.802, 0.838, 0.475, 0.688, 0.821, 0.665, 0.609, 0.690, 0.830. The average absolute difference between the empirical and model-based correlation matrix is 0.03, and the maximum absolute difference between the empirical and model-based correlation matrix is 0.21 (with two discrepancies with an absolute difference $> 0.10$), so the 1-factor structure is reasonable as a first-order approximation when considering that a $10 \times 10$ matrix with 45 correlations is approximated by a simple correlation matrix with 10 parameters. With a larger dimension (more stocks in the same sector), a 1-factor model with some weak conditional dependence (see [12]) could be a better dependence model.

Two parametric copula models are fitted to account for non-Gaussian dependence—1-factor with $d = 10$ linking copulas that are all BB1, or all reflected BB1 (abbreviated as BB1r). These are referred to briefly as 1-factor BB1 and 1-factor BB1r. The details of these models are summarized in Appendices A.1 and A.2 in Appendix A; in particular, Appendix A.1 has the definition of the 2-parameter bivariate BB1 copula and some of its dependence properties, and Appendix A.2 has the definition of the 1-factor copula for $d$ variables based on conditional independence of observed variables given a latent variable.

Table 1 has empirical and model-based lower and upper tail dependence measures: $\widehat{\lambda}_{jk,L}, \lambda_{jk,L}(\widehat{\boldsymbol{\vartheta}}), \widehat{\lambda}_{jk,U}, \lambda_{jk,U}(\widehat{\boldsymbol{\vartheta}})$. Model-based values are based on maximum likelihood estimates (MLEs) with 1-factor BB1r and 1-factor BB1. Table 2 has an empirical Spearman rank correlation as a central measure of dependence: $\widehat{\rho}_{jk,S}$. The values of $\rho_{jk,S}(\widehat{\boldsymbol{\vartheta}})$ for the two 1-factor copula models are quite close to the empirical values compared with some discrepancies for tail dependence measures. Table 3 has summaries, averaged over $d(d-1)/10 = 45$ bivariate margins. Tables 1 and 3 show that tail inferences from different models with lower and upper tail dependence can be quite different, but the models can have similar inferences for central quantities.

**Table 1.** Matrices of tail dependence measures for 10 stock GARCH-filtered returns: model-based 1-factor BB1r, empirical, model-based 1-factor BB1, respectively. Lower (upper) tail dependence below (above) diagonal. Bootstrap standard errors (SEs) for estimates of lower and upper tail dependence are mostly in the range 0.04 to 0.075.

| **Model-Based Tail-Dependence Based on MLE with 1-Factor BB1r** | | | | | | | | | |
|---|---|---|---|---|---|---|---|---|---|
| 1.000 | 0.258 | 0.193 | 0.017 | 0.176 | 0.093 | 0.135 | 0.037 | 0.039 | 0.233 |
| 0.400 | 1.000 | 0.267 | 0.022 | 0.242 | 0.126 | 0.184 | 0.049 | 0.051 | 0.326 |
| 0.449 | 0.470 | 1.000 | 0.018 | 0.181 | 0.096 | 0.139 | 0.038 | 0.040 | 0.240 |
| 0.257 | 0.268 | 0.298 | 1.000 | 0.016 | 0.009 | 0.013 | 0.004 | 0.004 | 0.021 |
| 0.353 | 0.369 | 0.413 | 0.239 | 1.000 | 0.088 | 0.127 | 0.035 | 0.037 | 0.218 |
| 0.449 | 0.471 | 0.533 | 0.299 | 0.414 | 1.000 | 0.069 | 0.020 | 0.020 | 0.114 |
| 0.334 | 0.349 | 0.390 | 0.227 | 0.310 | 0.391 | 1.000 | 0.027 | 0.029 | 0.167 |
| 0.328 | 0.342 | 0.382 | 0.223 | 0.304 | 0.383 | 0.288 | 1.000 | 0.008 | 0.045 |
| 0.383 | 0.401 | 0.450 | 0.258 | 0.354 | 0.451 | 0.335 | 0.329 | 1.000 | 0.047 |
| 0.434 | 0.455 | 0.513 | 0.289 | 0.400 | 0.514 | 0.378 | 0.370 | 0.435 | 1.000 |
| **Empirical Tail-Dependence Measures** | | | | | | | | | |
| 1.000 | 0.418 | 0.259 | 0.087 | 0.196 | 0.233 | 0.200 | 0.160 | 0.144 | 0.239 |
| 0.397 | 1.000 | 0.238 | 0.141 | 0.275 | 0.285 | 0.247 | 0.144 | 0.163 | 0.333 |
| 0.362 | 0.382 | 1.000 | 0.118 | 0.268 | 0.326 | 0.275 | 0.108 | 0.202 | 0.347 |
| 0.184 | 0.168 | 0.217 | 1.000 | 0.130 | 0.142 | 0.080 | 0.189 | 0.157 | 0.079 |
| 0.283 | 0.310 | 0.344 | 0.231 | 1.000 | 0.178 | 0.209 | 0.111 | 0.132 | 0.290 |
| 0.281 | 0.364 | 0.494 | 0.132 | 0.307 | 1.000 | 0.182 | 0.078 | 0.161 | 0.339 |
| 0.235 | 0.274 | 0.375 | 0.207 | 0.320 | 0.301 | 1.000 | 0.060 | 0.131 | 0.308 |
| 0.267 | 0.275 | 0.219 | 0.234 | 0.207 | 0.273 | 0.201 | 1.000 | 0.137 | 0.109 |
| 0.246 | 0.312 | 0.373 | 0.156 | 0.262 | 0.333 | 0.151 | 0.279 | 1.000 | 0.198 |
| 0.284 | 0.293 | 0.450 | 0.224 | 0.301 | 0.438 | 0.255 | 0.284 | 0.276 | 1.000 |
| **Model-Based Tail-Dependence Based on MLE with 1-Factor BB1** | | | | | | | | | |
| 1.000 | 0.385 | 0.363 | 0.172 | 0.317 | 0.335 | 0.279 | 0.223 | 0.273 | 0.385 |
| 0.308 | 1.000 | 0.416 | 0.195 | 0.363 | 0.383 | 0.317 | 0.253 | 0.311 | 0.442 |
| 0.394 | 0.397 | 1.000 | 0.184 | 0.342 | 0.361 | 0.300 | 0.240 | 0.294 | 0.416 |
| 0.169 | 0.170 | 0.211 | 1.000 | 0.163 | 0.172 | 0.144 | 0.117 | 0.142 | 0.194 |
| 0.263 | 0.265 | 0.336 | 0.147 | 1.000 | 0.316 | 0.264 | 0.211 | 0.258 | 0.362 |
| 0.396 | 0.399 | 0.525 | 0.212 | 0.337 | 1.000 | 0.278 | 0.223 | 0.272 | 0.383 |
| 0.260 | 0.262 | 0.332 | 0.146 | 0.225 | 0.333 | 1.000 | 0.187 | 0.228 | 0.317 |
| 0.263 | 0.266 | 0.336 | 0.147 | 0.228 | 0.338 | 0.225 | 1.000 | 0.183 | 0.253 |
| 0.317 | 0.320 | 0.410 | 0.174 | 0.273 | 0.412 | 0.270 | 0.273 | 1.000 | 0.311 |
| 0.358 | 0.362 | 0.469 | 0.194 | 0.307 | 0.471 | 0.303 | 0.307 | 0.373 | 1.000 |

**Table 2.** Empirical Spearman rank correlation matrix for 10 GARCH-filtered stock returns. Bootstrap SEs for Spearman are in the range 0.017 to 0.036. Model-based Spearman rhos based on 1-factor BB1r and 1-factor BB1 are quite close to the respective empirical values.

| **Empirical Spearman Rho Central Dependence Measures** | | | | | | | | | |
|---|---|---|---|---|---|---|---|---|---|
| 1.000 | 0.745 | 0.597 | 0.321 | 0.534 | 0.584 | 0.439 | 0.444 | 0.567 | 0.565 |
| 0.745 | 1.000 | 0.633 | 0.376 | 0.605 | 0.620 | 0.491 | 0.519 | 0.577 | 0.639 |
| 0.597 | 0.633 | 1.000 | 0.323 | 0.551 | 0.709 | 0.581 | 0.506 | 0.561 | 0.723 |
| 0.321 | 0.376 | 0.323 | 1.000 | 0.347 | 0.378 | 0.352 | 0.508 | 0.362 | 0.388 |
| 0.534 | 0.605 | 0.551 | 0.347 | 1.000 | 0.569 | 0.494 | 0.390 | 0.501 | 0.558 |
| 0.584 | 0.620 | 0.709 | 0.378 | 0.569 | 1.000 | 0.557 | 0.498 | 0.558 | 0.720 |
| 0.439 | 0.491 | 0.581 | 0.352 | 0.494 | 0.557 | 1.000 | 0.325 | 0.420 | 0.599 |
| 0.444 | 0.519 | 0.506 | 0.508 | 0.390 | 0.498 | 0.325 | 1.000 | 0.467 | 0.485 |
| 0.567 | 0.577 | 0.561 | 0.362 | 0.501 | 0.558 | 0.420 | 0.467 | 1.000 | 0.567 |
| 0.565 | 0.639 | 0.723 | 0.388 | 0.558 | 0.720 | 0.599 | 0.485 | 0.567 | 1.000 |

**Table 3.** Summaries to indicate how well model-based tail dependence and central dependence approximate respective empirical values. The averages and fractions are over $\binom{10}{2} = 45$ bivariate margins.

| **Summary** | **Value** |
|---|---|
| average $\lvert\widehat{\lambda}_{jk,L} - \lambda_{jk,L}(\widehat{\vartheta})\rvert$ for 1-factor BB1r | 0.088 |
| average $\lvert\widehat{\lambda}_{jk,U} - \lambda_{jk,U}(\widehat{\vartheta})\rvert$ for 1-factor BB1r | 0.101 |
| average $\lvert\widehat{\rho}_{jk,S} - \rho_{jk,S}(\widehat{\vartheta})\rvert$ for 1-factor BB1r | 0.035 |
| average $\lvert\widehat{\lambda}_{jk,L} - \lambda_{jk,L}(\widehat{\vartheta})\rvert$ for 1-factor BB1 | 0.043 |
| average $\lvert\widehat{\lambda}_{jk,U} - \lambda_{jk,U}(\widehat{\vartheta})\rvert$ for 1-factor BB1 | 0.088 |
| average $\widehat{\rho}_{jk,S} - \rho_{jk,S}(\widehat{\vartheta})$ for 1-factor BB1 | 0.036 |
| average $(\widehat{\lambda}_{jk,L} - \widehat{\lambda}_{jk,U})$ | 0.088 |
| average $(\lambda_{jk,L}(\widehat{\vartheta}) - \lambda_{jk,U}(\widehat{\vartheta}))$ for 1-factor BB1r | 0.275 |
| average $(\lambda_{jk,L}(\widehat{\vartheta}) - \lambda_{jk,U}(\widehat{\vartheta}))$ for 1-factor BB1 | 0.021 |
| fraction $\widehat{\lambda}_{jk,L} > \widehat{\lambda}_{jk,U}$ | 40/45 |
| fraction $\lambda_{jk,L}(\widehat{\vartheta}) > \lambda_{jk,U}(\widehat{\vartheta})$ for 1-factor BB1r | 45/45 |
| fraction $\lambda_{jk,L}(\widehat{\vartheta}) > \lambda_{jk,U}(\widehat{\vartheta})$ for 1-factor BB1 | 29/45 |

The tail asymmetry of financial returns, with commonly more dependence in the joint lower tail than in the joint upper tail, is explained and discussed in [13,14]. The 1-factor BB1r model has a smaller AIC value than 1-factor BB1, and it better matches the empirical property of lower tail dependence, being often larger than upper tail dependence. However, the 1-factor BB1r model tends to overestimate the difference in the lower and upper tail dependence, and the 1-factor BB1 model tends to underestimate the difference in lower and upper tail dependence. This motivates the tilted likelihood in Section 3 with an appropriate "prior" so that model-based tail dependence measures are closer to empirical counterparts.

It has been observed in many data examples (see [15] and Chapter 7 of [9]) that model-based assessment of tail dependence may not be accurate. The more recent development of tail-weighted dependence measures in [16] allows for better assessment on the reliability of a parametric copula model for tail inferences, by comparing empirical and model-based directional tail-weighted measures.

## 3. Tilted Likelihood for 1-Factor Copula Model with Tail Dependence

This section has a modified log-likelihood using a prior based on previous data for tail dependence parameters in a 1-factor copula model (as given in Appendix A.2). The starting point is the copula-based log-likelihood after univariate margins have been estimated.

Assume that satisfactory univariate models $\widehat{F}_j$ $(1 \le j \le d)$ have been fit to the random sample $\{(y_{i1}, \dots, y_{id}) : i = 1, \dots, n\}$ and then transform to the uniform scale to $\{\boldsymbol{u}_i = (u_{i1}, \dots, u_{id}) : i = 1, \dots, n\}$ with $u_{ij} = \widehat{F}_j(y_{ij})$ in the interval $(0, 1)$.

We consider mainly inference on dependence parameters for the data in the transformed uniform scale, considered as a realization of a random sample $\{\boldsymbol{U}_i\}$ for a copula cumulative distribution function (cdf) $C_U(\cdot;\boldsymbol{\vartheta})$, where $\boldsymbol{\vartheta} = (\boldsymbol{\vartheta}_1, \ldots, \boldsymbol{\vartheta}_d)$. The log-likelihood for a random sample of size $n$ is:

$$L(\boldsymbol{\vartheta}) = L(\boldsymbol{\vartheta}_j : j = 1, \ldots, d) = \sum_{i=1}^{n} \log c_U(\boldsymbol{u}_i; \boldsymbol{\vartheta}_1, \ldots, \boldsymbol{\vartheta}_d). \quad (1)$$

For the 1-factor copula based on BB1r (and other) linking copulas, there are lower bounds on components of the 2-dimensional $\boldsymbol{\vartheta}_j$.

For likelihood inference, there is invariance to 1-1 transforms of $\boldsymbol{\vartheta}_j$ to $\boldsymbol{\eta}_j$, with the latter being functions of lower and upper tail dependence parameters. Specifically, $\boldsymbol{\eta}_j = (\eta_{1j}, \eta_{2j}) = (\log[\lambda_{jL}/(1-\lambda_{jL}], \log[\lambda_{jU}/(1-\lambda_{jU})])$ with $\lambda_{jL}, \lambda_{jU}$ being the lower and upper tail dependence parameters for the bivariate copula linking variable $j$ to the latent variable. Note that $\boldsymbol{\eta}_j$ is unbounded. The tilted log-likelihood or log "posterior" is:

$$\widetilde{L}(\boldsymbol{\eta}_1, \ldots, \boldsymbol{\eta}_d) = \sum_{i=1}^{n} \log c_U(\boldsymbol{u}_i; \boldsymbol{\eta}_1, \ldots, \boldsymbol{\eta}_d) + \sum_{j=1}^{d} \log f_H(\boldsymbol{\eta}_j) \quad (2)$$

where the density $f_H$ does not depend on $j$. The above is called the tilted log-likelihood because the goal is to obtain parameter estimates that put less weight in the middle of the data space and more weight in the tails based on "prior" expected behavior of how the lower and upper tail dependence parameters are related.

With the appropriate transformation, the prior can be taken as multivariate normal. For bivariate BB1r or BB1, $\boldsymbol{\eta}_j$ is 2-dimensional, and $f_H$ is assumed to be bivariate normal. The latter is reasonable if the form of $\boldsymbol{\eta}_j$ is chosen so that (2) is closer to a quadratic in a neighborhood of its mode. Asymptotic likelihood theory (see [17]) implies that the log-likelihood is quadratic in a neighborhood of the mode, as $n \to \infty$, but the adequacy of the approximation for moderate sample size $n$ depends on the transform.

The justification of "independent" prior densities for different variables is based on some empirical checks for 1-factor copula construction with different bivariate linking copulas (with or without tail dependence). The inverse Hessian (roughly the covariance matrix of the sampling distribution of the MLE) of the negative log-likelihood in (1) for the 1-factor copula is close to the block diagonal, with a block for each $\boldsymbol{\eta}_j$. The product form of the "prior" is based on an assumption of a "super-population" for the variables linked to the latent variable (e.g., stocks in a market sector). The density $f_H$ can be considered a frequency density of $\boldsymbol{\eta}_j$ values over a large "super-population".

A method is described in Section 4 to decide on choices for $f_H$.

Similar ideas to the tilted log-likelihood have been used to obtain an adjusted log-likelihood that corrects some undesirable behavior of the MLE, given in [18,19]. There are also some connections with variational Bayes inference such as when the posterior density is assumed to be approximated by a multivariate Gaussian density after a suitable transform so that parameters are unconstrained. However, with copula applications [20,21], parsimonious and possibly unrealistic assumptions are made for the covariance matrix (such as diagonal or factor structure) of the Gaussian density. The optimization involves a Kullback–Leibler divergence of the Gaussian approximation and the posterior. This differs from optimizing (2) with no constraints on the form of the Hessian matrix at the mode.

*Numerical Optimization for Posterior Mode and Hessian at Mode*

The tilted log-likelihood has the penalized log-likelihood as an analogy so that standard numerical optimization methods can be used for estimating the mode and its Hessian.

The tilted log-likelihood in (2) and its log-likelihood counterpart in (1) are functions of $2d$ parameters for the 1-factor BB1r copula with $d$ variables. For the log-likelihood, Ref. [22] discusses an efficient numerical procedure where the log-likelihood, gradient, and

Hessian are analytically derived and coded in Fortran90, and all integrals are evaluated via Gauss–Legendre quadrature (see [23]).

The code is modified to handle the transform from BB1 parameters $(\theta_j, \delta_j)$ to $(\eta_{1j}, \eta_{2j})$, and this requires care in using the chain rule for partial derivatives. The code for (2) and its gradient and Hessian are inputted into an efficient modified Newton–Raphson algorithm, as summarized in Section 6.2 of [9]. This leads to much faster computations than coding the negative of (2) in R and using a quasi-Newton method for numerical minimization based on numerical gradients and Hessians because many more iterations are needed compared with the modified Newton–Raphson. With the use of Fortran90 (for loops), analytic derivatives, and modified Newton–Raphson iterations, the time to deduce the posterior mode is decreased by a factor larger than 20 for $2d = 40$ parameters. Without the increased speed, the simulation study reported in Section 6 would take too much time. Also numerical optimization with the quasi-Newton method performs much worse as the number of parameters increases beyond 40.

With the negative Hessian at the mode of the tilted log-likelihood, the inverse Hessian can be used to obtain interval estimates for functions of the parameters.

## 4. Closer Match of Empirical and Model-Based Tail Dependence

Suppose diagnostic plots suggest tail dependence for all pairs of variables. Maximum likelihood estimation with a parametric copula might not provide good model-based estimates of tail dependence parameters or reliable inferences for tail-based quantities. In this section, a least squares method is used to obtain parameter estimates for the 1-factor copula that will make the empirical and model-based tail dependence parameters closer to each other. That is, there is an objective function to find copula parameters to better match model-based and empirical tail dependence parameters.

Let $\boldsymbol{\theta}$ be the vector of all parameters $(\boldsymbol{\vartheta}_1, \ldots, \boldsymbol{\vartheta}_d)$. The $j$th component is $\boldsymbol{\vartheta}_j = (\theta_j, \delta_j)$ for the 1-factor BB1r or BB1 copula; see Appendix A.1 for the parametric BB1 family. The steps below assume that the 1-factor BB1r has lower AIC than 1-factor BB1 (empirical evidence from many applications of 1-factor copulas to GARCH-filtered stock returns).

1. Minimize negative of log-likelihood $L(\boldsymbol{\vartheta})$ in (1) to get MLE $\widehat{\boldsymbol{\vartheta}}$.
2. Get empirical matrix of lower tail dependence $\widehat{\lambda}_{jk,L}$, upper tail dependence $\widehat{\lambda}_{jk,U}$, central dependence Spearman rho $\widehat{\rho}_{jk,S}$.
3. Minimize

$$
\begin{aligned}
S(\boldsymbol{\vartheta}) \quad = \quad & \frac{1}{2d(d-1)}\Big\{\sum_{j<k}[\widehat{\lambda}_{jk,L} - \lambda_{jk,L}(\boldsymbol{\vartheta}_j, \boldsymbol{\vartheta}_k)]^2 + \sum_{j<k}[\widehat{\lambda}_{jk,U} - \lambda_{jk,U}(\boldsymbol{\vartheta}_j, \boldsymbol{\vartheta}_k)]^2 \\
& + \sum_{j\neq k}[\widehat{\rho}_{jk,S} - \rho_{jk,S}(\boldsymbol{\vartheta}_j, \boldsymbol{\vartheta}_k)]^2\Big\} \qquad (3)
\end{aligned}
$$

   with $\widehat{\boldsymbol{\vartheta}}$ as starting point. Let the result be $\widetilde{\boldsymbol{\vartheta}}$.
4. Convert $\widetilde{\boldsymbol{\vartheta}}_j$ to $\widetilde{\lambda}_{jV,L} = \lambda_{jV,L}(\widetilde{\boldsymbol{\vartheta}}_j)$, $\widetilde{\lambda}_{jV,U} = \lambda_{jV,U}(\widetilde{\boldsymbol{\vartheta}}_j)$ as defined in (A6), using the BB1r linking copula for variable $j$ and the latent variable $V$.
5. Transform to values in $(-\infty, \infty)$: $\log[\widetilde{\lambda}_{jV,L}/(1 - \widetilde{\lambda}_{jV,L})]$ and $\log[\widetilde{\lambda}_{jV,U}/(1 - \widetilde{\lambda}_{jV,U})]$ for $j = 1, \ldots, d$.
6. Get the sample mean vector and covariance matrix for a sample of size $d$ for the two transformed $\widetilde{\lambda}$'s. The mean vector and covariance matrix are used as parameters for the bivariate normal prior $f_H$ in (2). For the tilted likelihood, use the parametrization

$$
\boldsymbol{\eta}_j = \big(\log[\lambda_{jV,L}/(1 - \lambda_{jV,L})], \log[\lambda_{jV,U}/(1 - \lambda_{jV,U})]\big)
$$

   for $j = 1, \ldots, d$.

The data set mentioned in Section 2 as used in [10] has 64 stocks in the finance sector, 21 stocks in the energy sector and 60 stocks in the health sector of S&P 500 (years 2013–2015). The above procedure is applied to 20 random stocks from the finance sector, 10 random stocks from the energy sector, and 20 random stocks from the health sector. Below in (4) to (6) are the mean vector and covariance matrix for $f_H$ for three cases:

$$\mu_1 = \begin{pmatrix} 0.20 \\ -0.38 \end{pmatrix}, \quad \Sigma_1 = \begin{pmatrix} 0.163 & 0.134 \\ 0.134 & 0.231 \end{pmatrix}, \quad \rho_1 = 0.691; \tag{4}$$

$$\mu_2 = \begin{pmatrix} 0.04 \\ -0.74 \end{pmatrix}, \quad \Sigma_2 = \begin{pmatrix} 0.277 & 0.390 \\ 0.390 & 0.830 \end{pmatrix}, \quad \rho_2 = 0.813; \tag{5}$$

$$\mu_3 = \begin{pmatrix} -0.30 \\ -1.05 \end{pmatrix}, \quad \Sigma_3 = \begin{pmatrix} 0.121 & 0.140 \\ 0.140 & 0.365 \end{pmatrix}, \quad \rho_3 = 0.666. \tag{6}$$

They are used as the parameters of three bivariate normal distributions. The three cases are used in subsequent sections to allow a sensitivity analysis of the parameters in $f_H$.

All three cases in (4) to (6) indicate stronger tail dependence in the joint lower tail compared with the joint upper tail because of the larger value in the first component of $\mu$. Of the three cases, the first example has the strongest expected lower tail dependence because of largest first component of $\mu$. For the first two cases, the median lower tail dependence is larger than 0.5 because of the positive value. The median upper tail dependence is less than 0.5 for all three cases.

## 5. Data Example with Prior and Tilted Likelihood

This section summarizes the application of the tilted log-likelihood for GARCH-filtered stock returns. Initially, three 1-factor copula constructions, with BB1, BB1r and BB7 bivariate linking copulas to the latent variable, were fitted with maximum likelihood for different subsets of stocks. Here, as is common from many empirical applications, the 1-factor copula based on BB1r is best, based on the AIC.

The tilted log-likelihood in (2) was then used for analysis of random subsets of stocks from the finance, energy and health sectors; these were different subsets from those used to determine the prior parameters (4)–(6). The qualitative conclusions are similar for different random subsets, so below we report details for one case of 20 randomly chosen finance stocks, considered one representative application of the theory in the preceding sections.

The numerical details below are based on 20 stocks with the tickers LNC, PGR, MMC, C, KEY, CBOE, BK, BEN, AXP, ALL, BAC, RF, AFL, ZION, DFS, CMA, MCO, GL, TRV, and BRK-B, used to determine the prior $f_H$, and 20 other stocks with the tickers L, CME, MTB, MKTX, AIZ, MET, SCHW, FITB, STT, HBAN, PFG, BLK, SPGI, CB, COF, TFC, WRB, JPM, FRCB, and ICE for applying the procedure in Sections 3 and 4.

Inferences for tail dependence are compared for five cases below with summaries in Table 4.

1. 1-factor BB1r, $f_H$ based on finance sector stocks.
2. 1-factor BB1r, $f_H$ based on energy sector stocks.
3. 1-factor BB1r, $f_H$ based on health sector stocks.
4. 1-factor BB1, $f_H$ based on finance sector stocks.
5. 1-factor BB7, $f_H$ based on finance sector stocks.

The "parameters" of $f_H$ are $(\log \lambda_L/(1-\lambda_L), \log \lambda_U/(1-\lambda_U))$ and have different transformations to the parameters $(\theta, \delta)$ of BB1r, BBB1, BB7.

Table 4 shows that for BB1r, there is little sensitivity to the three priors (4)–(6). However, the worse fitting 1-factor BB1 and 1-factor BB7 models (based on last column of Table 4) do not lead to better matching with empirical dependence measures using the prior in (4). Overall, these latter two models fit worse in the middle of the data space, leading to smaller values for (2) at the mode.

**Table 4.** Closeness to corresponding empirical values to model-based ML or posterior modal $\eta_L.\eta_U$ values for lower tail dependence $\lambda_{jk,L}$, upper tail dependence $\lambda_{jk,U}$ and central dependence parameters $\rho_{jk,S}$ of $d(d-1)/2$ pairs; d = 10 GARCH-filter stock returns. The quantiles in columns 2 to 4 are from the average absolute difference over $d(d-1)/2$ pairs.

| Case | $\lambda_L$ | $\lambda_U$ | $\rho_S$ | **Objective** (2) |
|---|---|---|---|---|
| BB1r, MLE | 0.094 | 0.116 | 0.034 | – |
| BB1r, prior (4) | 0.077 | 0.043 | 0.034 | 5766 |
| BB1r, prior (5) | 0.081 | 0.054 | 0.034 | 5766 |
| BB1r, prior (6) | 0.074 | 0.046 | 0.035 | 5743 |
| BB1, prior (4) | 0.078 | 0.078 | 0.036 | 5737 |
| BB7, prior (4) | 0.140 | 0.134 | 0.062 | 5549 |

For 1-factor BB1 with the tilted log-likelihood (2), we looked at the negative inverse Hessian (covariance matrix of normal approximation) in posterior mode for row 2 of Table 4. There is almost zero correlation of the parameters for different variable indices $j$ (for different stocks). The inverse Hessian is too large to show in its entirety, but an extract of some entries is converted into standard deviations and correlations in Tables 5 and 6.

**Table 5.** Posterior mode and standard deviation (SD) of $\eta_{1j}, \eta_{2j}$ parameters. Note that $\mu_{\eta_{1j}} > \mu_{\eta_{2j}}$ implies strong lower tail dependence than upper tail dependence for variable $j$ with the latent variable. $\mu_{\eta_{1j}} > 0$ means that the estimated lower tail dependence with latent variable exceeds 0.5. The SD $\sigma$ values come from the square root of diagonal values of the negative inverse Hessian at the mode. The correlation values for each diagonal $2 \times 2$ block come from converting a covariance matrix to a correlation matrix.

| **Variable** $j$ | $\mu_{\eta_{1j}}$ | $\mu_{\eta_{2j}}$ | $\sigma_{\eta_{1j}}$ | $\sigma_{\eta_{2j}}$ | $\rho_{\eta_{1j},\eta_{2j}}$ |
|---|---|---|---|---|---|
| 1 | 0.292 | −0.351 | 0.081 | 0.202 | −0.398 |
| 2 | −0.308 | −0.797 | 0.101 | 0.217 | −0.315 |
| 3 | 0.447 | −0.010 | 0.081 | 0.186 | −0.442 |
| 4 | −0.771 | −1.422 | 0.119 | 0.243 | −0.163 |
| 5 | 0.250 | −0.904 | 0.076 | 0.227 | −0.274 |
| 6 | 0.758 | −0.261 | 0.068 | 0.215 | −0.373 |
| 7 | 0.435 | −0.390 | 0.076 | 0.209 | −0.379 |
| 8 | 0.560 | −0.165 | 0.075 | 0.200 | −0.411 |
| 9 | 0.553 | −0.137 | 0.075 | 0.200 | −0.422 |
| 10 | 0.657 | −0.314 | 0.070 | 0.213 | −0.372 |
| 11 | 0.803 | −0.255 | 0.067 | 0.215 | −0.366 |
| 12 | 0.460 | −0.755 | 0.071 | 0.224 | −0.292 |
| 13 | −0.108 | −1.312 | 0.086 | 0.234 | −0.197 |
| 14 | 0.134 | −0.859 | 0.081 | 0.226 | −0.292 |
| 15 | 0.253 | −0.637 | 0.079 | 0.219 | −0.336 |
| 16 | 0.600 | 0.101 | 0.078 | 0.186 | −0.450 |
| 17 | −0.149 | −1.240 | 0.089 | 0.233 | −0.216 |
| 18 | 0.533 | −0.036 | 0.078 | 0.192 | −0.437 |
| 19 | 0.107 | −0.734 | 0.083 | 0.221 | −0.323 |
| 20 | −0.393 | −1.228 | 0.101 | 0.235 | −0.215 |

**Table 6.** Part of negative inverse Hessian at posterior mode, that is, the posterior covariance for variables $\mu_{\eta_{1j}}, \mu_{\eta_{2j}}, j \in \{1,7,13\}$. Note that near the block diagonal form, the matrix is diagonal $2 \times 2$ block dominant.

| $j = 1$ | | $j = 7$ | | $j = 13$ | |
|---|---|---|---|---|---|
| 0.00662 | −0.00655 | −0.00002 | −0.00001 | 0.00005 | −0.00003 |
| −0.00655 | 0.04093 | −0.00002 | −0.00025 | 0.00001 | 0.00052 |
| −0.00002 | −0.00002 | 0.00570 | −0.00600 | 0.00005 | 0.00000 |
| −0.00001 | −0.00025 | −0.00600 | 0.04388 | 0.00002 | 0.00029 |
| 0.00005 | 0.00001 | 0.00005 | 0.00002 | 0.00737 | −0.00396 |
| −0.00003 | 0.00052 | 0.00000 | 0.00029 | −0.00396 | 0.05473 |

*Bayesian Computing with STAN*

Results based on the prior in (2) were also obtained via Bayesian computing with STAN (Hamiltonian Monte Carlo). Estimation for a 1-factor copula model via the Hamiltonian Monte Carlo is shown in [24], but their inferences do not include asymmetric tail dependence.

In Bayesian inference, the parameter vector $\Theta^*$ consists of both the (transformed) copula dependence parameters $\boldsymbol{\eta} = (\boldsymbol{\eta}_1, \boldsymbol{\eta}_2, \ldots, \boldsymbol{\eta}_d)$ and the latent variables $\boldsymbol{v} = (v_1, v_2, \ldots, v_n)$ in (A3). We assume a joint independent uniform prior distribution for the latent variables and a (product of) bivariate normal prior for the copula dependence parameters for the bivariate linking copulas. The prior density is given by

$$\pi_{\Theta^*}(\theta^*) = \pi_V(\boldsymbol{v})\, \pi_{H_1,\ldots,H_d}(\boldsymbol{\eta}) = \prod_{i=1}^{n} \mathbb{I}(-1 < v_i < 1) \prod_{j=1}^{d} f_H(\boldsymbol{\eta}_j),$$

where the mean and variance of the bivariate normal prior $f_H$ are given in (4)–(6). The "complete" likelihood function with the latent variables as parameters is

$$p_{\boldsymbol{U}|\Theta^*}(\boldsymbol{u}_1, \ldots, \boldsymbol{u}_n \mid \theta^*) = \prod_{i=1}^{n} p_{\boldsymbol{U}_i|V_i,H_1,\ldots,H_d}(\boldsymbol{u}_i \mid v_i, \boldsymbol{\eta}_{1:d}) = \prod_{i=1}^{n}\prod_{j=1}^{d} c_{jV}(u_j, v_i; \boldsymbol{\vartheta}_j(\boldsymbol{\eta}_j)), \tag{7}$$

where $c_{jV}$ is given in Appendix A.2. Since the Bayesian estimation treats the latent variables as additional parameters, the likelihood function consists of the conditional density function given the latent variables instead of the joint density function. The posterior density function of the parameters (up to a constant) is

$$\pi_{\Theta|\boldsymbol{U}}(\theta^* \mid \boldsymbol{u}_1, \ldots, \boldsymbol{u}_n) \propto p_{\boldsymbol{U},\Theta^*}(\boldsymbol{u}, \theta^*) = p_{\boldsymbol{U}|\Theta^*}\boldsymbol{u}_1, \ldots, \boldsymbol{u}_n \mid \theta^*)\, \pi_{\Theta^*}(\theta^*).$$

To perform Bayesian inference on the (transformed) copula dependence parameters of the 1-factor model, we use the No-U-Turn sampler (NUTS) proposed by [25]. NUTs is an extension of the Hamiltonian Monte Carlo algorithm, implemented within the STAN framework developed by [26]. The 1-factor copula models with BB1 and reflected BB1 copulas are fitted to the GARCH-filtered returns in STAN. For the data example with results summarized in Tables 5 and 6, the posterior statistics of $\boldsymbol{\eta}$ (including posterior means, standard deviations, and correlation matrix) are similar to the results obtained from maximizing the tilted likelihood function in (2). In comparison with Table 5, the median and maximum absolute differences are, respectively, (a) 0.006 and 0.033 for $\mu_\eta$'s, (b) 0.002 and 0.014 for $\sigma_\eta$'s, and (c) 0.023 and 0.059 for $\rho$'s.

From (7), it is seen that the log posterior is (up to a constant) equal to:

$$\widetilde{L}(\boldsymbol{\eta}_1, \ldots, \boldsymbol{\eta}_d, \boldsymbol{v}) = \sum_{i=1}^{n}\sum_{j=1}^{d} \log c_{jV}(u_j, v_i; \boldsymbol{\vartheta}_j(\boldsymbol{\eta}_j)) + \sum_{j=1}^{d} \log f_H(\boldsymbol{\eta}_j);$$

this is equivalent to the tilted log-likelihood in (2) after marginalizing over the latent variables $\boldsymbol{v}$. Therefore, the two approaches should yield essentially the same result.

With a flat prior on the $\eta_j$, the posterior estimates should align with the maximum likelihood estimates. However, in the case of estimating BB1 or reflected BB1 copulas, identifiability issues arise when using a flat prior. The two parameters of BB1 or reflected BB1 are negatively dependent, which can result in different combinations of parameter values producing similar likelihood values. This issue might be overlooked in maximum likelihood estimation since it converges to one of the maxima, with an appropriate starting point for numerical optimization. However, it becomes evident in Bayesian estimation, where the model struggles to distinguish between different parameter values in the posterior distributions. We found that incorporating informative priors can effectively mitigate this problem. These priors leverage tail dependence measures to provide additional information about the relationship between the parameters, thereby improving the model's ability to identify meaningful and interpretable parameter values.

## 6. Simulation Summary

This section has some simulation results for comparisons. Simulated data sets of size $n = 754$ and $d = 20$ are obtained to match the data example in Section 5; the algorithm for the simulation is in Algorithm 22 of [9]. For each simulated data set, $(\eta_{1j}, \eta_{2j})$ for $j = 1, \ldots, d$ are generated at random from (4) and then a random sample $\{(u_{i1}, \ldots, u_{id}) : i = 1, \ldots, n\}$ is generated from 1-factor BB1r based on the tail dependence parameters. For each simulated data set, as a sensitivity analysis, the log posterior in (2) for all three choices of $f_H$ based on (4)–(6) is maximized to obtain the mode and the approximate covariance matrix of the posterior density; also the MLE based on (1) is obtained.

The MLEs of the $\eta_{1j}, \eta_{2j}$ parameters are transformed to the estimated $\theta, \delta$ parameters of BB1r. Similarly, three sets of posterior modes for $\eta_{1j}, \eta_{2j}$ parameters are transformed to estimate the $\theta, \delta$ parameters. Then, the following root mean squares (rms) are computed:

$$\mathrm{rms}_m = \left[(2d)^{-1} \sum_{j=1}^{d} \left((\hat{\theta}_j^{(m)} - \theta_j)^2 + (\hat{\delta}_j^{(m)} - \delta_j)^2\right)\right]^{1/2} \tag{8}$$

for the four sets of estimators. The superscripts $m = 1, 2, 3$ indicate the three priors, and the superscript $m = 0$ indicates maximum likelihood. Over 100 simulated data sets, the rms summaries are given in Table 7.

**Table 7.** Values of average difference in values in (8) over 100 simulated data sets. Also included are the fraction of times that the posterior mode from (2) is closer to the "true" vector compared with the MLE, and lower/upper quartiles of (8).

| $m$ | **Average** $\mathbf{rms}_0 - \mathbf{rms}_m$ | **Fraction** $\mathbf{rms}_0 > \mathbf{rms}_m$ | **Q1** $\mathbf{rms}_m$ | **Q3** $\mathbf{rms}_m$ |
|---|---|---|---|---|
| 0 | | | 0.085 | 0.101 |
| 1 | [illegible] | 0.95 | 0.068 | 0.079 |
| 2 | 0.019 | 0.92 | 0.071 | 0.082 |
| 3 | 0.013 | 0.80 | 0.074 | 0.091 |

As expected, all three priors lead to closer estimates to the $(\theta, \delta)$ parameters used to generate the simulated data sets than the MLEs. The three sets of $\{(\hat{\theta}_j^{(m)}, \hat{\delta}_j^{(m)})\}$ for $m = 1, 2, 3$ are relatively much closer to each other than with the MLE. For all simulated data sets, the value of the tilted log-likelihood (2) at the posterior mode is largest for prior (4) and smallest for prior (6).

Another summary in Table 8 is the closeness to the empirical $\lambda_{jk,L}$ and $\lambda_{jk,U}$ over the $\binom{d}{2}$ pairs:

$$\Delta_{M,m} = [d(d-1)/2]^{-1} \sum_{j<k} |a^{(m)}_{jk,M} - a^{empirical}_{jk,M}| \quad (9)$$

where $m \in \{0,1,2,3\}$ as above, and $M \in \{L,U,C\}$ for lower tail dependence, upper tail dependence, and central dependence, with dependence measures $a \in \{\widehat{\lambda}_{jk,L}, \widehat{\lambda}_{jk,U}, \widehat{\rho}_{jk,S}\}$, respectively.

**Table 8.** Values of average difference for values of (9) in 100 simulated data sets. Also, the fraction of times that the posterior mode from (2) improves on the MLE based on (9), and lower/upper quartiles of (9).

| $m$ | $M$ | avg $\Delta_{M,0} - \Delta_{M,m}$ | Fraction $\Delta_{M,m} < \Delta_{M,0}$ | Q1 $\Delta_{M,m}$ | Q3 $\Delta_{M,m}$ |
|---|---|---|---|---|---|
| 0 | L | | | 0.059 | 0.078 |
| 1 | L | 0.001 | 0.46 | 0.060 | 0.077 |
| 2 | L | 0.001 | 0.48 | 0.060 | 0.077 |
| 3 | L | 0.000 | 0.37 | 0.060 | 0.079 |
| 0 | U | | | 0.073 | 0.129 |
| 1 | U | 0.011 | 0.87 | 0.065 | 0.116 |
| 2 | U | 0.004 | 0.70 | 0.070 | 0.122 |
| 3 | U | 0.011 | 0.92 | 0.065 | 0.114 |

From Table 8, there is better matching with the tilted log-likelihood for upper tail dependence but no improvement for lower tail dependence. The Spearman values $\rho_{jk,S}$ are much closer for empirical versus model based parameters.

In the comparison of the simulation results to those for the stock return data in Section 5, the improvements in using (2) are less. This can be explained as follows. For finance stock return data with stocks from one sector, the 1-factor structure with lower and upper tail dependence is reasonable, and BB1r linking copulas can be considered good approximations, and there might also be weak conditional dependence of some stock returns conditioned on the latent variable. That is, the 1-factor BB1r copula model has some small degree of model misspecification, and this can explain why tilting to obtain model-based tail dependence parameters to match empirical counterparts should lead to better tail inference.

## 7. Discussion

A method has been proposed for improved tail inference when preliminary data and likelihood analysis suggest asymmetric tail dependence. The approach of the tilted log-likelihood introduces a prior distribution involving lower and upper tail dependence parameters. Incorporating the prior places more weight on the behavior of the joint lower and upper tails compared with the center of the probability space, thereby improving the extreme value inference. This can account for a small degree of model misspecification in the parametric model. The prior is chosen so that model-based lower and upper tail dependence parameters can be a closer match to empirical counterparts for a previous data set that has some similar features to the data set under consideration.

For simpler exposition, the theory is applied to a 1-factor copula model that can handle non-Gaussian dependence structures with asymmetric tail dependence. The tilted log-likelihood approach can be extended to other structured factor copula models (e.g., bi-factor and1-factor with weak residual dependence) with asymmetric tail dependence, where a super-population assumption is reasonable for how observed variables are linked to latent variables.

Also, the approach can be applied to vine copula models with bivariate tail dependence for all pairs of variables by choosing bivariate copulas with lower and upper tail dependence in tree 1 of the vine. From [5], lower and upper upper tail dependence in the first vine tree lead to this property for all pairs of variables. By including a prior based on pairs of variables with stronger dependence and asymmetric tail dependence, there could be a better match of vine copula model based tail dependence measures and empirical counterparts.

The skew-t copula (see [27]) can also be used for asymmetric tail dependence. However, the functional relation of copula parameters and tail dependence parameters is much more complicated than with the BB1 copula (latter in Appendix A.1) such that the tilted log-likelihood approach would be have to implemented with a different transform of the copula parameters.

Bayesian computing methods can be used if there are latent variables. Alternatively, a tilted log-likelihood similar to (2) can be optimized via (a) a quasi-Newton method if the total number of parameters is not large (say, fewer than 40), (b) a modified Newton–Raphson method if the analytical gradient and Hessian can be obtained, or (c) sequential estimation of parameters if possible (Section 5.5 of [9]). For methods (b) and (c), numerical optimization of the tilted log-likelihood is used to obtain the (approximate) posterior mode, and then the Hessian in this mode, in order to obtain interval estimates of the functions of parameters.

**Author Contributions:** Conceptualization, H.J.; methodology, H.J. and X.L.; software, H.J. and X.L.; writing—original draft preparation, H.J.; writing—review and editing, X.L. All authors have read and agreed to the published version of the manuscript.

**Funding:** This research has been supported by NSERC Discovery Grant GR010293 and an NSERC Postgraduate Scholarship.

**Data Availability Statement:** The data presented in this study are available on request from the corresponding author.

**Acknowledgments:** Thanks to the referees for their valuable comments and to the editors for their encouragement.

**Conflicts of Interest:** The authors declare no conflict of interest.

## Appendix A. Background Results on Copulas and Dependence Concepts

The appendix consists of subsections of known results in order to make this article more self-contained. Details of individual topics are in [9] if there are no additional references.

### *Appendix A.1. BB1 Copula Family and Tail Dependence Properties*

If $(U,V) \sim C$ for a bivariate copula $C$, the reflected copula $\widehat{C}(u,v)$ is the distribution of the reflection $(1-U,1-V)$. Simple probability calculations lead to:

$$\widehat{C}(u,v) = u+v-1+C(1-u,1-v), \quad 0 \le u,v \le 1.$$

The survival function of $C$ is related, it is defined as

$$\overline{C}(u,v) = \Pr(U>u, V>v) = 1-u-v+C(u,v), \quad 0 \le u,v \le 1, \tag{A1}$$

so that $\widehat{C}(u,v) = \overline{C}(1-u,1-v)$.

The bivariate 2-parameter BB1 copula family is useful to handle asymmetric lower and upper tail dependence. Asymmetric here refers to copulas where $C$ is different from $\widehat{C}$. For $\theta > 0, \delta > 1$,

$$C_{\mathrm{BB1}}(u,v;\theta,\delta) = \left\{1+\left[(u^{-\theta}-1)^{\delta}+(v^{-\theta}-1)^{\delta}\right]^{1/\delta}\right\}^{-1/\theta}, \quad 0 \le u,v \le 1. \tag{A2}$$

The reflected copula is: $C_{\mathrm{BB1r}}(u,v;\theta,\delta) = u+v-1+C_{\mathrm{BB1}}(1-u,1-v;\theta,\delta)$.

The BB1 copula and its reflection are the most useful for handling asymmetric tail dependence. Other choices for this property are BB7 and skew-t (see [27]). The BB1 family has the nice property that there is increasing concordance or positive dependence as $\theta$ and $\delta$ increase with independence as the lower bound of the parameter space is reached and comonotonicity (perfect dependence) as one of $\theta$ or $\delta$ goes to infinity. The BB7 copula does not have the concordance property over the entire parameter space.

Tail dependence parameters (as functions of copula family) are $\lambda_L(C_{\text{BB1}}) = 2^{-1/(\delta\theta)}$ and $\lambda_U(C_{\text{BB1}}) = 2 - 2^{1/\delta}$ as functions of $\theta$ and $\delta$. Then, $\lambda_U(C_{\text{BB1r}}) = \lambda_L(C_{\text{BB1}})$ and $\lambda_L(C_{\text{BB1r}}) = \lambda_U(C_{\text{BB1}})$ because the reflection reverses the joint upper and lower tails. The range of $(\lambda_L, \lambda_U)$ is $(0,1)^2$. To go from tail dependence parameters to copula parameters, the transforms are:

$$\begin{aligned}
&\delta = [\log 2]/\log(2-\lambda_U), \quad \theta = \log(2-\lambda_U)/(-\log\lambda_L) \quad \text{for BB1},\\
&\delta = [\log 2]/\log(2-\lambda_L), \quad \theta = \log(2-\lambda_L)/(-\log\lambda_U) \quad \text{for BB1r},\\
&\delta = [\log 2]/[-\log -\lambda_L), \quad \theta = [\log 2]/\log(2-\lambda_U) \quad \text{for BB7}.
\end{aligned}$$

For the data example in Section 5, the BB7 1-factor copula is fitted much worse, but it is included to show that the "prior" in (2) is independent of the tail-dependent family used for linking copulas to the latent variable.

*Appendix A.2. 1-Factor Copula Construction*

For the 1-factor copula model, it assumes conditional independence of $\boldsymbol{U} = (U_1, \ldots, U_d)$, given a latent variable $V \sim \mathcal{U}(0,1)$. Let $C_{jV}(\cdot, \boldsymbol{\vartheta}_j)$ (for $j = 1, \ldots, d$) be the bivariate copula cdf for the $j$th variable with the latent variable $V$. The $d$-variate copula cdf and density for $\boldsymbol{U} = (U_1, \ldots, U_d)$ are:

$$C_{\boldsymbol{U}}(\boldsymbol{u}; \boldsymbol{\vartheta}_1, \ldots, \boldsymbol{\vartheta}_d) = \int_0^1 \prod_{j=1}^d C_{j|V}(u_j|v; \boldsymbol{\vartheta}_j)\, dv, \tag{A3}$$

$$c_{\boldsymbol{U}}(\boldsymbol{u}; \boldsymbol{\vartheta}_1, \ldots, \boldsymbol{\vartheta}_d) = \int_0^1 \prod_{j=1}^d c_{jV}(u_j, v; \boldsymbol{\vartheta}_j)\, dv, \tag{A4}$$

where $C_{j|V}(u_j|v; \boldsymbol{\vartheta}_j) = \partial C_{jV}(u_j, v; \boldsymbol{\vartheta}_j)/\partial v$ is the conditional distribution of $[U_j|V = v]$ and $c_{jV}(u_j, v, \boldsymbol{\vartheta}_j) = \partial^2 C_{jV}(u_j, v; \boldsymbol{\vartheta}_j)/\partial v \partial u_j$ is the corresponding copula density. The $(j,k)$ bivariate margin is

$$C_{jk}(u_j, u_k) = \int_0^1 C_{j|V}(u_j|v; \boldsymbol{\vartheta}_j) C_{k|V}(u_k|v; \boldsymbol{\vartheta}_k)\, dv. \tag{A5}$$

The Spearman's rho for $(U_j, U_k)$ is Cor $(U_j, U_k)$. It is numerically best to compute it via a 2-dimensional numerical integral

$$12 \int_0^1 \int_0^1 C_{jk}(u_u, u_k)\, du_j\, du_k - 3$$

to avoid a possible unbounded copula density $c_{jk}$. For (A5), this becomes

$$12 \int_0^1 \left( \int_0^1 C_{j|V}(u_j|v)\, du_j \right) \left( \int_0^1 C_{j|V}(u_k|v)\, du_k \right) dv - 3 =: 12 \int_0^1 a_j(v)\, a_k(v)\, dv - 3;$$

This can be computed via a 1-dimensional Gauss–Legendre quadrature over $n_q$ quadrature points $v_1, \ldots, v_{n_q}$ for $v$, and $a_j(v)$ and $a_k(v)$ (with respect to $u_j$ and $u_k$) can be separately evaluated via the Gauss–Legendre quadrature for $v_1, \ldots, v_{n_q}$. See [23] for Gaussian quadrature theory.

Suppose $C_{jV}$ has lower and upper tail dependence for all $j$, such as with BB1 or reflected BB1 copulas. Define the survival function $\overline{C}_{jV}$ as in (A1). Then, from Section 2.18 of [9], there are functions $b_{jV}$ and $b^*_{jV}$ for lower and upper tails, respectively, such that for $w_j > 0$ and $w > 0$,

$$\begin{aligned} C_{jV}(uw_j, uw)/u &\rightarrow b_{jV}(w_j, w), \quad u \rightarrow 0^+, \\ \overline{C}_{jV}(1-uw_j, 1-uw)/u &\rightarrow b^*_{jV}(w_j, w), \quad u \rightarrow 0^+, \\ C_{j|V}(uw_j|uw) &\rightarrow b_{j|V}(w_j, w) = \partial b_{jV}(w_j, w)/\partial w, \quad u \rightarrow 0^+, \\ \overline{C}_{j|V}(1-uw_j|1-uw) &\rightarrow b^*_{j|V}(w_j, w) = \partial b^*_{jV}(w_j, w)/\partial w, \quad u \rightarrow 0^+. \end{aligned}$$

Lower and upper tail dependence parameters are defined in Section 2. The conditions of Theorem 8.76 of [9] are satisfied with BB1 copulas, and it implies for variable $j$ and $k$ ($j \neq k$) that the lower and upper table dependence parameters for $(U_j, U_k)$ are

$$\lambda_{jk,L} = \int_0^\infty b_{j|V}(1|z) b_{k|V}(1|z)\, \mathrm{d}z, \quad \lambda_{jk,U} = \int_0^\infty b^*_{j|V}(1|z) b^*_{k|V}(1|z)\, \mathrm{d}z. \tag{A6}$$

For BB1,

$$\begin{aligned} b_{jV}(w_j, w) &= (w_j^{-\delta\theta} + w^{-\delta\theta})^{-1/(\delta\theta)}, \\ b^*_{jV}(w_j, w) &= w_1 + w - (w_j^\delta + w^\delta)^{1/\delta}, \\ b_{j|V}(1|v) &= (1 + v^{\delta\theta})^{-1-1/(\delta\theta)}, \\ b^*_{j|V}(1|v) &= 1 - (1 + v^{-\delta})^{1/\delta - 1}. \end{aligned}$$

For reflected BB1, the lower and upper quantities are reversed, as the reflection just changes the upper (lower) quadrant to the lower (upper) quadrant.

Reflected BB1 and BB1 copulas usually fit better than the BB7 copula for stock return data with factor or vine copulas. From the concordance property of the BB1 copula, there is more lower and upper tail dependence as either of the two parameters increase.

*Appendix A.3. Normal Scores and Use for Diagnostics*

Let $y_1, \ldots, y_n$ be a sample of size $n$ for a variable $y$. The rank transform to the standard normal is

$$\hat{z}_i = \Phi^{-1}((\mathrm{rank}(y_i) - 0.5)/n),$$

where a larger $y$ value attains a larger rank (rank 1 for smallest and rank $n$ for largest (among the sorted values of $y_1, \ldots, y_n$). We refer to the $\{\hat{z}_i\}$ as the normal scores for $y$.

If there are $d$ variables and a sample $\{(y_{i1}, \ldots, y_{id}) : i = 1, \ldots, n\}$, then one can obtain vectors of normal scores $\{(\hat{z}_{i1}, \ldots, \hat{z}_{id}) : i = 1, \ldots, n\}$ with ranking performed separately for each variable. Pairs of variables have strong monotone dependence if the correlation of their normal score transforms is large. Figure 1 has examples of bivariate normal scores plots for pairs of GARCH-filtered returns. The plots are used to check for departures from elliptically shaped clouds of points, which are expected if the Gaussian copula fits well.

*Appendix A.4. GARCH Time Series*

A summary of the copula-GARCH models is as follows. Let $P_t$ ($t = 0, 1, \ldots, n$) be the price time series of a financial asset such as a market index or stock; the time index could be day, week, or month. The (log) return $R_t$ is defined as $\log(P_t/P_{t-1})$. For $d$ assets, denote the returns as $R_{t1}, \ldots, R_{td}$ at time $t$. For each financial return variable, a common choice is the GARCH(1,1) time series filter, with innovation distribution being the symmetric (or asymmetric) Student $t_\nu$ distribution with variance 1 and $\nu > 2$; see Section 4.3.6 of [28].

Let $F_j(\cdot, \nu_j)$ be the distribution of the innovation for the $j$th univariate marginal model:

$$R_{tj} = \mu_j + \sigma_{tj} Z_{tj}, \quad \sigma_{tj}^2 = \omega_j + \alpha_j R_{t-1,j}^2 + \beta_j \sigma_{t-1,j}^2, \quad j = 1, \ldots, d, \ t = 1, \ldots, n, \qquad \text{(A7)}$$

where for each $j$, $\omega_j > 0$, $\alpha_j > 0$, $\beta_j > 0$, the $Z_{tj}$ are assumed to be innovations over $t$, and the random $\sigma_{tj}^2$ depends on $R_{t-1,j}^2$ and $\sigma_{t-1,j}^2$. For stationarity, $\alpha_j + \beta_j < 1$ for all $j$. The vectors $(Z_{t1}, \ldots, Z_{td})$ for $t = 1, \ldots, n$ are assumed to be independent and identically distributed with distribution:

$$F_{\mathbf{Z}}(\mathbf{z}; \nu_1, \ldots, \nu_d, \boldsymbol{\vartheta}) = C\big(F_1(z_1; \nu_1), \ldots, F_d(z_d; \nu_d); \boldsymbol{\vartheta}\big),$$

where $\boldsymbol{\vartheta}$ is a dependence parameter of a $d$-dimensional copula $C$. Sometimes, an autoregressive coefficient $\phi_j$ is also added when $\mu_j$ in (A7) is replaced by $\mu_j + \phi_j R_{t-1,j}$. The flexible choice of the copula families includes vine and factor copula constructions.

## References


1. McNeil, A.J. Estimating the tails of loss severity distributions using extreme value theory. *ASTiN Bull.* **1997**, *27*, 117–137. [CrossRef]
2. Sun, M. Modeling cyber loss severity using a spliced regression distribution with mixture components. *Open J. Stat.* **2023**, *13*, 425–452. [CrossRef]
3. Falk, M.; Padoan, S.; Wisheckel, F. Generalized Pareto copulas: A key to multivariate extremes. *J. Multivar. Anal.* **2019**, *174*, 104538. [CrossRef]
4. Jondeau, E.; Rockinger, M. The copula-GARCH model of conditional dependencies: An international stock market application. *J. Int. Money Financ.* **2006**, *25*, 827–853. [CrossRef]
5. Joe, H.; Li, H.; Nikoloulopoulos, A.K. Tail dependence functions and vine copulas. *J. Multivar. Anal.* **2010**, *101*, 252–270. [CrossRef]
6. Krupskii, P.; Joe, H. Factor copula models for multivariate data. *J. Multivar. Anal.* **2013**, *120*, 85–101. [CrossRef]
7. Lee, D.; Joe, H.; Krupskii, P. Tail-weighted dependence measures with limit being the tail dependence coefficient. *J. Nonparametr. Stat.* **2018**, *30*, 262–290. [CrossRef]
8. Coblenz, M.; Dyckerhoff, R.; Grothe, O. Nonparametric estimation of multivariate quantiles. *Environmetrics* **2018**, *29*, e2488. [CrossRef]
9. Joe, H. *Dependence Modeling with Copulas*; Chapman & Hall/CRC: Boca Raton, FL, USA, 2014.
10. Fan, X. Dependence Modeling in High Dimensions with Latent Variables. Ph.D. Thesis, University of British Columbia, Vancouver, BC, Canada, 2024.
11. Johnson, R.A.; Wichern, D.W. *Applied Multivariate Statistical Analysis*, 5th ed.; Prentice Hall: Englewood Cliffs, NJ, USA, 2002.
12. Joe, H. Parsimonious graphical dependence models constructed from vines. *Can. J. Stat.* **2018**, *46*, 532–555. [CrossRef]
13. Ang, A.; Chen, J. Asymmetric correlations of equity portfolios. *J. Financ. Econ.* **2002**, *63*, 443–494. [CrossRef]
14. Longin, F.; Solnik, B. Extreme correlations in international equity markets. *J. Financ.* **2001**, *56*, 649–676. [CrossRef]
15. Nikoloulopoulos, A.K.; Joe, H.; Li, H. Vine copulas with asymmetric tail dependence and applications to financial return data. *Comput. Stat. Data Anal.* **2012**, *56*, 3659–3673. [CrossRef]
16. Li, X.; Joe, H. Multivariate directional tail-weighted dependence measures. *J. Multivar. Anal.* **2024**, *203*, 105319. [CrossRef]
17. Serfling, R.J. *Approximation Theorems of Mathematical Statistics*; Wiley: New York, NY, USA, 1980.
18. Liseo, B.; N, L. A note on reference priors for the scalar skew-normal distribution. *J. Stat. Plan. Inference* **2006**, *136*, 373–389. [CrossRef]
19. Azzalini, A.; Arellano-Valle, R.B. Maximum penalized likelihood estimation for skew-normal and skew-t distributions. *J. Stat. Plan. Inference* **2013**, *143*, 419–433. [CrossRef]
20. Loaiza-Maya, R.; Smith, M.S. Variational Bayes estimation of discrete-margined copula models with application to time series. *J. Comput. Graph. Stat.* **2019**, *28*, 523–539. [CrossRef]
21. Nguyen, H.; Ausin, M.C.; Galeano, P. Variational inference for high dimensional structured factor copulas. *Comput. Stat. Data Anal.* **2020**, *151*, 107012. [CrossRef]
22. Krupskii, P.; Joe, H. Structured factor copula models: Theory, inference and computation. *J. Multivar. Anal.* **2015**, *138*, 53–73. [CrossRef]
23. Stroud, A.; Secrest, D. *Gaussian Quadrature Formulas*; Prentice-Hall: Englewood Cliffs, NJ, USA, 1966.
24. Kreuzer, A.; Czado, C. Bayesian inference for a single factor copula stochastic volatility model using Hamiltonian Monte Carlo. *Econom. Stat.* **2021**, *19*, 130–150. [CrossRef]
25. Hoffman, M.D.; Gelman, A. The No-U-Turn sampler: Adaptively setting path lengths in Hamiltonian Monte Carlo. *J. Mach. Learn. Res.* **2014**, *15*, 1593–1623.

26. Stan Development Team. *Stan Modeling Language Users Guide and Reference Manual*, Version 2.30.1; 2023. Available online: https://mc-stan.org/users/citations/ (accessed on 10 June 2024).
27. Yoshiba, T. Maximum likelihood estimation of skew-t copulas with its applications to stock returns. *J. Stat. Comput. Simul.* **2018**, *88*, 2489–2506. [CrossRef]
28. Jondeau, E.; Poon, S.H.; Rockinger, M. *Financial Modeling under Non-Gaussian Distributions*; Springer: London, UK, 2007.

entropy

MDPI

Perspective

# Statistics as a Social Activity: Attitudes toward Amalgamating Evidence

**Andrew Gelman [1,2,*] and Keith O'Rourke [3,†]**

1 Department of Statistics Columbia University, New York, NY 10027, USA
2 Department of Political Science, Columbia University, New York, NY 10027, USA
3 O'Rourke Consulting, Ottawa, ON K1P 6K7, Canada
* Correspondence: gelman@stat.columbia.edu
† Keith O'Rourke is deceased.

**Abstract:** Amalgamation of evidence in statistics is conducted in several ways. Within a study, multiple observations are combined by averaging, or as factors in a likelihood or prediction algorithm. In multilevel modeling or Bayesian analysis, population or prior information is combined with data using the weighted averaging derived from probability modeling. In a scientific research project, inferences from data analysis are interpreted in light of mechanistic models and substantive theories. Within a scholarly or applied research community, data and conclusions from separate laboratories are amalgamated through a series of steps, including peer review, meta-analysis, review articles, and replication studies. These issues have been discussed for many years in the philosophy of science and statistics, gaining attention in recent decades first with the renewed popularity of Bayesian inference and then with concerns about the replication crisis in science. In this article, we review the amalgamation of statistical evidence from different perspectives, connecting the foundations of statistics to the social processes of validation, criticism, and consensus building.

**Keywords:** Bayesian inference; foundations of statistics

## 1. Aggregating Information in a Social Context

Weighing and amalgamating evidence is a central problem in the process of science, giving rise to much debate on what methods are appropriate as well as exactly where, when, and for what purposes they should be used. Within statistics, a central area of controversy is how to incorporate prior information in the context of objective and reproducible science. On the other hand, the weighing and amalgamating of evidence within a single isolated study (the multiple observations) in many default approaches in statistics is (surprisingly) often just automatic and implicit.

Vigorous debate on basic approaches in statistics likely comes as no surprise to statisticians and, increasingly, almost everyone else. Although there is much agreement on the mathematical definitions of terms and procedures in statistics (what they are) and on discerning if particular instances meet these standards (is it this?), the appropriate roles for these terms and procedures in facilitating scientific inquiry—their very purposes and what to make of them—seem beyond agreement for the foreseeable future. The tools are largely agreed upon, but their appropriate use, where, and for what purposes, are not at all. For instance, there is a fair amount of agreement on what probabilities are, but not on what they can be used for. Many frequentists ban any use of probability in representing (uncertain) knowledge of unknown parameters. On the other hand, while nearly all Bayesians utilize probabilities to represent knowledge (or lack of it), some would oppose any form of testing or empirical assessment of these. In the case of a single study, some statisticians would be concerned about the properties of procedures that can be discerned if the procedure would be repeatedly applied infinitely often under similar kinds of studies or even exactly the same study conditions. Others argue this is not even sensible.

Gillies [1,2] discussed a "pluralist" or "intersubjective" interpretation of probability, which is related to the concept of "institutional decision analysis", for which an important aspect of inference is that decisions be justifiable, which motivates clear linkages between measurement, modeling assumptions, inferences, and decision recommendations. Once we situate science and data analysis in a social context, these challenges become clear. In the present paper, we do not set up any agent-based models; rather, our goal is to provide a broader perspective on the problem of aggregation of evidence in statistics.

Going beyond a single isolated study, the system of scientific publication, criticism, and meta-analysis provides more general avenues for the amalgamation of evidence rather than just within a study, and here, individual statistical analyses can be understood as (first) steps in this larger process. Perhaps unsurprisingly in this larger process, disagreements abound as opinions vary on what contextual (extra-study) information can be incorporated, where, and how. Should previous studies be amalgamated in a combined analysis, used to build a judgment-informed prior, or merely used qualitatively to refine the analysis, helping the study to stand on its own as much as possible? In this article, we present a general perspective on statistics as primarily about conjecturing, assessing, and adopting idealized representations of reality, predominantly using probability-generating models for both parameters and data. This approach involves using an explicit prior probability distribution to represent available but rough scientific conjectures about what values the unknown parameters might have been set to, and a data-generating probability distribution to represent how the recorded data likely came about if the unknown parameters' values were set to specific possible values. This contrasts with another perspective on statistics, which views it primarily as a way to discern procedures with good properties that are uniform across a wide range of possible underlying realities and restricts their use, especially in science, to just those procedures. Our perspective is more conducive to information aggregation, as reality likely contains many commonalities that can be discerned and profitably utilized. We believe this approach can unify seemingly distinct statistical philosophies and also offer guidance in resolving the current replication crisis in science. When claims fail to replicate, the methods used likely did not reflect reality well, if at all.

## 2. Statistics as Amalgamation of Evidence

One of the frustrating—and fascinating—aspects of statistics, compared to many other modern sciences, is its profusion of seemingly incompatible philosophies. The Neyman–Pearson approach focuses on defining procedures for discriminating between hypotheses, targeting uniform type I errors for all null hypotheses and uniformly minimum type II errors for all alternatives. The Fisherian $p$-value, in contrast, evaluates the strength of evidence against a single null hypothesis without explicit reference to any alternative, targeting a uniform (0,1) distribution of $p$-values for all nulls. Another Fisherian approach, maximum likelihood, provides estimates within a parametric model (see [3–5]); meanwhile, Neyman–Pearson testing can be interpreted in Bayesian terms [6,7]. Bayesian inference can be viewed as a generalization of maximum likelihood but is anathema to many because of its assignment of probability distributions to parameters that are not the products of random processes. It targets probability distributions that represent the current understanding of the realities and uncertainties involved. Nonparametric approaches such as bootstrap and lasso have traditionally been shoehorned into the frameworks of hypothesis testing and interval estimation, but in recent years, the machine learning approach has focused not on those classical problems but rather on pure prediction. They aim to reduce the assumptions (used to represent the current understanding of the realities and uncertainties) involved and to enhance the identification of procedures with seemingly good properties. The decision on what information to combine is often dictated by probability models or inferential algorithms that are largely chosen by convention. This occurs for basic users who are taught to use $t$-tests for continuous data (group variances assumed to be common, to give a combined variance estimate with more degrees of freedom), $\chi^2$ tests for discrete data (various choices about common parameters when defining expectations to test consistency with), linear regression models (assuming all observations have common slopes given that the explanatory variables fit as well as a common standard deviation), Cox models for survival data (common proportional hazard function assumed so that it cancels out), etc., but even experienced statisticians often seem unclear about the choices made regarding which information to combine in their data analysis.

Even amid the diversity of statistical methods and philosophies, all these approaches involve the amalgamation of evidence. This is true from the simplest models of random sampling and independent identically distributed data; to slightly more complex models with hierarchical, time-series, and spatial structures; to multistage deep learning algorithms that combine thousands of predictors or features. Even something as basic as Fisherian $p$-values or likelihood-ratio testing can be seen as ways to use the accumulation of data—that is, the piling-up of evidence—to draw increasingly certain conclusions; the integration of likelihood, although considered Bayesian, can also be interpreted more generally [8].

Modern data science has moved away from a mathematical framework of hypothesis testing and model building, toward a computationally focused environment of prediction, external validation, and reproducibility [9]. From this perspective, we can think of evidence being combined not to evaluate theories but to form more effective predictions; however, probability modeling can still be useful in constructing procedures that combine information efficiently while pointing to potential areas of sensitivity where predictions of interest are strongly influenced by particular decisions regarding pooling, partial pooling, or exclusion of evidence.

It has been said that the most important aspect of a statistical method is not what it does with the data but rather what data it uses. From this perspective, the power of Bayesian, regularization, and machine learning methods lies in their ability to incorporate large amounts of data into analysis and decision-making.

At the same time, as datasets become larger and more diverse, there is an increasing need to model and adjust for differences between samples (that is, available data) and populations, and between treatments and control groups in causal analysis. Amalgamation of evidence is important but it is not trivial; it is not just a matter of throwing data into a blender. One must evaluate data quality to decide what to include. Or, more generally, one must weigh and adjust data in light of what is known about the quality and representativeness of measurements and in light of the consistency of different data sources with available research hypotheses. Implicitly, these procedures can be seen as derived from different probabilistic data-generating models and prior distributions, but in our discussion, we focus on the information included in data analysis, not the algorithms used to construct inferences or the models underlying these algorithms.

Some of the fiercest debates in statistical theory and practice involve the use of prior information. For example, the well-respected statistician David Cox wrote the following:

> "There are situations where it is very clear that whatever a scientist or statistician might do privately in looking at data when they present their information to the public or government department or whatever, they should absolutely not use prior information because the prior opinions on some of these prickly issues of public policy can often be highly contentious with different people with strong and very conflicting views." [10]

We expressed disagreement, pointing to a problem on "the politically controversial problem of reconstructing historical climate from tree rings":

> "We have a lot of prior information on the processes under which tree rings grow and how they are measured. I don't think anyone would want to just take raw numbers from core samples as a climate estimate! All the tools from Statistical Methods for Research Workers won't take you from tree rings to temperature estimates. You need some scientific knowledge and prior information on where these measurements came from." [11]

Cox had decades of applied experience and would surely have agreed that prior information, in the form of physical/biological models, is essential to making climate-related decisions based on tree rings, and we are sure he would also have agreed that such models involve inevitable subjective choices. Rather, we believe Cox was concerned about the way that Bayesian methods can be abused, what one might call the "moral hazard" involved in a statistical method, in which all modeling decisions are up for grabs. In addition, there is concern that, in most settings, including the tree-ring example, expressing prior information as probability distributions can lead, paradoxically, to a false sense of certainty. Hence, the preference of Cox and others for the inclusion of prior information in a more piecemeal, case-by-case manner. From this perspective, the smoothness and apparent all-encompassing nature of Bayesian inference is itself a hazard.

The paradox is that flexibility is required to combine evidence from diverse sources, but if that flexibility is abused, the ultimate conclusions of the analysis can be dictated by the analyst rather than by the data. Perhaps default methods for combining evidence from diverse sources will be too hazardous. This is a concern with Bayesian inference with overconfident priors and with classical inference when "p-hacking", "researcher degrees of freedom", and "the garden of forking paths" allow users to find statistical significance from virtually any dataset [12]. And there is also the choice of what statistical method to use, a decision that is typically not based on statistical evidence [13]. We offer no general solution here but we think it useful to formulate all statistical methods as data aggregators of one sort or another and to be open about the evidence used to form any particular statistical conclusion—and also the available evidence that, for one reason or another, has been "left on the table" and is not yet incorporated into our inferences.

Beyond this, when we move beyond simple textbook examples of experimentation and sampling, there is typically no default analysis available. There is no general way to decide how to choose, combine, and transform regression predictors or features in a predictive model, and many scientific problems inherently involve the integration of information from different sources, for example, medical research interpreting clinical trial data in the light of biological models; or climate modeling combining data from tree rings, historical temperature data, and physical modeling; or election forecasting combining information from state polls, national polls, and forecasts based on economic and political conditions.

## 3. Amalgamation of Evidence in the Scientific Process

Statistical modeling typically focuses on a particular set or stream of data, which leads to some inference or decision. But it can also be helpful to think more "sociologically" of an evolution-like mechanism involving thousands of research hypotheses, millions of scientists, and processes of publication, publicity, career rewards, and replication, which lead not just to specific conclusions but also to strands of research, subfields, and allocations of research effort, as C. S. Peirce might have put it [14], communal science that is (and remains) profitable. In particular, in the field of psychology, there has been much recent discussion on the replicability (or lack thereof) of published research claims, and similar concerns have been raised in medical research. As Peirce [15] wrote,

> "The theory here given rests on the supposition that the object of the investigation is the ascertainment of truth. When the investigation is made to attain personal distinction, the economics of the problem are entirely different. But that seems to be well enough understood by those engaged in that sort of investigation."

But the current de facto procedure, in which studies are summarized by statistically significant estimates, has technical problems of bias and inefficiency even if we assume all researchers are acting altruistically.

Considering the entire academic research enterprise—the processes of peer reviews, publications, replications, and meta-analyses—as a grand collective effort of information aggregation, we join a long string of concerns from Peirce through [16] in seeing major problems with incentives and structure, and where simple technical fixes such as weighting studies by appraised quality can be disastrous [17]. Smaldino and McElreath [18] offer a simplified but suggestive model of problems with the current system of incentives and publications. On the one hand, the diversity of research labs must represent a strength, a potential escape from the groupthink that is associated with central planning. But, from the statistical standpoint, much information is lost by dividing our data into small pieces and summarizing each by a $p$-value. This would be an inefficient procedure even if $p$-values were computed as described in the textbooks based on pre-specified tests, but problems of drastic overestimation of effect sizes (type M or "magnitude" errors) become even worse given the documented ability of researchers at all levels to attain statistical significance virtually at will. Systematic overestimation of effect sizes creates a vicious cycle in which new studies are incorrectly anticipated as having a high probability of being successful [19], leading to further data whose significance is overstated.

A cleaner approach would be to analyze larger datasets directly, not by post-processing published estimates and $p$-values but by modeling larger and more diverse sets of raw data. This gives direct access to more efficient statistical analyses and also more ability to check model assumptions. Fisher unfortunately may have undermined the appreciation of this with his claim:

> "It is usually convenient to tabulate its [the likelihood's] logarithm, since for independent bodies of data such as might be obtained by different investigators, the "combination of observations" requires only that the log-likelihoods be added." [20]

This is technically correct if the data-generating model (which defines the likelihood) is never questioned or assessed—but it should be. To do this adequately, one needs all the individual raw data from all studies. Here, we quickly add that the prior's logarithm need only be added to the likelihood's logarithm to start a Bayesian analysis. Like the data-generating model, the prior also needs to be questioned or assessed. Again, we see a statistical and societal advantage to explicit recognition that inference arises from amalgamation of evidence, and more openness to the sources of this evidence and possible biases.

To step back from data analysis to the scientific enterprise more generally, various specific reforms of science have been proposed, including post-publication reviews, pre-registered replications, and publication/career credits for data quality (rather than just for novelty and statistical significance). We find it helpful to follow Peirce and think of these as steps in a larger process, rather than just merely attempts to minimize false positives in isolated studies. This quote from Peirce might suffice: "I [Peirce] do not call the solitary studies of a single man a science. It is only when a group of men, more or less in intercommunication, are aiding and stimulating one another by their understanding of a particular group of studies as outsiders cannot understand them, that I call their life a science." We also include two longer passages:

> "Science is to mean for us a mode of life whose single animating purpose is to find out the real truth, which pursues this purpose by a well-considered method, founded on thorough acquaintance with such scientific results already ascertained by others as may be available, and which seeks cooperation in the hope that the truth may be found, if not by any of the actual inquirers, yet ultimately by those who come after them and who shall make use of their results." (also in [21])

> "But what I mean by a "science" (...) is the life devoted to the pursuit of truth according to the best known methods on the part of a group of men who understand one another's ideas and works as no outsider can. It is not what they have already found out which makes their business a science; it is that they are pursuing a branch of truth according, I will not say, to the best methods, but according to the best methods that are known at the time. I do not call the solitary studies of a single man a science. It is only when a group of men, more

or less in intercommunication, are aiding and stimulating one another by their understanding of a particular group of studies as outsiders cannot understand them, that I call their life a science. It is not necessary that they should all be at work upon the same problem, or that all should be fully acquainted with all that it is needful for another of them to know; but their studies must be so closely allied that any one of them could take up the problem of any other after some months of special preparation and that each should understand pretty minutely what it is that each one of the other's work consists in; so that any two of them meeting together shall be thoroughly conversant with each other's ideas and the language he talks and should feel each other to be brethren."

## 4. Connections to the Philosophy of Science and the History of Statistics as a Quest for Principled Amalgamation

Statistical science has evolved from the growing awareness, extraction, and assessment of commonness amid diversity. Not only can physical laws (or, as social scientists say, "law-like relationships") be uncovered from noisy data, in the manner of Gauss, Laplace, and their followers, such as Airy [22], variations can be categorized and thought of as forms of commonality. This was a key insight of Galton, Pearson, and other statisticians who in the late 19th century applied the concept of probability distribution to biological variation. We have argued that, in recent years, this insight has been oversold, now that researchers have the demonstrated ability to extract large, statistically significant, spurious, and unreplicable findings from just about any dataset; that said, from a historical point of view, the idea that variation can itself be quantified is central to any statistical understanding of modern social and biological sciences.

Here, we focus on methods of quantifying commonness among different empirical studies and their reported observations. Commonness refers to studies aimed at the same target (aspect of reality) as well as qualitatively similar evidence of that target, hopefully varying only in precision, which can be readily assessed. On the other hand, qualitatively different data sources can vary in their biases, which may be very difficult to assess and properly correct so that something is actually common. Terms from psychometrics that make the same distinctions as bias and precision do here would be validity and reliability.

Awareness of commonness can lead to an increase in evidence regarding the target; disregarding commonness wastes evidence; and mistaken acceptance of commonness destroys otherwise available evidence. It is the tension between these last two processes that drives many of the theoretical and practical controversies within statistics. A concrete but simple example that demonstrates practical controversies nicely would be the situation depicted in the Wiki entry on Simpson's paradox [23]. The illustration of the quantitative version: a positive trend appears for two separate groups (blue and red), whereas a negative trend (black, dashed) appears when the groups are combined.

The illustration clearly depicts an underlying reality of exactly the same positive trend for two groups (both slopes equal to 1) that happen to have different intercepts, one at about 5 and the other at −7. A default application of regression modeling using the eight data points displayed in the illustration would likely specify a single intercept, slope, and standard deviation parameter. The incorrect single intercept here is a mistaken acceptance of commonness, which destroys the evidence for common positive slopes by providing a single negative slope estimate of roughly −0.6, in addition to providing a single incorrect intercept estimate of about 9. Specifying the correct commonness here—that of separate intercepts but a single common slope and single standard deviation parameter—captures (all the evidence for) the correct intercept and slope with no actual error, with the correct estimates of the intercepts of 5 and −7, the slope of 1, and the single standard deviation of 0. With realistic data, there are observation errors and the specification of separate intercepts, but incorrectly separate slopes and a common standard deviation parameter can waste evidence, providing two different slope estimates randomly varying around 1, and a biased-downward estimate of the standard deviation. One might further ask or question why the assumption of a common standard deviation was being made. Simply convenience?

This simple contrived example from Wiki illustrates a lack of concern regarding the need to accurately represent reality (correctly specifying common and non-common parameters) as accurately as possible, or at least well enough for statistical procedures to provide reasonable answers. The usual training in statistics likely suggests the default use of a common intercept in multivariate regression analysis as well as the occasional need to consider interactions (with the statistical custom of always specifying separate intercepts for interaction terms—the lower-order terms). But here, without interaction, evidence is destroyed, while with interaction, it is wasted. The result is misleading descriptive or predictive inference in the former scenario and inefficient descriptive or predictive inference in the latter.

Better descriptive or predictive inferences come from better underlying representations of reality. For descriptive or predictive inference, reality, as it is now (and likely to persist), is the only reality that needs to be represented well enough. On the other hand, for causal or transportable inference, both current realities and how those can be changed (causal) or local and remote realities (to transport between) need to be well represented [24]. For instance, randomization creates two similar realities, one of which can presumably be modified in a hopefully simple manner (though maybe not as simple as an additive effect). Causal and transportable inference is, of course, much more challenging, but this complexity should not lead to disregarding the importance of representing a single current reality accurately for descriptive or predictive inference.

Statistical science historically emerged out of the conjecture, assessment, and reasoned acceptance of the commonness of observations made by different members of the community of astronomers. Among a set of apparently related observations, some combination was conjectured to be better than just enumerating the set, but a justification for how to weigh observations, whether repeatedly made by the same astronomer or by different astronomers, was completely lacking and desperately sought. Astronomers and others would often reflect on how to determine which dataset was the best (thus implicitly assigning weights of 0 to all the remaining data); anticipating that was the obvious solution, but they had yet to learn that, as Stigler [25] put it, "the details of individual observations had to be, in effect, erased to reveal a better indication than any single observation could on its own". In the modern world of social media, we similarly speak of the wisdom of crowds, an idea which is often illustrated using an example by Galton [26].

The problem of information aggregation has attracted the attention of the brightest minds of the time, including mathematicians and philosophers such as Laplace and Gauss. Its resolution came from recognizing a common object being measured by all and the reasonableness of a common error probability model for all—regardless of whether the observations were made by the same or different astronomers. This involved a model for both the common target of reality (the aspect of reality the observation was attempting to capture) and a common observational error that is the same for all. According to [27], it was the idea of "dealing with observations made by various other observers under different conditions—that actually 'spurred' on the development". The probabilistic error model, along with the willingness to use it on data from multiple sources, was the key technological insight needed. In gambling, probability models provided a means to determine the best bet regarding outcomes from games and devices that had common chance outcome mechanisms; in contrast, in astronomy, the error probability model representing common errors provided a means to determine the best combination for a target taken as common and, hence, the best weights for the combination of observations [28,29]. In much of statistical practice, probability models provide a formal mathematical basis for amalgamating and assessing commonness, which then sets out the best combinations for various purposes. For overviews and historical accounts; see [25,30,31]. More recently, machine learning methods have shifted to more algorithmic, less model-based approaches—not from any perceived defect with the probability models but rather for computational reasons when dealing with "big data"—but, again, the principle remains that data from different sources can and will be pooled in a single procedure (unless trivially based on single observations).

A repeated broadening of what was considered common can be briefly outlined here, starting with the initial recognition of a common object being measured and the reasonableness of a common error model that implied the weights for the best combination. The next step involves extending or revising this to still include a common object being measured but now with a differing error model, i.e., one that allows for a source of error that affects all observations taken on that day, yet represented as being drawn from a common distribution of error distributions (a recognition of commonness at a higher level). This extension/revision implies different weights for the best combination. Earlier, in a different context than astronomy (ratios of male to female births in different cities), the reasonableness of a common error model was kept but the object being measured itself was not taken as common; instead, it was conjectured/represented as being a draw from a common distribution of objects. That is, the objects being measured were allowed to vary but were aligned with being drawn from a shared probability distribution. At this point, the purposeful design (or induction of commonness) in the observations' underlying distributions emerges. An early instance was Peirce's recognition that random sampling and random assignment of treatments induce a common distribution for the sample and population, or treatment and control group. Nowadays, we might frame all these issues using multilevel models with variance at the observation level and, in the astronomy context, variance components for individual measurement methods, astronomers, and other factors that could induce systematic error.

In Bayesian inference, the prior density is just multiplied by the factors of the likelihood, quantifying the information coming from the data (conditional on the assumed class of models). The prior can then be seen mathematically as just one more data point. To make this absolutely clear, each observation defines a likelihood (the probabilities of observing that very observation for the various parameter values the parameters can take), and the study likelihood is a product of those single observation likelihoods (conditioned on other observations if observations are not independent). The posterior is proportional to the prior multiplied by the combined study likelihood. This multiplication can be rearranged and re-expressed in any way that does not change it. Taking logarithms, the log posterior is proportional to the sum of the log prior and all the individual log-likelihoods—a "weighted combination" with the "weights" determined by the functional form of the prior density and individual likelihoods. Some authors object to the prior being in this combination, using what could be seen as an apples and oranges argument, arguing that now what is being amalgamated is of a different nature. Reid and Cox [32] expressed concerns with "merg[ing] seamlessly what may be highly personal assessments with evidence from data possibly collected with great care", instead using prior information "largely or entirely qualitatively". We disagree and see this seemingly outright refusal to consider possible representations of commonness between prior and observations as simply "blocking inquiry" by disallowing a potentially profitable scientific representation of the unknown that may well be a "powerful aid to the formation of true and fruitful conceptions", to paraphrase Peirce. For the present paper, it is not necessary to resolve this disagreement but just to point out that it can viewed as a question of amalgamation of evidence rather than as a dispute of objectivity vs. subjectivity, which is how Bayesian/non-Bayesian debates are often framed; for further discussion on this topic, see Gelman and Hennig [33].

From our perspective, one can "interpret the parameter prior in a frequentist way, as formalizing a more or less idealized data generating process generating parameter values" [33]. One of the earliest to concretely express this view was Francis Galton, who constructed a physical machine to clearly demonstrate both parameter and observation generation. It involved a two-stage quincunx. The top level represents the generation or setting of the unknown parameter (the prior) and the second level is the generation of a single noisy observation of each observed object's value (the data-generating model or likelihood). By tracing back from a chosen value of noisy observations (the slot the pellet ended up in) and identifying all the various values of unknown parameters that had generated them, a crude sample from the posterior is identified and obtained. Though clunky and limited (just a single unknown parameter with a single observation from each), it fully demonstrates how Bayesian inference uses probability-generating models, both for parameter values and observations, to amalgamate commonness between observations and then those observations and the prior).

There are real risks of taking things as common, in a sense that—in reality—they are not, whether between the parameter-generating process and the data-generating process or among the data-generating process for different observations themselves. We use the phrase "conjecture, assessment, and reasoned acceptance of the commonness" to emphasize that. But similar scientific judgment is required in deciding how to combine measurements—the "likelihood" part of the model—and we do not see the risks of model errors as being qualitatively different when considering data-combination rules, such as when considering how to express prior information; see Evans [34] on this point.

Bayesian models "domesticate" uncertainty by turning it into (probabilistically represented) variation; in economic jargon, they convert Knightian uncertainty into quantifiable risk. Such procedures gain statistical efficiency at the cost of making mathematical assumptions about distributions and, more importantly, the independence of error terms (strong replication), thus inducing skepticism among many potential users; however, alternative approaches that seem to avoid such assumptions typically perform information aggregation in some other way, for example, by avoiding pooling across data sources but then averaging over time. In nearly any situation where a decision needs to be made, *some* choices need to be made regarding the pooling of data.

Comparing the technique of nearest neighbors to linear regression will help clarify what we mean by unavoidable choices being made for pooling. For simplicity, consider a single $x$ variable and its role in predicting a single $y$ variable. A linear regression model conjectures a single common intercept and common slope for predicting the expected value of $y$ from all values of $x$ as well as a common standard deviation parameter. The probability model for all observations is taken to be normal$(a + bx, \sigma)$ and all observations provide evidence for just three parameters. In contrast, nearest neighbor regression tries to avoid specifying any commonality of expected values of $y$ for differing values of $x$, instead allowing expected values to vary arbitrarily by neighborhood. The technique identifies these neighborhoods from the observations and takes averages only within neighborhoods (never across). It usually specifies the sizes of these neighborhoods. Taking the size of the neighborhoods as 2 requires that a single nearest neighbor is found for every observation and assumed to have the same expectation—referred to as $NN_1$. Nearest neighbors do not actually avoid specifying some commonness, however, as $NN_0$ is not taken as an acceptable procedure (having no neighbors, all observations must be taken as islands on their own). So, commonness of expectation between at least two observations is enforced. Then, to achieve better "good" properties, commonness is allowed over a larger number of observations depending on the dataset—referred to as $NN_k$. Additionally, a common variance is usually assumed between neighborhoods (a secondary feature). To derive combinations based on more than one observation, and to obtain variance estimates from more than a few isolated points in each neighborhood, you treat non-common points and non-common parameters "grudgingly" as common—simply to improve the properties for estimating what you can.

This alternative approach to statistics avoids relying on probability models, instead aiming for procedures that work well under weak assumptions; for example, instead of assuming a distribution is Gaussian, you would just want the procedure to work well under some conditions on the smoothness of the second derivative of the log density function. These approaches have also evolved in astronomy, with Legendre developing least squares regression without requiring the probability-generating models that Gauss had assumed and used to obtain the exact same technique.

Instead of requiring probability model assumptions, this approach requires a choice of good properties (why minimize squared error?) over a class of problems to be dealt with (where values of unknowns are constrained in some way, such as being linear in regression or proportional hazards in survival analysis). Probability models make representations that aim to capture certain aspects of reality that cannot be directly assessed but do allow for indirect evaluations of their adequacy. On the other hand, alternative approaches choose properties to be optimal for a given class of applications (e.g., applications having linear expectations or proportional hazards) with no direct justification for the goodness of the property nor guarantees of a particular application belonging to that class; that is, with no way to assess the goodness of the property or belonging within that appropriate class, without making some representation of reality to average or maximize over.

Given sufficient flexibility, data aggregation can always be seen as appropriate, but if the data to be combined are too different—and if there is no good model to bridge these differences—there will be little or no practical gain from pooling, and indeed, there can be a risk if analysts use inappropriately strong models that do not sufficiently account for variation among data sources.

With regard to exactly when observations have something in common amongst them so that aggregation can be applied to useful effect, there is always some judgment involving "replication (or exchangeability) on some level by the statistician" (Gelman and Hennig, 2017). For a replication to be a true replication and not a mere duplication, there must not be complete dependence, and for a replication to be strong, there must be as much independence as possible. Often data-analytic procedures are set up in terms of observations that can be taken as independent under reasonable assumptions. It is through these unit-of-analysis contributions that we wish to understand how to conjecture, extract, and assess commonness. In astronomy, the units of analysis were simply individual observations and they were understood as being independent.

An extreme case often arising in social science is when differing scales (for example, aggressiveness, anger, etc.) are used for assessing treatment effects in different randomized experiments. It can be challenging, especially given what is reported in such studies, to specify probability-generating models for these different outcomes that have common parameters. This points to the interplay between the design of experiments, data collection, and analysis, as expressed for example by Cox [35]. Cleaner data collection puts less of an analysis burden; conversely, the sorts of "big data" that arise from social media, etc., are messy and require more assumptions in order to make causal inferences and generalize from sample to population. This in turn increases computational requirements, both from the sample size and model complexity, and helps explain why much of the work of modern applied and theoretical statistics centers on algorithms and computing. Again, this is all happening within the context of information aggregation; see, for example, Li, Srivastava, and [36].

By aiming to accurately represent reality, and recognizing that an aspect of this reality being common is part of what validates commonness, we align ourselves with the broader philosophical community as defined by Peirce, Ramsay, and others. As we stated elsewhere [33], "Although there is no objective access to observer-independent reality, we acknowledge that there is an almost universal human experience of a reality perceived as located outside the observer and as not controllable by the observer. We see this reality as a target of science, which makes observed reality a main guiding light for science. We are therefore 'active scientific realists' in the sense of [37], who writes: 'I take reality as whatever is not subject to one's will, and knowledge as an ability to act without being frustrated by resistance from reality' and 'Active scientific realism implies that finding out the truth about objective reality is not the ultimate aim of science, but that science rather aims at supporting human actions'". We add here that we strive for more than just not being frustrated by resistance from reality; rather, we want our findings and claims that aim at truth to be "beliefs which succeed for reasons connected to the way things are" [38].

The classical view of statistics, briefly mentioned before, primarily about procedures to obtain estimates, tests, confidence intervals, etc. with certain good properties (often common properties for all possible unknowns), has limitations when moving beyond simple settings. We believe scientific research would be more effective if statistics was viewed instead as primarily about conjecturing, assessing, and adopting idealized representations of reality, predominantly using probability-generating models for both parameters and data that can make the most out of commonness, for example, using hierarchical models with group-level predictors so that unexplained group-level variance is low and more information can be pooled from different sources. It seems to be already widely supported for probability-generating models for data "[providing an] explicit description in the idealized form of the physical, biological, ... data generating process", which is essentially "to hypothesize a data generating mechanism that produces observations as if from some physical probabilistic mechanisms" [32]. We have argued that limiting probability-generating models just for data while banning them for parameters is too restrictive for much of science.

Our belief in the efficacy of information aggregation, using continuous parameters to determine the level of partial pooling, is supported by a belief that reality—though never directly accessible—is continuous, in which different experiments, treatments, and outcomes are connected somehow rather than distinct severed islands on their own. Differing considerations and purposes can then be brought to bear on what best combinations (estimates, summaries) follow. From a slightly different direction, Tibshirani [39] argues that enforcing sparsity is not primarily motivated by beliefs about the world, but rather by benefits such as computability and interpretability, indicating how considerations other than correspondence to reality often play an important role in statistics and, more generally, in science. Tibshirani's view fits squarely within the alternative "classical" or non-Bayesian approach, in which techniques are chosen based on various robust operational properties rather than being viewed as approximations of reality. With this in mind, when we indicate that we consider generating models as an idealization, we need to point out that they could be, in fact, just 'fictions'—useful 'fictions' if they lead to an ability to act without being frustrated by resistance from reality. Sometimes, fiction does turn out to be connected with how things truly are. But, if their connections are accidental, with anything more than just in the short term, we suspect that they will not be as profitable for scientific practice, as, by definition, science (continuously) tries to represent reality accurately, or at least less wrong.

## 5. Conclusions

The foundations of statistics remain controversial, even among its leading practitioners, unlike fields such as biology, chemistry, or physics, which no longer experience such foundational disputes. In many ways, statistics looks more like social sciences, such as sociology, economics, and political science, which are riven by deep ideological divisions, but with the difference that statistics is a field of mathematics and computing in which ideology does not seem to play any obvious role. However, mathematics and computing just define and implement the tools (where there is much agreement), the purposes for which these tools should be used, and the interpretations of the results they produce in specific applications, extending beyond just mathematics and computing (and here, there is little agreement).

Whatever the historical sources and ultimate resolutions of the debates within the field of statistics, we see the combination of evidence as central to *any* statistical method, and we view methods as stronger to the extent that they can incorporate diverse sources of information, weighting, or adjusting appropriately to account for inevitable problems of data quality and representativeness.

Furthermore, we view statistical concepts of data integration, along with the quantification of uncertainty and variation, as central to understanding and reforming the currently broken system of scientific publication and promotion.

Finally, all these concerns relate to a longstanding skeptical tradition in the philosophy of science. Ironically, various modern abuses of statistics, such as the pursuit of statistical significance or, more generally, the deterministic thinking that leads researchers to establish certitude beyond the capabilities of their data, arise from skeptical ideas in statistics, such as

Fisher's warnings about over-interpreting chance variation or the Neyman–Pearson–Wald rigorizing of certain stylized statistical decision problems.

When amalgamating evidence, we typically are at least one step beyond the available theory—it only *feels* like amalgamation if it cannot be done automatically—but we should not let this stop us from trying. It is through recognizing, formalizing, and modeling our attempts at combining information—and by recording and learning from our failures—that we will do better.

**Funding:** This research received no external funding.

**Acknowledgments:** We thank three reviewers for helpful comments and the Office of Naval Research for grant N00014-15-1-2541.

**Conflicts of Interest:** Author Keith O'Rourke was employed by the company O'Rourke Consulting. The remaining author declares that the research was conducted in the absence of any commercial or financial relationships that could be construed as a potential conflict of interest.

## References

1. Gillies, D. Intersubjective probability and confirmation theory. *Br. J. Philos. Sci.* **1991**, *42*, 513–533. [CrossRef]
2. Gillies, D. *Philosophical Theories of Probability*; Routledge: London, UK, 2000.
3. Cox, D.R. Some remarks on likelihood factorization. In *Lecture Notes—Monograph Series*; Institute of Mathematical Statistics: Beachwood, OH, USA, 2001; pp. 165–172.
4. Fraser, D.F. *Probability and Statistics: Theory and Applications*; Duxbury Press: North Scituate, MA, USA, 1976.
5. Meng, X.L. Decoding the h-likelihood. *Stat. Sci.* **2009**, *24*, 280–293. [CrossRef]
6. Li, F.; Mealli, F. A conversation with Donald B. Rubin. *Stat. Sci.* **2014**, *29*, 439–457. [CrossRef]
7. Rubin, D.B. Bayes, Neyman, and calibration. Discussion of Berk, Western, and Weiss. *Sociol. Methodol.* **1995**, *25*, 473–479. [CrossRef]
8. Berger, J.O.; Liseo, B.; Wolpert, R.L. Integrated likelihood methods for eliminating nuisance parameters. *Stat. Sci.* **1999**, *14*, 1–28. [CrossRef]
9. Donoho, D. Data science at the singularity (with discussion). *Harvard Data Sci. Rev.* **2024**, *6*, 1–51. [CrossRef]
10. Cox, D.; Mayo, D. A statistical scientist meets a philosopher of science. *Ration. Mark. Morals* **2011**, *2*, 103–114.
11. Gelman, A. Ethics and the statistical use of prior information. *Chance* **2012**, *25*, 52–54. [CrossRef]
12. Simmons, J.; Nelson, L.; Simonsohn, U. False-positive psychology: Undisclosed flexibility in data collection and analysis allow presenting anything as significant. *Psychol. Sci.* **2011**, *22*, 1359–1366.
13. Gelman, A.; O'Rourke, K. Convincing evidence. In *Roles, Trust, and Reputation in Social Media Knowledge Markets*; Matei, S., Bertino, E., Eds.; Springer: Berlin/Heidelberg, Germany, 2015.
14. Wible, J.R. Charles Sanders Peirce's economy of research. *J. Econ. Methodol.* **1994**, *1*, 135–160.
15. Peirce, C.S. Note on the theory of the economy of research. *Coast Surv. Rep.* **1879**, *1876*, 197–201. [CrossRef]
16. Ioannidis, J.P.A. Evidence-based medicine has been hijacked: A report to David Sackett. *J. Clin. Epidemiol.* **2016**, *73*, 82–86. [CrossRef]
17. Greenland, S.; O'Rourke, K. On the bias produced by quality scores in meta-analysis, and a hierarchical view of proposed solutions. *Biostatistics* **2001**, *2*, 463–471. [CrossRef]
18. Smaldino, P.; McElreath, R. The natural selection of bad science. *R. Soc. Open Sci.* **2016**, *3*, 160384. [CrossRef]
19. Button, K.S.; Ioannidis, J.P.A.; Mokrysz, C.; Nosek, B.A.; Flint, J.; Robinson, E.S.J.; Munafo, M.R. Power failure: Why small sample size undermines the reliability of neuroscience. *Nat. Rev. Neurosci.* **2013**, *14*, 365–376. [CrossRef]
20. Fisher, R.A. *Statistical Methods and Scientific Inference*; Hafner: New York, NY, USA, 1956.
21. Peirce, C.S. The Charles S. Peirce Papers. *32 Microfilm Reels of the Manuscripts Kept in the Houghton Library*; Photographic Service 1966; Harvard University Library: Cambridge, UK, 1902.
22. Airy, G.B. *On the Algebraical and Numerical Theory of Errors of Observations and the Combination of Observations*; Macmillan: New York, NY, USA, 1861.
23. Schutz. Simpson's Paradox Continuous. 2017. Available online: https://en.wikipedia.org/wiki/Simpson's_paradox (accessed on 30 June 2024).
24. Pearl, J.; Bareinboim, E. External validity: From do-calculus to transportability across populations. *Stat. Sci.* **2014**, *29*, 579–595. [CrossRef]
25. Stigler, S.M. *The History of Statistics: The Measurement of Uncertainty before 1900*; Harvard University Press: Cambridge, MA, USA, 1986.
26. Galton, F. Vox populi. *Nature* **1907**, *75*, 450–451. [CrossRef]
27. Stigler, S.M.*The Seven Pillars of Statistical Wisdom*; Harvard University Press: Cambridge, MA, USA, 2016.
28. Keynes, J.M. The principal averages and the laws of error which lead to them. *J. R. Stat. Soc.* **1911**, *74*, 322–331. [CrossRef]

29. O'Rourke, K. Meta-analytical themes in the history of statistics: 1700 to 1938. *Pak. J. Stat.* **2002**, *18*, 285–300.
30. Cox, D.R. Combination of data. In *Encyclopedia of Statistical Science*; Kotz, S., Johnson, N.L., Eds.; Wiley: Hoboken, NJ, USA, 1982.
31. Hald, A. *A History of Mathematical Statistics from 1750 to 1930*; Wiley: Hoboken, NJ, USA, 1998.
32. Reid, N.; Cox, D.R. On some principles of statistical inference. *Int. Stat. Rev.* **2015**, *83*, 293–308. [CrossRef]
33. Gelman, A.; Hennig, C. Beyond subjective and objective in statistics (with discussion and rejoinder). *J. R. Stat. Soc. A* **2017**, *180*, 967–1033. [CrossRef]
34. Evans, M. Measuring statistical evidence using relative belief. *Comput. Struct. Biotechnol. J.* **2016**, *14*, 91–96. [CrossRef]
35. Cox, D.R. The design of empirical studies: Toward a unified view. *Eur. J. Epidemiol.* **2016**, *31*, 217–228. [CrossRef]
36. Li, C.; Srivastava, S.; Dunson, D.B. Simple, scalable and accurate posterior interval estimation. *Biometrika* **2017**, *104*, 665–680. [CrossRef]
37. Chang, H. *Is Water $H_2O$?: Evidence, Realism and Pluralism*; Springer: Berlin/Heidelberg, Germany, 2012.
38. Misak, C. *Cambridge Pragmatism: From Peirce and James to Ramsey and Wittgenstein*; Oxford University Press: Oxford, UK, 2016.
39. Tibshirani, R.J. In praise of sparsity and convexity. In *Past, Present, and Future of Statistical Science*; Lin, X., Genest, C., Banks, D.L., Molenberghs, G., Scott, D.W., Wang, J.L., Eds.; CRC Press: Boca Raton, FL, USA, 2014; pp. 497–505.

*entropy*

MDPI

*Article*

# Bayesian Modeling for Nonstationary Spatial Point Process via Spatial Deformations

**Dani Gamerman [1,*,†,‡], Marcel de Souza Borges Quintana [1,2,‡] and Mariane Branco Alves [1,‡]**

1 DME-Instituto de Matemática, Universidade Federal do Rio de Janeiro, Rio de Janeiro 21941-909, RJ, Brazil; marcel@dme.ufrj.br (M.d.S.B.Q.); mariane@im.ufrj.br (M.B.A.)

2 Instituto Nacional de Infectologia Evandro Chagas-FIOCRUZ, Rio de Janeiro 21040-360, RJ, Brazil

* Correspondence: dani@im.ufrj.br

† Current address: Departamento de Metodos Estatisticos (DME), Instituto de Matematica, Universidade Federal do Rio de Janeiro, Av. Athos da Silveira Ramos 149, Centro Tecnologico, P.O. Box 68530, Rio de Janeiro 21941-909, RJ, Brazil.

‡ These authors contributed equally to this work.

**Abstract:** Many techniques have been proposed to model space-varying observation processes with a nonstationary spatial covariance structure and/or anisotropy, usually on a geostatistical framework. Nevertheless, there is an increasing interest in point process applications, and methodologies that take nonstationarity into account are welcomed. In this sense, this work proposes an extension of a class of spatial Cox process using spatial deformation. The proposed method enables the deformation behavior to be data-driven, through a multivariate latent Gaussian process. Inference leads to intractable posterior distributions that are approximated via MCMC. The convergence of algorithms based on the Metropolis–Hastings steps proved to be slow, and the computational efficiency of the Bayesian updating scheme was improved by adopting Hamiltonian Monte Carlo (HMC) methods. Our proposal was also compared against an alternative anisotropic formulation. Studies based on synthetic data provided empirical evidence of the benefit brought by the adoption of nonstationarity through our anisotropic structure. A real data application was conducted on the spatial spread of the *Spodoptera frugiperda* pest in a corn-producing agricultural area in southern Brazil. Once again, the proposed method demonstrated its benefit over alternatives.

**Keywords:** spatial deformation; point process; Cox process; Gaussian process; Bayesian inference; MCMC; HMC

## 1. Introduction

A spatial point process is a stochastic process that governs the location of events in a geographic space (Diggle [1]). A point pattern is a collection of locations in a given area and is interpreted as the realization of a point process (Illian et al. [2]). This type of pattern can be analyzed when georeferenced data are available and the exact locations of the events of interest are known; for example, the geographic coordinates of trees infected by a particular pest or the location of occurrences of a disease. Unlike the applications in geostatistics, in which the locations are fixed and the interest lies on the measurement of some random response, the very location of the occurrences is the random object in point processes. In the early literature on spatial point processes, it was common to assume that patterns were realizations of stationary and isotropic point processes, which implies that the statistical properties of the point process are invariant under spatial translations and rotations. However, these assumptions are often unrealistic, since in many cases there may be local or directional influences in the correlation structure of the spatial random process.

Several authors have explored nonstationarity and anisotropy in point processes. Häbel et al. [3] introduced anisotropic pair-potential functions based on Ripley's $K$-function. Gabriel [4] proposed a similar extension in a spatiotemporal context. Hahn and Vedel Jensen [5]

unified nonstationary model classes under a framework of hidden second-order stationary processes. Konstantinou and Särkkä [6] extended Ripley's $K$-function to three dimensions using a pairwise interaction Markov field model to accommodate anisotropic data. Rajala et al. [7] devised a two-stage non-parametric method for quantifying geometric anisotropy. Sormani et al. [8] formulated a comprehensive framework for addressing geometric anisotropy, including directional versions of Ripley's $K$-function, wavelet transforms, and spectral analysis, along with a method based on projecting Fry points onto the unit sphere. Martin et al. [9] introduced a new family of geometric anisotropic random fields and derived anisotropic point processes from them. Kwon et al. [10] utilized Hawkes process models, a class of self-exciting point process capturing event-triggering effects, to analyze earthquake occurrences. Dong et al. [11] devised another non-stationary spatiotemporal self-exciting point process, incorporating a neural network-based kernel to capture spatially varying triggering effects. Biard and Saussereau [12] applied a fractional Poisson process to situations where variances increase over time according to a defined power law. Roveri et al. [13] introduced a method to analyze and synthesize point patterns with adaptive density and correlations using a locally stationary point process. Most of these methodologies have the advantage of not requiring specific model assumptions. However, they have the disadvantage of not indicating what the intensity function would be if inherent anisotropy were taken into account, and they do not allow for an evaluation of the influence of covariates.

In geostatistics, various methods address nonstationarity/anisotropy in spatial modeling, such as process convolution models (Higdon et al. [14], Risser and Calder [15]), kernel/smoothing methods (Fuentes [16]), and basis functions (Pintore and Holmes [17], Stephenson et al. [18]). Spatial deformation allows the data to control the behavior of the fitted process without specifying mechanisms. Sampson and Guttorp [19] proposed a non-parametric method for estimating spatial covariance globally using a deformation technique. It maps coordinates from the geographical $G$-space to the deformed $D$-space (where stationarity holds), locating monitoring stations with multidimensional scaling and interpolating via thin plate splines. The inclusion of a non-linear deformation in the correlation function necessarily implies the loss of stationarity of the process and allows for anisotropic formulation, encompassing a wider range of models for dependence between locations. Challenges include multiple mappings in $D$-space and non-bijective predictions. Schmidt and O'Hagan [20] introduced a bi-dimensional Gaussian process to handle uncertainty in spatial deformation estimation.

This paper aims to apply spatial deformation to spatial point processes in order to handle anisotropy and nonstationarity. Challenges arise when adapting deformation to point processes based on Cox processes (see, for example, Diggle [1]), such as the problem of dealing with infinite dimensionality and the intractability of likelihood functions for non-homogeneous Poisson processes. Discretizing the $G$-space to address this issue is a common approach, involving forming partitions with constant intensities and using the centroids as representative points of each partition fraction (Moller et al. [21]; Brix and Diggle [22]; Paez and Diggle [23]). The discretization procedure also impacts the use of the deformation process (DP), which inherently operates in continuous space but is well-defined in finite dimensions in discretized space.

The Log–Gaussian Cox process is a standard model in point process analysis where the logarithmic function links an intensity function to a Gaussian process (GP). Adams et al. [24] used a logistic link for isotropic scenarios, and Gonçalves and Gamerman [25] applied a probit link for efficient sampling. Both bounded link functions require an extra parameter to account for the maximal intensity. An evaluation of the effect of different link functions on the intensity function estimation in anisotropic/nonstationary situations is also carried out in this paper.

This study presents an extended spatial Cox process for point process analysis for estimating intensity function with consideration for anisotropy and nonstationarity through spatial deformation. The novelty lies in using deformations to handle anisotropy in spatial point processes. The research employs the geometry-aware Hamiltonian Monte Carlo (HMC) method for sampling and evaluates different link functions across various scenarios. The methodology allows for data-driven guidance for estimating spatial anisotropy/non-stationarity behavior. It incorporates a multi-dimensional Gaussian process as a prior specification for the DP, adopting a fully Bayesian approach that assigns a probability distribution to spatial deformation as a latent process and quantifying estimation uncertainty. The method resolves the non-identifiability of the deformation, and notably, the proposed model can also accommodate intensity regressors.

The presentation of the paper is organized as follows: Section 2 describes the proposed Cox process, considering the spatial deformation through the multi-dimensional Gaussian process. Section 3 presents an analysis of the performance of the proposed model and estimation method, considering both synthetic and real data. Section 3.1 presents the results of simulation exercises for the comparison of the proposed anisotropic formulation to an isotropic one. Section 3.2 shows the estimation through the proposed anisotropic model compared to an isotropic formulation for the *Spodoptera fruguperda* pest data in an agricultural area of corn production in the city of Cascavel, Brazil. Section 3.3 provides favourable comparative results of our formulation against an alternative anisotropic specification. Section 4 discusses the results and indicates current and future extensions of this work.

## 2. Methodology

As previously mentioned, the well-established deformation technique involves mapping geographic coordinates from the original space ($G$-space) to a new latent space ($D$-space), ensuring stationarity and isotropy. This work employs an approach similar to previous studies, such as Schmidt and O'Hagan [20] and Morales et al. [26], where the random function $d : G \rightarrow D$ transforms original coordinates from $G$-space to the new $D$-space, following a prior $l$-variate Gaussian process

$$d \mid \sigma_d^2, \phi \sim \mathrm{GP}(h, \sigma_d^2, \rho_\phi), \tag{1}$$

where $h$ is a prior mean function, $\sigma_d^2$ is a $l \times l$ covariance matrix and $\phi$ is the vector of parameters for any valid correlation function

$$Corr(d(s_i), d(s_j)) = \rho_\phi(\|s_i - s_j\|),\ \forall s_i \text{ and } s_j \in G. \tag{2}$$

The covariance structure of the GP is essential for representing the behavior of the function $d$. It controls the prior warping degree of the mapping. Details on the specification of GP hyperparameters will be discussed later in the text.

The hierarchical structure for the proposed extension for the Cox process is given by

$$Y \mid \lambda \sim \mathrm{PP}(\lambda) \tag{3}$$
$$\lambda(s) = \lambda^* g(\mu + \beta(s)),\ \forall s \in G \tag{4}$$
$$\beta \mid \delta, \theta, d \sim \mathrm{GP}(0, 1/\delta, \rho_\theta) \tag{5}$$
$$d \mid \sigma_d^2, \phi \sim \mathrm{GP}(h, \sigma_d^2, \rho_\phi), \tag{6}$$

where PP indicates a Poisson process with intensity function $\lambda$, $g^{-1}(\cdot)$ is an appropriate link function, $\lambda^* = \sup_{s \in G} \lambda(s)$ (if the supremum exists (for $g(\cdot)$ functions bounded to $[0,1]$, for example *probit* or *logit* link functions, it is necessary to estimate $\lambda^*$ because the intensity function can take values greater than 1. For upper unbounded $g(\cdot)$ functions such as the exponential, $\sup_{s \in G} \lambda(s) = \infty$ and we can fix $\lambda^* = 1$.)); $\mu$ is an intercept, $\beta$ is a GP with mean 0, the precision is $\delta$ and the vector of parameters is $\theta$ for any valid correlation function

$$Corr(\beta(s_i), \beta(s_j)) = \rho_\theta(\|d(s_i) - d(s_j)\|), \tag{7}$$

where $s_i$ and $s_j$ are any points, again, in $G$.

In this study, we will analyze the *probit* ($\Phi^{-1}(\cdot)$) and logarithmic link functions. The bounded range of the cumulative standard normal function $\Phi(\cdot)$ to $[0,1]$ requires estimating $\lambda^*$, whereas for the unbounded exponential function (logarithmic link), $\lambda^* = 1$ and its estimation is not required.

The prior mean for $d$ is assumed as the identity function ($h(s) = s$) to express prior indifference on how $D$ differs from $G$. The diagonal matrix $\boldsymbol{\sigma}_d^2 = \text{diag}(\sigma^2_{d_{11}}, \ldots, \sigma^2_{d_{ll}})$ indicates deformation variability across dimensions. For example, when $G$ denotes geographical coordinates ($k = 2$) and $D$ has the same dimension ($l = 2$), higher/lower $\sigma^2_{d_{ii}}$ values allow more/less deformation along the horizontal axis ($i = 1$) or vertical axis ($i = 2$). Additionally, increased correlation range in (2) implies smoother deformation among nearby regions. While both $\beta$ and $d$ are Gaussian processes, from now on we use "GP" for $\beta$ and "deformation process (DP)" for $d$, in order to clarify which process we are referring to.

The likelihood function of the PP in (3) is given by the Janossy density (see, for example, D. J. Daley [27], p. 122) and is expressed as

$$L(\beta, \mu, \lambda^*; N = n, \{s_i\}_{i=1}^n) \propto \prod_{i=1}^{n} \lambda^* g(\mu + \beta(s_i)) \exp\left\{ - \int_G \lambda^* g(\mu + \beta(s)) \mathrm{d}\nu(s) \right\}, \tag{8}$$

with respect to a PP dominating measure with a constant intensity function, the integral corresponds to a Lebesgue integral. As previously mentioned, the likelihood function in expression (8) depends on infinite-dimensional quantities like $\beta$ and $d$, which is a problem for making inferences mainly concerning the integral on all $G$-space.

When estimating model hyperparameters, fixing some or using informative priors might be necessary due to hierarchical complexity. The phenomenon being examined requires a complex, highly-structured hierarchical model, needing meticulous attention to fully comprehend and accurately elicit all its components. For $\boldsymbol{\sigma}_d^2$ and $\phi$, a balanced deformation degree is sought to avoid folding or a loss of anisotropy. It is well known that $\Phi(s) \approx 0$ for any $s < -3$ and $\Phi(s) \approx 1$ for any $s > -3$. Therefore, a reasonable strategy when using the *probit* link function is to set $\mu = 0$ and $\delta = 0.5$ to favor parameter identification in Equation (4). A Gamma prior is assigned to $\lambda^*$, possibly centered on some empirically-set intensity or with a non-informative specification. Under the *log* link, vague improper uniform prior for $\mu$ and non-informative Gamma prior for $\delta$ are used.

For the GP $\beta$, for the sake of simplicity, we adopted the exponential correlation function $\rho_\theta(\|d(s_i) - d(s_j)\|) = \exp(-(\|d(s_i) - d(s_j)\|)/\theta)$. $\theta$ follows a Gamma($a_\theta$, $b_\theta$) prior, centered on a value that produces low correlation only for higher distances in the geographic region. Defining the density of $(d, \theta, \lambda^*, \mu, \delta, \beta, N = n, \{s_i\}_{i=1}^n | G, \boldsymbol{\sigma}_d^2, \phi)$ as the Radon–Nikodym derivative of $\mathbb{P}$ with respect to a suitable dominating measure $\mathbb{W}$ we have

$$\begin{aligned} \pi(d, \theta, \lambda^*, \mu, \delta, \beta, N = n, \{s_i\}_{i=1}^n | G, \boldsymbol{\sigma}_d^2, \phi) = \pi_{GP_2}(d | \boldsymbol{\sigma}_d^2, \phi) \pi(\theta) \pi(\lambda^*) \times \\ \pi(\mu) \pi(\delta) \pi_{GP}(\beta | \delta, \theta, d) \times L(\beta, \lambda^*, \mu; N = n, \{s_i\}_{i=1}^n) \end{aligned} \tag{9}$$

with $\pi(\theta)$, $\pi(\lambda^*)$, $\pi(\mu)$, $\pi(\delta)$ denoting the prior densities described above, $\pi_{GP}(\beta|...)$ and $\pi_{GP_2}(d|...)$ as described in expressions (4) and (6), and $L(\beta, \lambda^*, \mu; N = n, \{s_i\}_{i=1}^n)$ as in expression (8). The joint posterior distribution is proportional to (9).

A usual approach to dealing with infinite-dimensional quantities $\beta$ and $d$ in this likelihood is to discretize the space of interest. By discretizing the geographical space into a partition $\cup_{z=1}^{Z} G_z = G$ where $G_k \cap G_{k'} = \emptyset$ for every $k \neq k'$, it is possible to define piece-wise constant intensities and assume that for each sub-region $G_z$ the centroid $s_z$ is a representative point. The greater the number of occurrences, the more refined the discretization could be in effectively disseminating information, leading to more accurate estimates to more adequately characterize the intensity function. Defining $\beta(s) := \beta(s_z)\ \forall s \in G_z, z = 1, ..., Z$, the integral in (8) can be rewritten as

$$\sum_{z=1}^{Z} \lambda^* g(\mu + \beta(s_z)) \nu(G_z)$$

where $\nu(G_z)$ is the Lebesgue measure (for $k = 2$, for example, it represents the area) of the $z$-th region; now it is possible to perform inferences for the discretized space.

Defining $y := [y_1, \ldots, y_Z]$ for $y_z$ the total count of events in $G_z$, $z = 1, \ldots, Z$, the posterior density for the model with space discretization based on expression (9) is given by

$$\begin{aligned}\pi(\boldsymbol{d_Z}, \theta, \lambda^*, \mu, \delta, \beta_Z, |G, y, \sigma_d^2, \phi) \propto \pi_{MVN}(\boldsymbol{d_Z}|\sigma_d^2, \phi)\pi(\theta)p(\lambda^*)\times \\ \pi(\mu)\pi(\delta)\pi_{MN}(\beta_Z|\delta, \theta, \boldsymbol{d_Z}) \times L(\beta_Z, \lambda^*, \mu; y)\end{aligned} \tag{10}$$

where $\beta_Z := [\beta(s_1), \ldots, \beta(s_Z)]_{Z\times 1}$, $\boldsymbol{d_Z} := \begin{bmatrix} d(s_1) & \ldots & d(s_Z)\end{bmatrix}_{l\times Z}$ (where $l \in \mathbb{N}$ is the dimension of $D$-space), $\pi_{MVN}(\boldsymbol{d_Z}|\ldots)$ is the matrix-variate normal density (see, for example, Morales et al. [26]), $\pi_{MN}(\beta_Z|\ldots)$ is the multivariate normal density with a zero mean vector and covariance matrix $\boldsymbol{\Sigma}_\beta$ with elements $[\boldsymbol{\Sigma}_\beta]_{ij} = \frac{1}{\delta}\rho_\theta(\|d(s_i) - d(s_j)\|)$ for $i = 1, \ldots, Z$ and $j = 1, \ldots, Z$ and $L(\beta_Z, \lambda^*, \mu; y)$ is the likelihood function (8) by applying the discretization method, resulting in

$$L(\beta_Z, \lambda^*, \mu; y) = \prod_{z=1}^{Z}(\lambda^*\Phi(\beta(s_z)))^{y_z} \exp\left\{-\sum_{z=1}^{Z}\lambda^* g(\mu + \beta(s_z))\nu(G_z)\right\}. \tag{11}$$

For the developments presented in Section 3, we focus on two-dimensional (2D) $G$-space (latitude and longitude), but the concepts presented here could naturally extend to other dimensions like time (1D) or 3D, when altitude is included. The $D$-space dimension is set as 2, as in Sections 3.1 and 3.2, balancing deformation and computational complexity.

The interpolation of the process $d$ at coordinates $s_W := \begin{bmatrix}\tilde{s}_1 & \ldots & \tilde{s}_W\end{bmatrix}$, $\tilde{s}_w \in G$, $\forall w = 1, \ldots, W$ may be required. This is carried out by applying the standard conditional distribution properties of multivariate normal combined with matrix-variate and multivariate normal relationships (e.g., Gupta and Nagar [28]). Suppose

$$\begin{bmatrix} vec(\boldsymbol{d_W}) \\ vec(\boldsymbol{d_Z}) \end{bmatrix} \sim \text{MN}\left(\begin{bmatrix} vec(\boldsymbol{s_W}) \\ vec(\boldsymbol{s_Z}) \end{bmatrix}, \begin{bmatrix} \boldsymbol{R_{11}} & \boldsymbol{R_{12}} \\ \boldsymbol{R_{21}} & \boldsymbol{R_{22}} \end{bmatrix} \otimes \sigma_d^2\right)$$

where $\boldsymbol{d_W} := \begin{bmatrix} d(\tilde{s}_1) & \ldots & d(\tilde{s}_W)\end{bmatrix}$; $[\boldsymbol{R_{11}}]_{ij} = \rho_\phi(\|[vec(\boldsymbol{s_W})]_i - [vec(\boldsymbol{s_W})]_j\|)$ for $i = 1, \ldots, W$ and $j = 1, \ldots, W$ where $[vec(\boldsymbol{s_W})]_i := \tilde{s}_i$ denotes each coordinate to be interpolated; $[\boldsymbol{R_{22}}]_{ij} = \rho_\phi(\|[vec(\boldsymbol{s_Z})]_i - [vec(\boldsymbol{s_Z})]_j\|)$ for $i = 1, \ldots, Z$ and $j = 1, \ldots, Z$, with $[vec(\boldsymbol{s_Z})]_i := s_i$ denoting each centroid coordinate from the partition; and $[\boldsymbol{R_{12}}]_{ij} = \rho_\phi(\|[vec(\boldsymbol{s_W})]_i - [vec(\boldsymbol{s_Z})]_j\|)$ for $i = 1, \ldots, W$ and $j = 1, \ldots, Z$; and finally $\boldsymbol{R_{21}} = \boldsymbol{R_{12}}^T$. Therefore, the distribution of $vec(\boldsymbol{d_W}) \mid vec(\boldsymbol{d_Z})$ is given by

$$vec(\boldsymbol{d_W}) \mid vec(\boldsymbol{d_Z}) \sim \text{MN}\left(\mu_{W|Z}, \Sigma_{W|Z}\right)$$

where

$$\mu_{W|Z} = vec(\boldsymbol{s_W}) + (\boldsymbol{R_{12}}\boldsymbol{R_{22}^{-1}} \otimes \boldsymbol{I_2})(vec(\boldsymbol{d_Z}) - vec(\boldsymbol{s_Z}))$$

and $\Sigma_{W|Z} = (\boldsymbol{R_{11}} - \boldsymbol{R_{12}}\boldsymbol{R_{22}}^{-1}\boldsymbol{R_{12}}^T) \otimes \sigma_d^2$. The codes provided in Appendix A can be used to obtain a sample of size $L$ from the posterior distribution of $vec(\boldsymbol{d_W})$. Specifically, for each $l$-th sample of $vec(\boldsymbol{d_Z})^{(l)}$, a sample from the posterior distribution of $vec(\boldsymbol{d_W})$ can be generated from:

$$vec(\boldsymbol{d_W}) \mid vec(\boldsymbol{d_Z}) \sim \text{MN}\left(\mu_{W|Z}, \Sigma_{W|Z}\right)$$

where $\mu_{W|Z}^{(l)} = vec(\boldsymbol{s_W}) + (\boldsymbol{R_{12}}\boldsymbol{R_{22}^{-1}} \otimes \boldsymbol{I_2})(vec(\boldsymbol{d_Z})^{(l)} - vec(\boldsymbol{s_Z}))$ and the interpolation is based on the mean distribution.

Function $d$ is unidentifiable, since all the transformations of the coordinates in $D$-space which keep the same distances between locations are observationally equivalent. Scaling all distances by a constant is also equivalent. For the practical application of the deformation model in the Bayesian paradigm, fixing the locations of two points in $D$-

space is recommended (Damian et al. [29], Morales et al. [26], Sampson and Meiring [30]). We anchor $d(s_1) := s_1$ and $d(s_Z) := s_Z$ to prevent translation or rotation.

Bayesian inference is implemented via Markov Chain Monte Carlo (MCMC). Sampling of the posterior samples was handled by applying Hamiltonian Monte Carlo (HMC). Non-centered parameterizations (see, for example, Papaspiliopoulos et al. [31]) were employed for both the Gaussian process $\beta$ and deformation process $d$. This choice also enhances favorable a posteriori geometry and computational efficiency. The analyses were accomplished on R version 4.0.3 (R Core Team (2020)) and some MCMC parts were developed on C++ and Rcpp library to make an interface between R and C++. The Rstan package (Carpenter et al. [32]) provided comparable results and was used to make an interface. The Stan codes used in all subsequent analyses are available in Appendix A.

## 3. Results

In this section, comparisons between our anisotropic proposal and isotropic formulations are presented, based on simulated and real data. The analyses were performed on a notebook with a Core i5 processor and 8 GB RAM. When the DP was considered, convergence times ranged from 1.5 to 4 hours, with a total number of iterations ranging from 1500 to 3000, and with burn-in ranging from 500 to 2000 and no thinning. When considering the isotropic covariance structure, convergence times ranged from 30 minutes to 1 hour. The convergence of the chains was evaluated by observing the trace plot and the statistics: effective sample size (ESS) and $\hat{R}$, available on Rstan library.

Anisotropic and isotropic formulations were fitted to both synthetic and real data. Their ability to recover patterns associated with the intensity function of the underlying point process was also evaluated. The adopted model comparison criteria consider different aspects such as predictive ability, the trade-off between fit quality and complexity, and estimation accuracy. Such criteria include the sum of the Conditional Predictive Ordinate (CPO) on the logarithmic scale (slCPO) (Pettit [33]), Deviance Information Criterion (DIC) (Spiegelhalter et al. [34]), averaged Interval Score (AIS) (Winkler [35]), and Mean Absolute Error (MAE).

### 3.1. Simulating the Process with a Deterministic Intensity

Point processes with a substantially varying intensity function favor anisotropic models. This assumption is tested with a PP with intensity function given by

$$f(x,y) = \begin{cases} 191\sin(22.8x^2(1-y)^2)e^{x^2+(1-y)^2} + 1150 & y < x < 1 \text{ and } 0 < y < 1 \\ 191\sin(22.8x^2(1-y)^2)e^{x^2+(1-y)^2} + 1150 + 450\cos(10y^{1.2}(1-x)^{1.2}) & 0 < x < y \text{ and } 0 < y < 1 \end{cases} \quad (12)$$

Figure 1 exhibits the intensity function generated by the deterministic expression (12). The anisotropy assumption is likely to be more adequate due to the varying level of oscillation of the intensity function as it gets close to the corners. The deformation should be significant and stretch the original space in the direction of the highest oscillation.

Figure 2 shows the discretized version of the original intensity function (12) and its resulting estimation with different link functions and deformation options (with/without). Panel (a) displays the true intensity function. It is clear that the estimation process considering anisotropy via DP, displayed in panels (c) and (e) (for the probit and log link functions, respectively) produced a better recovery of the intensity function patterns than the respective isotropic processes, displayed in panels (b) and (d), for the same link functions. The DP formulation performs better, especially for the region of higher variation, regardless of the choice of the link function. Figure 3 reports an exploratory analysis with a comparison between posterior intensity function point estimates along with their true values. Again, it confirms that better estimates were obtained also for the lowest and highest values for the models considering nonstationarity. The model selection criteria presented in Table 1 show that the scenarios where both the DP and the probit link function showed superior performance.

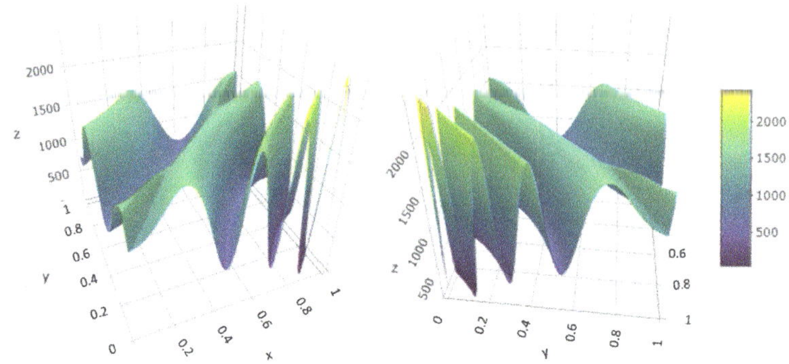


**Figure 1.** Intensity function given by expression (12) exhibited in different angles.

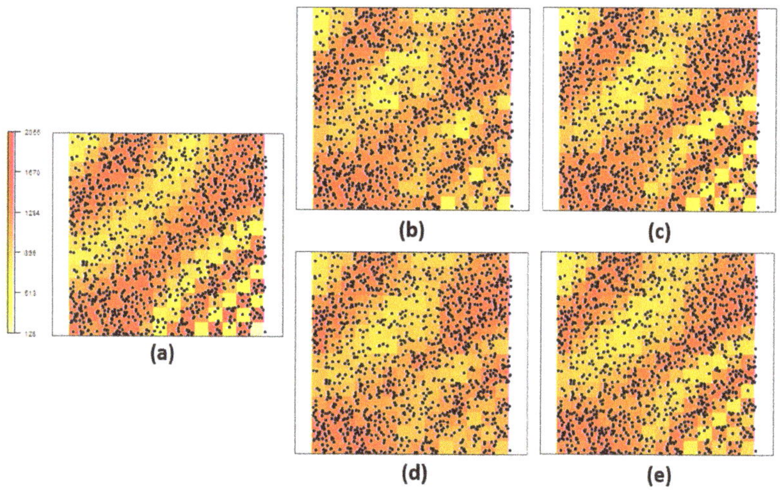


**Figure 2.** Estimation of the intensity function of expression (12): (**a**) True intensity function on the defined grid along with generated point process (dots), (**b**) estimated intensity function not considering and (**c**) considering the deformation for *probit* link function, (**d**) estimated intensity function not considering and (**e**) considering the deformation for *log* link function.

**Table 1.** Some model selection criteria comparing the estimation of the intensity function for the simulated data (12) considering or not considering the deformation using the *probit* or the *log* link function.

| Link | Deformation | MAE | AIS | slCPO | DIC |
|---|---|---|---|---|---|
| *probit* | without | 180.76 | 1463.83 | −507.68 | 988.25 |
| | with | **133.5** | **1163.06** | **−479.31** | **947.21** |
| *log* | without | 199.43 | 1588.27 | −508.09 | 1001.09 |
| | with | 154.67 | 1198.28 | −484.63 | 966.1 |

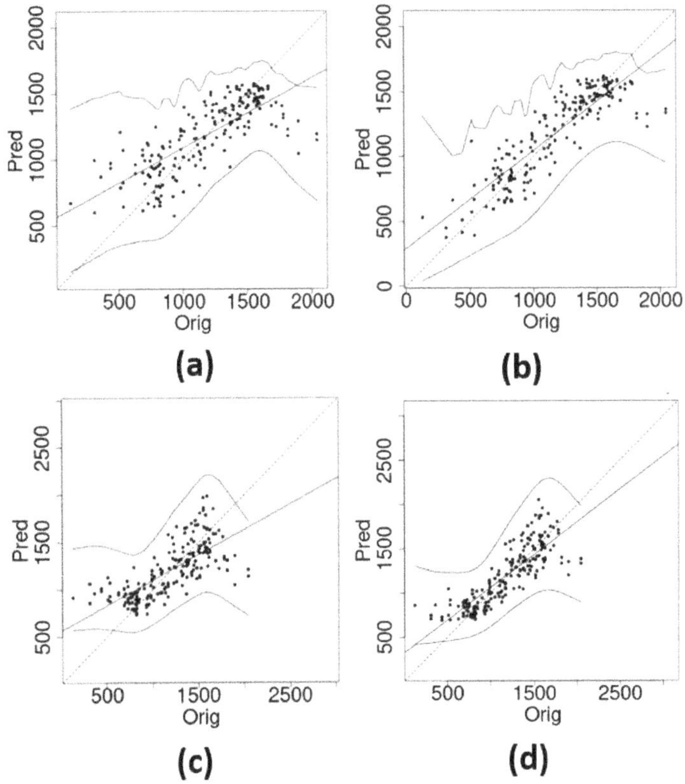


**Figure 3.** Further details of estimation of the intensity function (12). Scatter plot of true and estimated intensity function for different estimating scenarios: (**a**) intensity function not considering and (**b**) considering the deformation for *probit* link function, (**c**) intensity function not considering and (**d**) considering the deformation for *log* link function. The dots represent the pair of true and estimated intensity function values for all pixels. Full and dashed lines represent the identity and the exploratory regression lines, respectively. The latter is obtained by performing the fit of the estimated values based on the assumed true values as a covariate.

Figure 4 shows the interval score (IS) for the estimated intensity function from scenario (12) with and without the DP for the *probit* and *log* link function. It can be noted that both models where DP was estimated seem to have smaller IS, especially for the region with higher variation for both link functions.

Figure 5 compares intensity function posterior density for specific locations, revealing different intensity function prediction behaviors based on intensity function regimes. Locations 1 and 2 (in the low intensity function region) show an estimated intensity function closer to true values and CI, enclosing true value only when DP is assumed. Location 3 (in high-intensity region) exhibits CI, including true intensity with *log* link and DP assumption. Location 4 (in the smooth intensity function region) shows similar results for all models.

In order to avoid confusion due to the differences between hyperparameters associated with different link functions, and since results show an overall superior performance of the model with probit link, further results from Figure 6 present more details for the *probit* link only. Greater deformation from the original grid (near $(0,1)$ and $(1,0)$) resulted in higher SD variability. Our approach is fully Bayesian and Table 2 displays mean values and credibility intervals for hyperparameters that are estimated through the Hamiltonian Monte Carlo algorithm described in Appendix A.

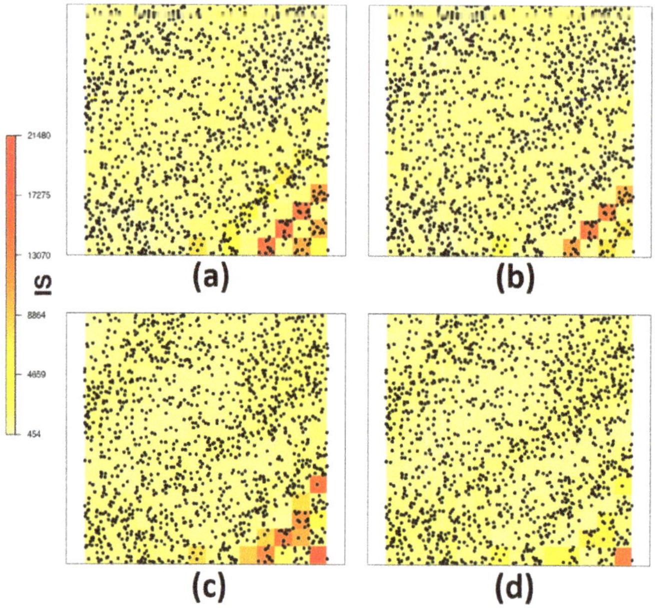


**Figure 4.** For the scenario of expression (12): (**a**) IS for the model not considering and (**b**) considering the deformation for *probit* link function, (**c**) IS for the model not considering and (**d**) considering the deformation for *log* link function.

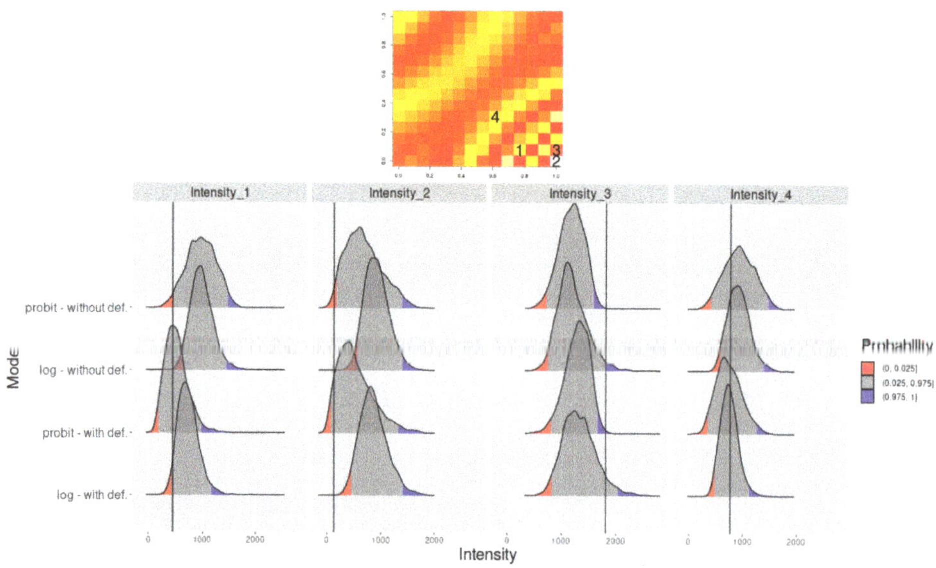


**Figure 5.** Intensity function estimation for the four selected locations: true intensity function (**top**) and density plot for the selected locations with their respective credibility interval of 95% (**bottom**) for the four models considered.

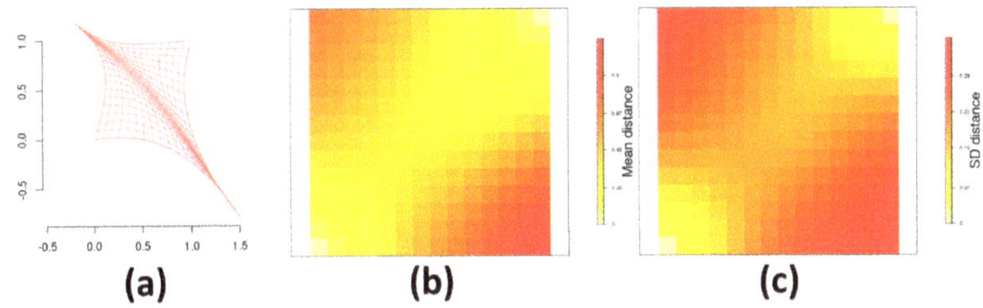

Figure 6. Estimation of the deformation $d$: (a) estimated mean deformation for the *probit* link function; (b) mean and (c) standard deviation for the posterior distribution of the distance between each centroid $s_z$ and $d(s_z)$ for $z \in \{1, \ldots, Z\}$ for the *probit* link function.

Table 2. The estimated mean and 95% credibility interval (CI) for the maximum intensity $\lambda^*$ and range parameter $\theta$ for the simulated data (12) considering or not considering the deformation using the *probit* link function.

| Deformation | $\widehat{\lambda^*}$ (CI95%($\lambda^*$)) | $\hat{\theta}$ (CI95%($\theta$)) |
|---|---|---|
| without | 1646.7 (1464; 1889.6) | 0.51 (0.21; 1.11) |
| with | 1697.4 (1518.5; 1933.2) | 0.65 (0.28; 1.36) |

A sensitivity analysis was carried out to examine the impact on estimated intensity function from fixed and estimated parameters. The analysis showed that intensity function estimates were robust to the proposed values for range $\phi$, covariance $\sigma_d^2$, precision $\delta$, and intercept $\mu$, within plausible parameter ranges. The sensitivity to the prior distribution for range parameter $\theta$ was low, while different priors for maximum intensity $\lambda^*$ had some impact, warranting careful consideration. Details about sensitivity studies are available at Quintana (2022) ([36], Sections 3.5 and 4.2).

This section presented the results of inference based on data generated from an intensity function with substantial variation. The overall message from the exercise of this section is that the use of deformation improved upon inference with isotropic models. A number of different aspects were considered in this comparison, and most of them showed substantial improvement, stemming from the incorporation of anisotropy. Another result that was somewhat unexpected is that the probit link compared favourably against the frequently used logarithmic link. This effect could be associated with the versatility of the probit transformation that enables it to mimic even the logarithmic function by adapting its seemingly unbounded first half to cover the entire logarithmic trajectory.

### 3.2. Real Data Application—*Spodoptera frugiperda* Pest in a Corn-Producing Agricultural Area

The analyses presented in this section concern a real data experiment on the effects of a pest over a corn plantation. The data collection was carried out in an agricultural commercial area of 27 ha located in the city of Cascavel, Paraná state, Brazil (approx. 24.95° S, 53.57° W and 650 m asl). An occurrence is defined by the location of a plant of corn attacked with the fall armyworm in the experimental area during the crop year 2015/2016. The location is defined by the geographical coordinates of the infected plant, which were obtained using a GEOEXPLORE 3 GPS positioning system receiver in a Universal Transverse Mercator (UTM) coordinate system. The study area included 9360 corn plants, of which 1303 were infected by the *S. frugiperda* (Figure 7a). The dataset was provided by the Spatial Statistics Laboratory of Unioeste.

Nava et al. [37] investigated the dominant infestation behavior of fall armyworm in that agricultural area. They assessed whether the point pattern showed aggregation or regularity using tests proposed by Guan et al. [38], Mateu and Nicolis [39] and Rajala et al. [7] to detect anisotropic spatial behavior. They found significant anisotropy in the original dataset, detected mainly along the 135- and 45-degree directions due to planter machine design and area shape. In a central subset after rotation, no dominant directions were detected, suggesting potential localized anisotropy near experimental area borders.

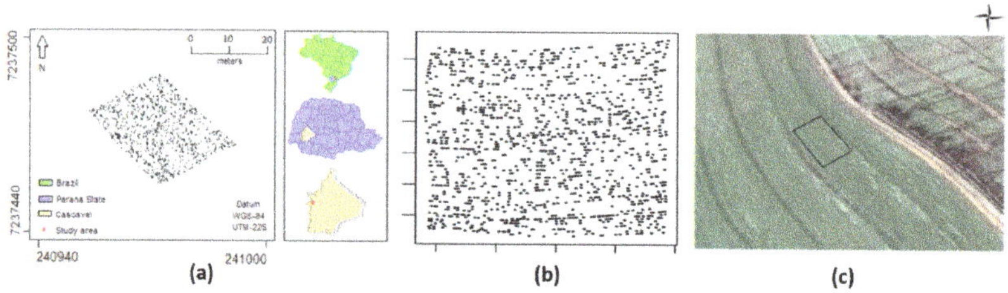


**Figure 7.** Point pattern for the corn plants infected by the *S. frugiperda* with (**a**) original and (**b**) rotated latitude and longitude and (**c**) a satellite image of the experimental area with the polygon of the study area. Adapted from Nava et al. [37].

Our methodology differs from Nava's approach in several ways. Firstly, their tests are limited to predefined angles, while our method adapts to structures at any angle or even different angles in various geographic regions. Secondly, their method evaluates geometric anisotropy, while ours applies to a broader class of anisotropy. Most importantly, while their approach tests indicative angles of anisotropy, our method estimates an intensity function that fully accounts for any kind of data-driven anisotropy.

Figure 8 displays infected plant locations and the estimated intensity function on a $17 \times 13$ grid for different link functions and DP considerations, while Table 3 shows the results of model comparison criteria. Our anisotropic formulation via DP shows better performance over the corresponding model without deformation. Additionally, the *probit* link function seems to provide better results over the corresponding model with logarithmic link.

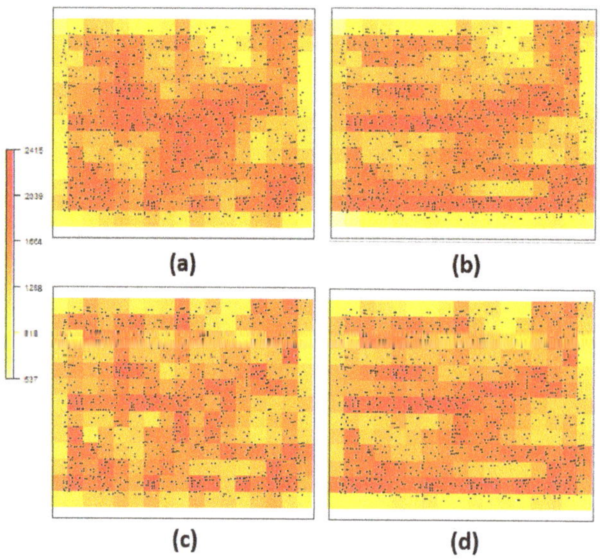


**Figure 8.** Estimation of the intensity function for *Spodoptera frugiperda* pest data: (**a**) not considering and (**b**) considering the deformation for probit link function, (**c**) not considering and (**d**) considering the deformation for log link function.

**Table 3.** Model selection criteria comparing the estimation of the intensity function for the *Spodoptera frugiperda* pest data for all models considered.

| Link | Deformation | slCPO | DIC |
|---|---|---|---|
| *probit* | without | −550.584 | 1075.75 |
| | with | **−537.145** | **1055.69** |
| *log* | without | −553.976 | 1087.62 |
| | with | −543.871 | 1069.05 |

Intensity function estimation with DP showed similar behavior for both link functions, as shown in Figure 8 (items (b) and (d)). Bands appeared near the horizontal direction, showing similarity in higher or lower intensity values. When stationarity/isotropy was assumed and DP was not used (items (a) and (c) in Figure 8), the intensity function appeared less smooth, lacking clear intensity bands horizontally.

Figure 9 displays the posterior standard deviation of intensity function for *Spodoptera frugiperda* pest data for all considered models. The *probit* link showed almost uniformly lower SD in intensity function estimates compared to the *log* link. Higher posterior SD for the intensity function along with higher SD variability were observed with deformation when the *log* link was considered.

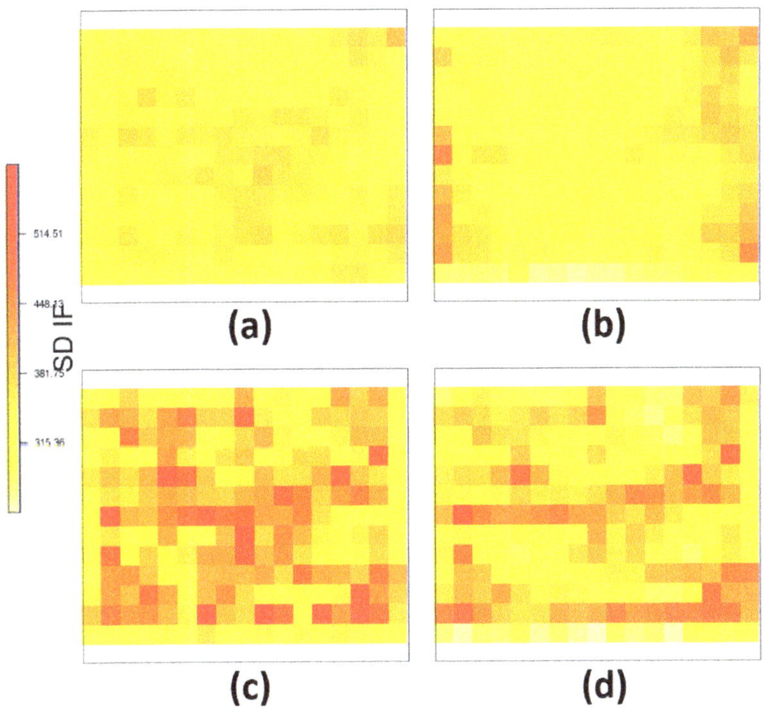


**Figure 9.** Standard deviation for the intensity function for the model for the *Spodoptera frugiperda* pest data: (**a**) not considering and (**b**) considering the deformation for *probit* link function, (**c**) not considering and (**d**) considering the deformation for *log* link function.

Figure 10 compares intensity function posterior density for specific locations by evaluating different intensity function predictions in areas with varying intensity. Locations #1, #2, #3 and #4 showed more concentrated posterior distributions for models considering DP when compared to the corresponding isotropic models. Table 4 displays *log* CPO values, indicating better predictive capacity in these regions for DP models.

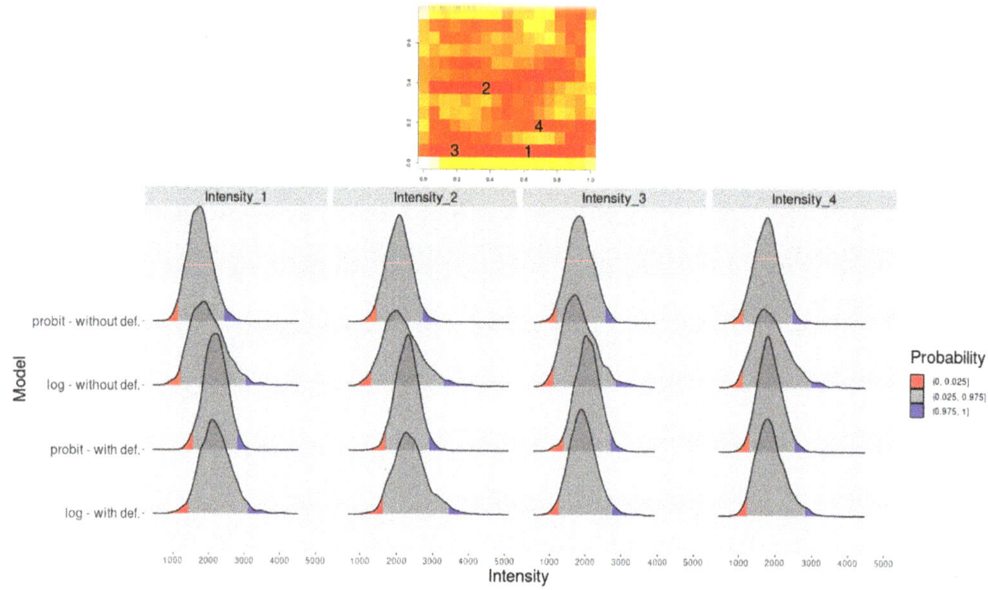


**Figure 10.** Estimated intensity function map for the *Spodoptera frugiperda* pest data showing the positions of intensity function selected for posterior density comparison across models (**top**) and density plot for the selected positions with their respective credibility interval of 95% (**bottom**).

**Table 4.** Estimated intensity function and CPO (in log scale) for locations of Figure 10.

| Deformation | Link | Mean Intensity Function(loc[1]) | lCPO[loc[1]] | Mean Intensity Function(loc[2]) | lCPO[loc[2]] |
|---|---|---|---|---|---|
| without | probit | 1743.21 | − 4.03 | 2048.23 | −3.54 |
| | log | 1973.68 | −3.72 | 2144.00 | −3.93 |
| with | probit | 2187.37 | −2.68 | 2285.29 | −2.90 |
| | log | 2205.25 | −2.94 | 2392.56 | −2.99 |
| Deformation | Link | mean intensity function(loc[3]) | lCPO[loc[3]] | mean intensity function(loc[4]) | lCPO[loc[4]] |
| without | probit | 1840.86 | −2.56 | 1754.79 | −3.35 |
| | log | 1821.05 | −2.75 | 1882.98 | −3.27 |
| with | probit | 2048.01 | −2.28 | 1846.86 | −2.91 |
| | log | 1939.08 | −2.43 | 1876.19 | −3.00 |

Figure 11 depicts the DP-estimated intensity function surface and the posterior mean and standard deviation for the distance between centroids $s_z$ and $d(s_z)$ for the *probit* link function. These statistics help assess uncertainty related to the estimated DP. We can see a compressing space near the horizontal direction, suggesting higher spatial correlation in that orientation. The bands detected in the intensity function also align with this correlation. Variability in estimates increased in regions farther from the original grid, observed in the SD plot.

Table 5 displays the mean values and credibility intervals for parameters $(\lambda^*, \theta)$ when *probit* link function is considered. Although there are differences in posterior point estimates, the associated posterior uncertainty in both cases prevents any distinction between the resulting inference for these hyperparameters.

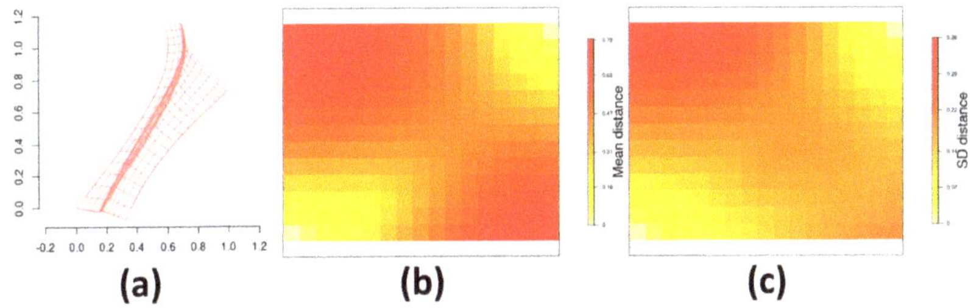


**Figure 11.** Estimation of the deformation $d$ for the *Spodoptera frugiperda* pest data: (**a**) estimated mean deformation for the *probit* link function; (**b**) mean and (**c**) standard deviation for the posterior distribution of the distance between each centroid $s_z$ and $d(s_z)$ for $z \in \{1, \ldots, Z\}$ for the *probit* link function.

**Table 5.** The estimated mean and credibility interval (CI) of 95% for the maximum intensity $\lambda^*$ and range parameter $\theta$ for the *Spodoptera frugiperda* pest data considering or not considering the deformation using the *probit* link function.

| Link | Deformation | $\widehat{\lambda^*}$ (CI95%($\lambda^*$)) | $\hat{\theta}$ (CI95%($\theta$)) |
|---|---|---|---|
| *probit* | without | 3648.1 (2895.8; 4526.0) | 1.88 (0.77; 4.01) |
| | with | 3698.7 (2993.7; 4506.2) | 1.71 (0.68; 3.59) |

Finally, Figure 12 illustrates the estimated intensity function and DP using the best fit scenario (*probit* link function with DP estimation) on the original, unrotated, and rescaled geographic region. Overall, this real data analysis showed results that coincide qualitatively with those from the analysis of synthetic data. Namely, in the presence of intensity functions with high variability, models incorporating deformation outperformed the corresponding isotropic versions across a variety of comparison criteria.

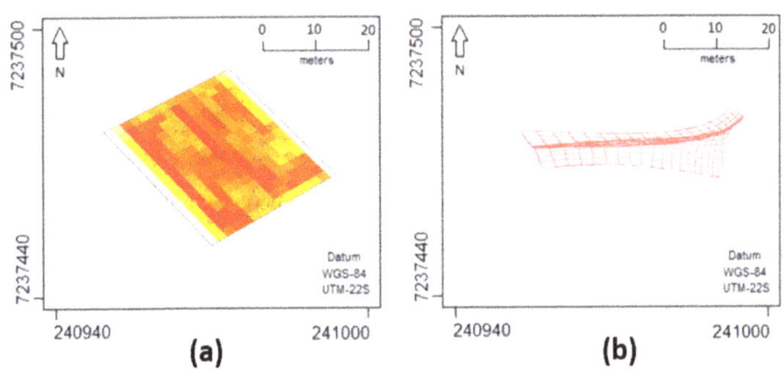


**Figure 12.** Estimated (**a**) intensity function and (**b**) DP for the model considering the *probit* link function for unrotated and rescaled *Spodoptera frugiperda* pest data.

### 3.3. Comparative Analysis of Spatial Deformation and Geometric Anisotropy

As mentioned in Section 1, alternative approaches exist to address the anisotropy of spatial processes, with geometric anisotropy being a commonly used methodology (see, for example, ref. [40]). This approach is relatively straightforward to implement, involving a linear transformation corresponding to the rotation and stretching of the geographic coordinate axes, and relies solely on the estimation of two parameters: the rotation angle and the anisotropic ratio between the axes. However, it restricts anisotropy to a predefined structure. This section compares several model selection criteria for the model considering geometric anisotropy with the proposed model that incorporates spatial deformation to address the inherent anisotropy in the data for both *probit* and *log* link functions.

For the simulated process shown in Section 3.1, the estimated rotation angle was $-43.23°$ and the anisotropic ratio was 1.41 when geometric anisotropy was considered. The model selection criteria presented in Table 6, comparing the results for the model considering geometric anisotropy and the model considering spatial deformation for both *probit* and *log* link functions, indicate that the scenarios where both spatial deformation and the *probit* link function were used showed superior performance.

**Table 6.** Some model selection criteria comparing the estimation of the intensity function for the simulated data (12) considering the geometric anisotropy and the DP using the *probit* or the *log* link function.

| Link | Anisotropy | MAE | AIS | slCPO | DIC |
|---|---|---|---|---|---|
| **probit** | Geometric | 198.82 | 1529.01 | − 505.94 | 985.27 |
| | Deformation | **133.5** | **1163.06** | **−479.31** | **947.21** |
| *log* | Geometric | 205.71 | 1639.04 | −507.24 | 997.5 |
| | Deformation | 154.67 | 1198.28 | −484.63 | 966.1 |

For the real data analysis presented in Section 3.2, the estimated rotation angle was 3.27°, and the anisotropic ratio was 1.21 when geometric anisotropy was considered. The model selection criteria shown in Table 7, which compare the results of the model considering geometric anisotropy with the model considering the DP for both *probit* and *log* link functions, again demonstrate that the scenarios where both the DP and the *probit* link function were employed exhibited superior performance.

**Table 7.** Model selection criteria comparing the estimation of the intensity function for the *Spodoptera frugiperda* pest data considering the geometric anisotropy and the DP using the *probit* or the *log* link function.

| Link | Anisotropy | slCPO | DIC |
|---|---|---|---|
| ***probit*** | Geometric | − 548.351 | 1072.98 |
| | **Deformation** | **−537.145** | **1055.69** |
| *log* | Geometric | −554.508 | 1087.49 |
| | Deformation | −543.871 | 1069.05 |

## 4. Discussion

The proposed point process analysis model, incorporating anisotropy and nonstationarity via DP, outperformed models lacking these considerations in both simulated and real data analyses. Criteria assessing fit quality showed marked improvements. Specifically, in a scenario observing varying oscillation frequencies, models accommodating deformation showed better discrimination between higher and lower frequency zones than those without. Models omitting deformation failed to distinguish the intensity regions accurately. Incorporating deformation notably enhanced all model selection criteria, favoring the model that accounted for it. This approach, addressing anisotropy and nonstationarity via spatial deformation (rather than other specific pattern across the entire space), proved beneficial because the change in the intensity function regime occurred mainly in the relevant subregions, by deforming the geographic space differently across regions. Moreover, specifying a parametrized anisotropy and/or nonstationarity formulation for these intensity function behavior would be insufficient to capture these types of changes in the intensity function. Comparisons between the proposed anisotropic model via deformation and the geometric anisotropic model indicated favorable results for the proposed formulation. This was observed in both artificially generated data and real data concerning the *Spodoptera frugiperda* pest.

Deformation behavior in *Spodoptera frugiperda* pest control data shows increased spatial correlation along the horizontal direction (in rotated coordinates), aligning with findings from Nava et al. [37], highlighting higher anisotropy at a 135° angle in non-rotated data. This is consistent with agricultural practices, mirroring the direction of planting machines. Estimated infestation levels enable targeted pesticide application, aiding environmental and consumer health by prioritizing doses in specific regions and prevailing directions.

Different link functions may suit each case, especially when assessing the behavior of the intensity function. In scenarios with low overall intensity but sudden spikes, the logarithm link function can better capture peaks. Alternatively, the *probit* link function might perform better for frequent sudden intensity function decays. When the intensity function behaves erratically, fitting both and selecting the best performance based on model criteria proves relevant in practical terms.

An extended model includes covariates influencing the point pattern by substituting $\{\beta(s) : s \in G\}$ with $\{W(s)\beta(s) : s \in G\}$ in expression (3), where $W(s)$ represents some form of square root precision matrices. Similarly, for some applications offsets $\{r(s) : s \in G\}$ might be needed for a comparison of varying population sizes across space. For instance, defining $\Lambda(s) := \lambda(s)r(s)$ in expression (3) allows the data $Y$ to be rewritten as $Y|\Lambda \sim \mathrm{PP}(\Lambda)$.

The isotropic model can be obtained as the special case of our DP when the main diagonal of $\sigma_d^2$ tends to zero. Model comparison may then be also obtained by a mixture model with prior weight $\alpha$ for isotropy and complementary prior weight $1-\alpha$ for the DP component. Posterior inference on $\alpha$ might prove useful for assessing the relevance of the anisotropic component.

The work of this paper considered only discretized space. Recent sampling methods using Poisson thinning offer crucial extensions towards inference in continuous space. Gonçalves and Gamerman [25] utilized Poisson thinning for non-homogeneous Poisson processes, employing a spatial Cox model driven by a Gaussian process. Their MCMC algorithm allowed for direct simulation, resembling our model with a *probit* link function. Extending the methods in this direction merges the benefits of continuous surfaces, improves the intensity estimation for nonstationary/anisotropic processes, and are the subject of our interest for future work.

**Author Contributions:** Conceptualization, D.G., M.d.S.B.Q. and M.B.A.; methodology, D.G., M.d.S.B.Q. and M.B.A.; software, M.d.S.B.Q.; validation, D.G., M.d.S.B.Q. and M.B.A.; formal analysis, D.G., M.d.S.B.Q. and M.B.A.; investigation, M.d.S.B.Q.; resources, M.d.S.B.Q.; data curation, M.d.S.B.Q.; writing—original draft preparation, M.d.S.B.Q.; writing—review and editing, D.G. and M.B.A.; visualization, M.d.S.B.Q.; supervision, D.G. and M.B.A.; project administration, D.G. and M.B.A.; funding acquisition, D.G. All authors have read and agreed to the published version of the manuscript.

**Funding:** The research of DG was supported by grants from Conselho Nacional de Desenvolvimento Científico e Tecnológico—CNPq and Fundação de Amaparo à Pesquisa do Estado de Minas Gerais—FAPEMIG, both from Brazil.

**Data Availability Statement:** Simulated data is freely available upon request from author MSBQ and real data is freely available from Unioeste's Spatial Statistics Laboratory—Campus Cascavel upon request.

**Acknowledgments:** This research was based on the development of the doctoral thesis of MSBQ under the joint supervision of DG and MBA. We thank Unioeste's Spatial Statistics Laboratory—Campus Cascavel for providing the data used in the application presented in Section 3.2.

**Conflicts of Interest:** The authors declare no conflicts of interest. The funders had no role in the design of the study; in the collection, analyses, or interpretation of data; in the writing of the manuscript; or in the decision to publish the results.

## Abbreviations

The following abbreviations are used in this manuscript:

| | |
|---|---|
| IS | Interval score |
| AIS | Averaged interval score |
| CI | Credibility interval |
| CPO | Conditional predictive ordinate |
| DIC | Deviance information criterion |
| DP | Deformation process |
| GP | Gaussian process |
| IS | Interval score |
| HMC | Hamiltonian Monte Carlo |
| LGCP | Log-Gaussian Cox process |
| MAE | Mean absolute error |
| MCMC | Markov Chain Monte Carlo |
| PP | Poisson process |
| slCPO | Sum of the *log* of the conditional predictive ordinate |
| SD | Standard deviation |

## Appendix A. Stan Codes

### *Appendix A.1. Isotropic Scenario with Log Link Function*

```
data {
  int<lower=1> Z;
  int<lower=1> D;
  vector[D] x[Z];
  int<lower=0> y[Z];
  real<lower=0> at;
  real<lower=0> bt;
  real<lower=0> argr;
  real<lower=0> gc;
}

transformed data {
  real eps = 1e-9;
}

parameters{
  vector[Z] eta;
  real mu;
  real<lower=0> delta;
  real<lower=0> theta;
}

model{
  vector[Z] beta;

  delta ~ gamma(0.01,0.01);
  theta ~ gamma(at,bt);

  {
    matrix[Z, Z] L_K;
    matrix[Z, Z] K;

    for (i in 1:(Z - 1)) {
      K[i, i] = (1.0/delta) + eps;
      for (j in (i + 1):Z) {
        K[i, j] = (1.0/delta)*exp(-(1.0/theta)* sqrt(sum(square(x[i,] - x[j,])))^
            gc);
        K[j, i] = K[i, j];
      }
    }
    K[Z, Z] = (1.0/delta) + eps;
    L_K = cholesky_decompose(K);
```

```
    beta = L_K * eta;
  }

  eta ~ std_normal(); //eta must be multivariate normal

  y ~ poisson(argr*exp(mu + beta)); //likelihood
}
```

*Appendix A.2. Deformation Process with Log Link Function*

```
data {
  int<lower=1> Z;
  int<lower=1> D;
  vector[2*Z-4] vd0a;
  vector[2] vecd00;
  vector[2] vecd11;
  matrix[2*Z-4,2*Z-4] Kvecda;
  int<lower=0> y[Z];
  real<lower=0> at;
  real<lower=0> bt;
  real<lower=0> argr;
  real<lower=0> gc;
}

transformed data{
  real eps = 1e-9;
  matrix[2*Z-4,2*Z-4] L_Kvecda;
  L_Kvecda = cholesky_decompose(Kvecda);
}

parameters{
  vector[Z] eta;
  vector[2*Z-4] eta_vecda;
  real mu;
  real<lower=0> delta;
  real<lower=0> theta;
}

model{
  vector[2*Z-4] vecda;
  vector[Z] beta;

  {
    vecda = vd0a + L_Kvecda * eta_vecda;
  }
  eta_vecda ~ std_normal();

  delta ~ gamma(0.01,0.01);
  theta ~ gamma(at,bt);

  {
    matrix[Z, Z] L_K;
    matrix[Z, Z] K;

    K[1,1] = (1.0/delta) + eps;
    for (i in 2:(Z-2)) {
      K[i, i] = (1.0/delta) + eps;
      for (j in (i+1):(Z-1)) {
        K[i, j] = (1.0/delta)*exp(-(1.0/theta)* sqrt(square(vecda[2*(i-1)-1] -
            vecda[2*(j-1)-1]) + square(vecda[2*(i-1)] - vecda[2*(j-1)]))^gc);
        K[j, i] = K[i, j];
      }
    }
    K[Z-1, Z-1] = (1.0/delta) + eps;
    for (j in 2:(Z-1)) {
        K[1, j] = (1.0/delta)*exp(-(1.0/theta)* sqrt(square(vecd00[1] - vecda[2*(j
            -1)-1]) + square(vecd00[2] - vecda[2*(j-1)]))^gc);
        K[j, 1] = K[1, j];
```

```
        K[Z, j] = (1.0/delta)*exp(-(1.0/theta)* sqrt(square(vecd11[1] - vecda[2*(j
            -1)-1]) + square(vecd11[2] - vecda[2*(j-1)]))^gc);
        K[j, Z] = K[Z, j];
      }
    K[1,Z] = (1.0/delta)*exp(-(1.0/theta)* sqrt(square(vecd00[1] - vecd11[1]) +
        square(vecd00[2] - vecd11[2]))^gc);
    K[Z,1] = K[1, Z];
    K[Z,Z] = (1.0/delta) + eps;

    L_K = cholesky_decompose(K);
    beta = L_K * eta;
  }

  eta ~ std_normal(); //eta must be multivariate normal

  y ~ poisson(argr*exp(mu + beta)); //likelihood

}
```

*Appendix A.3. Isotropic Scenario with Probit Link Function*

```
data {
  int<lower=1> Z;
  int<lower=1> D;
  vector[D] x[Z];
  int<lower=0> y[Z];
  real<lower=0> delta; //0.5
  real<lower=0> at;
  real<lower=0> bt;
  real<lower=0> argr;
}

transformed data {
  real eps = 1e-9;
}

parameters {
  vector[Z] eta;
  real<lower=0> lambdaA;
  real<lower=0> theta;
}

model {
  vector[Z] beta;
  real lambdaAargr;

  theta ~ gamma(at,bt);

  {
    matrix[Z, Z] L_K;
    matrix[Z, Z] K;

    //real lambdaAargr = lambdaA*argr;

    for (i in 1:(Z - 1)) {
      K[i, i] = (1.0/delta) + eps;
      for (j in (i + 1):Z) {
        K[i, j] = (1.0/delta)*exp(-(1.0/theta)* sqrt(sum(square(x[i,] - x[j,]))));
        K[j, i] = K[i, j];
      }
    }
    K[Z, Z] = (1.0/delta) + eps;
    L_K = cholesky_decompose(K);
    beta = L_K * eta;
  }

  eta ~ std_normal(); //eta must be multivariate normal
```

```
  lambdaAargr = lambdaA*argr;

  lambdaA ~ gamma(0.01,0.01);

  y ~ poisson(lambdaAargr*Phi(beta)); //likelihood
}
```

*Appendix A.4. Deformation Process with Probit Link Function*

```
data {
  int<lower=1> Z;
  int<lower=1> D;
  vector[2*Z-4] vd0a;
  vector[2] vecd00;
  vector[2] vecd11;
  matrix[2*Z-4,2*Z-4] Kvecda;
  int<lower=0> y[Z];
  real<lower=0> delta;
  real<lower=0> at;
  real<lower=0> bt;
  real<lower=0> argr;
}

transformed data{
  real eps = 1e-9;
  matrix[2*Z-4,2*Z-4] L_Kvecda;
  L_Kvecda = cholesky_decompose(Kvecda);
}

parameters{
  vector[Z] eta;
  vector[2*Z-4] eta_vecda;
  real<lower=0> lambdaA;
  real<lower=0> theta;
}

model{
  vector[2*Z-4] vecda;
  vector[Z] beta;
  real lambdaAargr;

  {
    vecda = vd0a + L_Kvecda * eta_vecda;
  }

  eta_vecda ~ std_normal();

  theta ~ gamma(at,bt);

  {
    matrix[Z, Z] L_K;
    matrix[Z, Z] K;

    K[1,1] = (1.0/delta) + eps;
    for (i in 2:(Z-2)) {
      K[i, i] = (1.0/delta) + eps;
      for (j in (i+1):(Z-1)) {
        K[i, j] = (1.0/delta)*exp(-(1.0/theta)* sqrt(square(vecda[2*(i-1)-1] -
            vecda[2*(j-1)-1]) + square(vecda[2*(i-1)] - vecda[2*(j-1)])));
        K[j, i] = K[i, j];
      }
    }
    K[Z-1, Z-1] = (1.0/delta) + eps;
    for (j in 2:(Z-1)) {
        K[1, j] = (1.0/delta)*exp(-(1.0/theta)* sqrt(square(vecd00[1] - vecda[2*(j
            -1)-1]) + square(vecd00[2] - vecda[2*(j-1)])));
        K[j, 1] = K[1, j];
```

```
            K[Z, j] = (1.0/delta)*exp(-(1.0/theta)* sqrt(square(vecd11[1] - vecda[2*(j
                -1)-1]) + square(vecd11[2] - vecda[2*(j-1)])));
            K[j, Z] = K[Z, j];
        }
        K[1,Z] = (1.0/delta)*exp(-(1.0/theta)* sqrt(square(vecd00[1] - vecd11[1]) +
            square(vecd00[2] - vecd11[2])));
        K[Z,1] = K[1, Z];
        K[Z,Z] = (1.0/delta) + eps;

        L_K = cholesky_decompose(K);
        beta = L_K * eta;
    }

    eta ~ std_normal(); //eta must be multivariate normal

    lambdaAargr = lambdaA*argr;

    lambdaA ~ gamma(0.01,0.01);

    y ~ poisson(lambdaAargr*Phi(beta)); //likelihood
}
```

## References


1. Diggle, P. *Statistical Analysis of Spatial and Spatiotemporal Point Patterns*; Taylor & Francis Inc.: London, UK , 2013.
2. Illian, J.; Penttinen, A.; Stoyan, H.; Stoyan, D. *Statistical Analysis and Modelling of Spatial Point Patterns (Statistics in Practice)*; Wiley-Interscience: Hoboken, NJ, USA, 2008; p. 560.
3. Häbel, H.; Rajala, T.; Marucci, M.; Boissier, C.; Schladitz, K.; Redenbach, C.; Särkkä, A. A three-dimensional anisotropic point process characterization for pharmaceutical coatings. *Spat. Stat.* **2017**, *22*, 306–320. [CrossRef]
4. Gabriel, E. Estimating Second-Order Characteristics of Inhomogeneous Spatio-Temporal Point Processes. *Methodol. Comput. Appl. Probab.* **2014**, *16*, 411–431. [CrossRef]
5. Hahn, U.; Vedel Jensen, E.B. Hidden Second-order Stationary Spatial Point Processes. *Scand. J. Stat.* **2016**, *43*, 455–475. [CrossRef]
6. Konstantinou, K.; Särkkä, A. Pairwise interaction Markov model for 3D epidermal nerve fibre endings. *J. Microsc.* **2022**, *288*, 54–67. [CrossRef] [PubMed]
7. Rajala, T.A.; Särkkä, A.; Redenbach, C.; Sormani, M. Estimating geometric anisotropy in spatial point patterns. *Spat. Stat.* **2016**, *15*, 100–114. [CrossRef]
8. Sormani, M.; Redenbach, C.; Särkkä, A.; Rajala, T. Second order analysis of geometric anisotropic point processes revisited. *Spat. Stat.* **2020**, *38*, 100456. [CrossRef]
9. Martin, J.S.; Murrell, D.J.; Olhede, S.C. Multivariate geometric anisotropic Cox processes. *Scand. J. Stat.* **2023**, *50*, 1420–1465. [CrossRef]
10. Kwon, J.; Zheng, Y.; Jun, M. Flexible spatio-temporal Hawkes process models for earthquake occurrences. *Spat. Stat.* **2023**, *54*, 100728. [CrossRef]
11. Dong, Z.; Zhu, S.; Xie, Y.; Mateu, J.; Rodríguez-Cortés, F.J. Non-stationary spatio-temporal point process modeling for high-resolution COVID-19 data. *J. R. Stat. Soc. Ser. C Appl. Stat.* **2023**, *72*, 368–386. [CrossRef]
12. Biard, R.; Saussereau, B. Fractional Poisson Process: Long-Range Dependence and Applications in Ruin Theory. *J. Appl. Probab.* **2014**, *51*, 727–740. [CrossRef]
13. Roveri, R.; Öztireli, A.C.; Gross, M. General Point Sampling with Adaptive Density and Correlations. *Comput. Graph. Forum* **2017**, *36*, 107–117. [CrossRef]
14. Higdon, D.M.; Swall, J.; Kern, J.C. Non-stationary spatial modeling. In *Bayesian Statistics 6, Proceedings of the Sixth Valencia International Meeting, Valencia, Spain, 6–10 June 1998*; Oxford University Press: Oxford, UK, 1999; pp. 761–768.
15. Risser, M.D.; Calder, C.A. Regression-based covariance functions for nonstationary spatial modeling. *Environmetrics* **2015**, *26*, 284–297. [CrossRef]
16. Fuentes, M. A high frequency kriging approach for nonstationary environmental processes. *Environmetrics* **2001**, *12*, 469–483. [CrossRef]
17. Pintore, A.; Holmes, C.C. *Constructing Localized Non-Stationary Covariance Functions Through the Frequency Domain*; Technical Report; Imperial College: London, UK, 2003.
18. Stephenson, J.; Holmes, C.; Gallagher, K.; Pintore, A. A Statistical Technique for Modelling Non-stationary Spatial Processes. In *Geostatistics Banff 2004*; Leuangthong, O., Deutsch, C.V., Eds.; Springer: Dordrecht, The Netherlands, 2005; pp. 125–134. [CrossRef]
19. Sampson, P.D.; Guttorp, P. Nonparametric Estimation of Nonstationary Spatial Covariance Structure. *J. Am. Stat. Assoc.* **1992**, *87*, 108–119. [CrossRef]
20. Schmidt, A.M.; O'Hagan, A. Bayesian inference for non-stationary spatial covariance structure via spatial deformations. *J. R. Stat. Society. Ser. B (Stat. Methodol.)* **2003**, *65*, 743–758. [CrossRef]

21. Moller, J.; Syversveen, A.R.; Waagepetersen, R.P. Log Gaussian Cox Processes. *Scand. J. Stat.* **1998**, *25*, 451–482. [CrossRef]
22. Brix, A.; Diggle, P.J. Spatiotemporal prediction for log-Gaussian Cox processes. *J. R. Stat. Society. Ser. B (Stat. Methodol.)* **2001**, *63*, 823–841. [CrossRef]
23. Paez, M.S.; Diggle, P.J. Cox processes for estimating temporal variation in disease risk. *Environmetrics* **2009**, 20, 981–1003. [CrossRef]
24. Adams, R.P.; Murray, I.; MacKay, D.J.C. Tractable nonparametric Bayesian inference in Poisson processes with Gaussian process intensities. In Proceedings of the 26th Annual International Conference on Machine Learning, ICML 2009, Montreal, QC, Canada, 14–18 June 2009; Danyluk, A.P., Bottou, L., Littman, M.L., Eds.; ACM International Conference Proceeding Series; ACM: New York, NY, USA, 2009; Volume 382, pp. 9–16. [CrossRef]
25. Gonçalves, F.B.; Gamerman, D. Exact Bayesian inference in spatio-temporal Cox processes driven by multivariate Gaussian processes. *J. R. Stat. Soc. Ser. B (Stat. Methodol.)* **2018**, *80*, 157–175. . [CrossRef]
26. Morales, F.E.C.; Gamerman, D.; Paez, M.S. State space models with spatial deformation. *Environ. Ecol. Stat.* **2012**, *20*, 191–214. [CrossRef]
27. Daley, D.J.; Vere-Jones, D. *An Introduction to the Theory of Point Processes*; Springer: New York, NY, USA, 2006.
28. Gupta, A.K.; Nagar, D.K. *Matrix Variate Distributions*; Taylor & Francis Group: London, UK, 2018; p. 384.
29. Damian, D.; Sampson, P.D.; Guttorp, P. Bayesian estimation of semi-parametric non-stationary spatial covariance structures. *Environmetrics* **2001**, *12*, 161–178. [CrossRef]
30. Sampson, P.D.; Meiring, W. *Nonstationary Spatial Covariance Modeling Through Spatial Deformation*; Pan-American Advanced Study Institute on Spatio-Temporal Statistics: Búzios, Brazil, 2014.
31. Papaspiliopoulos, O.; Roberts, G.O.; Sköld, M. A General Framework for the Parametrization of Hierarchical Models. *Stat. Sci.* **2007**, *22*, 59–73. [CrossRef]
32. Carpenter, B.; Gelman, A.; Hoffman, M.D.; Lee, D.; Goodrich, B.; Betancourt, M.; Brubaker, M.; Guo, J.; Li, P.; Riddell, A. Stan: A Probabilistic Programming Language. *J. Stat. Softw.* **2017**, *76*, 1–32. [CrossRef] [PubMed]
33. Pettit, L.I. The Conditional Predictive Ordinate for the Normal Distribution. *J. R. Stat. Society. Ser. B (Methodol.)* **1990**, *52*, 175–184. [CrossRef]
34. Spiegelhalter, D.J.; Best, N.G.; Carlin, B.P.; van der Linde, A. Bayesian measures of model complexity and fit. *J. R. Stat. Soc. Ser. B (Stat. Methodol.)* **2002**, *64*, 583–639. [CrossRef]
35. Winkler, R.L. A Decision-Theoretic Approach to Interval Estimation. *J. Am. Stat. Assoc.* **1972**, *67*, 187–191. [CrossRef]
36. Quintana, M.S.B. Bayesian Modeling for Spatial Point Process with Nonstationary Covariance Structure via Spatial Deformations. Unpublished D.Sc. Thesis, Graduate Program of Statistics, Universidade Federal do Rio de Janeiro, Rio de Janeiro, Brazil, 2022.
37. Nava, D.T.; Nicolis, O.; Uribe-Opazo, M.A.; De Bastiani, F. Statistical methods for identifying anisotropy in the Spodoptera frugiperda spatial distribution. *Span. J. Agric. Res.* **2018**, *16*, e1003. [CrossRef]
38. Guan, Y.; Sherman, M.; Calvin, J.A. Assessing Isotropy for Spatial Point Processes. *Biometrics* **2005**, *62*, 119–125. [CrossRef]
39. Mateu, J.; Nicolis, O. Multiresolution analysis of linearly oriented spatial point patterns. *J. Stat. Comput. Simul.* **2013**, *85*, 621–637. [CrossRef]
40. Banerjee, S.; Carlin, B.P.; Gelfand, A.E. *Hierarchical Modeling and Analysis for Spatial Data*; Chapman and Hall/CRC: New York, NY, USA, 2014. [CrossRef]

entropy

MDPI

Article

# Dose Finding in Oncology Trials Guided by Ordinal Toxicity Grades Using Continuous Dose Levels

**Mourad Tighiouart** [1,*,†,‡] **and André Rogatko** [2,†]

[1] Department of Computational Biomedicine, Cedars-Sinai Medical Center, Los Angeles, CA 90069, USA
[2] Independent Researcher, 2765-399 Monte Estoril, Portugal
* Correspondence: mourad.tighiouart@cshs.org
† These authors contributed equally to this work.
‡ Current address: Cedars-Sinai Medical Center, 700 N San Vicente Blvd., Pacific Design Center G-589, West Hollywood, CA 90069, USA.

**Abstract:** We present a Bayesian adaptive design for dose finding in oncology trials with application to a first-in-human trial. The design is based on the escalation with overdose control principle and uses an intermediate grade 2 toxicity in addition to the traditional binary indicator of dose-limiting toxicity (DLT) to guide the dose escalation and de-escalation. We model the dose–toxicity relationship using the proportional odds model. This assumption satisfies an important ethical concern when a potentially toxic drug is first introduced in the clinic; if a patient experiences grade 2 toxicity at the most, then the amount of dose escalation is lower relative to that wherein if this patient experienced a maximum of grade 1 toxicity. This results in a more careful dose escalation. The performance of the design was assessed by deriving the operating characteristics under several scenarios for the true MTD and expected proportions of grade 2 toxicities. In general, the trial design is safe and achieves acceptable efficiency of the estimated MTD for a planned sample size of twenty patients. At the time of writing this manuscript, twelve patients have been enrolled to the trial.

**Keywords:** cancer phase I trials; maximum tolerated dose; ordinal toxicity grade; proportional odds model; overdose control; continuous dose

## 1. Introduction

Phase 1 clinical trials in oncology are usually small studies to test the safety and tolerability of first-in-human cancer drugs or a combination of existing ones. These trials are generally open to a heterogeneous population of cancer patients with late-stage disease who have exhausted all standard therapy [1]. As a result, ethical issues have been raised by many authors due to targeting vulnerable patients [2–4], potential risks to patients with low therapeutic effects [5–7], and an improbable expectation of benefits from the patients' perspectives [8–11]. However, owing to the development of targeted agents and immune checkpoint inhibitors, a recent study analyzing 465 clinical protocols of cancer phase 1 trials showed that the response rate doubled over the past two decades, reaching 18% in the last 10 years, while the risk of treatment-related deaths remained unchanged, at less than 1% [12]. In this manuscript, we are concerned with cancer phase I trials whose primary endpoint is the determination of the maximum tolerated dose (MTD) or recommended phase 2 dose (RP2D). This is defined as the dose $\gamma$ that is expected to produce dose-limiting toxicity (DLT) within one or more cycles of treatment in a prespecified proportion $\theta$ of patients:

$$P(\text{DLT}|\text{Dose} = \gamma) = \theta. \tag{1}$$

The number of prespecified cycles of therapy to resolve the DLT status of a patient for the purpose of dose escalation and de-escalation depends on the nature of treatment and schedule of administration. For example, if only immunotherapy agents are used, then the DLT window of time to resolve toxicity is often taken as two cycles of treatment. For treatment involving radiation therapy with expected late-onset toxicity, an observation window of four to six cycles is taken instead.

The definition of DLT depends on the expected treatment-related side effects or toxicities graded according to the Common Terminology Criteria for Adverse Events (CTCAE) version 5 [13]. For safety and ethical reasons, these trials enroll successive cohorts of patients starting with the minimum dose available in the trial or a dose deemed safe by the investigator, and the dose allocated to the next cohort of patients depends on the doses and toxicity outcomes of the previously treated patients. To this end, statistical designs have been studied extensively over the last three decades and shown to be safe and efficient in estimating the MTD. These include parametric models such as the continual reassessment method (CRM) [14], escalation with overdose control (EWOC) [15–17], the Bayesian logistic regression model (BLRM) [18], semi-parametric design [19], and nonparametric dose finding methods including the modified toxicity probability interval (mTPI) [20], Bayesian optimal interval design (BOIN) [21], and the nonparametric overdose control method [22].

The vast majority of statistical designs for phase 1 trials that are used in practice assume that the DLT is a binary indicator of toxicity, typically taking the value 1 if a patient experiences a grade 3 or 4 non-hemathologic or grade 4 hemathologic toxicity, and zero otherwise, despite the fact that many authors extended these designs to account for multiple toxicity types and grades using ordinal toxicity and quasi-continuous grades (see, e.g., [23–33]). Indeed, some of these methods have shown that accounting for lower grade toxicities may result in less patients being overdosed when the true MTD is near the minimum dose level available in the trial. In this manuscript, we extend the design in [24] by allowing the MTD to be outside the dose range with positive probability a priori using the model reparameterization introduced in [34]. This design is based on the EWOC principle by guiding dose escalation using grade 2 toxicity in addition to the binary indicator of DLT. This extension was motivated by a conversation with a clinician for the purpose of designing a first-in-human trial where it is desirable to have a more careful dose escalation and there is high uncertainty regarding the maximum available dose in the trial obtained from preclinical experiments. We show that our design addresses the ethical concerns regarding dose escalation in the presence of low-grade toxicity and the absence of DLT; if a patient experiences grade 2 toxicity at the most, then the size of the dose escalation is lower relative to that which would've occurred had the current patient experienced a maximum of grade 1 toxicity. Moreover, the design is coherent in both escalation and de-escalation.

The article is organized as follows. In Section 2, we present the dose–toxicity model for ordinal toxicity grades and the dose escalation algorithm EWOC scheme. Properties of the design to address some of the ethical concerns in first-in-human trials are described in Section 3. In Section 4, we apply our methodology to design a real-life phase 1 trial with continuous dose levels and assess the performance of the design by simulating trials under several scenarios for the location of the true MTD and rates of grade 2 toxicity. We conclude our manuscript with a discussion in Section 5.

## 2. Materials and Methods

### 2.1. Model

Let $X_{\min}$ and $X_{\max}$ be the minimum and maximum doses available in the trial, $X_{\min} > 0$. We assume that all CTCAE toxicities and their respective grades are collected by the end of the first treatment cycle so that the DLT observation window is one cycle of treatment. Following the work of [24], let $G = 0, 1, \ldots, 4$ be the maximum grade of any type of toxicity experienced by a patient by the end of cycle 1. Define

$$Y = \begin{cases} 0 & \text{if } G = 0,1 \\ 1 & \text{if } G = 2 \\ 2 & \text{if } G = 3,4, \end{cases}$$

where the event $Y = 2$ corresponds to a DLT. The dose–toxicity association is modeled using a known strictly increasing cumulative distribution function (cdf) $F(\cdot)$ as follows:

$$P(Y \geq j|x) = F(\eta_j + \beta x), j = 1, 2, \quad (2)$$

where $x \in [X_{\min}, X_{\max}]$, $\eta_1, \eta_2$ are the model intercepts and $\beta$ is the slope parameters of a proportional odds model. The parameters $\eta_1, \eta_2$ represent the logarithm of the odds of grade 2 or more toxicity and logarithm of the odds of DLT in the absence of treatment, respectively. We further assume that the probability of DLT is a non-decreasing function of dose, i.e., $\beta \geq 0$. By definition, the MTD, $\gamma$, which is the parameter of interest, is the maximum dose that is expected to produce DLT in a prespecified proportion $\theta$ of patients:

$$P(\text{DLT}|x) = P(Y = 2|x = \gamma) = F(\eta_2 + \beta\gamma) = \theta. \quad (3)$$

The value of the target probability of DLT $\theta$ is set to be relatively high when the DLT is a transient, correctable, or nonfatal condition and low when it is lethal or life threatening; see [35–37] for examples of phase 1 trials with $\theta = 0.1, 0.25$, and 0.33, respectively.

### 2.2. Likelihood and Model Reparameterization

Let $D_n = \{(x_i, Yi), i = 1, \ldots, n\}$ be the data after $n$ patients complete the first cycle of therapy and their toxicity status has been resolved. The likelihood for the parameters $\eta_1, \eta_2, \beta$ is

$$\begin{aligned} L_n(\eta_1, \eta_2, \beta|D_n) = \prod_{i=1}^{n} &[1 - F(\eta_1 + \beta x_i)]^{I(Y_i=0)}[F(\eta_1 + \beta x_i) - F(\eta_2 + \beta x_i)]^{I(Y_i=1)} \\ &\times [F(\eta_2 + \beta x_i)]^{I(Y_i=2)}, \end{aligned} \quad (4)$$

where $I(\cdot)$ is the indicator function.

We reparameterize model (2) in terms of parameters clinicians can easily interpret. Unlike the reparameterization in [24], which assumes that the MTD is in $[X_{\min}, X_{\max}]$ with prior probability 1, we adopt the reparameterization in [34], which allows for a positive prior probability that $\gamma$ is outside the dose range $[X_{\min}, X_{\max}]$. Specifically, let $\rho_0$ be the probability of DLT at $X_{\min}$, $\rho_1$ be the probability of grade 2 or more toxicity at $X_{\min}$, and $\rho_2$ be the probability of DLT at $X_{\max}$. It follows that

$$\begin{cases} \eta_1 = & F^{-1}(\rho_1) - (F^{-1}(\rho_2) - F^{-1}(\rho_0))(X_{\min}/(X_{\max} - X_{\min})) \\ \eta_2 = & F^{-1}(\rho_2) - (F^{-1}(\rho_2) - F^{-1}(\rho_0))(X_{\max}/(X_{\max} - X_{\min})) \\ \beta = & (F^{-1}(\rho_2) - F^{-1}(\rho_0))/(X_{\max} - X_{\min}). \end{cases} \quad (5)$$

We standardize the doses to be in the interval $[0, 1]$ using the transformation $h(u) = (u - X_{\min})/(X_{\max} - X_{\min})$ and define

$$\begin{aligned} F_1(\rho_0, \rho_1, \rho_2; x) = & \; F\left[F^{-1}(\rho_1) + (F^{-1}(\rho_2) - F^{-1}(\rho_0))x\right] \\ F_2(\rho_0, \rho_1, \rho_2; x) = & \; F\left[F^{-1}(\rho_0) + (F^{-1}(\rho_2) - F^{-1}(\rho_0))x\right] \end{aligned} \quad (6)$$

It follows that the likelihood of the reparameterized model is

$$\begin{aligned} L_n(\rho_0, \rho_1, \rho_2|D_n) = \prod_{i=1}^{n} &[1 - F_1(\rho_0, \rho_1, \rho_2; x_i)]^{I(Y_i=0)}[F_1(\rho_0, \rho_1, \rho_2; x_i) - F_2(\rho_0, \rho_1, \rho_2; x_i)]^{I(Y_i=1)} \\ &\times [F_2(\rho_0, \rho_1, \rho_2; x_i)]^{I(Y_i=2)}. \end{aligned} \quad (7)$$

### 2.3. Prior Specification

The monotonicity assumption of the dose–toxicity relationship implies that $0 \leq \rho_0 \leq \rho_2 \leq 1$. Furthermore, the proportional odds model assumption (2) implies that $\eta_2 \leq \eta_1$. Using (5), this leads to $0 \leq \rho_0 \leq \rho_1 \leq 1$. We therefore specify a prior distribution $g(\rho_0, \rho_1, \rho_2)$ as follows: $\rho_1, \rho_2$ are independent, $\rho_j \sim \text{beta}(a_j, b_j), j = 1, 2$ and given $\{\rho_1, \rho_2\}$,

$\rho_0/\min(\rho_1,\rho_2) \sim \text{beta}(a_0,b_0)$. Using Bayes' rule, the posterior distribution of the model parameters is

$$\pi(\rho_0,\rho_1,\rho_2|D_n) \propto L(\rho_0,\rho_1,\rho_2|D_n) \times g(\rho_0,\rho_1,\rho_2). \quad (8)$$

Features of this posterior distribution can be estimated using JAGS [38].

### 2.4. Trial Design

In this section, we describe the general EWOC design for continuous dose levels. The criteria for dose allocation to successive cohorts of patients is based on controlling the posterior probability that the MTD $\gamma$ exceeds the recommended dose level for the next cohort of patients.

The parameter of interest $\gamma$ in the standardized scale can be obtained from (3):

$$\gamma = \frac{F^{-1}(\theta) - F^{-1}(\rho_0)}{F^{-1}(\rho_2) - F^{-1}(\rho_0)}\, I\left(\gamma > \frac{-X_{\min}}{X_{\max} - X_{\min}}\right), \quad (9)$$

where $I(\cdot)$ is the indicator function. The lower bound $l_b = -X_{\min}/(X_{\max} - X_{\min})$ results from the transformation $h(\cdot)$ and the fact that unstandardized doses $x$ are positive.

Let $n$ be the maximum number of patients to be enrolled in the trial. The first cohort of patients receive the dose $x = X_{\min}$. Denote by $\Pi_k(\gamma) = \Pi(\gamma|D_k)$ the marginal posterior cdf of the MTD, $k = 1,\ldots,n-1$. The next cohort of patients receive the dose $x_{k+1} = \Pi_k^{-1}(\alpha)$. In other words, the dose allocated to the next patient(s) is chosen such that the posterior probability that it exceeds the MTD, given the current data, is bounded by $\alpha$. This is known as the overdose protection property of EWOC, where at each dose allocation stage of the trial, we seek a dose that controls the posterior probability of exposing patients to toxic dose levels. At the end of the trial, we estimate the MTD as the median of the posterior distribution of $\gamma$, $\pi(\gamma|D_n)$. Other design considerations such as size of the cohorts, size of the dose escalation, and stopping rules for safety are described in the phase 1 trial example of DZ-002.

## 3. Design Properties

The design described in Section 2.4 has the following properties:

(i) Overdose Control: Each time patients are ready to be enrolled to the trial, we seek a dose to allocate to these patients while controlling the posterior probability of exposing them to toxic dose levels.

(ii) Toxicity-Dependent Dose Escalation: If the maximum grade of toxicity experienced by patient $k$ is grade 2, then the dose allocated to patient $k+1$ is lower than the dose that would have been given to patient $k+1$ had the maximum grade of toxicity experienced by patient $k$ been grade 0 or 1.

(iii) Coherence: If patient $k$ treated at dose level $x_k$ experiences DLT, then the dose $x_{k+1}$ allocated to patient $k+1$ satisfies $x_{k+1} \leq x_k$. Similarly, if patient $k$ does not experience DLT and has no grade 2 toxicity, then the dose $x_{k+1}$ allocated to patient $k+1$ satisfies $x_{k+1} \geq x_k$.

Property (i) is the overdose protection defining characteristic of EWOC and was first introduced in [15,39]. Under the one-parameter logistic link function $F(u) = (1+e^{-u})^{-1}$ and the assumption of bounded support for the MTD $\gamma$ a priori, ref. [39] showed that the sequence of doses generated by the EWOC algorithm minimizes the amount by which patients are underdosed and converges to $\gamma$ in probability. Property (ii) implies a cautious dose escalation and is particularly appealing for drugs used in first-in-human trials; if a patient experiences grade 2 toxicity, then it is ethical not to increase the dose by the same amount had this patient exhibited grade 1 toxicity at the most. The last property is the coherence principle introduced in [40], which states that it is ethical not to increase a dose for the next patient if the previously treated patient exhibited DLT when given the same dose level. Properties (ii) and (iii) are summarized in the following theorems.

**Theorem 1.** *Let $D_k = \{(x_i, Y_i), i = 1, \ldots, k\}$ be the data on the first k patients according to the EWOC algorithm and $D_k^{'} = D_{k-1} \cup \{(x_k, Y_k^{'})\}$. Let $x_{k+1} = \Pi_k^{-1}(\alpha|D_k)$ and $x_{k+1}^{'} = \Pi_k^{-1}(\alpha|D_k^{'})$, where $\Pi_k(\cdot|D_k)$ is the marginal posterior cdf of the MTD $\gamma$. Suppose that for all $x \in [X_{\min}, X_{\max}]$ and all $(\rho_0, \rho_1), 0 \leq \rho_0 \leq \rho_1 \leq 1, (F_1 - F_2)/(1 - F_1)$ is monotonically increasing in $\rho_2$. Then, $x_{k+1}^{'} \geq x_{k+1}$ whenever $Y_k^{'} = 0$ and $Y_k = 1$.*

**Theorem 2.** *Suppose that for all $x \in [X_{\min}, X_{\max}]$ and all $(\rho_0, \rho_1), 0 \leq \rho_0 \leq \rho_1 \leq 1, F_1$ and $F_2$ are monotonically increasing in $\rho_2$. Let $x_k$ be the dose allocated to patient k and $Y_k$ be the corresponding toxicity response. Then, if $Y_k = 2$, the dose $x_{k+1}$ allocated to the next patient satisfies $x_{k+1} \leq x_k$. Furthermore, if $Y_k = 0$, then $x_{k+1} \geq x_k$.*

The proofs of theorems 1 and 2 are similar to the proofs in [24] since (9) implies that $\gamma$ is a decreasing function of $\rho_2$ for fixed $\rho_0$ and the assumption of a bounded support for the MTD $\gamma$ in [24] was not used in the proof of those theorems.

## 4. Application to Real-Life Example

### 4.1. DZ-002 Phase 1 Trial

The methodology was applied to design and conduct a phase 1 trial using the drug DZ-002 in patients with advanced solid malignancies and lymphoma (see ClinicalTrials.gov NCT04970992). The active ingredient of DZ-002 is DZ-SIM, a heptamethine cyanine dye (HMCD)–simvastin conjugate aimed at specifically targeting cancer cells that have demonstrated superior cytotoxicity compared to SIM both in tumor cell cultures and xenograft models. The starting dose of DZ-002 is $X_{\min} = 0.8$ mg/kg IV, based on animal toxicity studies. The doses for subsequent patients will be based on the EWOC algorithm, taking into account grade 0 to 4 toxicities encountered in previously enrolled patients. The maximum planned dose will not exceed $X_{\max} = 15$ mg/kg IV. The MTD of DZ-002 is defined as the dose such that the probability of DLT at the MTD is $\theta = 0.33$. We used the logistic function $F(u) = (1 + e^{-u})^{-1}$ as the link function. It is easy to verify that this link function satisfies the monotonicity condition of theorem 1. The hyperparameters defining the prior distributions are $a_j = b_j = 1, j = 0, 1, 2$. The first cohort of up to 3 patients receives the minimum dose of 0.8 mg/kg and the dose for the subsequent cohort is determined according to the EWOC algorithm. Specifically, the dose for each subsequent cohort is determined so that, based on all available data, the posterior probability that the dose exceeds the MTD $\gamma$ is equal to a prespecified feasibility bound, $\alpha$. The feasibility bound starts at $\alpha = 0.1$, and increases to a maximum value of 0.5 by increments of 0.05 whenever a new dose allocation is computed, where this value is a compromise between the therapeutic aspect of the agent and its toxic side effects. Chu et al. [41] showed that in general, this design provides better protection in limiting higher doses for patients compared with four versions of CRM designs with a similar convergence rate. Note that the toxicity-dependent dose escalation condition (ii) in Section 3 will be satisfied when the feasibility bound $\alpha$ reaches 0.5 and may hold for $\alpha < 0.5$. If the EWOC algorithm recommends a dose lower than $X_{\min} = 0.8$ mg/kg, then 0.8 mg/kg is assigned to the next cohort of patients. Similarly, if the algorithm recommends a dose above $X_{\max} = 15$ mg/kg, then 0.8 mg/kg is assigned to the next cohort of patients. For ethical considerations, at any time during the trial, a patient may be enrolled if there are no more than two patients with unresolved DLT status in the study. In other words, if there are three patients under treatment who did not experience DLT and have not finished their cycle 1 therapy, then another patient cannot be enrolled. Further, the clinical investigator imposes a restriction on the increments of any dose escalation. Specifically, the increment of any dose escalation is restricted not to exceed 20% of the dose range (0.8, 15). The Food and Drug Administration (FDA) further imposed that dose escalation increments cannot exceed 2-fold of the current dose. In essence, our escalation scheme is more conservative than the FDA's recommendation for doses above 2.8 mg/kg IV. The trial plans to enroll a maximum of $n = 20$ patients. This study will be terminated if the posterior probability of the DLT at the minimum dose that exceeds $\theta$

is 0.8 or more. Furthermore, this study will be terminated if the posterior probability of the DLT at the maximum available dose that is less than $\theta$ is 0.9 or more. In this case, the recommended MTD is the maximum dose of 15 mg/kg. At the end of the study, the MTD will be estimated as the minimum of the median of the posterior distribution of the MTD, given the data and 15 mg/kg.

Figure 1 shows all the possible dose assignments to the first two patients and selected situations for patients 3 and 4, assuming that we treat successive cohorts of one patient and the toxicity status of a patient has been resolved before enrolling the next patient. The first patient is given a minimum dose of 0.8 mg/kg, and if this patient does not have grade 2 or more toxicity, patient # 2 will be given a dose of 1.6 mg/kg. The EWOC algorithm recommends a dose much higher than 1.6 mg/kg, but this dose satisfies the FDA 2-fold restriction. If the maximum grade of toxicity for patient # 1 is 2 ($G = 2$), than patient # 2 is assigned 1.2 mg/kg. If patients # 1, 2, and 3 do not experience grade 2 or more toxicities, then patient # 4 will be assigned 5.6 mg/kg according to the EWOC algorithm. On the other hand, if patient # 2 is treated with 1.6 mg/kg and experiences DLT, then the dose for patient # 3 decreases to 1.0 mg/kg according to the EWOC algorithm. This figure also shows that the next dose increment for a patient who experienced a maximum of grade 2 toxicity is smaller than the dose increment had this patient experienced no grade 2 or more toxicity. Furthermore, for doses greater than the minimum dose, the dose for the next patient is de-escalated form the current dose if the current patient experiences a DLT.

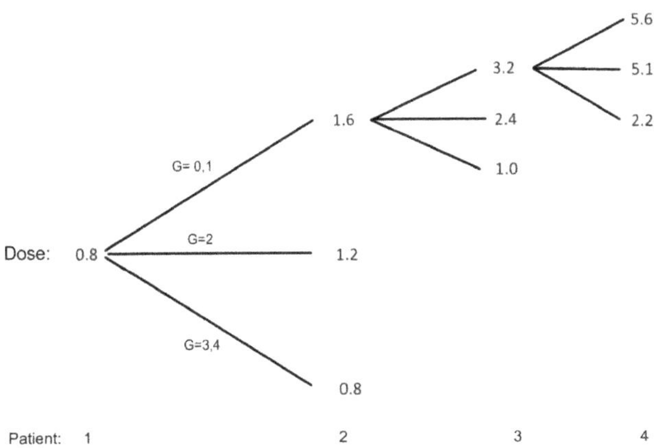


**Figure 1.** Possible dose allocation for patients 1 and 2 and selected situations for patients 3 and 4. G = 3, 4 corresponds to DLT.

## 4.2. Design Operating Characteristics

We evaluate the performance of this design under three scenarios for true MTD $\gamma$ and two values of $\rho_1$, the probability of grade 2 or more toxicity at $X_{\min}$ (see Table 1). An additional scenario # 7 was requested by the FDA. These scenarios reflect different locations for the true MTD in the interval $(0.8, 15.0)$ mg/kg and rates of grade 2 or more toxicities. The sample size used is $n = 20$ and $M = 2000$ trial replicates were simulated. DLTs and grade 2 or more toxicities were generated from the proportional odds model with logistic link function $F(u) = (1 + e^{-u})^{-1}$ so that the true and working models were the same. Operating characteristics under model misspecification were studied in [24] in the case of bounded support for the MTD $\gamma$ and Appendix A. Successive cohorts of one patient were treated starting with the minimum dose of 0.8 mg/kg and restrictions on dose escalation increments by the investigators and the FDA were implemented.

**Table 1.** Operating characteristics under seven scenarios.

| Scenarios | | Safety | | Efficiency | | |
|---|---|---|---|---|---|---|
| # I ($\rho_0, \rho_1, \rho_2$) | True MTD (mg/kg) | Ave DLT Rate | % Trials withDLT Rate > $\theta + 0.1$ | Estimated MTD | Average Bias | Percent Selection |
| 1: (0.12,0.50,0.95) | 4.53 | 0.38 | 22% | 5.04 | 1.30 | 65% |
| 2: (0.03,0.50,0.90) | 7.76 | 0.33 | 5% | 7.94 | 0.98 | 64% |
| 3: (0.01,0.50,0.40) | 14.02 | 0.22 | 0.0% | 13.6 | −0.36 | 78% |
| 4: (0.12,0.80,0.95) | 4.53 | 0.38 | 23% | 5.09 | 1.35 | 65% |
| 5: (0.03,0.80,0.90) | 7.76 | 0.34 | 5% | 7.96 | 0.99 | 63% |
| 6: (0.01,0.80,0.40) | 14.02 | 0.23 | 0% | 13.72 | −0.33 | 80% |
| 7: (0.20,0.30,0.70) | 5.21 | 0.35 | 12% | 6.56 | 1.98 | 74% |

Table 1 gives the operating characteristics in terms of safety and efficiency of the estimated MTD. The estimated MTD is obtained by averaging the 2000 estimated MTDs, and the average bias is across all simulated trials. The percent selection column is defined as the percent of trials that recommend a dose with probability of DLT within 10% of the target probability of DLT $\theta = 0.33$. The average DLT rate is around the target probability of DLT $\theta = 0.33$ in all scenarios except when the true MTD is near the maximum dose (scenarios 3 and 6). In these cases, the average DLT rate is about 10% lower than the target. The percent of trials with an excessive rate of DLT, defined as more than an absolute 10% above the target, is small in all scenarios except when the true MTD is near the minimum dose; when the true MTD is 4.53 mg/kg, the estimated probability that a prospective trial results in a DLT rate above $\theta + 0.1$ is about 0.23. In general, the trial is safe when the true MTD is not located near the minimum dose. This is consistent with model-based and nonparameteric designs of cancer phase 1 trials. With respect to efficiency, in all scenarios, the estimated MTD is reasonably close to the true MTD and the percent selection is very high when the true MTD is near the maximum dose (scenarios 3 and 6), i.e., scenarios that are expected by the clinician. We also note the contribution of using grade 2 toxicity to guide the dose escalation in addition to DLT. For instance, scenarios 4 and 7 are cases where the true MTD is low. However, the percent selection for scenario 7 is 74% compared to 65% for scenario 4. This is due to the small probability of grade 2 or more DLT for scenario 7 ($\rho_1 = 0.3$) compared to $\rho_1 = 0.8$ for scenario 4. With a high rate of grade 2 or more toxicity, dose escalation is slower.

The gray bar-plots in Figure 2 show the impact of the probability of grade 2 or more toxicity $\rho_2$ on the safety of the trial and efficiency of the estimated MTD. For fixed values of the true MTD, the maximum change in the absolute average bias is 0.15 mg/kg, which is negligible for practical purposes, as $\rho_2$ varies from 0.3 to 0.8. When the true MTD is small (1.6 mg/kg), the average DLT rate decreases by an absolute 2% when $\rho_2$ increases from 0.3 to 0.8. For a large value of the MTD (12.4 mg/kg), the percent of patients that were overdosed across all trials decreases by an absolute 6% from 23% to 17% when $\rho_2$ increases from 0.3 to 0.8. Here, a dose $x$ is defined as an overdose if $x > x^*$, where $x^*$ is defined as the dose for which $P(Y = 1|x^*) = \theta + 0.1$. This observation illustrates the importance of including grade 2 toxicities in the model for treatments that are expected to produce a high proportion of these toxicities. The differences may be larger for larger sample sizes. In conclusion, the design is reasonably safe and efficient for a sample size of $n = 20$.

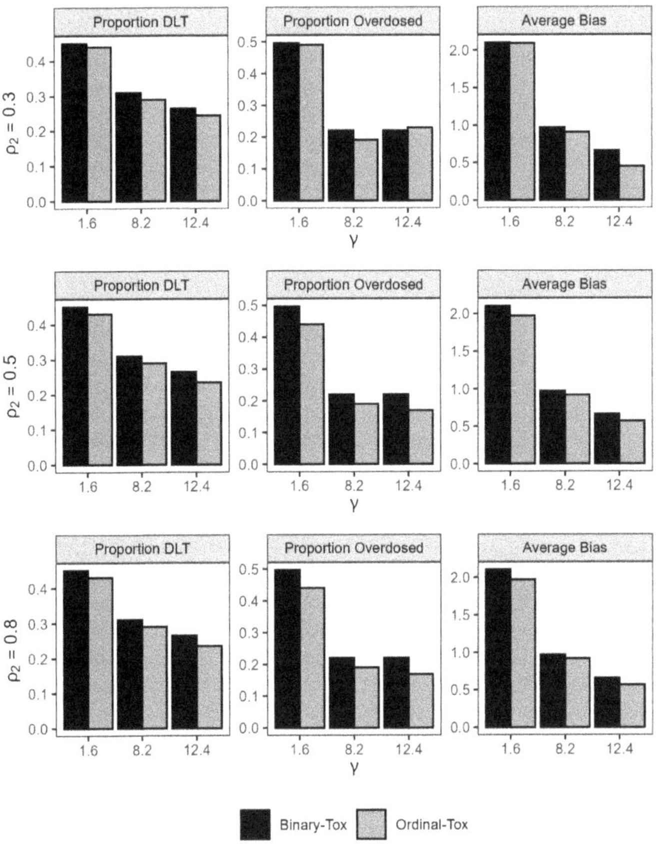


**Figure 2.** Summary statistics for trial safety and efficiency under ordinal toxicity and binary toxicity models under all scenarios.

## 4.3. Comparing Ordinal Toxicity to Binary Toxicity

We further compared the performance of the proportional odds model (2) (ordinal toxicity) to the traditional model that does not account for grade 2 toxicity (binary toxicity). Specifically, the binary toxicity model assumes that

$$Y = \begin{cases} 0 & \text{if } G = 0,1,2 \\ 1 & \text{if } G = 3,4, \end{cases}$$

where the event $Y = 1$ corresponds to a DLT. The dose–toxicity association is modeled using a known strictly increasing cumulative distribution function (cdf) $F(\cdot)$, as follows:

$$P(Y = 1|x) = F(\eta + \beta x). \tag{10}$$

The performance of these models was assessed by simulating 2000 trail replicates using the same settings of Section 4.2 under three scenarios for the true MTD $\gamma = 1.6, 8.2,$ 12.4 mg/kg and three probabilities of grade 2 or more toxicity $\rho_2 = 0.3, 0.5, 0.8$ for a total of nine scenarios. In addition to the average DLT rate and absolute average bias across all trials, we also compared the models with respect to the proportion of patients that were overdosed.

Figure 2 shows that the average rate of DLTs is always smaller for the model that accounts for a grade 2 toxicity relative to the binary toxicity model across all scenarios with the largest difference of 3% achieved when the true MTD is near the minimum dose and the true probability of grade 2 or more toxicity is high ($\rho_2 = 0.8$). Similarly, the proportion of patients that were overdosed is lower when we account for a grade 2 toxicity in eight out of the nine scenarios, with the highest difference achieved when the true MTD is 1.6 mg/kg and $\rho_2$ is high. As for efficiency of the estimated MTD, the absolute average bias is uniformly smaller for the ordinal toxicity model relative to the binary toxicity model across all scenarios. These results are generally consistent with the findings in [24].

## 5. Discussion

In this manuscript, we described a Bayesian adaptive scheme to design and conduct a first-in-human dose finding trial in oncology. To the best of our knowledge, this is the first application of a real phase 1 trial that uses continuous dose levels and is guided by DLT as well as grade 2 toxicity outcomes. Unlike phase 1 trials that use accelerated titration [42] for the first few patients in the trial, our design uses lower-grade toxicity outcomes throughout the trial. The grouping of toxicities into three categories was selected based on the discussion with the clinician, who felt that a grade 2 toxicity should inform us that the dose causing this type of toxicity is an indication that we may be close to reaching the MTD. Comparison of the performance of this model with the one that retains the original toxicity grades as a function of sample size will be investigated in future work. The trial is ongoing and at the time of writing this manuscript, about 12 patients have been enrolled to the trial. Our approach is appropriate for handling the ethical concern regarding dose escalation in the presence of low-grade toxicity and the absence of DLT. For instance, if a patient experiences grade 2 toxicity at the most, then it is ethical not to escalate the dose for the next patient by the same amount as the one had the current patient experienced a maximum of grade 1 toxicity. This is particularly important for first-in-human trials where a more careful dose escalation scheme is warranted. In addition, the coherence in escalation and de-escalation principles introduced by the authors of [40] holds under the proportional odds model assumption (2). Finally, an additional restriction on the size of dose escalation is imposed whenever the EWOC algorithm recommends an increase in dose for the next cohort of patients. The clinician selected an increase of no more than 20% of the dose range, which is more conservative than the 2-fold recommendation from the FDA for doses above 2.8 mg/kg. Our design achieves reasonable operating characteristics under the proportional odds model, a relatively small sample size, and three unknown parameters $\rho_0, \rho_1, \rho_2$ with vague prior distributions. In practice, it is important to calibrate the prior hyperparameters following conversations with the clinician regarding the uncertainty of the location of the true MTD. For instance, expert opinion from the clinician regarding the a priori probabilities that the true MTD is above the maximum and below the minimum doses, and effective sample size may be specified to determine the hyperparameters.

**Author Contributions:** Methodology, M.T. and A.R. All authors have read and agreed to the published version of the manuscript.

**Funding:** This work is partially funded by the National Center for Advancing Translational Sciences (NCATS) UCLA CTSI (UL1 TR001881-01), NCI grant P01 CA233452-02, U01 grant CA232859-05, and 3U01CA232859-05S1.

**Institutional Review Board Statement:** The study was conducted in accordance with the Declaration of Helsinki, and approved by the Institutional Review Board of Cedars-sinai Medical Center (IRB # 01430 on April 2021).

**Data Availability Statement:** The original contributions presented in the study are included in the article, further inquiries can be directed to the corresponding author.

**Conflicts of Interest:** Mourad Tighiouart is a consultant for Da Zen Theranostics Inc., the sponsor of the trial as of 05/2024. The remaining author declares that the research was conducted in the absence of any commercial or financial relationships that could be construed as a potential conflict of interest.

## Appendix A. Model Robustness

We assessed model misspecification with respect to the proportional odds model assumption (2) by generating the toxicity responses from a non-proportional odds model:

$$P(Y \geq j|x) = F(\eta_j + \beta_j x), j = 1, 2. \tag{A1}$$

Figure A1 shows the probability of DLT as a function of dose for the true proportional odds model $M_0$ shown by the black solid curve and the two misspecified non-proportional odds models $M_1$ and $M_2$ shown by the blue and red curves, respectively. The corresponding model parameters $\alpha_j, \beta_j, j = 1, 2$ are shown in Table A1. These parameters have been selected so that the three models have the same MTD $\gamma = 7.76$ mg/kg. The probability of grade 2 or more toxicity as a function of dose is shown by a dashed black curve. The operating characteristics were derived under the same settings of Section 4.2 using the logistic link function $F(u) = (1 + e^{-u})^{-1}$ in Equation (A1).

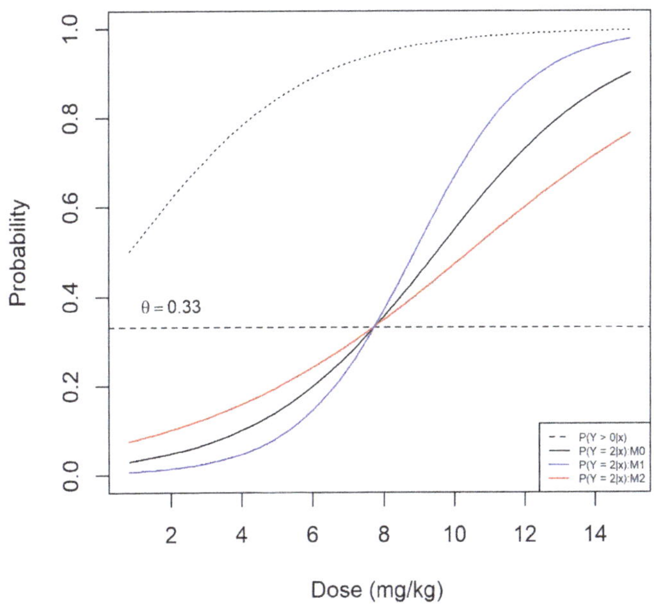


**Figure A1.** Dose–toxicity relationship under the proportional odds model (black solid curve) and non-proportional odds models $M_1$ and $M_2$ when the true MTD is $\gamma = 7.76$ mg/kg. The black dashed curve corresponds to the probability of grade 2 or more toxicity.

Table A1 shows that the average DLT rate across all 2000 simulated trials is 0.33 for models $M_0$ and $M_1$ and 0.32 for model $M_2$. The maximum difference in the percent of trials with an excessive rate of DLT between the true model $M_0$ and misspecified models is 2%. Similarly, the largest absolute difference in the average bias between the true and misspecified models is 0.25 mg/kg. Lastly, the percent selection of the misspecified models are within 3% of the true model $M_0$. We conclude that the proportional odds model are fairly robust to small deviations from the true model around the MTD.

**Table A1.** Operating characteristics under seven scenarios.

| Scenarios | | Safety | | | Efficiency | |
|---|---|---|---|---|---|---|
| Model | True MTD (mg/kg) | Ave DLT Rate | % Trials with DLT Rate > $\theta + 0.1$ | Estimated MTD | Average Bias | Percent Selection |
| $M_0$ $(\eta_1, \eta_2, \beta)$ $(0, -3.47, 5.67)$ | 7.76 | 0.33 | 5% | 7.94 | 0.98 | 64% |
| $M_1$ $(\eta_1, \eta_2, \beta_1, \beta_2)$ $(0, -3.47, 5.67, 8.78)$ | 7.76 | 0.33 | 2.0% | 7.79 | 0.82 | 61% |
| $M_2$ $(\eta_1, \eta_2, \beta_1, \beta_2)$ $(0, -3.47, 5.67, 3.68)$ | 7.76 | 0.32 | 3.3% | 8.19 | 1.23 | 67% |

## References


1. Roberts, T.G.; Goulart, B.H.; Squitieri, L.; Stallings, S.C.; Halpern, E.F.; Chabner, B.A.; Gazelle, G.S.; Finkelstein, S.N.; Clark, J.W. Trends in the risks and benefits to patients with cancer participating in phase 1 clinical trials. *J. Am. Med. Assoc.* **2004**, *292*, 2130–2140. [CrossRef] [PubMed]
2. Lipsett, M.B. On the nature and ethics of phase I clinical trials of cancer chemotherapies. *J. Am. Med. Assoc.* **1982**, *248*, 941–942. [CrossRef]
3. Emanuel, E.J. A phase I trial on the ethics of phase I trials. *J. Clin. Oncol.* **1995**, *13*, 1049–1051. [CrossRef] [PubMed]
4. Cox, K.; Avis, M. Ethical and practical problems of early anti-cancer drug trials: A review of the literature. *Eur. J. Cancer Care (Engl.)* **1996**, *5*, 90–95. [CrossRef]
5. Estey, E.; Hoth, D.; Simon, R.; Marsoni, S.; Leyland-Jones, B.; Wittes R. Therapeutic response in phase I trials of antineoplastic agents. *Cancer Treat. Rep.* **1986**, *70*, 1105–1115. [PubMed]
6. Decoster, G.; Stein, G.; Holdener, E.E. Responses and toxic deaths in phase I clinical trials. *Ann. Oncol.* **1990**, *1*, 175–181. [CrossRef] [PubMed]
7. Von Hoff, D.D.; Turner, J. Response rates, duration of response, and dose response effects in phase I studies of antineoplastics. *Investig. New Drugs* **1991**, *9*, 115–122. [CrossRef] [PubMed]
8. Daugherty, C.; Ratain, M.J.; Grochowski, E.; Stocking, C.; Kodish, E.; Mick, R.; Siegler, M. Perceptions of cancer patients and their physicians involved in phase I trials. *J. Clin. Oncol.* **1995**, *13*, 1062–1072. [CrossRef] [PubMed]
9. Meropol, N.J.; Weinfurt, K.P.; Burnett, C.B.; Balshem, A.; Benson, A.B.; Castel, L.; Corbett, S.; Diefenbach, M.; Gaskin, D.; Li, Y.; et al. Perceptions of patients and physicians regarding phase I cancer clinical trials: Implications for physician-patient communication. *J. Clin. Oncol.* **2003**, *21*, 2589–2596. [CrossRef]
10. Cheng, J.D.; Hitt, J.; Koczwara, B.; Schulman, K.A.; Burnett, C.B.; Gaskin, D.J.; Rowland, J.H.; Meropol, N.J. Impact of quality of life on patient expectations regarding phase I clinical trials. *J. Clin. Oncol.* **2000**, *18*, 421–428. [CrossRef]
11. Horng, S.; Emanuel, E.J.; Wilfond, B.; Rackoff, J.; Martz, K.; Grady, C. Descriptions of benefits and risks in consent forms for phase 1 oncology trials. *N. Engl. J. Med.* **2002**, *347*, 2134–2140. [CrossRef]
12. Chihara, D.; Lin, R.; Flowers, C.R.; Finnigan, S.R.; Cordes, L.M.; Fukuda, Y.; Huang, E.P.; Rubinstein, L.V.; Nastoupil, L.J.; Ivy, S.P.; et al. Early drug development in solid tumours: Analysis of National Cancer Institute-sponsored phase 1 trials. *Lancet* **2022**, *400*, 512–521. [CrossRef]
13. U.S. Department of Health and Human Services. *Common Terminology Criteria for Adverse Events (CTCAE)*, Version 5.0; U.S. Department of Health and Human Services: Washington, DC, USA, 2017.
14. O'Quigley, J.; Pepe, M.; Fisher, L. Continual reassessment method: A practical design for phase 1 clinical trials in cancer. *Biometrics* **1990**, *46*, 33–48. [CrossRef]
15. Babb, J.S.; Rogatko, A.; Zacks, S. Cancer Phase I clinical trials: Efficient dose escalation with overdose control. *Stat. Med.* **1998**, *17*, 1103–1120. [CrossRef]
16. Tighiouart, M.; Rogatko, A.; Babb, J.S. Flexible Bayesian methods for cancer phase I clinical trials. Dose escalation with overdose control. *Stat. Med.* **2005**, *24*, 2183–2196. [CrossRef]
17. Tighiouart, M.; Rogatko, A. Dose finding with escalation with overdose control (EWOC) in cancer clinical trials. *Stat. Sci.* **2010**, *25*, 217–226. [CrossRef]
18. Neuenschwander, B.; Branson, M.; Gsponer, T. Critical aspects of the Bayesian approach to phase I cancer trials. *Stat. Med.* **2008**, *27*, 2420–2439. [CrossRef]
19. Clertant, M.; O'Quigley, J. Semiparametric dose finding methods. *J. R. Stat. Ser. B (Stat. Methodol.)* **2017**, *79*, 1487–1508. [CrossRef]

20. Ji, Y.; Wang, S.J. Modified toxicity probability interval design: a safer and more reliable method than the 3+3 design for practical phase I trials. *J. Clin. Oncol.* **2013**, *31*, 1785–1791. [CrossRef]
21. Liu, S.; Yuan, Y. Bayesian optimal interval designs for phase I clinical trials. *J. R. Stat. Ser. C (Appl. Stat.)* **2015**, *64*, 507–523. [CrossRef]
22. Lin, R.; Yin, G. Nonparametric overdose control with late-onset toxicity in phase I clinical trials. *Biostatistics* **2017**, *18*, 180–194. [CrossRef]
23. Iasonos, A.; Zohar, S.; O'Quigley, J. Incorporating lower grade toxicity information into dose finding designs. *Clin. Trials* **2011**, *8*, 370–379. [CrossRef]
24. Tighiouart, M.; Cook-Wiens, G.; Rogatko, A. Escalation with overdose control using ordinal toxicity grades for cancer phase I clinical trials. *J. Probab. Stat.* **2012**, *2012*, 317634. [CrossRef]
25. Chen, Z.; Tighiouart, M.; Kowalski, J. Dose escalation with overdose control using a quasi-continuous toxicity score in cancer phase I clinical trials. *Contemp. Clin. Trials* **2012**, *33*, 949–958. [CrossRef]
26. Gordon, N.H.; Willson, J.K.V. Using toxicity grades in the design and analysis of cancer phase I clinical trials. *Stat. Med.* **1992**, *11*, 2063–2075. [CrossRef]
27. Wang, C.; Chen, T.T.; Tyan, I. Designs for phase I cancer clinical trials with differentiation of graded toxicity. *Commun. Stat.* **2000**, *29*, 975–987. [CrossRef]
28. Bekele, B.N.; Thall, P.F. Dose-finding based on multiple toxicities in a soft tissue sarcoma trial. *J. Am. Stat. Assoc.* **2004**, *99*, 26–35. [CrossRef]
29. Yuan, Z.; Chappell, R.; Bailey, H. The continual reassessment method for multiple toxicity grades: A Bayesian quasi-likelihood approach. *Biometrics* **2007**, *63*, 173–179. [CrossRef]
30. Potthoff, R.F.; George, S.L. Flexible phase I clinical trials: Allowing for nonbinary toxicity response and removal of other common limitations. *Stat. Biopharm. Res.* **2009**, *1*, 213–228. [CrossRef]
31. Van Meter, E.M.; Garrett-Mayer, E.; Bandyopadhyay, D. Proportional odds model for dose finding clinical trial designs with ordinal toxicity grading. *Stat. Med.* **2011**, *30*, 2070–2080. [CrossRef]
32. Lee, S.M.; Cheng, B.; Cheung, Y.K. Continual reassessment method with multiple toxicity constraints. *Biostatistics* **2011**, *12*, 386–398. [CrossRef]
33. Diniz, M.A.; Kim, S.; Tighiouart, M. A Bayesian adaptive design in cancer phase I trials using dose combinations with ordinal toxicity grades. *Stats* **2020**, *3*, 221–238. [CrossRef]
34. Tighiouart, M.; Cook-Wiens, G.; Rogatko, A. A Bayesian Adaptive Design for Cancer Phase I Trials Using a Flexible Range of Doses. *J. Biopharm. Stat.* **2018**, *28*, 562–574. [CrossRef]
35. Babb, J.S.; Rogatko, A. Patient specific dosing in a cancer phase I clinical trial. *Stat. Med.* **2001**, *20*, 2079–2090. [CrossRef]
36. Tuli, R.; Shiao, S.L.; Nissen, N.; Tighiouart, M.; Kim, S.; Osipov, A.; Bryant, M.; Ristow, L.; Placencio-Hickok, V.R.; Hoffman, D.; et al. A phase 1 study of veliparib, a PARP-1/2 inhibitor, with gemcitabine and radiotherapy in locally advanced pancreatic cancer. *EBioMedicine* **2019**, *40*, 375–381. [CrossRef]
37. Gong, J.; Thomassian, S.; Kim, S.; Gresham, G.; Moshayedi, N.; Ye, J.; Yang, J.; Jacobs, J.; Lo, S.; Nissen, N.; et al. Phase I Trial of Bermekimab with Nanoliposomal Irinotecan and 5-Fluorouracil/Folinic Acid in Advanced Pancreatic Ductal Adenocarcinoma. *Sci. Rep.* **2022**, *12*, 15013. [CrossRef]
38. Plummer, M. A program for analysis of Bayesian graphical models using Gibbs sampling. In Proceedings of the 3rd International Workshop on Distributed Statistical Computing, Vienna, Austria, 20–22 March 2003; Volume 124, pp. 1–10.
39. Zacks, S.; Rogatko, A.; Babb, J. Optimal Bayesian-feasibile dose escalation for cancer phase I trials. *Stat. Probab. Lett.* **1998**, *38*, 215–220. [CrossRef]
40. Cheung, Y.K. Coherence principles in dose-finding studies. *Biometrika* **2005**, *92*, 863–873. [CrossRef]
41. Chu, P.L.; Lin, Y.; Shih, W.J. Unifying CRM and EWOC designs for phase I cancer clinical trials. *J. Stat. Plan. Inference* **2009**, *139*, 1146–1163. [CrossRef]
42. Simon, R.; Rubinstein, L.; Arbuck, S.G.; Christian, M.C.; Freidlin, B.; Collins, J. Accelerated titration designs for phase I clinical trials in oncology. *J. Natl. Cancer Inst.* **1997**, *89*, 1138–1147. [CrossRef]

entropy

MDPI

Article

# Relative Belief Inferences from Decision Theory

**Michael Evans** [1,*,†] **and Gun Ho Jang** [2,†]

[1] Department of Statistical Sciences, University of Toronto, Toronto, ON M5G 1Z5, Canada
[2] Ontario Institute for Cancer Research, MaRS Centre, 661 University Avenue, Suite 510, Toronto, ON M5G 0A3, Canada; gjang@oicr.on.ca
[*] Correspondence: mevansthree.evans@utoronto.ca
[†] These authors contributed equally to this work.

**Abstract:** Relative belief inferences are shown to arise as Bayes rules or limiting Bayes rules. These inferences are invariant under reparameterizations and possess a number of optimal properties. In particular, relative belief inferences are based on a direct measure of statistical evidence.

**Keywords:** Bayesian inference; evidential inference; statistical evidence; relative belief; loss functions; Bayesian-unbiasedness; Bayes rules; admissibility; limits of Bayes rules

## 1. Introduction

We consider a sampling model for data $x$, as given by a collection of densities $\{f(\cdot \,|\, \theta) : \theta \in \Theta\}$ with respect to a support measure $\mu$ on a sample space $\mathcal{X}$, and a proper prior, given by density $\pi$ with respect to support measure $\nu$ on $\Theta$. When the data $x \in \mathcal{X}$ are observed, these ingredients lead to the posterior distribution on $\Theta$ with density given by $\pi(\theta \,|\, x) = \pi(\theta) f(x \,|\, \theta)/m(x)$ with respect to support measure $\nu$, where

$$m(x) = \int_\Theta \pi(\theta) f(x \,|\, \theta)\, \nu(d\theta)$$

is the prior predictive density of the data. In addition, there is a quantity of interest $\psi = \Psi(\theta)$, where

$$\Psi : \Theta \to \Psi(\Theta) = \{\psi : \psi = \Psi(\theta) \text{ for some } \theta \in \Theta\},$$

for which inferences, such as an estimate $\psi(x)$ or a hypothesis assessment $H_0 : \Psi(\theta) = \psi_0$, are required. Let $\pi_\Psi$ denote the marginal prior density of $\psi$ and

$$m(x \,|\, \psi) = \int_\Theta f(x \,|\, \theta)\, \Pi(d\theta \,|\, \psi)$$

be the conditional prior predictive of the data after integrating out the nuisance parameters via the prior conditional distribution of $\theta$ given $\Psi(\theta) = \psi$. Bayesian inferences for $\psi$ are then based on the ingredients $(\{m(\cdot \,|\, \psi) : \psi \in \Psi(\Theta)\}, \pi_\Psi, x)$ alone or by adding a loss function $L$. Note that the probability measure associated with $m$ will be denoted by $M$ and the probability measure associated with $m(\cdot \,|\, \psi)$ will be denoted by $M(\cdot \,|\, \psi)$ when these are used in the paper.

A natural question arises, namely, how are we to determine the inferences for $\psi$, namely, an estimate $\psi(x)$, or assess the hypothesis $H_0 : \Psi(\theta) = \psi_0$ based upon these ingredients? Several approaches have been put forward to answering this question. Two broad categories can be described, namely, the evidential/inferential approach and the behavioristic/decision-theoretic approach.

The evidential approach can be characterized as having the goal of letting the evidence in the data $x$ determine the inferences and can be subdivided into frequentist, pure likelihood, and Bayesian theories. Central to this is the need to somehow characterize the concept of statistical evidence. The frequentist theory only uses the ingredients $(\{f(\cdot\,|\,\theta) : \theta \in \Theta\}, x)$ together with the idea that inferences are to be graded based on their behavior in hypothetical repeated sampling experiments. Despite the impressive accomplishments of Alan Birnbaum in attempting to formulate a definition of statistical evidence, (see [1]), it is fair to say that there is still no such generally acceptable definition within the frequentist context. The pure likelihood theory is also based on the ingredients $(\{f(\cdot\,|\,\theta) : \theta \in \Theta\}, x)$ but the idea of using repeated sampling characteristics to determine the inferences is dropped and the likelihood function $L(\cdot\,|\,x) : \Theta \to [0, \infty)$, as defined by $L(\theta\,|\,x) = cf(x\,|\,\theta)$ for any positive constant $c$, is taken to be the proper characterization of statistical evidence. All inferences are then determined by the likelihood; for example, see the discussion in [2]. Again, there are gaps in this treatment, as it is unclear when the likelihood function provides evidence in favor of or against a particular value of $\theta$ being the true value, and it is unclear how the likelihood is to be used for marginal parameters $\psi = \Psi(\theta)$. The Bayesian approach based on the ingredients $(\{m(\cdot\,|\,\psi) : \psi \in \Psi(\Theta)\}, \pi_\Psi, x)$ is more successful at characterizing statistical evidence concerning $\psi$ through the principle of evidence, which, loosely speaking, suggests that if the data lead to the posterior probability of an event being greater than (less than) the corresponding prior probability, then there is evidence in favor of (against) the event being true. A precise statement of the principle of evidence is provided in Section 2.3. A full theory of inference based on this idea, and called relative belief, has been developed over a number of years (see [3]), and is sketched in Section 2.3. A much fuller discussion of the issues and developments within the context of the evidential approach to developing statistical theory can be found in [4].

The decision-theoretic approach can also be divided into frequentist and Bayesian theories. The frequentist approach is based on the ingredients $(\{f(\cdot\,|\,\theta) : \theta \in \Theta\}, x)$ together with a loss function $L : \Theta \times \Psi(\Theta) \to [0, \infty)$ where $L(\theta, \Psi(\theta)) = 0$ for all $\theta$ and, generally, $L(\theta, \psi)$ represents the loss or penalty incurred when $\psi$ is chosen as the true value of $\Psi(\theta)$. The idea then is to look for a decision procedure $\delta(x)$ that performs well with respect to the average loss or risk $R(\theta, \delta) = \int_{\mathcal{X}} L(\theta, \delta(x)) f_\theta(x)\, \mu(dx)$, namely, choose a $\delta$ that makes $R(\theta, \delta)$ small uniformly in $\theta$. The frequentist decision theory, however, is not always successful in determining a suitable $\delta$. The Bayesian theory of decision considers the prior risk $r(\delta) = \int_\Theta R(\theta, \delta)\pi(\theta)\, \nu(d\theta)$ and is generally successful in determining a $\delta$ that minimizes $r(\delta)$; this is referred to as the Bayes rule. The Bayesian theory of decision has been axiomatized (see [5]); this provides considerable support for this approach.

If the various approaches to determining inferences all lead to more or less the same answers, then there would be little controversy, but unfortunately, this is not the case. The goal of this paper is to show that relative belief inferences can also be developed within the context of decision theory even though their primary motivation is through the characterization of statistical evidence. It is of historical relevance and interest that two of the founders of the statistical discipline, Fisher and Neyman, disagreed profoundly on the purpose of statistical analyses. Fisher saw the purpose of statistics as summarizing what the evidence in the observed data says about questions of scientific interest, while Neyman described the purpose in behavioristic or decision-theoretic terms, where the goal is to minimize average losses in repeated performances. Ref. [6] described this debate, which continues to be part of the statistical profession. The significance of the results of this paper is that it demonstrates that relative belief inference allows for a possible resolution of this conflict and, as we will now discuss, also resolves a general criticism of decision theory.

A natural requirement for statistical analysis is that all the ingredients chosen by the statistician need to be checkable against the observed data to ensure they align with the objective data (or, at least, are correctly collected). The choice of the model, prior, and loss functions are typically subjective decisions made by the analyst, and many consider such subjectivity to be at odds with the demands of science. However, both the model and the prior can be checked against the observed data to determine whether the choices made are contradicted by the data. Model checking has long been an acceptable, even necessary, part of statistical practice. In recent years, methods have been developed to check for a conflict between the prior and data. These methods determine if the prior placed the bulk of its mass in a region of the parameter space unsupported by the data as containing the true value of the parameter. Ref. [7] contained a discussion about checking for prior-data conflicts and also on what to do when a prior fails its checks. While such checking does not establish the objectivity of these elements, it at least allows the objective data to comment on the relevance of the choices made. However, it is unclear how one can check the loss function $L$ using the data, and this ambiguity may be considered a flaw in decision theory, particularly for scientific applications.

There are, however loss functions that are considered intrinsic and that avoid this criticism. For example, Ref. [8] proposed using the intrinsic loss function based on a measure of distance between sampling distributions. Ref. [9] proposed using the intrinsic loss function based on the Kullback–Leibler divergence $KL(f(\cdot\,|\,\theta)\;\|\;f(\cdot\,|\,\theta'))$ between $f(\cdot\,|\,\theta)$ and $f(\cdot\,|\,\theta')$. When $\psi=\theta$, the intrinsic loss function is given by

$$L(\theta,\theta') = \min(KL(f(\cdot\,|\,\theta)\;\|\;f(\cdot\,|\,\theta')), KL(f(\cdot\,|\,\theta')\;\|\;f(\cdot\,|\,\theta))).$$

For a marginal parameter $\psi$, the intrinsic loss function is $L(\theta,\psi) = \inf_{\theta'\in\Psi^{-1}\{\psi\}} L(\theta,\theta')$. These loss functions are intrinsic because they are based on the sampling model, allowing their suitability to be verified through model checking. The loss functions used to derive relative belief inferences for $\psi=\Psi(\theta)$ are based upon the prior $\pi_\Psi$, see Section 3 for the definitions, and so are also intrinsic and checkable against the data while checking for prior-data conflict.

In some contexts, relative belief inferences are Bayes rules, but in a general context, they are seen to arise as the limits of Bayes rules. This approach has some historical antecedents. For example, in [10], it is shown that the MLE is asymptotically a Bayes rule, but this conclusion is drawn under a fixed loss function, with increasing amounts of data and a sequence of priors. In the context discussed here, however, the data amount is fixed, as are the model and prior, but there is a sequence of loss functions, all based on a single fixed prior. The loss functions relevant for deriving relative belief inferences are similar to those used to justify maximum a posteriori (MAP) inferences. It can be demonstrated that under certain conditions, MAP inferences emerge as the limits of Bayes rules through a sequence of loss functions,

$$L_\lambda(\theta,\psi) = I_{B^c_\lambda(\psi)}(\Psi(\theta)) \tag{1}$$

where $\lambda>0$, $B_\lambda(\Psi(\theta))$ is the ball of radius $\lambda$ centered at $\psi$, $I_A$ denotes the indicator function for set $A$ and, in the continuous case, the support measure on $\Psi(\Theta)$ is volume measure (see [11]). MAP inferences are not invariant under reparameterizations and such invariance can be considered as a desirable property of any inference method. Relative belief inferences, however, are invariant under reparameterizations.

Section 2 is concerned with describing the general characteristics of three approaches to deriving Bayesian inferences. Sections 3 and 4 show how relative belief estimation and prediction inferences can be seen to arise from decision theory and Section 5 does this for credible regions and hypothesis assessment. In particular, it is shown here that relative belief estimators, as used in practice, are admissible. The contents of Sections 3–5 are original contributions by the authors that were derived some years ago but not published. Some of this discussion has appeared in Ref. [3] and is included here to provide a complete exposition of the relationship between relative belief and decision theory. All proofs of theorems and corollaries are in Appendix A, except for cases where $\Psi(\Theta)$ is finite, as these are quite straightforward and provide motivation for the more complicated contexts.

It should be emphasized that the authors do not consider the fact that relative belief inferences can be derived within the context of decision theory as the primary justification for the approach. Rather, the justification lies within the Bayesian context, which leads—via the principle of evidence—to a clear characterization of statistical evidence. The specific loss functions used, while appealing, are not essential to this characterization. The fact that relative belief inferences are consistent with two of the major themes of statistical research pursued over the years, in our view, provides substantial support for their appropriateness.

## 2. Bayesian Inference

Some approaches to deriving Bayesian inferences will now be described in detail.

### 2.1. Bayesian Decision Theory

An ingredient that is commonly added to $(\{f(\cdot\,|\,\theta) : \theta \in \Theta\}, \pi, x)$ is a loss function, namely, $L : \Theta \times \Psi(\Theta) \to [0, \infty)$, satisfying $L(\theta, \psi) = L(\theta', \psi)$ whenever $\Psi(\theta) = \Psi(\theta')$ and $L(\theta, \psi) = 0$ only when $\psi = \Psi(\theta)$. The goal is to find a procedure, say $\delta(x) \in \Psi(\Theta)$, which in some sense minimizes the loss $L(\theta, \delta(x))$ based on the joint distribution of $(\theta, x)$. Given the assumptions on $L$, the loss function can instead be thought of as a map $L : \Psi(\Theta) \times \Psi(\Theta) \to [0, \infty)$ with $L(\psi, \psi') = 0$ iff $\psi = \psi'$ and the ingredients can be represented as $(\{m(\cdot\,|\,\psi) : \psi \in \Psi(\Theta)\}, \pi_\Psi, L, x)$.

The goal of a decision analysis is then to find a decision function $\delta : \mathcal{X} \to \Psi(\Theta)$ that minimizes the *prior risk*,

$$r(\delta) = \int_{\Psi(\Theta)} \int_{\mathcal{X}} L(\psi, \delta(x))\, M(dx\,|\,\psi)\, \Pi_\Psi(d\psi) = \int_{\mathcal{X}} r(\delta\,|\,x)\, M(dx),$$

where $r(\delta\,|\,x) = \int_{\Psi(\Theta)} L(\psi, \delta(x))\, \Pi_\Psi(d\psi\,|\,x)$ is the *posterior risk*. Such a $\delta$ is called a Bayes rule and clearly a $\delta$ that minimizes $r(\delta\,|\,x)$ for each $x$ is a Bayes rule. Further discussion of the Bayesian decision theory can be found in [12].

As noted in [9], a decision formulation also leads to credible regions for $\psi$, namely, a $\gamma$-*lowest posterior loss-credible region* is defined by

$$D_\gamma(x) = \{\psi : r(\psi\,|\,x) \le d_\gamma(x)\}, \tag{2}$$

where $d_\gamma(x) = \inf\{k : \Pi_\Psi(\{\psi : r(\psi\,|\,x) \le k\}\,|\,x) \ge \gamma$. Note that $\psi$ in (2) is interpreted as the decision function that takes the value $\psi$ constantly in $x$. Clearly, as $\gamma \to 0$, set $D_\gamma(x)$ converges to the value of a Bayes rule at $x$. For example, with quadratic loss, the Bayes rule is given by the posterior mean and a $\gamma$-lowest posterior loss region is the smallest sphere centered at the mean containing (at least) $\gamma$ of the posterior probability.

### 2.2. MAP Inferences

The highest posterior density (HPD) or MAP-based approach to determining inferences constructs credible regions of the following form

$$H_\gamma(x) = \{\psi : \pi_\Psi(\psi\,|\,x) \ge h_\gamma(x)\}, \tag{3}$$

where $\pi_\Psi(\cdot\,|\,x)$ is the marginal posterior density with respect to a support measure $\nu_\Psi$ on $\Psi(\Theta)$, and $h_\gamma(x)$ is chosen so that $h_\gamma(x) = \sup\{k : \Pi_\Psi(\{\psi : \pi_\Psi(\psi\,|\,x) \ge k\}\,|\,x) \ge \gamma\}$. It follows from (3) that, to assess the hypothesis $H_0 : \Psi(\theta) = \psi_0$, we can use the tail probability given by $1 - \inf\{\gamma : \psi_0 \in H_\gamma(x)\}$. Furthermore, the class of sets $H_\gamma(x)$ is naturally "centered" at the posterior mode (when it exists uniquely) as $H_\gamma(x)$ converges to this point as $\gamma \to 0$. The use of the posterior mode as an estimator is commonly referred to as MAP estimation. We can then think of the size of set $H_\gamma(x)$, say for $\gamma = 0.95$, as a measure of how accurate the MAP estimator is in a given context. Furthermore, when $\Psi(\Theta)$ is an open subset of Euclidean space, then $H_\gamma(x)$ minimizes the volume among all $\gamma$-credible regions.

It is well-known that HPD inferences suffer from a defect. In particular, in the continuous case, MAP inferences are not invariant under reparameterization. For example, this means that, if $\psi_{MAP}(x)$ is the MAP estimate of $\psi$, then it is not necessarily true that $\Upsilon(\psi_{MAP}(x))$ is the MAP estimate of $\tau = \Upsilon(\psi)$ when $\Upsilon$ is a 1-1 smooth transformation.

The non-invariance of a statistical procedure seems very unnatural as it implies that the statistical analysis depends on the parameterization and typically there does not seem to be a good reason for this. Note too that estimates based upon taking posterior expectations will also suffer from this lack of invariance. It is also the case that MAP inferences are not based on a direct characterization of statistical evidence. Both of these issues motivate the development of relative belief inferences.

One justification for MAP inference is decision-theoretic via the loss functions defined in (1). It is common, however, to also consider posterior probabilities of events as expressions of evidence and so think of this approach as evidential in nature. Posterior probabilities, however, express beliefs rather than evidence. For instance, the posterior probability of an event may be very small yet larger than its prior probability, indicating that the data have increased belief in the event's occurrence. This would suggest that the data provide evidence in favor of the event being true, rather than evidence against it, even though the posterior probability remains small. It appears that evidence is better characterized by how the data change beliefs, rather than by the beliefs themselves.

### 2.3. *Relative Belief Inferences*

Relative belief inferences, like MAP inferences, are based on the ingredients $(\{m(\cdot\,|\,\psi) : \psi \in \Psi(\Theta)\}, \pi_\Psi, x)$. Note that underlying both approaches is the principle (axiom) of conditional probability that says that initial beliefs about $\psi$, as expressed by the prior $\pi_\Psi$, must be replaced by conditional beliefs as expressed by the posterior $\pi_\Psi(\cdot\,|\,x)$. In this approach, however, a measure of statistical evidence is used given by the relative belief ratio,

$$RB_\Psi(\psi\,|\,x) = \frac{\pi_\Psi(\psi\,|\,x)}{\pi_\Psi(\psi)} = \frac{m(x\,|\,\psi)}{m(x)}. \tag{4}$$

The relative belief ratio produces the following conclusions: if $RB_\Psi(\psi\,|\,x) > 1$, then there is evidence in favor of $\psi$ being the true value, if $RB_\Psi(\psi\,|\,x) < 1$, there is evidence against $\psi$ being the true value, and if $RB_\Psi(\psi\,|\,x) = 1$, then there is no evidence either way. These implications follow from a very simple principle of inference.

> Principle of evidence: for probability model $(\Omega, \mathcal{F}, P)$, if $C \in \mathcal{F}$ is observed to be true, where $P(C) > 0$, then there is evidence in favor of $A \in \mathcal{F}$ being true if $P(A\,|\,C) > P(A)$, evidence against $A \in \mathcal{F}$ being true if $P(A\,|\,C) < P(A)$, and no evidence either way if $P(A\,|\,C) = P(A)$.

This principle seems obvious when $\Pi_\Psi$ is a discrete probability measure. For the continuous case, where $\Pi_\Psi(\{\psi\}) = 0$, let $N_\epsilon(\psi)$ be a sequence of neighborhoods of $\psi$ converging nicely to $\psi$ as $\epsilon \to 0$ (see [13]), then under weak conditions, e.g., $\pi_\Psi$ is continuous and positive at $\psi$,

$$\lim_{\epsilon\to 0} RB_\Psi(N_\epsilon(\psi)\,|\,x) = \lim_{\epsilon\to 0} \frac{\Pi_\Psi(N_\epsilon(\psi)\,|\,x)}{\Pi_\Psi(N_\epsilon(\psi))} = \frac{\pi_\Psi(\psi\,|\,x)}{\pi_\Psi(\psi)} = RB_\Psi(\psi\,|\,x)$$

and this justifies the general interpretation of $RB_\Psi(\psi\,|\,x)$ as a measure of evidence. The relative belief ratio determines the inferences.

A natural estimate of $\psi$ is the *relative belief estimate*,

$$\psi_{RB}(x) = \arg\sup_{\psi} RB_\Psi(\psi\,|\,x)$$

as it has maximum evidence in favor. To assess the accuracy of $\psi_{RB}(x)$, consider the *plausible region* $Pl_\Psi(x) = \{\psi : RB_\Psi(\psi\,|\,x) > 1\}$, which is the set of $\psi$ values with evidence supporting them as the true value. The size of $Pl_\Psi(x)$ along with its posterior content $\Pi_\Psi(Pl_\Psi(x)\,|\,x)$, which measures the belief that the true value is in $Pl_\Psi(x)$, provides an assessment of accuracy.

So, if $Pl_\Psi(x)$ is "small" and $\Pi_\Psi(Pl_\Psi(x)\,|\,x) \approx 1$, then $\psi_{RB}(x)$ is to be considered an accurate estimate of $\psi$ but not otherwise. A relative belief $\gamma$-credible region is given by

$$C_{\Psi,\gamma}(x) = \{\psi : RB_\Psi(\psi\,|\,x) \geq c_\gamma(x)\},$$

where $c_\gamma(x) = \sup\{c : \Pi_\Psi(RB_\Psi(\psi\,|\,x) \geq c\,|\,x) \geq \gamma\}$, for $\psi$ can also be quoted provided $C_{\Psi,\gamma}(x) \subset Pl_\Psi(x)$. The containment is necessary, as otherwise, $C_{\Psi,\gamma}(x)$ would contain a value $\psi$ for which there is evidence against $\psi$ being the true value.

To assess the hypothesis $H_0 : \Psi(\theta) = \psi_0$, the value $RB_\Psi(\psi_0\,|\,x)$ indicates whether there is evidence in favor of or against $H_0$. The strength of this evidence can be measured by the posterior probability $\Pi_\Psi(\{\psi_0\}\,|\,x)$, as this measures the belief in what the evidence says. So, if $RB_\Psi(\psi_0\,|\,x) > 1$ and $\Pi_\Psi(\{\psi_0\}\,|\,x) \approx 1$, then there is strong evidence that $H_0$ is true, while when $RB_\Psi(\psi_0\,|\,x) < 1$ and $\Pi_\Psi(\{\psi_0\}\,|\,x) \approx 0$, there is strong evidence that $H_0$ is false. Since $\Pi_\Psi(\{\psi_0\})$ can be small, even 0 in the continuous case, it makes more sense to measure the strength of the evidence in such a case by

$$Str_\Psi(\psi_0\,|\,x) = \Pi_\Psi(RB_\Psi(\psi\,|\,x) \leq RB_\Psi(\psi_0\,|\,x)\,|\,x).$$

If $RB_\Psi(\psi_0\,|\,x) > 1$ and $Str_\Psi(\psi_0\,|\,x) \approx 1$, then the evidence is strong that $\psi_0$ is the true value as there is little belief that the true value of $\psi$ has more evidence in its favor than $\psi_0$. If $RB_\Psi(\psi_0\,|\,x) < 1$ and $Str_\Psi(\psi_0\,|\,x) \approx 0$, then the evidence is strong that $\psi_0$ is not the true value as there is a widespread belief that the true value of $\psi$ has more evidence in its favor than $\psi_0$. There is no reason to quote a single number to measure the strength; both $\Pi_\Psi(\{\psi_0\}\,|\,x)$ and $Str_\Psi(\psi_0\,|\,x)$ can be quoted when relevant.

An important aspect of both $Str_\Psi(\psi_0\,|\,x)$ and $\Pi_\Psi(Pl_\Psi(x)\,|\,x)$ is what happens as the data increase. To ensure that these behave appropriately, namely, $Str_\Psi(\psi_0\,|\,x) \to 0(\text{or}1)$ when $H_0$ is false (or true) and $\Pi_\Psi(Pl_\Psi(x)\,|\,x) \to 1$, it is necessary to take into account the difference that matters, $\delta$. By this, we mean that there is a distance measure $d_\Psi$ on $\Psi(\Theta) \times \Psi(\Theta)$ such that if $d_\Psi(\psi,\psi') \leq \delta$, then in terms of the application, these values are considered equivalent. Such a $\delta$ always exists because measurements are always taken to finite accuracy. For example, if $\psi$ is real-valued, then there is a grid of values $\ldots\psi_{-2},\psi_{-1},\psi_0,\psi_1,\psi_2,\ldots$ separated by $\delta$, and inferences are determined using the relative belief ratios of the intervals $[\psi_i - \delta/2, \psi_i + \delta/2)$. In effect, $H_0$ is now $H_0 : \Psi(\theta) \in [\psi_0 - \delta/2, \psi_0 + \delta/2)$. When the computations are carried out in this way, then $Str_\Psi(\psi_0\,|\,x)$ and $\Pi_\Psi(Pl_\Psi(x)\,|\,x)$ do what is required. As a particular instance of this, see the results in Section 4, where such discretization plays a key role.

It is easy to see that the class of relative-belief credible regions $\{C_{\Psi,\gamma}(x) : \gamma \in [0,1]\}$ for $\psi$ is independent of the marginal prior $\pi_\Psi$. When a value $\gamma \in [0,1]$ is specified, however, set $C_{\Psi,\gamma}(x)$ depends on $\pi_\Psi$ through $c_\gamma(x)$. So, the form of relative belief inferences about $\psi$ is completely robust to the choice of $\pi_\Psi$ but the quantification of the uncertainty in the inferences is not. For example, when $\psi = \Psi(\theta) = \theta$, then $\theta_{RB}(x)$ is the MLE; however, in general, $\psi_{RB}(x)$ is the maximizer of the integrated likelihood $m(x\,|\,\psi)$. Similarly, relative belief regions are likelihood regions in cases of the full parameter and integrated likelihood regions. As such, likelihood regions can be seen as essentially Bayesian in character with a clear and precise characterization of evidence through the relative belief ratio, and now have probability assignments through the posterior. A relative belief ratio, $RB_\Psi(\psi\,|\,x)$, while proportional to an integrated likelihood, cannot be multiplied by an arbitrary positive constant—as with a likelihood—without losing its interpretation in measuring statistical evidence. It has been established in [14] that relative belief inferences for $\psi$ are optimally robust to the prior $\pi_\Psi$.

As can be seen from (4), relative belief inferences are always invariant under smooth reparameterizations; this is at least one reason why they are preferable to MAP inferences. Any rule for measuring evidence, which satisfies the principle of evidence, also produces valid estimates, as these lie in $Pl_\Psi(x)$ and so will have the same "accuracy" as $\psi_{RB}(x)$. For example, if instead of the relative belief ratio, the difference $\pi_\Psi(\psi\,|\,x) - \pi_\Psi(\psi)$ is used as the measure of evidence with a cut-off of 0, then this satisfies the principle of evidence, but the estimate is no longer necessarily invariant under reparameterizations. The Bayes factor with a cut-off of 1 is also a valid measure of evidence but there are a number of reasons why the relative belief ratio is to be preferred to the Bayes factor for general inferences (see [15]).

We will now consider a simple example that illustrates the various concepts just discussed.

**Example 1.** *Location normal*

*Suppose that we have a sample $x = (x_1, \ldots, x_n)$ from a $N(\theta, \sigma_0^2)$ where the mean $\theta \in \Theta = \mathbb{R}^1$ is unknown and the variance $\sigma_0^2$ is assumed known. Suppose interest lies in making inferences about $\psi = \Psi(\theta) = \theta$, and the prior $\pi$ on $\theta$ is given by a $N(\theta_0, \tau_0^2)$ distribution. In this context, $\bar{x}$ serves as a minimal sufficient statistic, allowing the focus to be restricted to the $N(\theta, \sigma_0^2/n)$ model while ignoring the remaining aspects of the data, at least for inference. Certainly the residuals $(x_1 - \bar{x}, \ldots, x_n - \bar{x})$ are relevant for model checking. The prior predictive density $m$ of $\bar{x}$ is then given by the density of a $N(\theta_0, \tau_0^2 + \sigma_0^2/n)$ distribution and, as discussed in [7], this is relevant for checking for prior-data conflicts via the tail probability $M(m(\bar{X}) \leq m(\bar{x}))$ with small values indicating the existence of a conflict.*

*The posterior $\Pi(\cdot \,|\, x)$ of $\theta$ is given by*

$$\theta \,|\, \bar{x} \sim N\left(\left(n/\sigma_0^2 + 1/\tau_0^2\right)^{-1}(n\bar{x}/\sigma_0^2 + \theta_0/\tau_0^2), \left(n/\sigma_0^2 + 1/\tau_0^2\right)^{-1}\right).$$

*As such, $\theta_{MAP}(\bar{x}) = \left(n/\sigma_0^2 + 1/\tau_0^2\right)^{-1}(n\bar{x}/\sigma_0^2 + \theta_0/\tau_0^2)$. If, as is common, squared error loss is employed, then the Bayes rule for estimating $\theta$ is given by $\theta_{MAP}(\bar{x})$, as this is also the posterior mean. On the other hand, the relative belief ratio is given by*

$$\begin{aligned} RB(\theta \,|\, \bar{x}) &= \frac{\pi(\theta \,|\, \bar{x})}{\pi(\theta)} = \frac{m(\bar{x} \,|\, \theta)}{m(\theta)} \\ &= \left(\frac{\tau_0^2 + \sigma_0^2/n}{\sigma_0^2/n}\right)^{1/2} \frac{\exp(-n(\bar{x} - \theta)^2/2\sigma_0^2)}{\exp(-(\tau_0^2 + \sigma_0^2/n)^{-1}(\bar{x} - \theta_0)^2/2)} \end{aligned}$$

*as, since there are no nuisance parameters, $m(\cdot \,|\, \theta)$ equals the sampling density of $\bar{x}$.*

*From this, it is immediate that $\theta_{RB}(\bar{x}) = \bar{x}$, which is the MLE, a result that is generally true for relative belief when estimating the full model parameter. The plausible interval for $\theta$ is then, putting $r_0 = (\sigma_0^2/n)/(\tau_0^2 + \sigma_0^2/n)$, given by*

$$Pl(\bar{x}) = \{\theta : RB(\theta \,|\, \bar{x}) > 1\} = \left(\bar{x} \pm \sigma_0 \sqrt{\frac{(\tau_0^2 + \sigma_0^2/n)^{-1}(\bar{x} - \theta_0)^2 - \log(r_0)}{n}}\right)$$

*and note that $-\log(r_0) > 0$, so this interval is always defined. The length of $Pl(\bar{x})$ and its posterior content, computed using $\Pi(\cdot \,|\, \bar{x})$, provide a measure of the accuracy of $\theta_{RB}(\bar{x})$. Notice that $Pl(\bar{x})$ converges almost surely to the degenerate interval consisting of the true value of $\theta$ and the posterior content of the interval converges to 1 as $n \to \infty$.*

*To assess a hypothesis, say $H_0 : \theta = \theta_0$, the relevant relative belief ratio is as follows:*

$$RB(\theta_0 \,|\, \bar{x}) = r_0^{1/2} \exp\left(-\frac{r_0 - 1}{r_0} \frac{n}{\sigma_0^2} \frac{(\bar{x} - \theta_0)^2}{2}\right).$$

*This gives evidence in favor (or against) $H_0$ when*

$$\frac{n(\bar{x} - \theta_0)^2}{\sigma_0^2} < (>) \frac{r_0 \log r_0}{r_0 - 1}$$

*and note that the right-hand side is always positive. The strength of this evidence is given by*

$$\begin{aligned}
&Str(\theta_0 \mid x) = \Pi(RB(\theta \mid x) \leq RB(\theta_0 \mid x) \mid x) = \Pi(|\bar{x} - \theta| \geq |\bar{x} - \theta_0| \mid x) \\
&= F(\bar{x} + |\bar{x} - \theta_0|; \left(n/\sigma_0^2 + 1/\tau_0^2\right)^{-1}(n\bar{x}/\sigma_0^2 + \theta_0/\tau_0^2), \left(n/\sigma_0^2 + 1/\tau_0^2\right)^{-1}) - \\
&F(\bar{x} - |\bar{x} - \theta_0|; \left(n/\sigma_0^2 + 1/\tau_0^2\right)^{-1}(n\bar{x}/\sigma_0^2 + \theta_0/\tau_0^2), \left(n/\sigma_0^2 + 1/\tau_0^2\right)^{-1}),
\end{aligned}$$

*where $F(\cdot\,; \mu, \lambda)$ denotes the $N(\mu, \lambda)$ cdf. As $n \to \infty$, the strength converges to 0 (the strongest possible evidence against) when $H_0$ is false and converges to 1 (the strongest possible evidence in favor) when $H_0$ is true.*

## 3. Estimation: Discrete Parameter Space

The following theorem presents the basic definition of the loss function for the parameter of interest $\psi = \Psi(\theta)$ when the set of possible values of $\psi$, namely, $\Psi(\Theta) = \{\psi : \psi = \Psi(\theta) \text{ for some } \theta \in \Theta\}$, is finite. This establishes an important optimality result. The indicator function for the set $A$ is denoted as $I_A$.

**Theorem 1.** *Suppose that $\pi_\Psi(\psi) > 0$ for every $\psi \in \Psi(\Theta)$, $\Psi(\Theta)$ is finite with $\nu_\Psi$ equal to counting measure on $\Psi(\Theta)$. Then for the loss function*

$$L_{RB}(\theta, \psi) = \frac{I_{\{\psi\}^c}(\Psi(\theta))}{\pi_\Psi(\Psi(\theta))}, \tag{5}$$

*the relative belief estimator $\psi_{RB}$ is a Bayes rule.*

**Proof.** We have that

$$\begin{aligned}
r(\delta \mid x) &= \int_{\Psi(\Theta)} \frac{I_{\{\delta(x)\}^c}(\psi)}{\pi_\Psi(\psi)} \Pi_\Psi(d\psi \mid x) \\
&= \int_{\Psi(\Theta)} RB_\Psi(\psi \mid x)\, \nu_\Psi(d\psi) - RB_\Psi(\delta(x) \mid x).
\end{aligned} \tag{6}$$

Since $\Psi(\Theta)$ is finite, the first term in (6) is finite and a Bayes rule at $x$ is given by the value $\delta(x)$ that maximizes the second term. Therefore, $\psi_{RB}$ is a Bayes rule. □

The loss function $L_{RB}$ seems very natural. Beliefs about the true value of $\psi$ are expressed by the prior $\pi_\Psi$. As such, consider values where $\pi_\Psi(\psi)$ is very low and $\psi$ is indeed false. It would then be misleading if inferences suggested such a value as being true. So it is appropriate for such values to bear large losses. In a sense, the statistician is acknowledging what such values are by the choice of the prior. Of course, the prior may be wrong in the sense that the bulk of its mass is placed in a region where the true value of $\psi$ does not lie. This is why checking for prior-data conflict, before conducting inference, is always recommended. Procedures for checking priors were discussed in [16,17], and an approach to replacing priors found to be at fault was developed in [7]. The loss function $L_{RB}$ motivates the other losses for relative belief discussed here, making this comment relevant to those losses as well.

The prior risk of $\delta$ satisfies the following,

$$r(\delta) = \int_{\Psi(\Theta)} \int_{\mathcal{X}} \frac{I_{\{\delta(x)\}^c}(\psi)}{\pi_\Psi(\psi)} M(dx \mid \psi)\, \Pi_\Psi(d\psi) = \sum_{\psi \in \Psi(\Theta)} M(\delta(x) \neq \psi \mid \psi), \tag{7}$$

where $M(\cdot \mid \psi)$ is the conditional prior predictive probability measure of the data given $\psi$, so (7) is the sum of the conditional prior error probabilities over all $\psi$ values. If instead the loss function is taken to be $L_{MAP}(\theta, \psi) = I_{\{\psi\}^c}(\Psi(\theta))$, as in (1), then the same proof used in Theorem 1 establishes that $\psi_{MAP}$ is a Bayes rule with respect to this loss, and the prior risk is given by,

$$\sum_{\psi} M(\delta(x) \neq \psi \,|\, \psi)\pi_{\Psi}(\psi), \tag{8}$$

which represents the prior probability of making an error. Both $L_{MAP}$ and $L_{RB}$ are two-valued loss functions but, when an incorrect decision is made, the loss is constant in $\Psi(\theta)$ for $L_{MAP}$, while it equals the reciprocal of the prior probability of $\Psi(\theta)$ for $L_{RB}$. So, $L_{RB}$ penalizes an incorrect decision much more severely when the true value of $\Psi(\theta)$ is in the tails of the prior. Note that $\psi_{MAP} = \psi_{RB}$ when $\Pi_{\Psi}$ is uniform. It is evident that (7) serves as an upper bound to (8), indicating that controlling losses based on $L_{RB}$ automatically controls the losses based on $L_{MAP}$.

As already noted, $RB_{\Psi}(\psi \,|\, x)$ is proportional to the integrated likelihood of $\psi$. So, under the conditions of Theorem 1, the maximum integrated likelihood estimator is a Bayes rule. Furthermore, the Bayes rule is the same for every choice of $\pi_{\Psi}$ and only depends on the full prior through the conditional prior $\Pi(\cdot \,|\, \psi)$ placed on the nuisance parameters. When $\psi = \theta$, then $\theta_{RB}(x)$ is the MLE of $\theta$ and so the MLE of $\theta$ is a Bayes rule for every prior $\pi$.

Note that when $\Psi(\Theta) = \{\psi_0, \psi_1\}$, then $RB_{\Psi}(\psi_0 \,|\, x) > (<)1$ iff $RB_{\Psi}(\psi_1 \,|\, x) < (>)1$, so $\psi_{RB}(x) = \psi_0$ when $RB_{\Psi}(\psi_0 \,|\, x) > 1$, and $\psi_{RB}(x) = \psi_1$ otherwise. This is the classical context for hypothesis testing, where $\psi_{RB}(x) = \psi_0$ can be viewed as acceptance of the hypothesis $H_0 : \theta \in \Psi^{-1}\{\psi_0\}$, and $\psi_{RB}(x) = \psi_1$ as rejection of $H_0$. Theorem 1 establishes that relative belief offers a Bayes rule for the hypothesis testing problem.

The loss function (5) does not provide meaningful results when $\Psi(\Theta)$ is infinite as (7) shows that $r(\delta)$ will be infinite. So, we modify (5) via a parameter $\eta > 0$ and define the loss function as follows,

$$L_{RB,\eta}(\theta, \psi) = \frac{I_{\{\psi\}^c}(\Psi(\theta))}{\max(\eta, \pi_{\Psi}(\Psi(\theta)))}. \tag{9}$$

Note that $L_{RB,\eta}$ is bounded by $1/\eta$. This loss function is like (5) but does not allow for arbitrarily large losses. The following result shows that we can restrict attention to values of $\eta$ that are sufficiently small.

**Theorem 2.** *Suppose that $\pi_{\Psi}(\psi) > 0$ for every $\psi \in \Psi(\Theta)$, where $\Psi(\Theta)$ is countable with $\nu_{\Psi}$ equal to counting measure, and that $\psi_{RB}(x)$ is the unique maximizer of $RB_{\Psi}(\psi \,|\, x)$ for all $x$. For the loss function (9) and Bayes rule $\delta_{\eta}$, then $\delta_{\eta}(x) \to \psi_{RB}(x)$ as $\eta \to 0$, for every $x \in \mathcal{X}$.*

The proof of Theorem 2 also establishes the following result.

**Corollary 1.** *For all sufficiently small $\eta$, the value of a Bayes rule at $x$ is given by $\psi_{RB}(x)$.*

The following is an immediate consequence of Theorem 1 and Corollary 1 as $\psi_{RB}$ is a Bayes rule.

**Corollary 2.** *$\psi_{RB}$ is an admissible estimator with respect to the loss function $L_{RB}$ when $\Psi(\Theta)$ is finite, and with respect to loss $L_{RB,\eta}$, when $\eta$ is sufficiently small, and $\Psi(\Theta)$ is countable.*

In a general estimation problem, $\delta$ is risk-unbiased with respect to a loss function $L$ if $E_{\theta}(L(\theta', \delta(x))) \geq E_{\theta}(L(\theta, \delta(x)))$ for all $\theta', \theta \in \Theta$. This says that, on average, $\delta(x)$ is closer to the true value than any other value when we interpret $L(\theta, \delta(x))$ as a measure of distance between $\delta(x)$ and $\Psi(\theta)$. A definition of *Bayesian-unbiasedness* for $\delta$ with respect to $L$ is given by the inequality,

$$\int_{\Theta} \int_{\Theta} E_{\theta}(L(\theta', \delta(x)))\, \Pi(d\theta)\, \Pi(d\theta') \geq \int_{\Theta} E_{\theta}(L(\theta, \delta(x)))\, \Pi(d\theta) = r(\delta),$$

as this retains the idea of being closer, on average, to the true value than a false value. We will now consider a family of loss functions defined as follows,

$$L(\theta, \psi) = I_{\{\psi\}^c}(\Psi(\theta))h(\Psi(\theta)) \tag{10}$$

where $h$ is a nonnegative function satisfying $\int_\Theta h(\Psi(\theta))\,\Pi(d\theta) < \infty$ . This includes $L_{RB}$ and $L_{MAP}$ when $\Psi(\Theta)$ is finite and $L_{RB,\eta}$.

**Theorem 3.** *If $\Psi(\Theta)$ is finite or countable, then $\psi_{RB}(x)$ is Bayesian-unbiased under the loss function (10).*

Suppose after observing $x$, there is a need to predict a future (or concealed) value $y \in \mathcal{Y}$, where $y \sim g_{\delta(\theta)}(y \mid x)$, a density with respect to the support measure $\mu_{\mathcal{Y}}$ on $\mathcal{Y}$, and it is assumed that the true value of $\theta$ in the model for $x$, gives the true value of $\delta(\theta)$. The prior predictive density of $y$ is given by $q(y) = \int_\Theta \int_{\mathcal{X}} \pi(\theta) f_\theta(x) g_{\delta(\theta)}(y \mid x)\, \mu(dx)\, \nu(d\theta)$ while the posterior predictive density is $q(y \mid x) = \int_\Theta \pi(\theta \mid x) g_{\delta(\theta)}(y \mid x)\, \nu(d\theta)$. The relative belief ratio for a future value of $y$ is, thus, $RB_Y(y \mid x) = q(y \mid x)/q(y)$, and the relative belief prediction, namely, the value that maximizes $RB_Y(\cdot \mid x)$, is denoted as $y_{RB}(x)$. When $\mathcal{Y}$ is finite, using the same argument as in Theorem 1, $y_{RB}$ is a Bayes rule under the loss function $L_{RB}(y, y') = I_{\{y\}^c}(y')/q(y)$. Also, it can be demonstrated that $y_{RB}$ is a limit of the Bayes rule when $\mathcal{Y}$ is countable.

We will now consider a common application where $\Psi(\Theta)$ is finite.

**Example 2.** *Classification*

*For a classification problem, there are k categories $\{\psi_1, \ldots, \psi_k\}$, prescribed by a function $\Psi$, where $\pi_\Psi(\psi_i) > 0$ for each i. Estimating $\psi$ is then equivalent to classifying the data as having come from one of the distributions in the classes specified by $\Psi^{-1}\{\psi_i\}$. The standard Bayesian solution to this problem is to use $\psi_{MAP}(x)$ as the classifier. From (8), we have that $\psi_{MAP}(x)$ minimizes the prior probability of misclassification, while from (7), $\psi_{RB}(x)$ minimizes the sum of the probabilities of misclassification. The essence of the difference is that $\psi_{RB}(x)$ treats the misclassification errors equally while $\psi_{MAP}(x)$ weights the errors by their prior probabilities.*

*The following shows that minimizing the sum of error probabilities is often more appropriate than minimizing the weighted sum. Suppose that $k = 2$ and $x \sim$ Bernoulli($\psi_0$) or $x \sim$ Bernoulli($\psi_1$) with $\pi(\psi_0) = 1 - \epsilon$ and $\pi(\psi_1) = \epsilon$ representing the known proportions of individuals coming from population 0 or 1. For example, consider $\psi_0$ as the probability of a positive diagnostic test for a disease in the non-diseased population while $\psi_1$ is this probability for the diseased population. Suppose that $\psi_0/\psi_1$ is very small, indicating that the test is successful at identifying the disease while not yielding many false positives and that $\epsilon$ is very small, so the disease is rare. The challenge then becomes assigning a randomly chosen individual to a population based on their test results.*

*The posterior is given by $\pi(\psi_0 \mid 1) = \psi_0(1-\epsilon)/(\psi_0(1-\epsilon) + \psi_1\epsilon)$ and $\pi(\psi_0 \mid 0) = (1-\psi_0)(1-\epsilon)/((1-\psi_0)(1-\epsilon) + (1-\psi_1)\epsilon)$. Therefore,*

$$\psi_{MAP}(1) = \begin{cases} \psi_0 & \text{if } \psi_0/\psi_1 > \epsilon/(1-\epsilon) \\ \psi_1 & \text{otherwise} \end{cases}$$

$$\psi_{MAP}(0) = \begin{cases} \psi_0 & \text{if } (1-\psi_0)/(1-\psi_1) > \epsilon/(1-\epsilon) \\ \psi_1 & \text{otherwise} \end{cases}$$

*This implies that $\psi_{MAP}$ will always classify a person to the non-diseased population when $\epsilon$ is small enough, e.g., when $\psi_0 = 0.05, \psi_1 = 0.80$, and $\epsilon < 0.0625$. In contrast, in this situation, $\psi_{RB}$ always classifies an individual with a positive test to the diseased population and the non-diseased* *population for a negative test. Since $M(\cdot \mid \psi_i)$ is the Bernoulli$(\psi_i)$ distribution, when $\psi_0 < \psi_1$ and $\epsilon$ are small enough, we have the following:*

$$\begin{aligned} M(\psi_{MAP} \neq \psi_0 \mid \psi_0) + M(\psi_{MAP} \neq \psi_1 \mid \psi_1) &= 0 + 1 = 1, \\ M(\psi_{RB} \neq \psi_0 \mid \psi_0) + M(\psi_{RB} \neq \psi_1 \mid \psi_1) &= \psi_0 + (1 - \psi_1) = 0.25. \end{aligned}$$

*This clearly illustrates the difference between these two procedures as $\psi_{RB}$ does better than $\psi_{MAP}$ on the diseased population when $\psi_0$ is small and $\psi_1$ is large, as would be the case for a good diagnostic. Of course, $\psi_{MAP}$ minimizes the overall error rate, but at the price of ignoring the most important class in this problem, namely, those who have the disease. Note that this example can be extended to the situation where we need to estimate the $\psi_i$ based on samples from the respective populations, but this will not materially affect the overall conclusions.*

*We will now consider a situation where $(x, c)$ is such that $x \mid c \sim f_c, c \mid \epsilon \sim$ Bernoulli$(\epsilon)$, where $f_0$ and $f_1$ are known but $\epsilon$ is unknown with a prior $\pi$. This is a generalization of the previous discussion, where $\epsilon$ is assumed to be known. Then, based on a sample $(x_1, c_1), \ldots, (x_n, c_n)$ from the joint distribution, the goal is to predict the value $c_{n+1}$ for a newly observed $x_{n+1}$.*

*The prior of c is $q(c) = \int_0^1 (1-\epsilon)^{1-c} \epsilon^c \pi(\epsilon)\, d\epsilon$ , and if $\epsilon \sim$ beta$(\alpha, \beta)$, the prior predictive of $c_{n+1}$ is Bernoulli$(\alpha/(\alpha+\beta))$. The posterior predictive density of $c_{n+1}$ equals, where $\bar{c} = n^{-1} \sum_{i=1}^n c_i$,*

$$\begin{aligned} &q(c \mid (x_1, c_1), \ldots, (x_n, c_n), x_{n+1}) \\ &\propto (f_0(x_{n+1}))^{1-c} (f_1(x_{n+1}))^c \int_0^1 \epsilon^{n\bar{c}+c} (1-\epsilon)^{n(1-\bar{c})+(1-c)} \pi(\epsilon)\, d\epsilon \\ &= f_c(x_{n+1}) \Gamma(\alpha + n\bar{c} + c) \Gamma(\beta + n(1-\bar{c}) + 1 - c). \end{aligned}$$

*It follows that, suppressing the dependence on the data, we have the following,*

$$\begin{aligned} c_{MAP} &= \begin{cases} 1 & \textit{if } \frac{f_1(x_{n+1})}{f_0(x_{n+1})} \frac{(\alpha+n\bar{c})}{(\beta+n(1-\bar{c}))} > 1 \\ 0 & \textit{otherwise,} \end{cases} \\ c_{RB} &= \begin{cases} 1 & \textit{if } \frac{f_1(x_{n+1})}{f_0(x_{n+1})} \frac{\beta(\alpha+n\bar{c})}{\alpha(\beta+n(1-\bar{c}))} < 1 \\ 0 & \textit{otherwise} \end{cases} \end{aligned} \tag{11}$$

*Note that $c_{MAP}$ and $c_{RB}$ are identical whenever $\alpha = \beta$.*

*From these formulas, it is apparent that a substantial difference will arise between $c_{MAP}$ and $c_{RB}$ when either $\alpha$ or $\beta$ is much bigger than the other. As in Example 2, these correspond to situations where we believe that $\epsilon$ or $1 - \epsilon$ is very small. Suppose we take $\alpha = 1$ and let $\beta$ be relatively large, as this corresponds to knowing a priori that $\epsilon$ is very small. Then (11) implies that $c_{MAP} \leq c_{RB}$ and so $c_{RB} = 1$ whenever $c_{MAP} = 1$. A similar conclusion arises when we take $\beta = 1$ and $\alpha < 1$.*

*To see what kind of improvement is possible, we consider a simulation study. Let $f_0$ be a $N(0,1)$ density, $f_1$ be a $N(\mu, 1)$ density, and $n = 10$ and the prior on $\epsilon$ be beta$(1, \beta)$. Table 1 presents the Bayes risks for $c_{MAP}$ and $c_{RB}$ for various choices of $\beta$ when $\mu = 1$. When $\beta = 1$, they are equivalent, but we see that as $\beta$ rises, the performance of $c_{MAP}$ deteriorates while $c_{RB}$ improves. Large values of $\beta$ correspond to having information where $\epsilon$ is small. When $\beta = 14$, about 0.50 of the prior probability is to the left of 0.05; with $\beta = 32$, about 0.80 of the prior probability is to the left of 0.05; and with $\beta = 100$, about 0.99 of the prior probability is to the left of 0.05. We see that the misclassification rates for the small group ($c = 1$) stay about the same for $c_{RB}$ as $\beta$ increases while they deteriorate markedly for $c_{MAP}$ as the MAP procedure basically ignores the small group.*

*We also investigated other choices for n and $\mu$. There is very little change as n increases. When $\mu$ moves toward 0 and $\mu$ moves away from 0, the error rates go up and go down, as one would expect; $c_{RB}$ always dominates $c_{MAP}$.*

**Table 1.** Conditional prior probabilities of misclassification for $c_{MAP}$ and $c_{RB}$ for various values of $\beta$ in Example 2 when $\alpha = 1$, $\mu = 1$, and $n = 10$.

| $\beta$ | $M_0(c_{MAP} \neq 0) + M_1(c_{MAP} \neq 1)$ | $M_0(c_{RB} \neq 0) + M_1(c_{RB} \neq 1)$ |
|---|---|---|
| 1 | $0.386 + 0.390 = 0.776$ | $0.386 + 0.390 = 0.776$ |
| 14 | $0.002 + 0.975 = 0.977$ | $0.285 + 0.380 = 0.665$ |
| 32 | $0.000 + 0.997 = 0.997$ | $0.292 + 0.349 = 0.641$ |
| 100 | $0.000 + 1.000 = 1.000$ | $0.300 + 0.324 = 0.624$ |

## 4. Estimation: Continuous Parameter Space

When $\psi$ has a continuous prior distribution, the argument in Theorem 2 does not work, as $\Pi_\Psi(\{\delta(x)\} \mid x) = 0$. There are several possible ways to proceed but one approach is to use a discretization of the problem that uses Theorem 2. For this, we will assume that the spaces involved are locally Euclidean, the mappings are sufficiently smooth, and take the support measures to be the analogs of Euclidean volume on the respective spaces. While the argument presented is broadly applicable, it has been simplified in this context by assuming that all spaces are open subsets of Euclidean spaces, with the support measures being the Euclidean volume on these sets.

For each $\lambda > 0$, suppose there is a discretization $\{B_\lambda(\psi) : \psi \in \Psi(\Theta)\}$ of $\Psi(\Theta)$ into a countable number of subsets with the following properties: $\psi \in B_\lambda(\psi), \Pi_\Psi(B_\lambda(\psi)) > 0$ and $\sup_{\psi \in \Psi} \text{diam}(B_\lambda(\psi)) \to 0$ as $\lambda \to 0$. So, if $\psi' \in B_\lambda(\psi)$, then $B_\lambda(\psi') = B_\lambda(\psi)$. For example, $B_\lambda(\psi)$ could be equal volume rectangles in $R^k$. Further, we assume that $\Pi_\Psi(B_\lambda(\psi))/\nu_\Psi(B_\lambda(\psi)) \to \pi_\Psi(\psi)$ as $\lambda \to 0$ for every $\psi$. This will hold whenever $\pi_\Psi$ is continuous everywhere and $B_\lambda(\psi)$ converges nicely to $\{\psi\}$ as $\lambda \to 0$. Let $\psi_\lambda(\psi)$ denote a point in $B_\lambda(\psi)$ such that $\psi_\lambda(\psi) = \psi_\lambda(\psi')$ whenever $\psi, \psi' \in\in B_\lambda(\psi)$ and put $\Psi_\lambda = \{\psi_\lambda(\psi) : \psi \in \Psi(\Theta)\}$. So, $\Psi_\lambda$ is a discretized version of $\Psi(\Theta)$. We will call this a *regular discretization* of $\Psi(\Theta)$. The discretized prior on $\Psi_\lambda$ is $\pi_{\Psi,\lambda}(\psi_\lambda(\psi)) = \Pi_\Psi(B_\lambda(\psi))$ and the discretized posterior is $\pi_{\Psi,\lambda}(\psi_\lambda(\psi) \mid x) = \Pi_\Psi(B_\lambda(\psi) \mid x)$.

The loss function for the discretized problem is defined in Theorem 2 as follows,

$$L_{RB,\lambda,\eta}(\theta, \psi_\lambda(\psi)) = \frac{I_{\{\psi_\lambda(\psi)\}}(\psi_\lambda(\Psi(\theta)))}{\max(\eta, \pi_{\Psi,\lambda}(\psi_\lambda(\Psi(\theta))))} \quad (12)$$

and let $\delta_{\lambda,\eta}(x)$ denote a Bayes rule for this problem.

**Theorem 4.** *Suppose that $\pi_\Psi$ is positive and continuous and we have a regular discretization of $\Psi$. Furthermore, suppose that $\psi_{RB}(x)$ is the unique maximizer of $RB_\Psi(\psi \mid x)$ and for any $\epsilon > 0$,*

$$\sup_{\{\psi: ||\psi - \psi_{RB}(x)|| \geq \epsilon\}} RB_\Psi(\psi \mid x) < RB_\Psi(\psi_{RB}(x) \mid x).$$

*Then, there exists $\eta(\lambda) \downarrow 0$ as $\lambda \to 0$ such that a Bayes rule $\delta_{\lambda,\eta(\lambda)}(x)$, under the loss $L_{RB,\lambda,\eta(\lambda)}$, converges to $\psi_{RB}(x)$ as $\lambda \to 0$ for all $x$.*

Theorem 4 states that $\psi_{RB}(x)$ is a limit of Bayes rules. So, when $\Psi(\theta) = \theta$, we have the result that the MLE is a limit of the Bayes rule, and more generally, the MLE from an integrated likelihood is a limit of Bayes rules. The regularity conditions stated in Theorem 4 hold in many common statistical problems.

Now let $\hat{\psi}_\lambda(x)$ be the relative belief estimate from the discretized problem, i.e., $\hat{\psi}_\lambda(x)$ maximizes $RB_\Psi(B_\lambda(\psi) \mid x)$ as a function of $\psi \in \Psi_\lambda$. The following is immediate from the proof of Theorem 4, Theorem 3, and Corollary 2:

**Corollary 3.** *$\hat{\psi}_\lambda$ is admissible and Bayesian-unbiased for the discretized problem, and $\hat{\psi}_\lambda(x) \to \psi_{RB}(x)$ as $\lambda \to 0$ for every $x$.*

By similar arguments, an analog of Theorem 4 for $\psi_{MAP}$ can be established. In this case, a simpler development can be followed in certain situations by using the loss function $I_{B^c_\lambda(\psi)}(\Psi(\theta))$. For this, the posterior risk of $\delta$ in the discretized problem, is given by $1 - \Pi_\Psi(B_\lambda(\delta(x)) \,|\, x) = 1 - \pi_\Psi(\delta'(x) \,|\, x)\nu_\Psi(B_\lambda(\delta(x)))$ for some $\delta'(x) \in B_\lambda(\delta(x))$. Now suppose $B_\lambda(\psi)$ is a cube centered at $\psi$ of edge length $\delta$. Suppose that for each $\epsilon > 0$, there exists $\lambda(\epsilon) > 0$, such that, when $||\psi - \psi_{MAP}(x)|| > \lambda(\epsilon)$, then

$$pi_\Psi(\psi \,|\, x) < \inf_{\psi' \in B_{\lambda(\epsilon)}(\psi_{MAP}(x))} \pi_\Psi(\psi' \,|\, x).$$

Since $\nu_\Psi(B_\lambda(\psi))$ is constant, a Bayes rule $\delta_{\lambda(\epsilon)}$ must then satisfy $||\delta_{\lambda(\epsilon)}(x) - \psi_{MAP}(x)|| < \epsilon$. This proves that $\psi_{MAP}$ is a limit of the Bayes rules. By contrast, for the loss

$$I_{B^c_\lambda(\psi)}(\Psi(\theta))/\Pi_\Psi(B_\lambda(\Psi(\theta))),$$

the posterior risk of $\delta$ is given by,

$$\int_\Psi \{\Pi_\Psi(B_\lambda(\psi))\}^{-1}\Pi_\Psi(d\psi \,|\, x) - \int_{B_\lambda(\delta(x))} \{\Pi_\Psi(B_\lambda(\psi))\}^{-1}\Pi_\Psi(d\psi \,|\, x)$$

and the first term is generally unbounded unless $\Psi(\Theta)$ is compact.

We will now consider an important example.

**Example 3.** *Regression*

*Suppose that $y = X\beta + e$, where $y \in R^n, X \in R^{n\times k}$ is fixed of rank k, $\beta \in R^{n\times k}$, and $e \sim N_n(0, \sigma^2 I)$. To simplify the discussion, we will assume that $\sigma^2$ is known but this is not necessary. Let $\pi$ be a prior density for $\beta$. For every $\pi$, having observed $(X, y)$, then $\beta_{RB}(y) = b = (X'X)^{-1}X'y$, the MLE of $\beta$.*

*It is interesting to contrast this result with more standard Bayesian estimates such as MAP or the posterior mean. For example, suppose that $\beta \sim N_k(0, \tau^2 I)$. Then the posterior distribution of $\beta$ is $N_k(\beta_{post}(y), \Sigma_{post})$, where*

$$\beta_{post}(y) = \Sigma_{post}(\sigma^{-2}X'Xb),\ \Sigma_{post} = (\tau^{-2}I + \sigma^{-2}X'X)^{-1}$$

*and note that $\beta_{MAP}(y) = \beta_{post}(y)$. Writing the spectral decomposition of $X'X$ as $X'X = Q\Lambda Q'$, we have that*

$$||\beta_{MAP}(y)|| = ||(I + (\sigma^2/\tau^2)\Lambda^{-1})^{-1}Q'b||.$$

*Since $||b|| = ||Q'b||$ and $1/(1 + \tau^2\lambda_i/\sigma^2) < 1$ for each i, this implies that $\beta_{MAP}(y)$ shrinks the MLE toward the prior mean of 0. When the columns of X are orthonormal, then $\beta_{MAP}(y) = r(1+r)^{-1}b$, where $r = \tau^2/\sigma^2$, and so the shrinkage is substantial unless $\tau^2$ is much larger than $\sigma^2$. This shrinkage is often cited as a positive attribute of these estimates. Consider now the situation where the true value of $\beta$ is some distance from the mean. In this case, it seems wrong to move $\beta$ toward the prior mean; thus, it is not clear whether shrinking the MLE is necessarily a good thing, particularly as this requires giving up invariance.*

*Suppose that estimating the mean response $\psi = \Psi(\beta) = w'\beta$ at $w$ for the predictors is required. The prior distribution of $\psi$ is $N(0, \sigma^2_\psi) = N(0, \tau^2 w'w)$ and the posterior distribution is $N(\psi_{MAP}(y), \sigma^2_{\psi,post}) = N(w'\beta_{MAP}(y), w'\Sigma_{post}(\beta)w)$. Note the following relationships,*

$$\sigma^2_\psi - \sigma^2_{\psi,post} = w'(\tau^2 I - \Sigma_{post})w = \tau^2 w'Q'(I - (I + (\tau^2/\sigma^2)\Lambda)^{-1})Qw > 0$$

*since $1/(1 + \tau^2\lambda_i/\sigma^2) < 1$ for each i. Therefore, maximizing the ratio of the posterior to prior densities leads to*

$$\psi_{RB}(y) = (1 - \sigma^2_{\psi,post}/\sigma^2_\psi)^{-1}\psi_{MAP}(y). \tag{13}$$

*Then $\sigma_{\psi}^2 > \sigma_{\psi,post}^2$ implies $|\psi_{RB}(y)| > |\psi_{MAP}(y)|$. Note that when $\sigma_{\psi,post}^2$ is much smaller than $\sigma_{\psi}^2$, in other words, the posterior is much more concentrated than the prior, then $\psi_{RB}(y)$ and $\psi_{MAP}(y)$ are very similar. In general, $\psi_{RB}(y)$ is not equal to $w'b$, the plug-in MLE of $\psi$, although it is the MLE from the integrated likelihood. Moreover, $\psi_{RB}(y) \to w'b$ as $\tau^2 \to \infty$, and when X has orthonormal columns, $\psi_{RB}(y) = w'b$.*

*Suppose predicting a response z at the predictor value $w \in R^k$ is required. When $\beta \sim N_k(0, \tau^2 I)$, the prior distribution of z is $z \sim N(0, \sigma^2 + \tau^2 w'w) = N(0, \sigma_z^2)$ and the posterior distribution is $N(\mu_{post}(z), \sigma_{post}^2(z))$, where we have that*

$$\mu_{post}(z) = w'\beta_{post}(y),\ \sigma_{post}^2(z) = \sigma^2 + w'\Sigma_{post}w.$$

*To obtain $z_{RB}(y)$, it is necessary to maximize the ratio of the posterior to the prior densities of z; this leads to*

$$z_{RB}(y) = (1 - \sigma_{post}^2(z)/\sigma_{prior}^2(z))^{-1}\mu_{post}(z). \tag{14}$$

*Note that $\sigma_z^2 - \sigma_{post}^2(z) = \sigma_z^2(w'\beta) - \sigma_{post}^2(w'\beta) > 0$; thus, $|z_{RB}(y)| > |\mu_{post}(z)|$, and $z_{RB}$ is further from the prior mean than $z_{MAP}(y) = \mu_{post}(z)$. Also, when $\sigma_{post}^2(z)$ is small, then $z_{RB}(y)$ and $z_{MAP}(y)$ are very similar. Finally, comparing (13) and (14), we have that*

$$z_{RB}(y) = (\sigma_{prior}^2(z)/\sigma_{post}^2(\psi))w'\psi_{RB}(y) = (1 + \sigma^2/\tau^2)\psi_{RB}(y)$$

*and so $\psi_{RB}(y)$ at w is more dispersed than the $z_{RB}(y)$ estimate of the mean at w; this makes good sense as we have to take into account the additional variation due to prediction. By contrast, $w_{MAP}(y) = \psi_{MAP}(y)$.*

## 5. Credible Regions and Hypothesis Assessment

Recall that a $\gamma$-relative-belief credible region for $\psi = \Psi(\theta)$ is given by $C_{\Psi,\gamma}(x) = \{\psi : RB_{\Psi}(\psi \mid x) \geq c_{\gamma}(x)\}$, where $c_{\gamma}(x) = \sup\{c : \Pi_{\Psi}(RB_{\Psi}(\psi \mid x) \geq c \mid x) \geq \gamma\}$. There is some arbitrariness in the choice of the greater than or equal sign to define the credible region as it could have been defined as $C_{\Psi,\gamma}(x) = \{\psi : RB_{\Psi}(\psi \mid x) > c_{\gamma}(x)\}$, where $c_{\gamma}(x) = \inf\{c : \Pi_{\Psi}(RB_{\Psi}(\psi \mid x) \leq c \mid x) \leq 1 - \gamma\}$. In the latter case, $c_{\gamma}(x)$ is the $(1-\gamma)$-th quantile of the posterior distribution of the relative belief ratio. This definition has some advantages as using this implies that the plausible region satisfies $Pl_{\Psi}(x) = C_{\Psi,\gamma}(x)$, where $\gamma = \Pi_{\Psi}(Pl_{\Psi}(x) \mid x)$. Also, the strength of the evidence concerning the hypothesis $H_0 : \Psi(\theta) = \psi_0$ satisfies $Str_{\Psi}(\psi_0 \mid x) = 1 - \Pi_{\Psi}(C_{\Psi,\gamma}(x) \mid x)$ where $\gamma = 1 - Str_{\Psi}(\psi_0 \mid x)$. The key point here is the close relationship between relative-belief credible regions, the plausible region, and the strength calculation. Thus, any decision-theoretic interpretation applicable to relative-belief credible regions also pertains to the plausible region and the strength of the evidence. Throughout this section, we will retain the definition for $C_{\Psi,\gamma}(x)$ provided in Section 2.3.

Now consider the lowest posterior loss $\gamma$-credible regions that arise from the prior-based loss functions considered here.

**Theorem 5.** *Suppose that $\pi_{\Psi}(\psi) > 0$ for every $\psi \in \Psi(\Theta)$, where $\Psi(\Theta)$ is finite with $\nu_{\Psi}$ equal to the counting measure. Then $C_{\Psi,\gamma}(x)$ is a $\gamma$-lowest posterior loss-credible region for the loss function $L_{RB}$.*

**Proof.** From (2) and (6), the $\gamma$-lowest posterior loss-credible region is given by

$$D_{\gamma}(x) = \left\{\psi : RB_{\Psi}(\psi \mid x) \geq \int_{\Psi} RB_{\Psi}(\zeta \mid x)\, \nu_{\Psi}(d\zeta) - d_{\gamma}(x)\right\}$$

and $d_{\gamma}(x) = \sup\{d : \Pi_{\Psi}(\{\psi : r(\psi \mid x) \leq d \mid x) \geq \gamma\}$. As $\int_{\Psi} RB_{\Psi}(z \mid x)\, \nu_{\Psi}(dz)$ is independent of $\psi$ it is clearly equivalent to define this region via $C_{\Psi,\gamma}(x) = \{\psi : RB_{\Psi}(\psi \mid x) \geq c_{\gamma}(x)\}$, namely, $D_{\gamma}(x) = C_{\Psi,\gamma}(x)$. $\square$

Now consider the case where $\Psi$ is countable and we use the loss function $L_{RB,\eta}$. Following the proof of Theorem 5, we see that a $\gamma$-lowest posterior loss region takes the form,

$$D_{\eta,\gamma}(x) = \{\psi : \pi_\Psi(\psi \,|\, x)/\max(\eta, \pi_\Psi(\psi)) \geq d_{\eta,\gamma}(x)\},$$

where $d_{\eta,\gamma}(x) = \sup\{d : \Pi_\Psi(\{\psi : \pi_\Psi(\psi \,|\, x)/\max(\eta, \pi_\Psi(\psi)) \geq d \,|\, x)\} \geq \gamma\}$.

**Theorem 6.** *Suppose that $\pi_\Psi(\psi) > 0$ for every $\psi \in \Psi$, the $\Psi$ is countable with $\nu_\Psi$ equal to counting measure. For the loss function $L_{RB,\eta}$, $C_{\Psi,\gamma}(x) \subset \liminf_{\eta\to 0} D_{\eta,\gamma}(x)$ whenever $\gamma$ is such that $\Pi_\Psi(C_{\Psi,\gamma}(x) \,|\, x) = \gamma$, and $\limsup_{\eta\to 0} D_{\eta,\gamma}(x) \subset C_{\Psi,\gamma'}(x)$ whenever $\gamma' > \gamma$ and $\Pi_\Psi(C_{\Psi,\gamma'}(x) \,|\, x) = \gamma'$.*

While Theorem 6 does not establish the exact convergence $\lim_{\eta\to 0} D_{\eta,\gamma}(x) = C_\gamma(x)$, it is likely that this does hold under quite general circumstances due to the discreteness. Theorem 6 shows that limit points of the class of sets $D_{\eta,\gamma}(x)$ always contain $C_{\Psi,\gamma}(x)$ and their posterior probability content differs from $\gamma$ by at most $\gamma' - \gamma$, where $\gamma' > \gamma$ is the next largest value for which we have exact content.

Now, consider the continuous case with a regular discretization. For $S^* \subset \Psi_\lambda = \{\psi_\lambda(\psi) : \psi_\lambda(\psi) \in B_\lambda(\psi)\}$, namely, $S^*$ is a subset of a discretized version of $\Psi(\Theta)$, we define the *un-discretized* version of $S^*$ to be $S = \cup_{\psi\in S^*} B_\lambda(\psi)$. Now, let $C^*_{\Psi,\lambda,\gamma}(x)$ be the $\gamma$-relative belief region for the discretized problem and let $C_{\Psi,\lambda,\gamma}(x)$ be its un-discretized version. Note that in a continuous context, we will consider two sets as equal if they differ only by a set of measure 0 with respect to $\Pi_\Psi$. The following result says that a $\gamma$-relative belief-credible region for the discretized problem, after un-discretizing, converges to the $\gamma$-relative belief region for the original problem.

**Theorem 7.** *Suppose that $\pi_\Psi$ is positive and continuous, there is regular discretization of $\Psi(\Theta)$ and $RB_\Psi(\psi \,|\, x)$ has a continuous posterior distribution. Then, $\lim_{\lambda\to 0} C_{\Psi,\lambda,\gamma}(x) = C_{\Psi,\gamma}(x)$.*

While Theorem 7 is interesting in its own right, it can also be used to prove that relative belief regions are limits of the lowest posterior loss regions.

Let $D^*_{\eta,\lambda,\gamma}(x)$ be the $\gamma$-lowest posterior loss region obtained for the discretized problem using loss function (12), and let $D_{\eta,\lambda,\gamma}(x)$ be the un-discretized version.

**Theorem 8.** *Suppose that $\pi_\Psi$ is positive and continuous, we have a regular discretization of $\Psi$, and $RB_\Psi(\psi \,|\, x)$ has a continuous posterior distribution. Then, we have that*

$$C_{\Psi,\gamma}(x) = \lim_{\lambda\to 0}\liminf_{\eta\to 0} D_{\Psi,\gamma}(x) = \lim_{\lambda\to 0}\limsup_{\eta\to 0} D_{\Psi,\gamma}(x).$$

In [18,19], additional properties of relative belief regions are developed. For example, it has been shown that a $\gamma$-relative belief region $C_{\Psi,\gamma}(x)$ for $\psi$, satisfying $\Pi_\Psi(C_{\Psi,\gamma}(x) \,|\, x) = \gamma$, minimizes $\Pi_\Psi(B)$ among all (measurable) subsets of $\Psi$ satisfying $\Pi_\Psi(B \,|\, x) \geq \gamma$. So, a $\gamma$-relative belief region is the smallest among all $\gamma$-credible regions for $\psi$, where the size is measured using the prior measure. This property has several consequences. For example, the prior probability that a region $B(x) \subset \Psi(\Theta)$ contains a false value from the prior is given by $\int_\Theta \int_\Psi F_\theta(\psi \in B(x))\,\Pi_\Psi(d\psi)\,\Pi(d\theta)$, where a false value is a value of $\psi \sim \Pi_\Psi$ generated independently of $(\theta, x) \sim \Pi_\Psi \times F_\theta$. It can be demonstrated that a $\gamma$-relative belief region minimizes this probability among all $\gamma$-credible regions for $\psi$ and is always unbiased in the sense that the probability of covering a false value is bounded above by $\gamma$. Furthermore, a $\gamma$-relative belief region maximizes the relative belief ratio $\Pi_\Psi(B \,|\, x)/\Pi_\Psi(B)$ and the Bayes factor $\Pi_\Psi(B \,|\, x)\Pi_\Psi(B^c)/\Pi_\Psi(B^c \,|\, x)\Pi_\Psi(B)$ among all regions $B \subset \Psi$ with $\Pi_\Psi(B) = \Pi_\Psi(C_{\Psi,\gamma}(x) \,|\, x)$.

While the results in this section focus on obtaining credible regions for parameters, similar results can be proven for the construction of prediction regions.

## 6. Conclusions

Relative belief inferences are based on a clear characterization of statistical evidence and are closely related to likelihood inferences. This, along with their invariance and optimality properties, positions these as prime candidates for appropriate inferences in Bayesian contexts. This paper shows that relative belief inferences also arise naturally in a decision-theoretic formulation using loss functions based on the prior. So, relative belief inferences represent a degree of unification between the evidential and decision-theoretic approaches to deriving statistical inferences.

**Author Contributions:** Conceptualization, M.E. and G.H.J.; Formal analysis, M.E. and G.H.J.; Writing—original draft, M.E.; Writing—review & editing, G.H.J. All authors have read and agreed to the published version of the manuscript.

**Funding:** This research was funded by the Natural Sciences and Engineering Research Council of Canada, grant RGPIN-2024-03839.

**Data Availability Statement:** Data is contained within the article.

**Conflicts of Interest:** The authors declare no conflicts of interest.

## Appendix A

**Proof of Theorem 2 and Corollary 1.** We have the following,

$$\begin{aligned} r_\eta(\delta\,|\,x) &= \int_\Psi L_{RB,\eta}(\theta,\delta(x))\pi_\Psi(\psi\,|\,x)\,\nu_\Psi(d\psi) \\ &= \int_\Psi \frac{\pi_\Psi(\psi\,|\,x)}{\max(\eta,\pi_\Psi(\psi))}\nu_\Psi(d\psi) - \frac{\pi_\Psi(\delta(x)\,|\,x)}{\max(\eta,\pi_\Psi(\delta(x)))}. \end{aligned} \tag{A1}$$

The first term in (A1) is bounded above by $1/\eta$ and does not depend on $\delta(x)$, so the value of the Bayes rule at $x$ is obtained by finding $\delta(x)$, which maximizes the second term. Note that,

$$\frac{\pi_\Psi(\delta(x)\,|\,x)}{\max(\eta,\pi_\Psi(\delta(x)))} = \begin{cases} \frac{\pi_\Psi(\delta(x)\,|\,x)}{\eta} & \text{if } \eta > \pi_\Psi(\delta(x)), \\ RB_\Psi(\delta(x)\,|\,x) & \text{if } \eta \le \pi_\Psi(\delta(x)). \end{cases} \tag{A2}$$

There are, at most, finitely many values of $\psi$ satisfying $\eta \le \pi_\Psi(\psi)$, and so $RB_\Psi(\psi\,|\,x)$ assumes a maximum on this set, say at $\psi_\eta(x)$, and $\psi_\eta(x) = \psi_{RB}(x)$ when $\eta \le \pi_\Psi(\psi_{RB}(x))$. If $\eta > \pi_\Psi(\delta(x))$, then $\pi_\Psi(\delta(x)\,|\,x)/\eta < RB_\Psi(\delta(x)\,|\,x) \le RB_\Psi(\psi_{RB}(x)\,|\,x)$. This proves that, for all $\eta \le \eta_0 = \pi_\Psi(\psi_{RB}(x)) > 0$, the maximizer of (A2) is given by $\delta(x) = \psi_{RB}(x)$, and the results are established. □

**Proof of Theorem 3.** The prior risk of $\delta$ is given by

$$\begin{aligned} r(\delta) &= \int_\Theta \int_\mathcal{X} L(\theta,\delta(x))\,F(dx\,|\,\theta)\,\Pi(d\theta) \\ &= \int_\Theta \int_\mathcal{X} [h(\Psi(\theta)) - I_{\{\delta(x)\}}(\Psi(\theta))h(\Psi(\theta))]\,F(dx\,|\,\theta)\,\Pi(d\theta) \\ &= \int_\Theta h(\Psi(\theta))\,\Pi(d\theta) - \int_\mathcal{X}\int_\Theta I_{\{\delta(x)\}}(\Psi(\theta))h(\Psi(\theta))\,\Pi(d\theta\,|\,x)\,M(dx) \\ &= \int_\Theta h(\Psi(\theta))\,\Pi(d\theta) - \int_\mathcal{X} h(\delta(x))\pi_\Psi(\delta(x)\,|\,x)\,M(dx) \end{aligned}$$

and

$$
\begin{aligned}
&\int_\Theta \int_\Theta \int_\mathcal{X} L(\theta', \delta(x))\, F(dx \,|\, \theta)\, \Pi(d\theta)\, \Pi(d\theta') \\
&= \int_\Theta \int_\Theta \int_\mathcal{X} [h(\Psi(\theta')) - I_{\{\delta(x)\}}(\Psi(\theta'))h(\Psi(\theta'))]\, F(dx \,|\, \theta)\, \Pi(d\theta)\, \Pi(d\theta') \\
&= \int_\Theta h(\Psi(\theta))\, \Pi(d\theta) - \int_\mathcal{X} h(\delta(x))\pi_\Psi(\delta(x))\, M(dx).
\end{aligned}
$$

Therefore, $\delta$ is Bayesian-unbiased if and only if

$$
\int_\mathcal{X} h(\delta(x))[\pi_\Psi(\delta(x) \,|\, x) - \pi_\Psi(\delta(x))]\, M(dx) \geq 0. \tag{A3}
$$

This inequality holds when $\delta(x) = \psi_{RB}(x)$ because $\pi_\Psi(\cdot \,|\, x)/\pi_\Psi(\cdot)$ is the density of $\Pi_\Psi(\cdot \,|\, x)$ with respect to $\Pi_\Psi$, which implies that the maximum of this density is greater than or equal to 1. □

**Proof of Theorem 4 and Corollary 3.** Just as in Theorem 2, a Bayes rule $\delta_{\lambda,\eta}(x)$ maximizes $\pi_{\Psi,\lambda}(\delta(x) \,|\, x)/\max(\eta, \pi_{\Psi,\lambda}(\delta(x)))$ for $\delta(x) \in \Psi_\lambda$. Furthermore, as in Theorem 2, such a rule exists. Now, we define $\eta(\lambda)$ so that $0 < \eta(\lambda) < \Pi_\Psi(B_\lambda(\psi_{RB}(x)))$, and note that $\eta(\lambda) \to 0$ as $\lambda \to 0$. As $\lambda \to 0$, we have that

$$
\frac{\pi_{\Psi,\lambda}(\psi_\lambda(\psi_{RB}(x)) \,|\, x)}{\max(\eta(\lambda), \pi_{\Psi,\lambda}(\psi_\lambda(\psi_{RB}(x)))} = \frac{\pi_{\Psi,\lambda}(\psi_\lambda(\psi_{RB}(x)) \,|\, x)}{\pi_{\Psi,\lambda}(\psi_\lambda(\psi_{RB}))} \to RB_\Psi(\psi_{RB}(x) \,|\, x). \tag{A4}
$$

Let $\epsilon > 0$. Let $\lambda_0$ be such that $\sup_{\psi \in \Psi} \mathrm{diam}(B_\lambda(\psi)) < \epsilon/2$ for all $\lambda < \lambda_0$. Then, for $\lambda < \lambda_0$, and any $\delta(x)$ satisfying $||\delta(x) - \psi_{RB}(x)|| \geq \epsilon$, we have

$$
\begin{aligned}
&\frac{\pi_{\Psi,\lambda}(\psi_\lambda(\delta(x)) \,|\, x)}{\pi_{\Psi,\lambda}(\psi_\lambda(\delta(x)))} = \frac{\int_{B_\lambda(\psi_\lambda(\delta(x)))} \pi_\Psi(\psi \,|\, x)\, \nu_\Psi(d\psi)}{\int_{B_\lambda(\psi_\lambda(\delta(x)))} \pi_\Psi(\psi)\, \nu_\Psi(d\psi)} \\
&= \frac{\int_{B_\lambda(\psi_\lambda(\delta(x)))} RB_\Psi(\psi \,|\, x)\pi_\Psi(\psi)\, \nu_\Psi(d\psi)}{\int_{B_\lambda(\psi_\lambda(\delta(x)))} \pi_\Psi(\psi)\, \nu_\Psi(d\psi)} \\
&\leq \sup_{\{\psi: ||\psi - \psi_{RB}(x)|| > \epsilon/2\}} RB_\Psi(\psi \,|\, x) < RB_\Psi(\psi_{RB}(x) \,|\, x).
\end{aligned} \tag{A5}
$$

By (A4) and (A5), there exists $\lambda_1 < \lambda_0$, such that, for all $\lambda < \lambda_1$, then

$$
\frac{\pi_{\Psi,\lambda}(\psi_\lambda(\psi_{RB}(x)) \,|\, x)}{\pi_{\Psi,\lambda}(\psi_\lambda(\psi_{RB}(x)))} > \sup_{\{\psi: ||\psi - \psi_{RB}(x)|| > \epsilon/2\}} RB_\Psi(\psi \,|\, x). \tag{A6}
$$

Therefore, when $\lambda < \lambda_1$, a Bayes rule, $\delta_{\lambda,\eta(\lambda)}(x)$ satisfies

$$
\begin{aligned}
&\frac{\pi_{\Psi,\lambda}(\delta_{\lambda,\eta(\lambda)}(x) \,|\, x)}{\pi_{\Psi,\lambda}(\delta_{\lambda,\eta(\lambda)}(x))} \geq \frac{\pi_{\Psi,\lambda}(\delta_{\lambda,\eta(\lambda)}(x) \,|\, x)}{\max(\eta(\lambda), \pi_{\Psi,\lambda}(\delta_{\lambda,\eta(\lambda)}(x)))} \\
&\geq \frac{\pi_{\Psi,\lambda}(\psi_\lambda(\psi_{RB}(x)) \,|\, x)}{\max(\eta(\lambda), \pi_{\Psi,\lambda}(\psi_\lambda(\psi_{RB}(x)))} = \frac{\pi_{\Psi,\lambda}(\psi_\lambda(\psi_{RB}(x)) \,|\, x)}{\pi_{\Psi,\lambda}(\psi_\lambda(\psi_{RB}(x)))}.
\end{aligned} \tag{A7}
$$

By (A5), (A6), and (A7) this implies that $||\delta_{\lambda,\eta(\lambda)}(x) - \psi_{RB}(x)|| < \epsilon/2$ and the convergence is established.

Now, $\pi_{\Psi,\lambda}(\hat{\psi}_\lambda(x) \,|\, x)/\pi_{\Psi,\lambda}(\hat{\psi}_\lambda(x)) \geq \pi_{\Psi,\lambda}(\delta_{\lambda,\eta(\lambda)}(x) \,|\, x)/\pi_{\Psi,\lambda}(\delta_{\lambda,\eta(\lambda)}(x))$, and so (A5), (A6), and (A7) imply that $||\hat{\psi}_\lambda(x) - \psi_{RB}(x)|| < \epsilon$ and the convergence of $\hat{\psi}_\lambda(x)$ to $\psi_{RB}(x)$ is established. □

**Proof of Theorem 6.** For $c > 0$ let $S_c(x) = \{\psi : RB_\Psi(\psi \,|\, x) \geq c\}$ and $S_{\eta,c}(x) = \{\psi : \pi_\Psi(\psi \,|\, x)/\max(\eta, \pi_\Psi(\psi)) \geq c\}$. Note that $S_{\eta,c}(x) \uparrow S_c(x)$ as $\eta \to 0$.

Suppose $c$ is such that $\Pi_\Psi(S_c(x)\,|\,x) \leq \gamma$. Then, $\Pi_\Psi(S_{\eta,c}(x)\,|\,x) \leq \gamma$ for all $\eta$, and so $S_{\eta,c}(x) \subset D_{\eta,\gamma}(x)$. This implies that $S_c(x) \subset \liminf_{\eta\to 0} D_{\eta,\gamma}(x)$ and since $\Pi_\Psi(C_{\Psi,\gamma}(x)\,|\,x) = \gamma$, this implies that $C_{\Psi,\gamma}(x) \subset \liminf_{\eta\to 0} D_{\eta,\gamma}(x)$.

Now suppose $c$ is such that $\Pi_\Psi(S_c(x)\,|\,x) > \gamma$. Then there exists $\eta_0$, such that for all $\eta < \eta_0$, we have $\Pi_\Psi(S_{\eta,c}(x)\,|\,x) > \gamma$. Since $D_{\eta,\gamma}(x) \subset S_{\eta,c}(x)$ when $\eta < \eta_0$, then $\limsup_{\eta\to 0} D_{\eta,\gamma}(x) \subset S_c(x)$. Choosing $c = c_{\gamma'}(x)$ for $\gamma' > \gamma$ implies $\limsup_{\eta\to 0} D_{\eta,\gamma}(x) \subset C_{\Psi,\gamma'}(x)$. □

**Proof of Theorem 7.** Let $S_c(x) = \{\psi : RB_\Psi(\psi\,|\,x) \geq c\}$ and

$$S_{\lambda,c}(x) = \{\psi : \Pi_\Psi(B_\lambda(\psi)\,|\,x)/\Pi_\Psi(B_\lambda(\psi)) \geq c\}.$$

Recall that $\lim_{\lambda\to 0}\Pi_\Psi(B_\lambda(\psi)\,|\,x)/\Pi_\Psi(B_\lambda(\psi)) = \lim_{\lambda\to 0} RB_\Psi(B_\lambda(\psi)\,|\,x) = RB_\Psi(\psi\,|\,x)$ for every $\psi$. If $RB_\Psi(\psi\,|\,x) > c$, there exists $\lambda_0$ such that for all $\lambda < \lambda_0$, then $\Pi_\Psi(RB_\Psi(B_\lambda(\psi)\,|\,x) > c$ and this implies that $\psi \in \liminf_{\lambda\to 0} S_{\lambda,c}(x)$. Now $\Pi_\Psi(RB_\Psi(\psi\,|\,x) = c) = 0$ and so $S_c(x) \subset \liminf_{\lambda\to 0} S_{\lambda,c}(x)$ (after possibly deleting a set of $\Pi_\Psi$-measure 0 from $S_c(x)$). If $\psi \in \limsup_{\lambda\to 0} S_{\lambda,c}(x)$, then $RB_\Psi(B_\lambda(\psi)\,|\,x) \geq c$ for infinitely many $\lambda \to 0$, which implies that $RB_\Psi(\psi\,|\,x) \geq c$ and, therefore, $\psi \in S_c(x)$. This proves $S_c(x) = \lim_{\lambda\to 0} S_{\lambda,c}(x)$ (up to a set of $\Pi_\Psi$-measure 0) so that $\lim_{\lambda\to 0}\Pi_\Psi(S_{\lambda,c}(x)\Delta S_c(x)\,|\,x) = 0$ for any $c$.

Let $c_{\lambda,\gamma}(x) = \sup\{c \geq 0 : \Pi_\Psi(S_{\lambda,c}(x)\,|\,x) \geq \gamma\}$ so $S_{c_\gamma(x)}(x) = C_{\Psi,\gamma}(x)$, $S_{\lambda,c_{\lambda,\gamma}(x)}(x) = C_{\Psi,\lambda,\gamma}(x)$ and

$$\begin{aligned}&\Pi_\Psi(C_{\Psi,\gamma}(x)\Delta C_{\Psi,\lambda,\gamma}(x)\,|\,x) = \Pi_\Psi(S_{c_\gamma(x)}(x)\Delta S_{\lambda,c_{\lambda,\gamma}(x)}(x)\,|\,x)\\ &\leq \Pi_\Psi(S_{c_\gamma(x)}(x)\Delta S_{\lambda,c_\gamma(x)}(x)\,|\,x) + \Pi_\Psi(S_{\lambda,c_{\lambda,\gamma}(x)}(x)\Delta S_{\lambda,c_\gamma(x)}(x)\,|\,x).\end{aligned} \tag{A8}$$

Since $S_{c_\gamma(x)}(x) = \lim_{\lambda\to 0} S_{\lambda,c_\gamma(x)}(x)$ then

$$\Pi_\Psi(S_{c_\gamma(x)}(x)\Delta S_{\lambda,c_\gamma(x)}(x)\,|\,x) \to 0$$

and $\Pi_\Psi(S_{\lambda,c_\gamma(x)}(x)\,|\,x) \to \Pi_\Psi(S_{c_\gamma(x)}(x)\,|\,x) = \gamma$ as $\lambda \to 0$. Now consider the second term in (A8). Since $RB_\Psi(\psi\,|\,x)$ has a continuous posterior distribution, $\Pi_\Psi(RB_\Psi(\psi\,|\,x) \geq c\,|\,x)$ is continuous in $c$. Let $\epsilon > 0$ and note that for all $\lambda$ small enough, $\Pi_\Psi(S_{\lambda,c_{\gamma-\epsilon}(x)}(x)\,|\,x) < \gamma$ and $\Pi_\Psi(S_{\lambda,c_{\gamma+\epsilon}(x)}(x)\,|\,x) > \gamma$, which implies that $c_{\gamma+\epsilon}(x) \leq c_{\lambda,\gamma}(x) \leq c_{\gamma-\epsilon}(x)$ and, therefore, $S_{\lambda,c_{\gamma+\epsilon}(x)}(x) \subset S_{\lambda,c_{\lambda,\gamma}(x)} \subset S_{\lambda,c_{\gamma-\epsilon}(x)}(x)$. As $S_{\lambda,c_{\lambda,\gamma}(x)}(x) \subset S_{\lambda,c_\gamma(x)}(x)$ or $S_{\lambda,c_{\lambda,\gamma}(x)}(x) \supset S_{\lambda,c_\gamma(x)}(x)$ then

$$\Pi_\Psi(S_{\lambda,c_{\lambda,\gamma}(x)}(x)\Delta S_{\lambda,c_\gamma(x)}(x)\,|\,x) = |\Pi_\Psi(S_{\lambda,c_{\lambda,\gamma}(x)}(x)\,|\,x) - \Pi_\Psi(S_{\lambda,c_\gamma(x)}(x)\,|\,x)|.$$

For all $\lambda$ small, then $|\Pi_\Psi(S_{\lambda,c_{\lambda,\gamma}(x)}(x)\,|\,x) - \Pi_\Psi(S_{\lambda,c_\gamma(x)}(x)\,|\,x)|$ is bounded above by

$$\begin{aligned}\max\{&|\Pi_\Psi(S_{\lambda,c_{\gamma+\epsilon}(x)}(x)\,|\,x) - \Pi_\Psi(S_{\lambda,c_\gamma(x)}(x)\,|\,x)|,\\ &|\Pi_\Psi(S_{\lambda,c_{\gamma-\epsilon}(x)}(x)\,|\,x) - \Pi_\Psi(S_{\lambda,c_\gamma(x)}(x)\,|\,x)|\}\end{aligned}$$

and this upper bound converges to $\epsilon$ as $\lambda \to 0$. Since $\epsilon$ is arbitrary, this implies that the second term in (A8) goes to 0 as $\lambda \to 0$ and this proves the result. □

**Proof of Theorem 8.** Without loss of generality suppose that $0 < \gamma < 1$. Let $\epsilon > 0$ and $\delta > 0$ satisfy $\gamma + \delta \leq 1$. Put $\gamma'(\lambda,\gamma) = \Pi_\Psi(C_{\Psi,\lambda,\gamma}(x)\,|\,x)$, $\gamma''(\lambda,\gamma) = \Pi_\Psi(C_{\Psi,\lambda,\gamma+\delta}(x)\,|\,x)$ and note that $\gamma'(\lambda,\gamma) \geq \gamma$, $\gamma''(\lambda,\gamma) > \gamma + \delta$. By Theorem 7, we have $C_{\Psi,\lambda,\gamma}(x) \to C_{\Psi,\gamma}(x)$ and $C_{\Psi,\lambda,\gamma+\delta}(x) \to C_{\Psi,\gamma+\delta}(x)$ as $\lambda \to 0$ so $\gamma'(\lambda,\gamma) \to \gamma$ and $\gamma''(\lambda,\gamma) \to \gamma + \delta$ as $\lambda \to 0$. This implies that there is a $\lambda_0(\delta)$ such that for all $\lambda < \lambda_0(\delta)$ then $\gamma'(\lambda,\gamma) < \gamma''(\lambda,\gamma)$. Therefore, by Theorem 6, we have that for all $\lambda < \lambda_0(\delta)$,

$$C_{\Psi,\lambda,\gamma}(x) \subset \liminf_{\eta\to 0} D_{\eta,\lambda,\gamma'(\lambda,\gamma)}(x) \subset \limsup_{\eta\to 0} D_{\eta,\lambda,\gamma'(\lambda,\gamma)}(x) \subset C_{\Psi,\lambda,\gamma+\delta}(x). \tag{A9}$$

From (A9) and Theorem 7, we conclude that

$$C_{\Psi,\gamma}(x) \subset \liminf_{\lambda\to 0}\liminf_{\eta\to 0} D_{\eta,\lambda,\gamma'(\lambda,\gamma)}(x) \subset \limsup_{\lambda\to 0}\limsup_{\eta\to 0} D_{\eta,\lambda,\gamma'(\lambda,\gamma)}(x) \subset C_{\Psi,\gamma+\delta}(x).$$

Since $\lim_{\delta\to 0} C_{\Psi,\gamma+\delta}(x) = C_{\Psi,\gamma}(x)$ this establishes the result. □

## References


1. Birnbaum, A. On the foundations of statistical inference (with discussion). *J. Am. Stat. Assoc.* **1962**, *57*, 269–326. [CrossRef]
2. Royall, R.M. *Statistical Evidence: A Likelihood Paradigm*; Chapman & Hall: London, UK, 1997.
3. Evans, M. *Measuring Statistical Evidence Using Relative Belief. Chapman & Hall/CRC Monographs on Statistics & Applied Probability*; Chapman and Hall/CRC: Boca Raton, FL, USA, 2015.
4. Evans, M. The concept of statistical evidence: Historical roots and current developments. *Encyclopedia* **2024**, *4*, 1201–1216. [CrossRef]
5. Savage, L.J. *The Foundations of Statistics*; Dover Publications: Mineola, NY, USA, 1971.
6. Lehmann, E.L. Neyman's statistical philosophy. In *Selected Works of E. L. Lehmann*; Springer: Boston, MA, USA, 1995; pp. 1067–1073.
7. Evans, M.; Jang, G.-H. Weak informativity and the information in one prior relative to another. *Stat. Sci.* **2011**, *26*, 423–439. [CrossRef]
8. Robert, C.P. Intrinsic losses. *Theory Decis.* **1996**, *40*, 191–214. [CrossRef]
9. Bernardo, J.M. Intrinsic credible regions: An objective Bayesian approach to interval estimation. *Test* **2005**, *14*, 317–384. [CrossRef]
10. Le Cam, L. On some asymptotic properties of maximum likelihood estimates and related Bayes' estimates. *Univ. Calif. Publ. Statist.* **1953**, *1*, 277–329.
11. Bernardo, J.M.; Smith, A.F.M. *Bayesian Theory. Wiley Series in Probability and Statistics*; John Wiley & Sons Ltd.: New York, NY, USA, 2000.
12. Berger, J.O. *Statistical Decision Theory and Bayesian Analysis*; Springer: New York, NY, USA, 1985.
13. Rudin, W. *Real and Complex Analysis*; McGraw Hill: New York, NY, USA, 1974.
14. Al-Labadi, L.; Evans, M. Optimal robustness results for some Bayesian procedures and the relationship to prior-data conflict. *Bayesian Anal.* **2017**, *12*, 702–728. [CrossRef]
15. Al-Labadi, L.; Alzaatreh, A.; Evans, M. How to measure evidence and its strength: Bayes factors or relative belief ratios? *arXiv* **2024**, arXiv:2301.08994.
16. Nott, D.; Wang, X.; Evans, M.; Englert, B.-G. Checking for prior-data conflict using prior to posterior divergences. *Stat. Sci.* **2020**, *35*, 234–253. [CrossRef]
17. Evans, M.; Moshonov, H. Checking for prior-data conflict. *Bayesian Anal.* **2006**, *1*, 893–914. [CrossRef]
18. Evans, M.; Shakhatreh, M. Optimal properties of some Bayesian inferences. *Electron. J. Stat.* **2008**, *2*, 1268–1280. [CrossRef]
19. Evans, M.; Guttman, I.; Swartz, T. Optimality and computations for relative surprise inferences. *Canad. J. Statist.* **2006**, *34*, 113–129. [CrossRef]

entropy

MDPI

Article

# A Bayesian Approach for Modeling and Forecasting Solar Photovoltaic Power Generation

**Mariana Villela Flesch [1], Carlos Alberto de Bragança Pereira [2] and Erlandson Ferreira Saraiva [3,*]**

1 Faculty of Engineering, Architecture and Urbanism and Geography, Federal University of Mato Grosso do Sul, Campo Grande 79070-900, MS, Brazil; mariflesch@hotmail.com
2 Institute of Matematics and Statistics, University of São Paulo, São Paulo 05508-090, SP, Brazil; cadebp@gmail.com
3 Institute of Matematics, Federal University of Mato Grosso do Sul, Campo Grande 79070-900, MS, Brazil
* Correspondence: erlandson.saraiva@ufms.br; Tel.: +55-67-3345-7511

**Abstract:** In this paper, we propose a Bayesian approach to estimate the curve of a function $f(\cdot)$ that models the solar power generated at $k$ moments per day for $n$ days and to forecast the curve for the $(n+1)$th day by using the history of recorded values. We assume that $f(\cdot)$ is an unknown function and adopt a Bayesian model with a Gaussian-process prior on the vector of values $\mathbf{f}(\mathbf{t}) = (f(1), \ldots, f(k))$. An advantage of this approach is that we may estimate the curves of $f(\cdot)$ and $f_{n+1}(\cdot)$ as "smooth functions" obtained by interpolating between the points generated from a $k$-variate normal distribution with appropriate mean vector and covariance matrix. Since the joint posterior distribution for the parameters of interest does not have a known mathematical form, we describe how to implement a Gibbs sampling algorithm to obtain estimates for the parameters. The good performance of the proposed approach is illustrated using two simulation studies and an application to a real dataset. As performance measures, we calculate the absolute percentage error, the mean absolute percentage error (MAPE), and the root-mean-square error (RMSE). In all simulated cases and in the application to real-world data, the MAPE and RMSE values were all near 0, indicating the very good performance of the proposed approach.

**Keywords:** photovoltaic solar power forecasting; statistical modeling; Bayesian inference; Gaussian process; MCMC; Gibbs sampling algorithm

## 1. Introduction

In recent years, there has been a significant increase in solar energy generation, from both photovoltaic plants and residences with photovoltaic panels installed on their roofs. This has been driven by societal and governmental interest in clean and renewable energy, with an important aspect of "clean" being lower $CO_2$ emission compared to fossil fuels. Because of this, more photovoltaic plants are being connected to local electric-supply systems every day.

However, according to [1], this causes instability in the grid, which is one of the greatest challenges to the energy industry. Electrical operators need to know how much energy will be added to the system in order to balance it with consumption and ensure that the system is capable of meeting consumer demand. For [2], the ability to predict photovoltaic solar power output is very important for secure grid operation, scheduling, and the effectiveness of power-grid management.

In this context, statistical models emerge as important tools for modeling and predicting photovoltaic power generation. Some statistical approaches used for modeling the solar photovoltaic power generation include linear regression models [3–6], autoregressive models [7–9], and artificial-neural-network models [10–12], that is, parametric models are still commonly employed due to their ease of use.

However, parametric models have at least three limitations: (i) the analysis is limited to the function (or functions) previously chosen by the analyst; (ii) the complexity and/or flexibility of the functions considered is limited by the number of parameters in the functions; and (iii) there may exist several functions that can fit the recorded values equally well. A common solution adopted in much statistical analysis is to fit a set of candidate models and then choose the best model using some model-selection criterion, such as AIC [13] or BIC [14]. Even in those cases, issues (ii) and (iii) still remain.

In this paper, in order to give models more flexibility instead of restricting them to a function $f(\cdot)$ chosen previously, we adopt a semi-parametric Bayesian approach, in which the curve of the function $f(\cdot)$ is estimated from the observed data. For this, we assume that cumulative solar photovoltaic power generation, measured at $k$ time instants per day, is modeled by an additive model composed of a nonlinear growth function $f(\cdot)$ evaluated at $k$ time instants plus a random error $\varepsilon$. However, instead of setting up $f(\cdot)$ as a known mathematical function, we assume that $f(\cdot)$ is an unknown function whose vector of values $\mathbf{f}(\mathbf{t}) = (f(1), \ldots, f(k))$ is treated as a set of parameters that must be estimated based on recorded data for $\mathbf{t} = (1, \ldots, k)$. To jointly estimate $\mathbf{f}(\mathbf{t})$ and the other parameters in the proposed model, we adopt a Bayesian approach with a Gaussian-process prior over $\mathbf{f}(\mathbf{t})$. An advantage of this approach is that we may estimate the curve of function $f(\cdot)$ using "smooth functions" that are obtained by linking points generated from a $k$-variate normal distribution with an appropriate mean vector and covariance matrix. Additionally, we present a forecasting procedure for the value of the curve on the $(n+1)$th day, conditioned on the values recorded over the first $n$ days.

Since the joint posterior distribution for the parameters and the predictive distribution of the proposed model do not have known mathematical forms, we describe how to implement a Gibbs sampling algorithm [15–17] to generate random values from these two distributions. This algorithm generates values from the distributions of interest in an indirect way, using the conditional posterior distributions, as long as those are known, which is the case for the model proposed here.

To illustrate the performance of the proposed model, we include two simulation studies. In the first one, we examine the performance of the proposed model in the estimation of the curve of $f(\cdot)$. As performance measures, we calculate the absolute percentage error (APE) and the mean absolute percentage error (MAPE). In all simulated cases, the proposed approach presents MAPE values near 0, indicating that the estimated values are close to the real values. In the second simulation study, we evaluate the performance of predictions made with the proposed approach. Analogously to the first simulation study, the proposed approach presents satisfactory performance, as indicated by MAPE values near zero. In addition to APE and MAPE values, we also evaluate the performance of predictions in terms of the root-mean-square error (RMSE). The RMSE values were all near zero, indicating a very good performance of the proposed approach. We also apply the proposed approach to a real dataset. Like in the simulation studies, the results obtained in this application were very accurate, with MAPE and RMSE values near zero.

The main novelty that we bring in this paper is in the way that we model the generation of solar photovoltaic power over time. First, we consider the photovoltaic power generated on each day as having its own behavior, and the behavior is taken to be proportional to the average behavior of the measurements over the last $n$ days. Second, the function $f(\cdot)$ that models the generation of solar power as a function of time is considered unknown, but with its curve estimated from the observed data. We highlight the following four advantages of this approach: (i) the proposed hierarchical Bayesian model is very flexible and adapts to the number of values recorded; (ii) the inference procedure is based on a Gibbs sampling algorithm, which can be easily implemented in statistical software such as R; (iii) the predicted growth curve for day $(n+1)$ is obtained directly using only the history of the first $n$ measurements; and (iv) there is no need to fit a set of models and afterwards compare them using some model-selection criterion.

The remainder of the paper is organized as follows. In Section 2, we present the dataset that has motivated us to develop the proposed modeling, the hierarchical Bayesian model, and the estimation procedure for the parameters of interest. In Section 2, we also present the results of the first simulation study. In Section 3, we present the prediction procedure and the second simulation study. In Section 4, we apply the proposed approach to a real dataset. Finally, in Section 5, we conclude with some final remarks.

## 2. Dataset and Statistical Modeling

A critical component of any statistical analysis is the dataset used to make inferences on the parameters of interest. The dataset used in this paper was obtained from a photovoltaic plant installed on the campus of the Brazilian Federal University of Mato Grosso du Sul. This dataset is freely available on the website https://github.com/lscad-facom-ufms/Solar2 (accessed on 3 June 2024), and more details on the experiment can be found in [18]. The dataset used to make inferences on the parameters of the proposed model contains measurements of solar photovoltaic power generation taken at $k = 74$ time instants each day over a period of $N = 19$ days. In other words, the dataset is a spreadsheet composed of 3 columns and $k \times n = 74 \times 19 = 1406$ lines. Figure 1 shows a clipping from the data spreadsheet, showing that the first column contains the day (1–19), the second column the time instant (TI, 1-74), and the third column the observed values for photovoltaic solar power (PSP) generated.

| 1 | Day | TI | PSP |
|---|---|---|---|
| 2 | 1 | 1 | 63.15 |
| 3 | 1 | 2 | 140.31 |
| 4 | 1 | 3 | 273.65 |
| 5 | 1 | 4 | 435.1 |

**Figure 1.** Clipping of the data spreadsheet.

Let $W_{it}$ be the solar power recorded at the $i$th time instant of the $i$th day and $\mathbf{W}_i = (W_{i1}, \ldots, W_{ik})$ the vector of values recorded on the $i$th day, for $i = 1, \ldots, N$ and $t = 1, \ldots, k$. Figure 2 shows the values recorded over the first two days of the experiment. As one can note, the recorded data on these two days present great variability, which makes the modeling process difficult. For the other days, the recorded values present similar behavior. Due to this, we opt to model the accumulated values.

Consider $W_{it}^{ac} = \sum_{t'=1}^{t} W_{it'}$ to be the accumulated values of the photovoltaic power generated through the $t$th time instant of the $i$th day and $\mathbf{W}_i^{ac} = \left(W_{it}^{ac}, \ldots, W_{ik}^{ac}\right)$ to be the vector of accumulated values, for $i = 1, \ldots, n$ and $t = 1, \ldots, k$. Figure 3a shows the accumulated values recorded over the first four days of the experiment. As one can note, the accumulated values present more stable and predictable behavior. However, many values in the vectors $\mathbf{W}_i^{ac}$ are on the scale of 100,000, which could cause computational problems in the inference process. To avoid this problem, we opt to model the *logarithm* of the accumulated values, denoted by $Y_{it} = \log\left(W_{it}^{ac}\right)$, for $i = 1, \ldots, N$ and $t = 1, \ldots, k$. Additionally, let $\mathbf{Y}_i = (Y_{i1}, \ldots, Y_{ik})$ be the vector of values recorded on the $i$th day, for $i = 1, \ldots, N$.

Figure 3b, shows the graph of $\mathbf{Y}$ values recorded over the first four days of the experiment. The symbols • in black connected by black lines represent the average values $\bar{\mathbf{y}} = (\bar{y}_1, \ldots, \bar{y}_k)$. For the other days, the recorded $\mathbf{Y}$ values present similar behavior. From this point forward, and without loss of generality, consider the modeling of $\mathbf{y} = (\mathbf{y}_1, \ldots, \mathbf{y}_n)$, that is, the data recorded over the first $n$ days of the experiment, for $n < N$, where the primary interest is in in the prediction of the values that will be generated on day $(n+1)$. That is, $\mathbf{y}$ is an $n \times k$ matrix in which row $i$ contains the $y$ values generated on day $i$, for $i = 1, \ldots, n$.

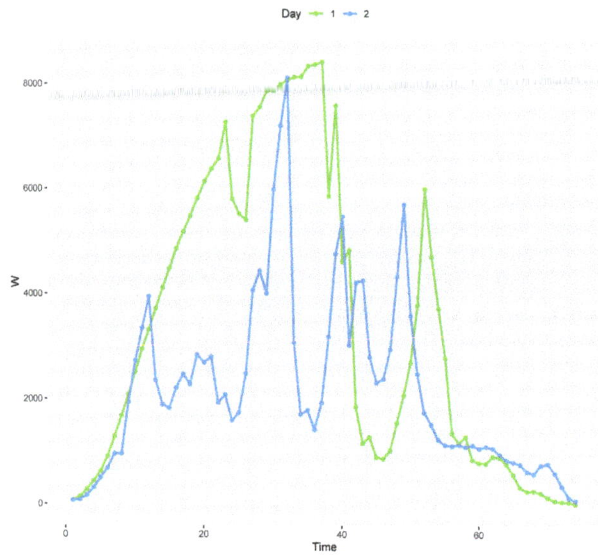


Figure 2. Solar power generated over time for days 1 and 2.

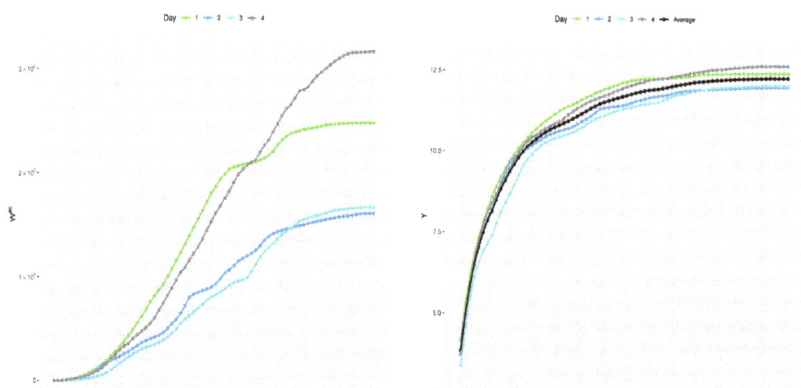


(a) (b)

**Figure 3.** Solar power generated over time. (**a**) $\mathbf{W}_1$, $\mathbf{W}_2$, $\mathbf{W}_3$, and $\mathbf{W}_4$. (**b**) $\mathbf{W}_1^{ac}$, $\mathbf{W}_2^{ac}$, $\mathbf{W}_3^{ac}$, and $\mathbf{W}_4^{ac}$.

### 2.1. Hierarchical Bayesian Model

Based on Figure 3b, consider the average curve (black line) to be a nonlinear growth function $f(t)$, where $\mathbf{f}(\mathbf{t}) = (f(1), \ldots, f(k))$ is a vector composed of the values of $f(\cdot)$ at $k$ instants of time, $\mathbf{t} = (1, \ldots, k)$. Assume that the growth function for the $i$th day is proportional to $f(\cdot)$, i.e., $f_i(\cdot) = C_i f(\cdot)$, for $C_i > 0$ and $i = 1, \ldots, n$ with $n \leq N$. In other words, we are assuming that there is a growth function $f(\cdot)$ whose curve represents the average curve from $n$ curves, with the curve on the $i$th day proportional to the average curve.

Consider recorded values on the $i$th day to be generated according to the following additive model:

$$\mathbf{Y}_i = (Y_{i1}, \ldots, Y_{ik}) \sim C_i \cdot \mathbf{f}(\mathbf{t}) + \boldsymbol{\varepsilon}_i, \tag{1}$$

with $C_i > 0$, where $\boldsymbol{\varepsilon}_i = (\varepsilon_{i1}, \ldots, \varepsilon_{ik})$ is a vector of random errors, for $i = 1, \ldots, n$. Assume that $\boldsymbol{\varepsilon}_i$ is generated according to a $k$-dimensional multivariate normal distribution with mean vector $\mathbf{0} = (0, \ldots, 0)$ and covariance matrix $\Sigma$ (dimension $k \times k$) composed of the elements $\sigma_\varepsilon(t,t') = \mathbb{C}ov(\varepsilon_{it}, \varepsilon_{it'})$, for $t,t' = 1, \ldots, k$ and $i = 1, \ldots, n$.

To complete Model (1), we could fix $f(\cdot)$ as a known mathematical function, such as the logistic or Gompertz growth functions, among others. However, three problems with this parametric approach are (i) the analysis is limited to the function (or functions) previously chosen by the analyst; (ii) the complexity and/or flexibility of the considered functions is limited by the number of parameters in the functions; and (iii) there may exist several functions that can fit the recorded values equally well. A common solution to problem (i) is to fit a set of candidate models and then choose the best model using some model selection criterion, such as AIC [13] or BIC [14]. However, issues (ii) and (iii) still remain.

In order to avoid restricting our model to a specific parametric function, from this point onward, we assume that $f(\cdot)$ is an unknown function and that the values $\mathbf{f}(\mathbf{t}) = (f(1), \ldots, f(k))$ are model parameters that need to be estimated from observed data. Under this scenario and with the model given by (1), the parameters of interest are $\boldsymbol{\theta} = (\mathbf{f}(\mathbf{t}), \Sigma, \mathbf{C})$, where $\mathbf{f}(\mathbf{t}) = (f(1), \ldots, f(k))$, $\Sigma$ is the covariance matrix of the vector of random errors, and $\mathbf{C} = (C_1, \ldots, C_n)$.

To estimate $\boldsymbol{\theta}$, we take a hierarchical Bayesian approach with a Gaussian-process prior on $\mathbf{f}(\mathbf{t})$, denoted by $\mathbf{f}(\mathbf{t})|\mathbf{m}, \Sigma_\mathbf{f} \sim \mathcal{GP}(\mathbf{m}, \Sigma_\mathbf{f})$. This means that we are considering $f(\cdot)$ as an unknown function, but with the vector of values $\mathbf{f}(\mathbf{t}) = (f(1), \ldots, f(k))$ generated by a $k$-variate normal distribution with mean vector $\mathbf{m}$ and covariance matrix $\Sigma_\mathbf{f}$ composed of the elements $\sigma_\mathbf{f}(t,t') = \mathbb{C}\text{ov}(f(t), f(t'))$, for $t,t' = 1, \ldots, k$. For $\Sigma$, we assume a conjugated inverse-Wishart prior distribution with parameter $(\delta, \mathbb{V})$, and, for $C_i$, we assume a prior distribution given by a truncated normal distribution (with the left-of-zero part removed) with parameters $\mu_\mathbf{c}$ and $\sigma^2_\mathbf{c}$, for $i = 1, \ldots, n$. The proposed model is then represented hierarchically:

$$\begin{aligned} \mathbf{Y}_i = (Y_{i1}, \ldots, Y_{ik})|\mathbf{f}(\mathbf{t}), \Sigma, \mathbf{C} &\sim \mathcal{N}_k(C_i\mathbf{f}(\mathbf{t}), \Sigma) \\ \mathbf{f}(\mathbf{t})|\mathbf{m}, \Sigma_\mathbf{f} &\sim \mathcal{GP}(\mathbf{m}, \Sigma_\mathbf{f}) \\ \Sigma|\delta, \mathbb{V} &\sim \mathcal{IW}(\delta, \mathbb{V}) \\ C_i|\mu_\mathbf{c}, \sigma^2_\mathbf{c} &\sim \mathcal{N}_{\text{trunc}}\left(0; \mu_\mathbf{c}, \sigma^2_\mathbf{c}\right), \end{aligned} \tag{2}$$

where $\mathcal{N}_k(\cdot)$, $\mathcal{GP}(\cdot)$, $\mathcal{IW}(\cdot)$, and $\mathcal{N}_{\text{trunc}}(0; \cdot)$ represent, respectively, a $k$-variate Gaussian distribution, the Gaussian process, the inverse-Wishart distribution, and the truncated normal distribution with values only on the right half-line; additionally, $\mathbf{m}$, $\Sigma_\mathbf{f}$, $\delta$, $\mathbb{V}$, $\mu_\mathbf{c}$, and $\sigma^2_\mathbf{c}$ are known hyperparameters, for $i = 1, \ldots, n$.

We complete the modeling by setting the following:

(i) $\mathbf{m} = \mathbf{0}$ in order to represent our lack of informative prior knowledge about the expected value of $\mathbf{f}(\mathbf{t})$;

(ii) $\Sigma_\mathbf{f} = \lambda\mathbb{W}$, with $\lambda > 0$ and $\mathbb{W}$ a matrix of dimension $k \times k$ composed of elements $\kappa(t,t')$, calculated according to the squared exponential kernel, i.e.,

$$\kappa(t,t') = \eta^2 \exp\left\{-\frac{(t-t')^2}{2\nu^2}\right\}, \tag{3}$$

with $\eta, \nu > 0$. The parameter $\eta$ controls how far the generated values are from the average. Small values for $\eta$ characterize functions that are close to their average value, whereas larger values allow greater variation. The parameter $\nu$ controls the smoothness of the function obtained by connecting the points. Small values of $\nu$ mean that function values may change quickly, and large values characterize functions that change more slowly (are smoother). We set $\lambda = 100$, $\eta = 1$, and $\nu = 1$ in order to obtain a weakly informative prior distribution;

(iii) We finalize the model by setting $\delta = k$, $\mathbb{V} = 0.01 \cdot \mathbb{I}_k$, where $\mathbb{I}$ is the identity matrix of dimension $k \times k$, and $\mu_\mathbf{c} = \sigma^2_\mathbf{c} = 1$.

Applying Bayes's theorem, the joint posterior distribution for $\boldsymbol{\theta} = (\mathbf{f}(\mathbf{t}), \Sigma, \mathbf{C})$ is given by

$$\pi(\boldsymbol{\theta}|\mathbf{y}, \mathbf{t}) \propto \mathcal{L}(\boldsymbol{\theta}|\mathbf{y}, \mathbf{t})\pi(\mathbf{f}(\mathbf{t})|\mathbf{m}, \Sigma_{\mathbf{f}})\pi(\Sigma|\delta, \mathbb{V})\pi\left(\mathbf{C}|\mu_{c}, \sigma_{c}^{2}\right), \tag{4}$$

where $\mathcal{L}(\boldsymbol{\theta}|\mathbf{y}, \mathbf{t})$ is the likelihood function of a $k$-variate normal distribution with parameters $\mathbf{f}(\mathbf{t})$ and $\Sigma$, and $\pi(\cdot)$ represents the probability density functions of the prior distributions, for $\mathbf{y} = (\mathbf{y}_1, \ldots, \mathbf{y}_n)$ and $\mathbf{t} = (1, \ldots, k)$.

However, the joint posterior distribution does not have a known mathematical form that allows us to generate random values from this distribution directly. Due to this, we need to use an algorithm that generates the random numbers of this joint distribution in an indirect way. In this paper, we opt to generate random values from $\pi(\boldsymbol{\theta}|\mathbf{y}, \mathbf{t})$ using the Gibbs sampling algorithm [15,17] due to its simplicity of implementation and efficiency. This algorithm generates values from the joint posterior distribution indirectly, using the conditional posterior distributions, as long as they are known.

For the proposed hierarchical Bayesian model, the conditional posterior distributions are known and given by

$$\mathbf{f}(\mathbf{t})|\mathbf{y}, \mathbf{t}, \bullet \sim \mathcal{GP}\left(\Sigma^{-1}\left(\sum_{i=1}^{n} C_i\Sigma^{-1} + \Sigma_{\mathbf{f}}^{-1}\right)^{-1}\sum_{i=1}^{n} C_i\mathbf{y}_i, \left(\sum_{i=1}^{n} C_i\Sigma^{-1} + \Sigma_{\mathbf{f}}^{-1}\right)^{-1}\right) \tag{5}$$

$$\Sigma|\mathbf{y}, \mathbf{t}, \bullet \sim \mathcal{IW}\left(\delta + k + n, \mathbb{V} + \sum_{i=1}^{n}(\mathbf{y}_i - C_i\mathbf{f}(\mathbf{t}))^{\top}(\mathbf{y}_i - C_i\mathbf{f}(\mathbf{t}))\right) \tag{6}$$

$$C_i|\mathbf{y}, \mathbf{t}, \bullet \sim \mathcal{N}_{\text{trunc}}\left(0, \frac{\mathbf{f}(\mathbf{t})^{\top}\Sigma^{-1}\mathbf{y}_i + 1)}{\mathbf{f}(\mathbf{t})^{\top}\Sigma^{-1}\mathbf{f}(\mathbf{t}) + 1}, \frac{\sigma_{\mathbf{c}}^2}{\mathbf{f}(\mathbf{t})^{\top}\Sigma^{-1}\mathbf{f}(\mathbf{t}) + \mu}\right), \tag{7}$$

where the symbol $\bullet$ represents all other parameters.

Using the conditional posterior distributions, we implement a Gibbs sampling algorithm according to the steps described in Algorithm 1.

**Algorithm 1** Gibbs sampling algorithm.

1: Let the state of the Markov chain consist of $\boldsymbol{\theta} = (\mathbf{f}(\mathbf{t}), \Sigma, \mathbf{C})$.
2: Initialize the algorithm with a configuration $\boldsymbol{\theta}^{(0)} = \left(\mathbf{f}(\mathbf{t})^{(0)}, \Sigma^{(0)}, \mathbf{C}^{(0)}\right)$.
3: **procedure** For the $l$th iteration of the algorithm, $l = 1, \ldots, L$:
4: generate $\mathbf{f}(\mathbf{t})^{(l)}$ from conditional distribution (5), given $\Sigma^{(l-1)}$ and $\mathbf{C}^{(l-1)}$;
5: generate $\Sigma^{(l)}$ from conditional distribution (6), given $\mathbf{f}(\mathbf{t})^{(l)}$ and $\mathbf{C}^{(l-1)}$;
6: generate $C_i^{(l)}$ from conditional distribution (7), given $\mathbf{f}(\mathbf{t})^{(l)}$ and $\Sigma^{(l)}$, for $i = 1, \ldots, n$.

After running $L$ iterations of the Gibbs sampling algorithm, we discard the first $B$ iterations as a burn-in. We also consider jumps of size $J$, i.e., only 1 drawn from every $J$ was extracted from the original sequence in order to obtain a sub-sequence of size $S = [(L - B)/J]$ to make inferences. The estimates for the parameters of interest are given by the average of the generated values, i.e.,

$$\hat{\mathbf{f}}(\mathbf{t}) = \frac{1}{S}\sum_{l=1}^{S}\mathbf{f}(\mathbf{t})^{(M(l))}, \ \hat{\Sigma} = \frac{1}{S}\sum_{l=1}^{S}\Sigma^{(M(l))} \text{ and } \hat{C}_i = \frac{1}{S}\sum_{l=1}^{S}C_i^{(M(l))}$$

where $\mathbf{f}(\mathbf{t})^{(M(l))}$, $\Sigma^{(M(l))}$, and $\mathbf{C}^{(M(l))}$ are the generated values for parameters $\mathbf{f}(\mathbf{t})$, $\Sigma$, and $\mathbf{C}$, respectively, in the $M(l) = (B + 1 + (l-1)\cdot J)$th iteration of the algorithm, for $l = 1, \ldots, S$. The 95% credibility interval for each of the parameters is given by the 2.5% and 97.5%

percentiles of the sampled values. The estimated curve of $f(\cdot)$ is obtained by plotting the points $\left(t, \hat{f}(t)\right)$ connected by lines, for $t = 1, \ldots, k$.

## 2.2. First Simulation Study

To illustrate the performance of the proposed approach, we develop a simulation study. To generate the dataset, we consider $f(\cdot)$ as the log-Gompertz function of parameters $\alpha_1$, $\alpha_2$, and $\alpha_3$ with the parametrization $f(t) = \log(\alpha_1) - \exp\{\alpha_2 - \alpha_3 t\}$, for $t > 0$. We set $\alpha_1 = 12$, $\alpha_2 = 2$, and $\alpha_3 = 0.1$. For the covariance matrix $\Sigma$, we calculate each term according to the squared-exponential kernel given in Equation (3) with $\eta^2 = 0.01$ and $\nu^2 = 10$.

The procedure to generate the artificial dataset is given by the following four steps:

(i) Fix the number of days $n$ and the number of time instants per day $k$;
(ii) With $\mathbf{t} = (1, \ldots, k)$, calculate $\mathbf{f}(\mathbf{t}) = (f(1), \ldots, f(k))$, where $f(t)$ is given by the log-Gompertz function described above;
(iii) Fix the values $\mathbf{C} = (C_1, \ldots, C_n)$, with $C_i > 0$ and $i = 1, \ldots, n$;
(iv) Generate $\mathbf{Y}_i = (Y_{i1}, \ldots, Y_{ik}) \sim \mathcal{N}_k(\mathbf{f}(\mathbf{t})^\top, \Sigma)$, for $i = 1, \ldots, n$

To simplify the visualization of the results, our first simulation study considers $n = 4$ and $k = 50$. We set $\mathbf{C} = (C_1, C_2, C_3, C_4) = (0.8, 0.9, 1.1, 1.2)$. Figure 4a shows the curve of $f(t)$, which we call the "average curve", and the curve for the $i$th day is given by $C_i\mathbf{f}(\mathbf{t})$, for $i = 1, 2, 3, 4$. Figure 4b shows the curves and actual $\mathbf{y}$ values generated for each day (coloured • symbols), in which black • symbols are the average values $\bar{\mathbf{y}}$.

With the dataset generated, we apply the proposed Gibbs sampling algorithm with $L$=55,000 iterations, $B = 5000$, and $J = 10$. In this way, we obtain a posterior sample of size $S = 5000$ to make inferences. To verify how far the estimates $\hat{f}(t)$ are from the real values $f(t)$, we calculate the absolute percentage error:

$$\mathrm{APE}(d_t) = \frac{|f(t) - \hat{f}(t)|}{f(t)} \cdot 100,$$

for $t = 1, \ldots, k$.

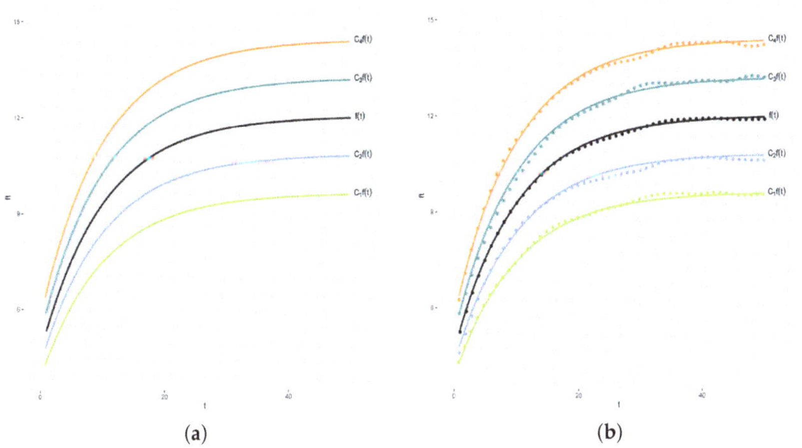

**Figure 4.** Real curves and generated values. (**a**) Real curves. (**b**) Generated values.

Figure 5a shows $f(t)$ (black line) and the estimated curve by the proposed method (red line) with a credibility band of 95% (red region). Figure 5b shows $\mathrm{APE}(\mathbf{d}) = (\mathrm{APE}(d_1), \ldots, \mathrm{APE}(d_k))$. $\mathrm{APE}(\mathbf{d})$ values ranged from a minimum of 0.0145 to a maximum of 1.4481, with a mean absolute percentage error (MAPE) of 0.4568. The small values of APE indicate that the estimated values $\hat{f}(t)$ are very close to the real values of $f(t)$, for $t = 1, \ldots, k$.

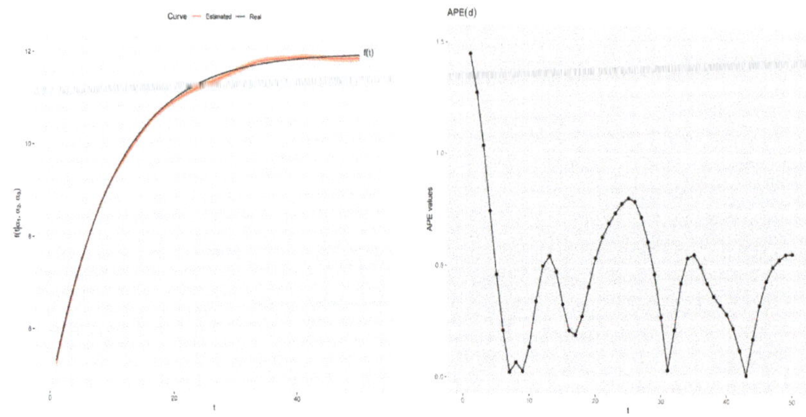


**(a)** **(b)**

**Figure 5.** Real and estimated curve and APE($\mathbf{d}$) values. (**a**) Real and estimated $f(t)$. (**b**) APE($\mathbf{d}$).

Similarly, we obtained the estimated curve for the $i$th day by plotting the pairs $(t, \hat{y}_{it})$ connected by lines, for $\hat{y}_{it} = \hat{C}_i \hat{f}(t), i = 1, \ldots, n$, and $t = 1, \ldots, k$. For this case, we calculate two different kinds of error: the APE for comparison between the real value $C_i f(t)$ and the estimated value $\hat{y}_{it}$; and the APE for comparison between the generated values $y_{it}$ and the estimated $\hat{y}_{it}$ values. They are calculated as follows:

$$\text{APE}(d_{it}) = \frac{|C_i f(t) - \hat{y}_{it}|}{C_i f(t)} \cdot 100 \quad \text{and} \quad \text{APE}(e_{it}) = \frac{|y_{it} - \hat{y}_{it}|}{y_{it}} \cdot 100$$

for $i = 1, \ldots, n$ and $t = 1, \ldots, k$.

Table 1 shows the estimates and 95% credibility intervals for parameters $C_i, i = 1, 2, 3, 4$. As one can note, the estimated values are very close to the real values, and the real values are inside the credibility intervals.

**Table 1.** Real value, estimated value, and 95% credibility interval for $C_i, i = 1, 2, 3, 4$.

| Parameter | Real Value | Estimated Value | Credibility Interval of 95% |
|---|---|---|---|
| $C_1$ | 0.8 | 0.8060 | (0.7997, 0.8080) |
| $C_2$ | 0.9 | 0.8955 | (0.8913, 0.9003) |
| $C_3$ | 1.1 | 1.0998 | (1.0939, 1.1057) |
| $C_4$ | 1.2 | 1.2006 | (1.1949, 1.2071) |

Figure 6a shows $C_i f(t)$ (black line) and the estimated curves by the proposed method (red lines), where the symbols • are the generated values for each day. Figure 6b shows the values of APE($\mathbf{d}_i$), and Table 2 shows the summary measures of APE($\mathbf{d}_i$) values, for $i = 1, \ldots, n$. As one can note, the estimated curves for each one of the four days is satisfactorily close to the real curves, as indicated by APE($\mathbf{d}_i$) values near zero, $i = 1, \ldots, n$.

**Table 2.** Summary measures of APE($\mathbf{d}_i$) values, for $i = 1,2,3,4$.

| Measure | Min | $1^oQ$ | Median | Mean | $3^oQ$ | Max |
|---|---|---|---|---|---|---|
| APE($\mathbf{d}_1$) | 0 | 0.2100 | 0.4450 | 0.5212 | 0.7675 | 1.3100 |
| APE($\mathbf{d}_2$) | 0 | 0.4825 | 0.8350 | 0.7972 | 1.0575 | 1.9400 |
| APE($\mathbf{d}_3$) | 0.0100 | 0.2400 | 0.4650 | 0.4650 | 0.5775 | 1.4600 |
| APE($\mathbf{d}_4$) | 0.0100 | 0.2375 | 0.4250 | 0.4364 | 1.5750 | 1.4000 |

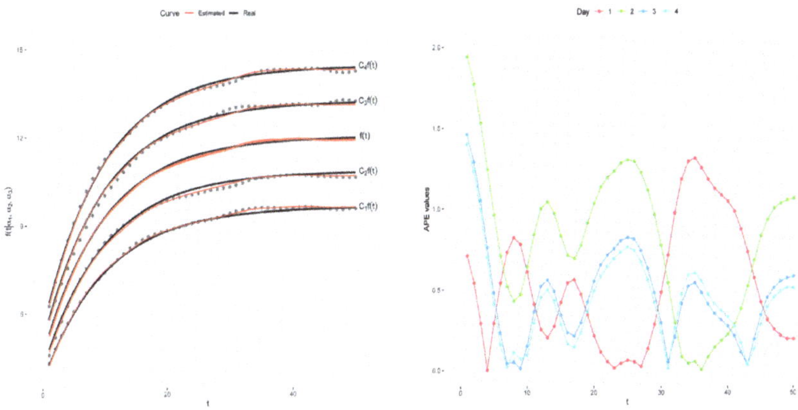


(**a**) (**b**)

**Figure 6.** Real and estimated curves and APE($\mathbf{d}_i$) values, for $i = 1,2,3,4$. (**a**) Real and estimated curves. (**b**) APE($\mathbf{d}_i$) values.

Figure 7 shows the graphic of the values of APE($\mathbf{e}_i$) $=$ (APE($e_1$), …, APE($e_k$)), and Table 3 shows the summary measures of APE($\mathbf{e}_i$) values, for $i = 1, \ldots, n$. APE($\mathbf{e}_i$) values are near zero, indicating that the estimated values $\hat{y}_{it}$ are satisfactorily close to the generated values $y_{it}$, for $i = 1, \ldots, n$ and $t = 1, \ldots, k$.

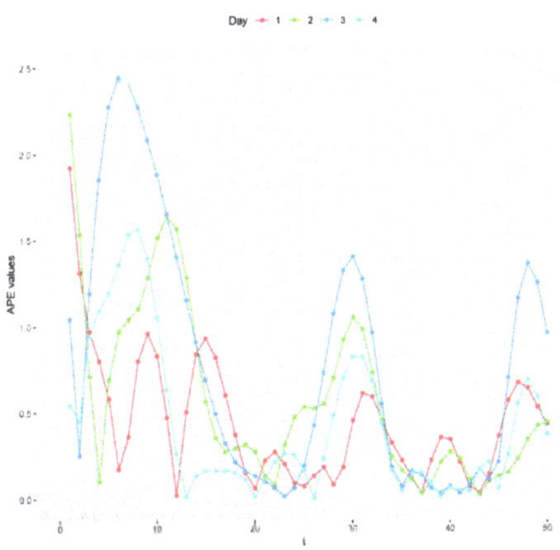


**Figure 7.** APE($e_i$) values, for $i = 1,2,3,4$.

**Table 3.** Summary measures of APE($e_i$) values, for $i = 1,2,3,4$.

| Measure | Min | $1^oQ$ | Median | Mean | $3^oQ$ | Max |
|---|---|---|---|---|---|---|
| APE($\mathbf{e}_1$) | 0.0200 | 0.1775 | 0.3600 | 0.4446 | 0.6075 | 1.9200 |
| APE($\mathbf{e}_2$) | 0.0200 | 0.2150 | 0.4300 | 0.5860 | 0.9175 | 2.2300 |
| APE($\mathbf{e}_3$) | 0.0100 | 0.1450 | 0.6200 | 0.7934 | 1.2650 | 2.4400 |
| APE($\mathbf{e}_4$) | 0 | 0.1325 | 0.2400 | 0.4330 | 0.3675 | 1.5600 |

Since the inferences were made from a posterior sample obtained from an MCMC algorithm, it is important to check the convergence of the sampled values. As is usual, we verify the convergence of the sampled values empirically, using the ergodic mean (ErM) of the sampled values. Figure 8 shows the graphic of the ErM for the sampled values for $f(1)$ and $f(30)$. As one can note, there is no reason to doubt the convergence of the sampled values since the ErM values present satisfactory stabilization. The graphs of ErM for the sampled values for other parameters are similar.

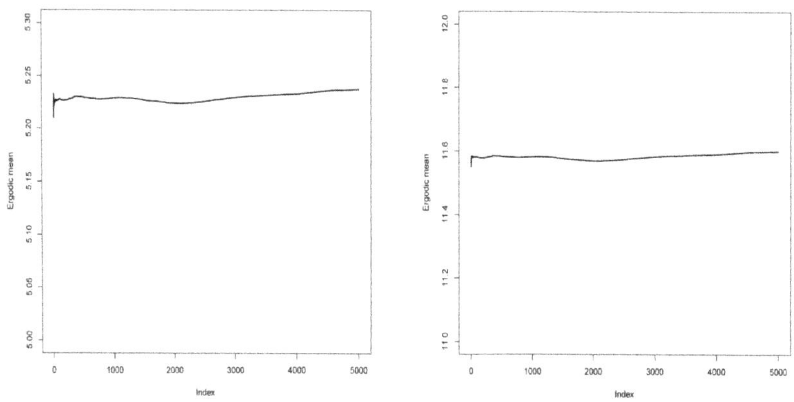


(**a**) (**b**)

**Figure 8.** Ergodic mean (ErM) for sampled values for $f(1)$ and $f(30)$. (**a**) $f(1)$. (**b**) $f(30)$.

## 3. Predictions

In addition to obtaining the estimates $\hat{\boldsymbol{\theta}} = \left(\hat{\mathbf{f}}(\mathbf{t}), \hat{\Sigma}, \hat{\mathbf{C}}\right)$ for the parameters $\boldsymbol{\theta} = (\mathbf{f}(\mathbf{t}), \Sigma, \mathbf{C})$, the modeling used in the previous section may also be used to predict the values that will be recorded on the $(n+1)$th day, i.e., $\mathbf{Y}_{n+1} = \left(Y_{1(n+1)}, \ldots, Y_{k(n+1)}\right)$. This can be performed by using the predictive distribution, given by

$$\pi(\mathbf{Y}_{n+1}|\mathbf{y}, \mathbf{t}) = \int \pi(\mathbf{Y}_{n+1}|\mathbf{y}, \mathbf{t}, \boldsymbol{\theta})\pi(\boldsymbol{\theta}|\mathbf{y}, \mathbf{t})d\boldsymbol{\theta}, \tag{8}$$

where $\pi(\boldsymbol{\theta}|\mathbf{y}, \mathbf{t})$ is the joint posterior distribution for $\boldsymbol{\theta}$, given in Equation (4). However, this integral does not have a known analytic solution. Due to this, we present in the following an MCMC algorithm for obtaining an approximation for this integral.

From Model (1), the marginal distribution for $\mathbf{Y}_i$ is given by a $k$-variate normal distribution with mean vector $\mathbf{0} = (0, \ldots, 0)^\top$ and covariance matrix $C_i^2\Sigma_\mathbf{f} + \Sigma$, for $i = 1, \ldots, n$. Thus,

$$\mathbf{Y} = (\mathbf{Y}_1, \ldots, \mathbf{Y}_n)|\Sigma_\mathbf{y} \sim \mathcal{N}_{nk}(\mathbf{0}, \Sigma_\mathbf{y}),$$

where $\mathcal{N}_{nk}(\cdot)$ represents an $nk$-variate normal distribution with mean vector $\mathbf{0}$ and a covariance matrix of dimension $nk \times nk$, given by

$$\Sigma_{\mathbf{y}} = \begin{bmatrix} C_1^2\Sigma_{\mathbf{f}} + \Sigma & \Sigma_{12} & \Sigma_{13} & \dots & \Sigma_{1n} \\ \Sigma_{21} & C_2^2\Sigma_{\mathbf{f}} + \Sigma & \Sigma_{23} & \dots & \Sigma_{2n} \\ \vdots & \vdots & \vdots & \vdots\vdots\vdots & \vdots \\ \Sigma_{n1} & \Sigma_{n2} & \Sigma_{n3} & \dots & C_n^2\Sigma_{\mathbf{f}} + \Sigma \end{bmatrix},$$

where $\Sigma_{ii'} = C_iC_{i'}\Sigma_{\mathbf{f}}$ are the covariance matrices (of dimension $k \times k$) among the measurements $\mathbf{Y}_i$ and $\mathbf{Y}_{i'}$, for $i, i' = 1, \dots, n$ and $i \neq i'$. Similarly, $\mathbf{Y}_{n+1} \sim \mathcal{N}_k(\mathbf{0}, C_{n+1}^2\Sigma_{\mathbf{f}} + \Sigma)$. Therefore, the joint distribution for $(\mathbf{Y}, \mathbf{Y}_{n+1})$ is

$$\begin{bmatrix} \mathbf{Y} \\ \mathbf{Y}_{n+1} \end{bmatrix} | \boldsymbol{\theta}, \mathbf{y}, \mathbf{t} \sim \mathcal{N}_{(n+1)k}\left( \begin{bmatrix} \mathbf{0} \\ \mathbf{0} \end{bmatrix}, \begin{bmatrix} \Sigma_{\mathbf{y}} & \mathbb{B}^T \\ \mathbb{B} & C_{n+1}^2\Sigma_{\mathbf{f}} + \Sigma \end{bmatrix} \right),$$

where $\mathbb{B} = \begin{bmatrix} \Sigma_{(n+1)1} \, \Sigma_{(n+1)2} \, \cdots \, \Sigma_{(n+1)n} \end{bmatrix}$ is a block of matrices, in which $\Sigma_{(n+1)i}$ are the covariance matrices among the values of $\mathbf{Y}_{n+1}$ and $\mathbf{Y}_i$ given by $\Sigma_{(n+1)i} = C_{n+1}C_i\Sigma_{\mathbf{f}}$, for $i = 1, \dots, n$.

Using the properties of the multivariate normal distribution, the conditional posterior distribution for $\mathbf{Y}_{n+1}$ is given by

$$\mathbf{Y}_{n+1} | \mathbf{y}, \mathbf{t}, \boldsymbol{\theta} \sim \mathcal{N}_k\left( \mathbb{B}\Sigma_{\mathbf{y}}^{-1}\mathbf{y}, \left(C_{n+1}^2\Sigma_{\mathbf{f}} + \Sigma\right) - \mathbb{B}^\top \left(C_{n+1}^2\Sigma_{\mathbf{f}} + \Sigma\right)^{-1} \mathbb{B} \right); \tag{9}$$

with $C_{n+1}$ generated from

$$C_{n+1} | \mathbf{C} \sim \mathcal{N}trunc(0, \overline{C}, S_{\mathbf{c}}^2), \tag{10}$$

where $\overline{C}$ and $S_{\mathbf{c}}^2$ are, respectively, the average and the variance of $\mathbf{C} = (C_1, \dots, C_n)$.

Thus, a sample from the conditional posterior distribution of $(Y_{n+1}, \boldsymbol{\theta})$ can be generated according to the steps in Algorithm 2.

**Algorithm 2** Prediction.

1: Let the state of the Markov chain consist of $\boldsymbol{\theta} = (\mathbf{f}(\mathbf{t}), \Sigma, \mathbf{C})$ and $\mathbf{Y}_{n+1}$.
2: Initialize the algorithm with a configuration $\boldsymbol{\theta}^{(0)} = \left(\mathbf{f}(\mathbf{t})^{(0)}, \Sigma^{(0)}, \mathbf{C}^{(0)}\right)$ and $C_{n+1}^{(0)}$.
3: **procedure** For the $l$th iteration of the algorithm, $l = 1, \dots, L$:
4: Update $\boldsymbol{\theta}$ according to Algorithm 1;
5: Generate $Y_{n+1}^{(l)}$ from conditional posterior distribution in (9) given $C_{n+1}^{(l-1)}$;
6: Generate $C_{n+1}$ from probability distribution in (10).

After running the algorithm for the same $L$ iterations, burn-in $B$, and jump $J$ as we used for algorithm (1), an approximation for the integral in (8) is given by

$$\tilde{\pi}(\mathbf{Y}_{n+1}|\mathbf{y}) = \frac{1}{S}\sum_{l=1}^{L} \mathbf{Y}_{n+1}^{(M(l))},$$

where $M(l)$ is the $(B + 1 + l \cdot J)$th iteration of the algorithm, for $l = 1, \dots, S$.

*Second Simulation Study*

To illustrate the performance of the prediction procedure, we present a second simulation study. Like in the first simulation study, we fix $n = 4$, $k = 50$, and $f(t)$ as the log-Gompertz function of parameters $\alpha_1 = 12$, $\alpha_2 = 2$, and $\alpha_3 = 0.1$. Here, the main objective is to predict the curve for the $(n + 1)$ = 5th day.

To obtain the curves of the first four days with the curve of $f(t)$ being the average curve, we adopt the following procedure:

(i) Let $C_i < n$ and define $\mathbf{p} = (p_1, p_2, p_3, p_4)$ with $p_i = \frac{C_i}{n}$, for $i = 1, 2, 3, 4$;
(ii) Generate $\mathbf{p} \sim \text{Dirichlet}(\boldsymbol{\alpha})$, where Dirichlet($\boldsymbol{\alpha}$) is the Dirichlet distribution with parameter $\boldsymbol{\alpha}$. We set up $\boldsymbol{\alpha} = (50, 50, 50, 50)$;
(iii) Obtain $C_i = n \cdot p_i$ and generate $\mathbf{Y}_i = (Y_{i1}, \ldots, Y_{ik}) \sim \mathcal{N}_k(C_i\mathbf{f}(\mathbf{t}), \Sigma)$, for $i = 1, \ldots, n$, where $\Sigma$ is obtained as described in simulation study 1.

The generated values for $\mathbf{C} = (C_1, C_2, C_3, C_4)$ were $(0.9187, 0.8767, 1.0126, 1.1919)$, respectively. Figure 9a shows the real curves for days 1 to 4, denoted by $C_i f(t)$ for $i = 1, 2, 3, 4$, and Figure 9b shows the same graphs as Figure 9a with the generated values for each day as correspondingly coloured • symbols, the black • symbols being the average values.

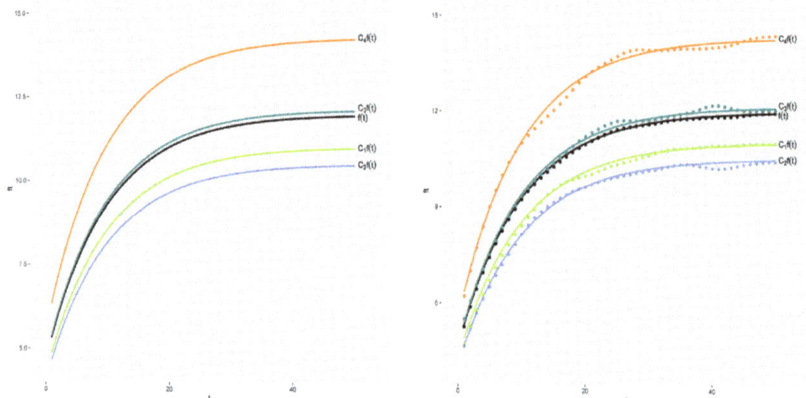


(a) (b)

**Figure 9.** Real curves and generated values. (**a**) Real curves. (**b**) Generated values.

With $(\mathbf{Y}_1, \ldots, \mathbf{Y}_n)$ values generated, we generate the data for the $(n+1)$th day as follows:

(i) Generate $C_{n+1} \sim \mathcal{N}_{\text{trunc}}(0, \overline{C}, S_c^2)$, where $\overline{C} = \frac{1}{n}\sum_{i=1}^{n} C_i$ and $S_c^2 = \frac{1}{n-1}\sum_{i=1}^{n}(C_i - \overline{C})^2$. From the generated $\mathbf{C} = (0.9187, 0.8767, 1.0126, 1.1919)$ values, the generated value for $C_{n+1}$ was 0.9823;
(ii) Generate $\mathbf{Y}_{n+1} = (Y_{(n+1)1}, \ldots, Y_{(n+1)k}) \sim \mathcal{N}_k(C_{n+1}\mathbf{f}(\mathbf{t}), \Sigma)$.

We then use the generated values for $(\mathbf{Y}_1, \ldots, \mathbf{Y}_n)$ in the the prediction procedure (Algorithm 2) and obtain the estimates for $\hat{\mathbf{Y}}_{n+1}$. For this, we apply the prediction procedure for the same $L$=55,000 iterations with a burn-in $B = 5000$ and jump of size $J = 10$ as we used in Algorithm 1. The estimated curve for the $(n+1)$th day is obtained by plotting the pairs $(t, \hat{y}_{(n+1)t})$ connected by lines, where, $\hat{y}_{(n+1)t}$ is the predicted value for $Y_{(n+1)t}$, for $t = 1, \ldots, k$.

Figure 10a shows $f(t)$ and the estimated curve by the proposed method, and Figure 10b shows the graph of APE($\mathbf{d}$) values. As in the first simulation study, the results show a very satisfactory performance of the proposed method, with the estimated curve very close to the real curve of $f(t)$, as indicated by APE($\mathbf{d}$) values all being less than 1.

Figure 11a shows $C_i f(t)$ (black line) and the estimated curves by the proposed method (red lines), with the symbols • representing the generated values for each day. Figure 11b shows APE($\mathbf{d}_i$), for $i = 1, \ldots, n$. As one can note, the estimated curves for each one of the four days are satisfactorily near the real curves, as indicated by APE($\mathbf{d}_i$) values near zero, for $i = 1, 2, 3, 4$. We also verify the convergence of the sampled values. Analogously to results presented in the first simulation study, there is no reason to doubt the convergence of the sampled values since the ErM values present satisfactory stabilization.

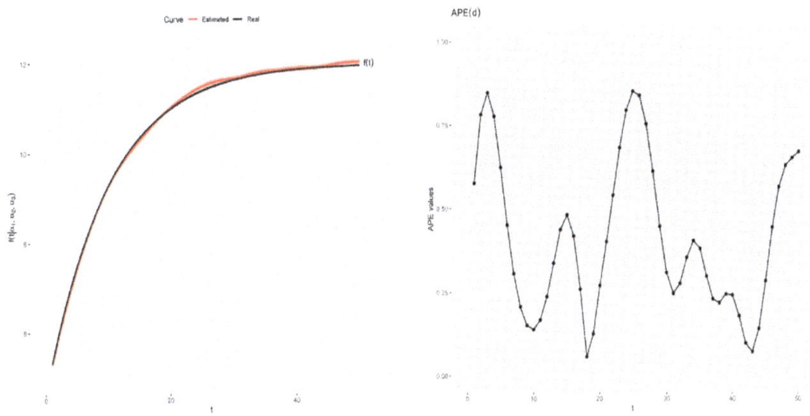


(a) (b)

**Figure 10.** Real and estimated $f(t)$ and APE($\mathbf{d}$) values. (**a**) Real and estimated curves. (**b**) APE($\mathbf{d}$) values.

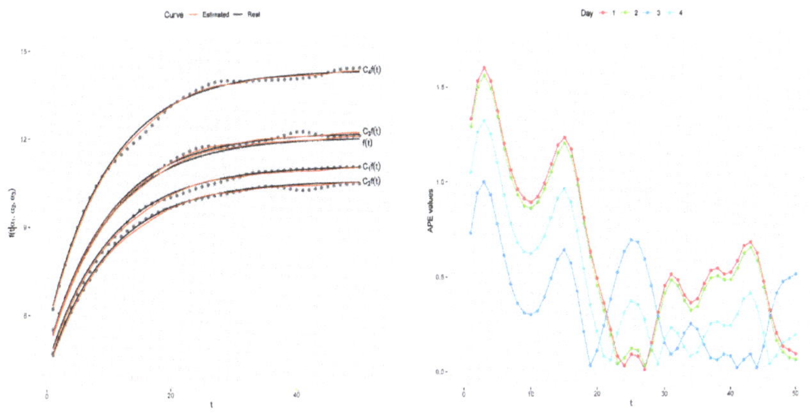


(a) (b)

**Figure 11.** Real and estimated curves and APE($\mathbf{d}_i$) values, for $i = 1,2,3,4$. (**a**) Real and estimated curves. (**b**) APE($\mathbf{d}_i$) values.

Figure 12a shows the curve for the $(n+1)$th day (green line), with the green • symbols representing the generated data for the $(n+1)$th day, the predicted curve (red line), and a posterior prediction 95% credibility band (red region). The estimate for $C_{n+1}$ is $\hat{C}_{n+1}$ = 0.9936 with a 95% credibility interval given by $(0.7207, 1.2716)$, that is, the real value $C_i = 0.9823$ is inside the credibility interval. Additionally, the real curve is completely inside the 95% posterior prediction band. Figure 12b shows the graph of APE($\mathbf{d}$) and APE($\mathbf{e}$) in relation to predicted values. All APE values are smaller than 3, indicating that predicted values are close to real values $C_{n+1}f(t)$ and to the generated values for $\mathbf{Y}_{n+1}$.

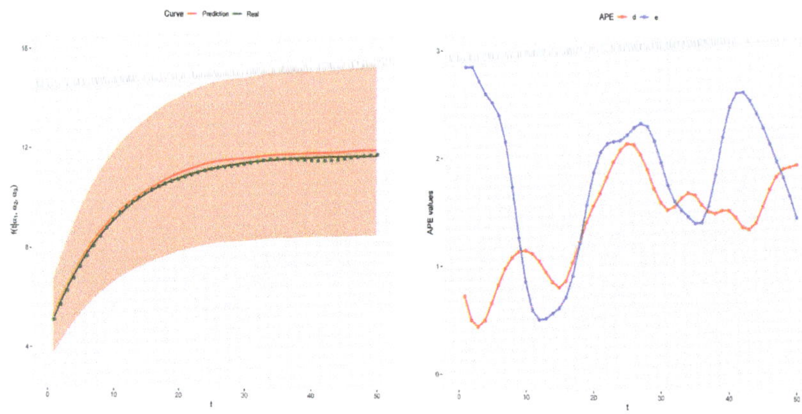


**(a)** **(b)**

**Figure 12.** Real and predicted curves and APE values. (**a**) Real and predicted curves. (**b**) APE values.

In addition to APE values, we also calculate the root-mean-square error (RMSE) in order to have one more performance measure of the predictions, given by

$$RMSE = \sqrt{\frac{1}{k}\sum_{t=1}^{k}\left(y_{(n+1)t} - \hat{y}_{(n+1)t}\right)^2},$$

where $y_{(n+1)t}$ is the value generated for the $t$-th time instant of the $(n+1)$-th day, and $\hat{y}_{(n+1)t}$ is the respective predicted value, for $t = 1, \ldots, k$. The RMSE value obtained was 0.2021, that is, similar to the APE values, the RMSE value also indicates that the predicted values are satisfactorily close to the generated values.

In order to avoid restricting the model to the results of just one artificial dataset, we repeat the second simulation study $M = 100$ times and calculate the percentage of times that the real curve for the $(n+1)$th day is completely inside the prediction band of 95% and the average of the APE and RMSE values. Overall, in 96% of simulated cases, the real curve of $C_{n+1}f(t)$ is completely inside the posterior prediction band, the average of the MAPE values is 0.9550, and the average of the RMSE values is 0.1534. Figure 13 shows the APE and RMSE values for the $M = 100$ simulations. Note that both results show a very satisfactory performance of the proposed method. As an illustration of the predictions results, Figure 14 shows the predicted curve with a 95% posterior prediction band (red region) and the real curve for the 18th and 27th simulations. For these two simulations, the MAPE values were 0.6115 and 4.0017, respectively; and the RMSE values were 0.0622 and 0.4996, respectively.

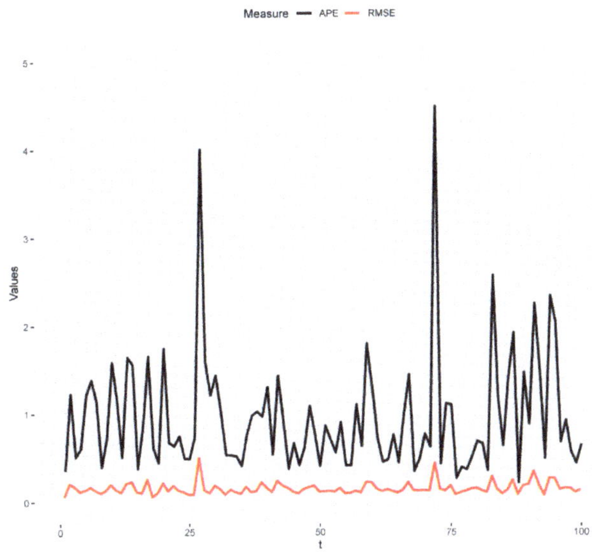


**Figure 13.** APE and RMSE values.

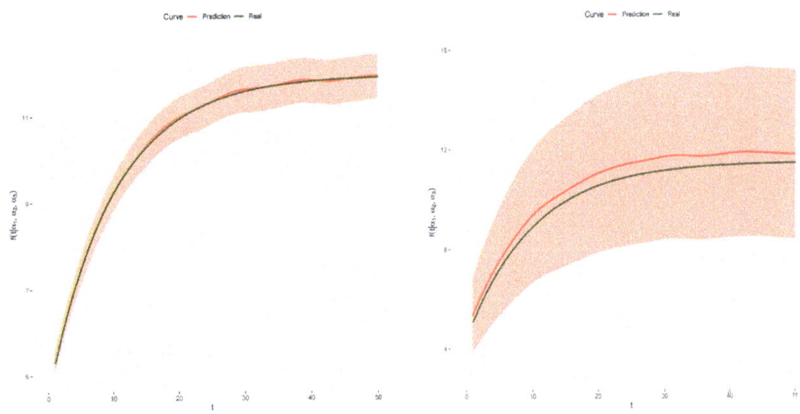


(a) (b)

**Figure 14.** Real and predicted curves for the 18th and 27th simulations. (**a**) 18th. (**b**) 27th.

## 4. Application

We now apply the proposed approach to the real dataset described in Section 2. For this application, we use the same hyperparameter values and the same $L$, $B$, and $J$ values used in the two simulation studies. Additionally, we use $n = 4$, i.e., we apply the proposed approach for estimating the curve of $f(t)$ using the dataset of four days, and then we predict the curve for the $(n+1)$th day. This procedure was applied for the data recorded over the first 19 days of the experiment, always using a window of 4 days, to obtain the estimated curve of $f(t)$ and to predict the curve for the $(n+1)$th day. Thus, overall, 15 analyses were carried out with predictions for days 5 to 19.

Our first application considers the recorded data on the first four days of the experiment to estimate the curve of $f(t)$, and then we predict the curve for the fifth day $(n+1=5)$. Figure 15a shows the average values recorded in the first four days (symbols •), the estimated curve of $f(t)$ (red line) and a 95% credibility band (red region). Figure 15b shows APE values for comparison between $\overline{\mathbf{y}}$ and the estimated values $\hat{\mathbf{y}} = (\hat{y}_1, \ldots, \hat{y}_n)$. The MAPE value is 0.2590. These results shows that the estimated values are very close to the recorded average values. In other words, the proposed approach presented a very satisfactory performance in estimating the average values recorded over the first four days on which the experiment was carried out.

Table 4 shows MAPE and RMSE values for the 15 analyses. MAPE values range from a minimum of 0.0095 for day 13 to a maximum of 0.5360 for day 11, with an average value of 0.2349. RMSE values range from 0.0011 for day 13 to a maximum of 0.0612 for day 11, with an average value of 0.0265. As one can see, all MAPE and RMSE values are near zero, indicating that the estimated values $\hat{\mathbf{y}}$ are close to the recorded $\overline{\mathbf{y}}$ for the 15 analyses.

**Table 4.** MAPE and RMSE values for analyses 1 to 15.

| Analysis | MAPE | RMSE | Analysis | MAPE | RMSE | Analysis | MAPE | RMSE |
|---|---|---|---|---|---|---|---|---|
| 1 | 0.2590 | 0.0292 | 6 | 0.2038 | 0.0228 | 11 | 0.5360 | 0.0612 |
| 2 | 0.1395 | 0.0155 | 7 | 0.3670 | 0.0393 | 12 | 0.1815 | 0.0208 |
| 3 | 0.0500 | 0.0061 | 8 | 0.2378 | 0.0273 | 13 | 0.0095 | 0.0011 |
| 4 | 0.0753 | 0.0085 | 9 | 0.2157 | 0.0243 | 14 | 0.3445 | 0.0394 |
| 5 | 0.3996 | 0.0450 | 10 | 0.4903 | 0.0542 | 15 | 0.0146 | 0.0017 |

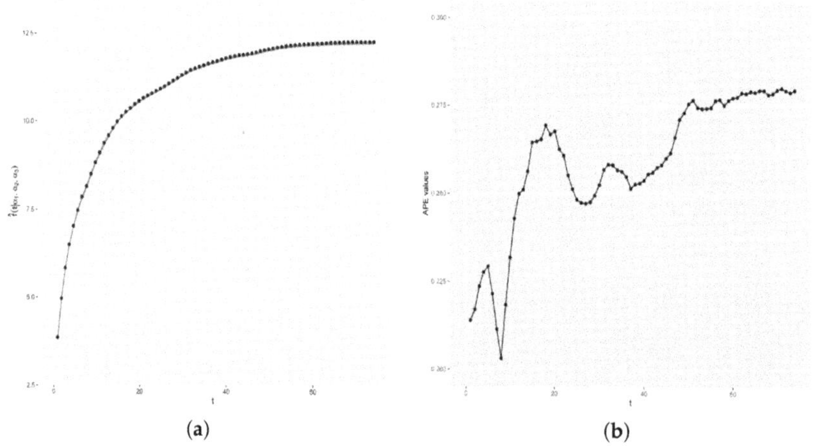

(a) (b)

**Figure 15.** Estimated curve of $f(t)$ and APE($\mathbf{e}$) values. (**a**) Estimated curve of $f(t)$. (**b**) APE($\mathbf{e}$) values.

Table 5 shows MAPE and RMSE values for the 15 predictions. As one can note, MAPE values vary from a minimum of 0.3344 for day 19 to a maximum of 7.1648 for day 13. The average value of MAPE over the 15 days was 2.5719. Similarly, RMSE values range from 0.0382 for day 19 to a maximum of 0.7410 for day 13, with an average value of 0.2895. Overall, these results show that the predicted values $\hat{\mathbf{y}}_i^{pred}$ are close to the recorded values $\mathbf{y}_i$, for $i = 5, \ldots, 19$.

As an illustration of the good performance of the proposed approach in predictions, Figure 16 shows the recorded values (symbols •), the predicted curve (red line), and a 95% prediction credibility band (red region) for the recorded values on days 9 and 19, which are the two days with the smallest MAPE and RMSE values. Figure 17 shows the prediction results for days 13 and 14, which are the two days with the greatest MAPE and RMSE values. Although predictions for days 13 and 14 present the two highest MAPE values, most of the recorded values are inside the 95% prediction credibility band. Overall, the proposed approach presented very satisfactory performance, as indicated by the small MAPE and RMSE values.

**Table 5.** MAPE and RMSE values for the predictions for days 5 to 19.

| Day | MAPE | RMSE | Day | MAPE | RMSE | Day | MAPE | RMSE |
|---|---|---|---|---|---|---|---|---|
| 5 | 2.8659 | 0.3180 | 10 | 2.8855 | 0.3323 | 15 | 0.6193 | 0.07321 |
| 6 | 2.3021 | 0.2628 | 11 | 5.1500 | 0.5780 | 16 | 0.5880 | 0.0677 |
| 7 | 5.1190 | 0.5321 | 12 | 3.6303 | 0.4415 | 17 | 0.5753 | 0.0786 |
| 8 | 1.0693 | 0.1222 | 13 | 7.1648 | 0.7410 | 18 | 0.7374 | 0.1128 |
| 9 | 0.3507 | 0.0409 | 14 | 5.1875 | 0.6027 | 19 | 0.3344 | 0.0382 |

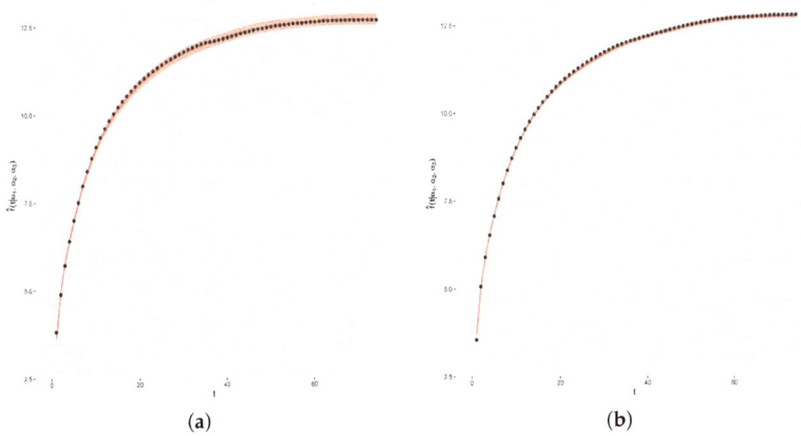

**Figure 16.** Recorded and predicted values for days 9 and 19. (**a**) Day 9. (**b**) Day 19.

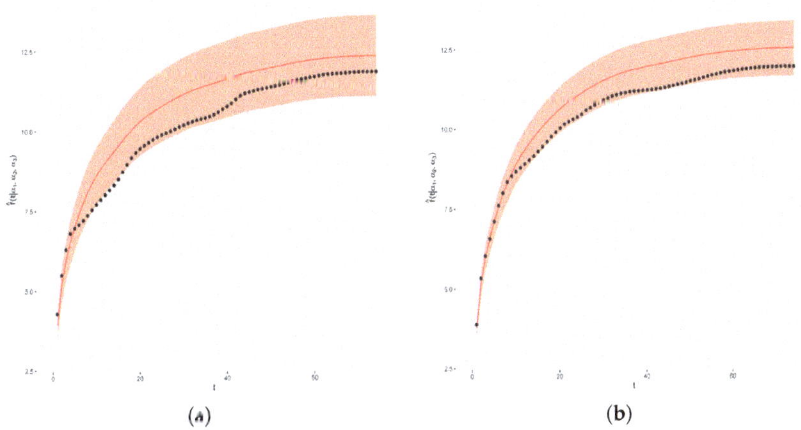

**Figure 17.** Recorded and predicted values for days 13 and 14. (**a**) Day 13. (**b**) Day 14.

## 5. Final Remarks

In this paper, we propose a Bayesian approach for modeling and forecasting photovoltaic solar power generation. For this, we assume that the growth curve of the generated power over the time of day is proportional to an average curve whose associated function is denoted by $f(t)$. However, instead of taking a parametric approach by setting up $f(t)$ as a known mathematical function, we assume that $f(t)$ is an unknown function, but with the vector of values $\mathbf{f}(\mathbf{t}) = (f(1), \ldots, f(k))$ generated a priori from a Gaussian process. To perform inference for the parameters of interest $\boldsymbol{\theta}$, we use a Gibbs sampling algorithm.

The good performance of the proposed approach and its four advantages as described in Section 1 were illustrated by means of two simulation studies and an application to a real dataset. The results obtained show that the proposed approach is an efficient alternative for modeling the solar power generated on the days considered in the study and also for forecasting next-day solar power generation.

From a practical point of view, the results show that the proposed modeling and the estimation procedure were very accurate in predicting energy generation for the next day. Although the proposed approach has been described as forecasting the growth curve for the next day, it can also be used to forecast power generation for short intervals, such as hourly power generation. An extension of the approach presented here is the inclusion of explanatory variables in the modeling since power generation is influenced by environmental variables such as temperature and irradiance. All computational implementations were carried out using the R software [19], and the code can be obtained by e-mailing the authors.

**Author Contributions:** Conceptualization, E.F.S. and C.A.d.B.P.; Data curation, M.V.F. and E.F.S.; Formal analysis, M.V.F. and E.F.S.; Methodology, M.V.F., E.F.S. and C.A.d.B.P.; Project administration, E.F.S.; Software, M.V.F. and E.F.S.; Supervision, E.F.S. and C.A.d.B.P.; Writing—review and editing, M.V.F., C.A.d.B.P. and E.F.S. All authors have read and agreed to the published version of the manuscript.

**Funding:** This study was financially supported by the Brazilian institutions CNPq (Conselho Nacional de Desenvolvimento Científico e Tecnológico), process number 402154/2023-1, and Fundect (Fundação de Apoio ao Desenvolvimento do Ensino, Ciência, e Tecnologia do Estado de Mato Grosso do Sul), TO number 120/2024, SIAFIC 818, process number 83/026.835/2024.

**Institutional Review Board Statement:** Not applicable.

**Data Availability Statement:** The real dataset is freely available on the websites cited in the article. It also can be obtained by emailing the authors.

**Acknowledgments:** The authors acknowledge the Universidade Federal de Mato Grosso do Sul for all support.

**Conflicts of Interest:** The authors declare no conflicts of interest.

## References


1. AlKandari, M.; Ahmad, I. Solar power generation forecasting using ensemble approach based on deep learning and statistical methods. *Appl. Comput. Inform.* **2024**, *20*, 231–250. [CrossRef]
2. Sharadga, H.; Hajimirza, S.; Balog, R.S. Time series forecasting of solar power generation for large-scale photovoltaic plants. *Renew. Energy* **2020**, *150*, 797–807. [CrossRef]
3. Ibrahim, S.; Daut, I.; Irwan, Y.M.; Irwanto, M.; Gomesh, N.; Farhana, Z. Linear Regression Model in Estimating Solar Radiation in Perlis. *Energy Procedia* **2012**, *18*, 1402–1412. [CrossRef]
4. Asri, R.; Friansa, K.; Siregar, S. Predicting Solar Irradiance Using Regression Model (Case Study: ITERA Solar Power Plant). *IOP Conf. Ser. Earth Environ. Sci.* **2021**, *830*, 012080. [CrossRef]
5. Erten, M.Y.; Aydilek, H. Solar Power Prediction using Regression Models. *Int. J. Eng. Res. Dev.* **2022**, *14*, s333–s342. [CrossRef]
6. El-Aal, S.A.; Alqabli, M.A.; Naim, A.A. Forecasting solar photovoltaic energy production using linear regression-based techniques. *J. Theor. Appl. Inf. Technol.* **2023**, *101*, 3326–3337.
7. Bimenyimana, S.; Osarumwense, G.N.; Lingling, L. Output Power Prediction of Photovoltaic Module Using Nonlinear Autoregressive Neural Network. *J. Energy, Environ. Chem. Eng.* **2017**, *2*, 32–40.
8. Pamain, A.; Rao, P.V.K.; Tilya, F.N. Prediction of photovoltaic power output based on different non-linear autoregressive artificial neural network algorithms. *Glob. Energy Interconnect.* **2022**, *5*, 226–235. [CrossRef]
9. Rogier, J.K.; Nawaz, M. Forecasting Photovoltaic Power Generation via an IoT Network Using Nonlinear Autoregressive Neural Network. *Procedia Comput. Sci.* **2019**, *151*, 643–650. [CrossRef]

10. Mellit, A.; Saglam, S.; Kalogirou, S.A. Artificial neural network-based model for estimating the produced power of a photovoltaic module. *Renew. Energy* **2013**, *60*, 71–78. [CrossRef]
11. Amer, H.N.; Dahlan, N.Y.; Azmi, AMLatip, M.F.A.; Onn, M.S.; Tumian, A. Solar power prediction based on Artificial Neural Network guided by feature selection for Large-scale Solar Photovoltaic Plant. *Energy Rep.* **2023**, *9* (Suppl. 12), 262–266. [CrossRef]
12. Abdelhak, K.; Razika, I.; Ali, B.; Abdelmalek, A.; Müslüm, A.; Nacer, L.; Nabila, I. Solar photovoltaic power prediction using artificial neural network and multiple regression considering ambient and operating conditions. *Energy Convers. Manag.* **2023**, *288*, 117186. [CrossRef]
13. Akaike, H. A new look at the statistical model identification. *IEEE Trans. Autom. Control* **1974**, *19*, 716–723. [CrossRef]
14. Schwarz, G. Estimating the dimension of a model. *Ann. Stat.* **1978**, *6*, 461–464. [CrossRef]
15. Gelf, A.E.; Smith, A.F.M. Sampling-Based Approaches to Calculating Marginal Densities. *J. Am. Stat. Assoc.* **1990**, *85*, 398–409. [CrossRef]
16. Gelman, A.; Carlin, J.B.; Stern, H.S.; Dunson, D.B.; Vehtari, A.; Rubin, D.B. *Bayesian Data Analysis*; CRC Press: Boca Raton, FL, USA, 1995; Volume 2.
17. Geman, S. and Geman, D. Stochastic Relaxation, Gibbs Distributions, and the Bayesian Restoration of Images. *IEEE Trans. Pattern Anal. Mach. Intell.* **1984**, *6*, 721–741. [CrossRef] [PubMed]
18. Souza, G.; Santos, R.R.; Saraiva, E.F. A Log-logistic predictor for power generation in photovoltaic systems. *Energies* **2022**, *15*, 5973. [CrossRef]
19. R Core Team. R: A Language and Environment for Statistical Computing. Available online: https://www.R-project.org/(accessed on 15 January 2024).

*entropy*

MDPI

*Article*

# Bayesian Assessment of Corrosion-Related Failures in Steel Pipelines

**Fabrizio Ruggeri [1,*], Enrico Cagno [2], Franco Caron [2], Mauro Mancini [2] and Antonio Pievatolo [1]**

1 Consiglio Nazionale delle Ricerche-Istituto di Matematica Applicata e Tecnologie Informatiche, I-20133 Milano, Italy; antonio.pievatolo@cnr.it
2 Department of Management, Economics and Industrial Engineering, Politecnico di Milano, I-20156 Milano, Italy; enrico.cagno@polimi.it (E.C.); franco.caron@polimi.it (F.C.); mauro.mancini@polimi.it (M.M.)
* Correspondence: fabrizio@mi.imati.cnr.it

**Abstract:** The probability of gas escapes from steel pipelines due to different types of corrosion is studied with real failure data from an urban gas distribution network. Both the design and maintenance of the network are considered, identifying and estimating (in a Bayesian framework) an elementary multinomial model in the first case, and a more sophisticated non-homogeneous Poisson process in the second case. Special attention is paid to the elicitation of the experts' opinions. We conclude that the corrosion process behaves quite differently depending on the type of corrosion, and that, in most cases, cathodically protected pipes should be installed.

**Keywords:** analytic hierarchy process; Poisson process; reliability of gas distribution networks

## 1. Introduction

This paper deals with the assessment of the probability of gas escape (hereinafter referred to as "failure") from the steel pipelines in a gas distribution network, in order to support the estimation of its dependability and to the implementation of the maintenance and renewal policy. The problem of the failure analysis of pipelines, especially due to corrosion, has been the subject of several studies in the literature, especially in engineering. For example, ref. [1] considered corrosion in offshore and onshore oil and gas pipelines, and used a numerical analytical approach based on first-order reliability method and Monte Carlo simulation to assess uncertainty. Ref. [2] used numerical and analytical methods for limit state functions, with a particular interest in burst limit pressures, considering their relevance for oil and gas standards. The assessment of burst pressure standards for a pipeline was also considered in [3], using numerical analysis methods like finite elements and applying them to Algerian data. Our approach differs from those, since we are adopting a statistical approach based on stochastic models. Probabilistic methods, including those based on the Bayesian approach, have been used in the field. Indeed, stochastic modeling of consequences of corrosion of materials is an important aspect of structural reliability analysis, which has attracted a significant interest, especially in engineering. There are works on corrosion in reinforced concrete components, where our approach might be adapted and applied. Ref. [4] studied the reliability over the design life of a reinforced concrete beam, while ref. [5] was interested in corrosion-induced cracks, and applied advanced Bayesian simulation techniques, based on Hamiltonian Markov chain Monte Carlo methods. The importance of those studies is evident in [6], where the authors addressed the issue of the behavior of the reinforced concrete when subject to seismic events.

Furthermore, the corrosion process is a particular example of degradation, another field of reliability with rich literature, including books like [7] and applications like the one in [8] about the wear of cylinder liners in ships.

We are considering a Bayesian approach to the problem, since we are able to combine actual data with experts' opinions. The Bayesian approach is widely used in reliability, with early works including the very influential book [9], followed by many others like [10], which strongly differs from the former not only because of the new areas of application but also because of the simulation techniques, mostly known as Markov Chain Monte Carlo, which were developed in the last 35 years.

In the paper a case study of a urban low pressure network laid in a metropolis of 1.5 million citizens is presented. Steel pipelines have very strong mechanical properties (failures are very rare), but they are easy prey for corrosive agents unless they are correctly protected.

After a brief description of the technical problem in Section 2, a Bayesian analysis based only on the observed number of failures during the period 1978–1997 is presented in Section 3. There, we focus on the probability that a failure occurs in a certain location, and that it is due to one among various types of corrosion processes. This information can be used as a quick reference to decide the kind of protection needed by a pipe for design purposes.

A more detailed analysis is carried out in Sections 4 and 5, where we relate the corrosion process to the occurrence of failures, by taking into account both the times of occurrence of failures and the evolution of the network over time. The result is the possibility of following the temporal evolution of the reliability of a portion of network subject to a given corrosive agent for maintenance purposes.

In all cases, information provided by the experts is incorporated into the models according to the Bayesian paradigm.

## 2. Factors Related to the Probability of Failure

In the case under examination, the number of failures of the steel pipelines due to corrosion is very small (33 failures in the period 1978–1997 over a network of 275 km as of 1997). The scarceness of historical data has led us to use a methodology that takes into account all possible kinds of information. The principal source of information is the experts' knowledge (grown inside the company that manages the gas distribution network), and the Bayesian framework [11] offers the tools to combine the historical data with the corporate memory.

From the available historical data inside the company and the interviews with experts, three principal elements that may be related to the failures of steel pipelines have been identified: the age of the pipe, the type of corrosion that led to the rupture of pipe, and the lay location of the pipe.

### 2.1. Age of the Pipe

Since corrosion is a process that develops progressively, time is an important factor of the corrosive phenomenon. Steel pipelines are subject to an electrolytic process that tends to reduce in thickness the walls of the pipe. Then, the pipe weakens and breaks because of the loss of its mechanical properties, with the consequent and extremely dangerous gas leak. Therefore, the age of the pipe, which can be correctly approximated by the lay date, is very important, because it represents the period of time the pipe has been exposed to this electrolytic phenomenon.

### 2.2. Type of Corrosion

Three types of corrosion have been determined: natural, galvanic, and by interference. Each of them is characterized by specific causes, and develops in fully different ways. This relates to their different relationships with the failure of the pipe.

2.2.1. Natural Corrosion ($N$)

It is principally caused by the aggressive properties of the ground. For example, very wet ground is a good conductor and, as such, facilitates the development of the electrolytic phenomenon on the steel.

2.2.2. Galvanic Corrosion ($G$)

A gas distribution network is very inhomogeneous because it is made up of very different materials (treated cast iron, spheroid graphite, traditional cast iron, polyethylene and so on). When a steel pipe is connected to a cast iron pipe, if the insulating material, that constitutes the principal protection of the pipe, is not perfectly efficient, a galvanic corrosion caused by the contact of the two materials can take place. In particular, there is a potential difference between cast iron and steel, where the latter assumes the anodic behavior and corrodes, while the former assumes the cathodic one.

2.2.3. Corrosion by Interference ($I$)

This is also called corrosion by stray current, because it is due to the presence of stray currents in the ground coming from other badly isolated electrical plants (for example, streetcar substations or train stations). These currents discharge themselves on the steel pipe, increasing the corrosion rate by various orders of magnitude. In other cities, other corrosive agents also hidden in the ground can be very important (especially near the sea), but not in the present case.

### *2.3. Lay Location*

The propensity to a particular type of corrosion is not the same all over the city, but changes according to the place where the pipe is laid. In fact, in some places, stray currents in the ground are significantly higher than in other places, which increases the propensity to a failure due to corrosion by interference. Therefore, two different areas can be determined: zone A, characterized by the presence of streetcar substations or rail stations, and zone B, without them.

## 3. Bayesian Inference on the Probability of Failure by Zone and by Type of Corrosion

### *3.1. Comparing the Observed Number of Failures by Zone and by Type of Corrosion*

The geometry of the failures across the city is not uniform. In Section 2.3, we have argued that the probability of a failure is higher where stray currents are present, which especially happens near streetcar substations, rail stations, and so on.

3.1.1. Closeness of Streetcar Substations

Near streetcar substations, the trunk of negative electric cables used to feed the streetcar line is hidden underground. The streetcar-feeding current is generated in the substation, goes through the aerial line (positive cables), and is transformed into power by the streetcar; then, it goes through the steel streetcar tracks (negative cables) to close the circuit in the substation.

The circuit is actually closed, in the last hundred meters, by underground cables connected to the steel streetcar tracks and to the generator of the substation. These cables generate stray currents because of the bad isolation.

3.1.2. Closeness of Rail Stations and Lines

In the case of rail stations, the stray currents derive not only by the bad isolation of the tracks, but also by the strong electric field coming from the passage of the train. Therefore, the train traffic is proportional to the mean intensity of the stray currents.

In conclusion, we determined two areas: zone A, where there is a trunk of negative electric cables used to feed the streetcar line or near rail stations or rails, and zone B, which is all other areas.

In order to compare the number of failures by zone, the number of observed failures must be divided by the lengths of the gas distribution networks in zone A and in zone B, respectively. Since this datum is unavailable, we approximate it by the area (in squared kilometers) of the two zones.

The observed number of failures by zone and by type of corrosion per kilometer and per year (named here "failure rate") is summarized in Table 1.

**Table 1.** Failure rate by zone and by type of corrosion.

| | Natural ($N$) | Galvanic ($G$) | By Interference ($I$) |
|---|---|---|---|
| Zone A (12 $km^2$) | 0.583 | 0.083 | 0.500 |
| Zone B (88 $km^2$) | 0.068 | 0.057 | 0.091 |

It is reasonable to expect that the "failure rate" by natural corrosion in zone A is comparable to that in zone B, but this is not the case for the observed failures, probably because of incorrect classifications made by the repairing teams. This will not affect the estimate of the marginal probability that a failure occurs in zone A, whereas it will bias the estimates of the marginal probabilities that a corrosion occurs of a given type, as well as the estimates of some conditional probabilities. Therefore, some care must be taken in interpreting the result, even if the misclassification bias will be partially counterbalanced by the prior opinion of the experts.

### 3.2. Prior Probability Assessment: The Analytic Hierarchy Process

Experts' prior estimates of the zone probability (from now on, we will use the shorthand "zone probability" to stand for "probability that a failure occurs in a given zone") have been achieved by means of the pairwise comparison technique of the Analytic Hierarchy Process (AHP) [12,13]. AHP is, at the same time, a useful and widely used methodology, and a controversial one, as recognized by many authors, including the proposer [14]. Ref. [15] presented a non-exhaustive list of 150 papers using AHP up to that time, illustrating critical and positive aspects of the methodology.

On the positive side, AHP helps in specifying prior probabilities when the experts are able to provide only qualitative judgments and not quantitative ones, like mean and variance of a prior distribution. Given a set of $n$ events, the experts are asked to compare them pairwise, making linguistic statements about the likelihood of occurrence of one with respect to the other. Each judgment is transformed into a number, and a square matrix of order $n$ is obtained with all the comparisons. The eigenvector of dimension $n$, corresponding to the largest eigenvalue of the matrix, is then normalized so that its elements sum to 1, and they represent the probabilities of occurrence of each of the $n$ events. Mathematical details can be found in the books mentioned earlier.

As anticipated, there are some controversial aspects about AHP. First, of all, the scale of linguistic judgments has to be clearly specified, especially regarding the increased order of the possible sentences. For example, all of the experts should understand that "much more likely" means that it is less likely than "clearly more likely". Training with simple examples is strongly suggested so that all of the experts agree on the scale and each statement, like that "clearly more likely" has more-or-less the same meaning for all of them. The assignment of numbers to statements is arbitrary, from their range to the value assigned to each judgment. The matrix could also have some inconsistencies, like values $a_{ij}$ and $a_{jk}$ assigned to comparisons between events $i$ and $j$ and between $j$ and $k$, respectively, but $a_{ik} \neq a_{ij}a_{jk}$ when comparing events $i$ and $k$. Measures of inconsistency have been proposed, as well as methods to attenuate the problem. Ref. [16] considered propensity to gas escape in cast iron pipelines laid under different conditions, like diameter, depth, and location. They used AHP to obtain opinions from the experts about the propensity for each condition (eight, given that each feature was taking two possible values). They considered a homogeneous Poisson process for the failure times, since cast iron is not subject to corrosion, as steel pipes, and propensity to fail can be assumed constant over time. Following the Bayesian approach, gamma priors were considered for the parameters of the different conditions and their parameters were chosen so that their mean and variance were given by the sample mean and variance of the opinions of the experts. Those priors were then validated by the company's experts. We are taking a similar approach here.

The team of experts was formed by two technicians and two engineers: the technicians assess the conditions of the pipes after an excavation and decide what action to take; the engineers have an overall knowledge of the technical and information management problems that arise inside the company.

Two types of assessments were requested: the probability of a failure in the two zones, and the probability of a type of corrosion conditioned to the zone. All questions were phrased in terms of relative probabilities. For example, the first one was: "In your opinion is a failure more likely to happen in zone A or in zone B? How much more likely?".

In order to fully exploit the answers, a linguistic judgment scale has been referred to the numerical scale $\{1,3,5,7,9\}$, and the judgments have been used to obtain the prior probability assessment. The five degrees of the linguistic judgment scale were: "equally likely", "a little more likely", "much more likely", "clearly more likely", "definitely more likely".

The experts answered considering the number of failures observed and that the areas near streetcar substations or rail stations are under close control. In spite of this, the subjective probability of failure in zone A was assessed as about four times greater than that in zone B.

The second part of the questionnaire regarded the comparison among the three types of corrosion by zone. The typical question was: "In an area with (without) streetcar substations or rail stations is it more likely to have natural or galvanic corrosion? How much more likely?".

From the questionnaire, $P(N|A)$, $P(G|A)$, $P(I|A)$, $P(N|B)$, $P(G|B)$, and $P(I|B)$ were obtained, while the zone probabilities conditioned to the type of corrosion were derived as follows:

$$\begin{aligned} P(C) &= P(C|A)P(A) + P(C|B)P(B) \\ P(A|C) &= \frac{P(C|A)P(A)}{P(C)} \end{aligned}$$

where $C \in \{I, N, G\}$ and the indicated probabilities have an obvious meaning.

The prior estimates and their standard deviations are shown in Table 2.

**Table 2.** Subjective assessments of zone probabilities and type of corrosion.

| | **Mean** | **Std. Dev.** |
|---|---|---|
| $P(A)$ | 0.7938 | 0.1962 |
| $P(B)$ | 0.2063 | 0.1962 |
| $P(A\|N)$ | 0.6133 | 0.2114 |
| $P(A\|G)$ | 0.6221 | 0.2168 |
| $P(A\|I)$ | 0.9581 | 0.0574 |
| $P(N)$ | 0.1636 | 0.0403 |
| $P(G)$ | 0.2767 | 0.1298 |

### 3.3. *Posterior Probabilities Distinguishing the Zone*

So far, from the expert judgments, it has emerged that the propensity to failure due to different types of corrosion is not the same for the two zones (in particular for the corrosion by interference). In the next two paragraphs, we derive the posterior zone probability, both marginal and conditioned to the type of corrosion.

#### 3.3.1. Zone Probability

Let us denote by $p$ the probability that a failure occurs in zone A, so $P(A) = p$. Denoting by $n_A$ the number of failures in zone A, and conditioning upon the total number of failures $n$, the phenomenon is described by a binomial distribution with $n$ trials and parameter $p$,

$$p(n_A|n,p) = \binom{n}{n_A} p^{n_A}(1-p)^{n-n_A} \tag{1}$$

The Beta distribution is conjugate to the binomial, so we take $p \sim \text{Beta}(a,b)$ a priori, where $a$ and $b$ are chosen consistently with the prior assessments in Table 2. Then, $p \sim \text{Beta}(a',b')$ a posteriori, with $a' = a + n_A$ and $b' = b + n - n_A$.

The expected loss, under quadratic loss function, is minimized by the posterior mean of $p$,

$$\text{E}(p|n,n_A) = a'/(a'+b') = 27.460/(27.460+29.866) = 0.4790.$$

The results are compared in Table 3.

**Table 3.** Comparison of historical, prior and posterior mean of $p$.

| | | Historical (MLE) | Prior | Posterior |
|---|---|---|---|---|
| $p$ | (zone A, 12 km$^2$) | 0.4528 | 0.7938 | 0.4790 |
| $1-p$ | (zone B, 88 km$^2$) | 0.5472 | 0.2062 | 0.5210 |

The strong influence of the streetcar substations and rail stations on the probability of failure of the steel pipelines is confirmed a posteriori. In fact, on average, around 48% of the failures is concentrated on 12% of the city area. The small difference between posterior means and MLEs gives us confidence that the failures have been classified correctly by zone.

#### 3.3.2. The Zone Probability Conditioned to the Type of Corrosion

Since the way to obtain the zone probability conditioned to the type of corrosion is the same as the previous paragraph, here, we report only the results in Table 4.

**Table 4.** Comparison of historical, prior and posterior mean of $p$ conditioned to the type of corrosion.

| | Historical (MLE) | Prior Mean | Prior Std. Dev. | Posterior Mean | Posterior Std. Dev. |
|---|---|---|---|---|---|
| $P(A\|N)$ | 0.5385 | 0.6133 | 0.2114 | 0.5662 | 0.1065 |
| $P(A\|G)$ | 0.1667 | 0.6221 | 0.2168 | 0.4125 | 0.0351 |
| $P(A\|I)$ | 0.4286 | 0.9581 | 0.0574 | 0.6700 | 0.0909 |

### 3.4. *Type of Corrosion: Marginal Posterior Probabilities*

The progress of the electrolytic phenomenon depends strictly on the type of corrosion, thus it is necessary to study which type of corrosion is more frequent. A corrosion of a given type occurs according to the probabilities $p_I \equiv P(I)$, $p_G \equiv P(G)$, and $p_N \equiv P(N)$.

As in Section 3.3.1, conditional upon $n$, the number of failures by type of corrosion $(n_I, n_G, n_N)$ has a multinomial distribution with parameters $p_I$, $p_G$, and $p_N = 1 - p_I - p_G$. Then, we have

$$p(n_N, n_G|n, p_N, p_G) = \binom{n}{n_N\ n_G} p_N^{n_N} p_G^{n_G} (1-p_N-p_G)^{n-n_N-n_G}$$

The generalization of the Bayesian procedure followed in Section 3.3.1 is obtained by giving a Dirichlet prior distribution to $(p_N, p_G)$ (which becomes a Beta distribution when there are only two classes),

$$p(p_N, p_G; a_N, a_G, a_I) = \frac{\Gamma(a_{\text{tot}})}{\Gamma(a_N)\Gamma(a_G)\Gamma(a_I)} p_N^{a_N-1} p_G^{a_G-1} (1 - p_N - p_G)^{a_I-1}$$

where $a_{\text{tot}} = a_N + a_G + a_I$, and where the hyperparameters are determined by matching the prior mean and variances in Table 2 to those given by the model as $c$ varies within $\{I, G, N\}$,

$$\begin{aligned} \mathrm{E}(p_c) &= \frac{a_c}{a_{\text{tot}}} \\ \mathrm{Var}(p_c) &= \frac{a_c(a_{\text{tot}} - a_c)}{a_{\text{tot}}^2(a_{\text{tot}} + 1)} \end{aligned}$$

The posterior distribution of $(p_N, p_G)$ is again Dirichlet with parameters

$$\begin{aligned} a_c' &= a_c + n_c \quad c \in \{I, G, N\} \\ a_{\text{tot}}' &= a_{\text{tot}} + n \end{aligned}$$

The comparison of the various means is reported in Table 5.

**Table 5.** Comparison of the historical, prior and posterior mean of $p_c$, $c \in \{I, G, N\}$.

| | Historical (MLE) | Prior Mean | Prior Std. Dev. | Posterior Mean | Posterior Std. Dev. |
|---|---|---|---|---|---|
| $P(N)$ | 0.3940 | 0.1636 | 0.0403 | 0.2290 | 0.0388 |
| $P(G)$ | 0.1818 | 0.2767 | 0.1298 | 0.2498 | 0.0400 |
| $P(I)$ | 0.4242 | 0.5597 | 0.1565 | 0.5212 | 0.0461 |

Here, the posterior means differ from the MLE's much more markedly than those in Table 3, showing that the experts' opinions do not agree with the classification of the failures by type of corrosion, which reinforces our suspects of misclassifications.

## 4. A Model for the Occurrence of Failures

### 4.1. Available Data and Notation

The introduction of the age of the pipes in the analysis requires considering additional data: the times of occurrence of the failures, the installation dates, and the lengths of subnetworks laid in different periods. Because the network existing in 1978–1997 (the period for which the records are reliable) is also composed of subnetworks laid very early, the periodic growth of the network since its outset must be considered. A yearly record of the increments in kilometers of the network is available from the gas company, regardless of the zone, because no systematic attempt to distinguish zone A from zone B was ever made by the company.

We set out the mathematical notation at this point, in order not to interrupt the flow of ideas in the following. Since we are examining a corrosion process, it makes sense to partition the networks into subnetworks whose components have been laid in the same period (e.g., in the same year). Suppose that there are $r$ subnetworks. Denote these subnetworks by their installation year $\{s_i, i = 1, \ldots, r\}$ and their lengths (in kilometers) by $l_i$. When we refer to a generic subnetwork, we index it by $s$ only without subscript, and we denote its length by $l_s$.

The time of the $k$-th observed failure in subnetwork $s_i$ is denoted by $t_{ick}$, where $c \in \{I, G, N\}$ indicates the type of corrosion that caused the failure: by interference, galvanic, or natural. The index $k$ ranges from 1 to $n_{ic}$.

The observation interval for the subnetwork is denoted by $[\max\{T_0, s_i\}, T_1]$, where $T_0$ is 1 January 1978 and $T_1$ is 31 December 1997.

### 4.2. Modeling a Single Failure

We build a stochastic model for the observed failures in the whole network, starting from the modeling of the time of occurrence of a single failure. A failure in a subnetwork $s$ occurs as the final result of a sequence of events: first, some external intervention causes a damage to the protection of a pipe after a random time $u$ since the installation of the pipe; second, because of the damage, a corrosion process of type $c$, according to the location, takes place until the failure of the pipe after a random time $v$, independently of $u$. The actual time of failure can then be written as $t = s + u + v$, so that the probability density of $t$ is the convolution of the probability densities of $u$ and of $v$. Denote these densities by $h(\cdot|\lambda, l_s)$ and $g(\cdot|M_c, \beta_c)$, respectively, where the subscript $c$ indicates the dependence of the distribution of the corrosion time $v$ on the type of corrosion that has taken place. The probability density of $t$ is then

$$\begin{aligned} f(t|\lambda, M_c, \beta_c, l_s, s) &= \int_0^{t-s} g(t-s-u|M_c, \beta_c)h(u|\lambda, l_s)\,du \\ &= \int_s^t g(t-z|M_c, \beta_c)h(z-s|\lambda, l_s)\,dz \end{aligned} \quad (2)$$

where we have set $z = s + u$.

We chose $h(\cdot|\lambda, l_s)$ to be negative exponential, because the absence of damages up to a given time does not change the probability of occurrence, i.e., the hazard function is constant. Then,

$$h(u|\lambda, l_s) = l_s \lambda e^{-l_s \lambda u},$$

where the presence of the factor $l_s$ implies that the mean time to damage is shorter for longer subnetworks. The density of $v$ must belong to a family of densities that allow for increasing hazard functions, because of the presence of the corrosion process. The Weibull family is widely used in this kind of situation, so we set

$$g(v|M_c, \beta_c) = M_c \beta_c v^{\beta_c - 1} e^{-M_c v^{\beta_c}}.$$

The integral in (2) cannot be solved explicitly, so we will use numerical integration when $f(\cdot|\lambda, M_c, \beta_c, l_s, s)$ is needed.

### 4.3. Combining the Single Failure Models

When corrosion has led to the rupture of a pipeline section having a certain lay date $s_i$, it is replaced by a new section. Therefore, subnetwork $s_i$ becomes shorter at every rupture event until all of its parts are substituted, hence its life span is finite. During its life, a random number $N_{ic}$ of failures due to corrosion of type $c$ occur. Conditional upon $N_{ic}$, we can regard the failure times as independent random variables, all with density (2), because the subnetworks are large and the failures occur at different locations. In our case, $N_{ic}$ is unknown, and we have observed the failures only in the interval $[\max\{T_0, s_i\}, T_1]$, so the joint density function of $t_{ic} = \{t_{ick}, k = 1, \ldots, n_{ic}\}$ and $n_{ic}$ must be found by averaging the conditional density over $N_{ic}$, which takes the following form, as shown in Appendix A:

$$\begin{aligned} f(t_{ic}, n_{ic}|N_{ic}, \lambda, M_c, \beta_c, l_i, s_i) &= \prod_{k=1}^{n_{ic}} f(t_{ick}|\lambda, M_c, \beta_c, l_i, s_i) \\ &\quad \cdot [1 - D_{ic}]^{N_{ic} - n_{ic}} \cdot \frac{N_{ic}!}{(N_{ic} - n_{ic})!} \end{aligned} \quad (3)$$

where

$$D_{ic} = \int_{\max\{T_0, s_i\}}^{T_1} f(t|\lambda, M_c, \beta_c, l_i, s_i)\,dt. \quad (4)$$

Suppose now that $N_{ic}$ is Poisson distributed with parameter $l_i\nu_c$, where $l_i$ accounts for the different lengths of the subnetworks, then the marginal joint density of $t_{ic}$ and $n_{ic}$ is

$$f(t_{ic}, n_{ic}|\lambda, M_c, \beta_c, l_i, s_i) = \prod_{k=1}^{n_{ic}} f(t_{ick}|\lambda, M_c, \beta_c, l_i, s_i) \cdot e^{-l_i\nu_c D_{ic}} (l_i\nu_c)^{n_{ic}}. \quad (5)$$

In a nutshell, Equation (5) is the probability density for what is observed in the window $[\max\{T_0, s_i\}, T_1]$ from a Poisson process on $[s_i, +\infty)$ with intensity function given by $l_i\nu_c f(\cdot|\lambda, M_c, \beta_c, l_i, s_i)$. The fact that the intensity function decays to zero as time goes on is an approximation of the limited life span of the subnetwork $s_i$. Of course, the marginal distribution of $n_{ic}$ is Poisson with parameter $l_i\nu_c D_{ic}$. For the theory of Poisson processes and its applications see, e.g., [17], while [18] provide a thorough Bayesian analysis.

### 4.4. The Likelihood Function and the Bayesian Inference

The likelihood function for the unknown parameter vector $\theta = (\lambda, M, \beta, \nu)$, where $M = (M_I, M_G, M_N)$, and a similar definition holds for $\beta$ and $\nu$, is obtained from (5) by taking the product over the indices $i$ and $c$,

$$L(\theta; t_I, t_G, t_N) \propto \lambda^{n_{\cdot\cdot}} e^{-\sum_i \sum_c l_i\nu_c D_{ic}} \prod_c \Bigg\{ (M_c\beta_c)^{n_{\cdot c}} \prod_{i=1}^{r} \left[ (l_i^2\nu_c)^{n_{ic}} \prod_{k=1}^{n_{ic}} \int_{s_i}^{t_{ick}} (t_{ick} - z)^{\beta_c - 1} e^{-M_c(t_{ick}-z)^{\beta_c}} e^{-l_i\lambda(z - s_i)} \, dz \right] \Bigg\} \quad (6)$$

The vectors $t_c$, $c \in \{I, G, N\}$, appearing on the left-hand side of (6), contain the times of observed failures after a corrosion of type $c$; the dot subscripts indicate that the subscript in that position has been summed over; when $n_{ic} = 0$, the product with index $k$ in the second line is set to 1.

For the Bayesian inference, we assign prior distributions to all of the parameters in $\theta$, and assume they are a priori independent, since they describe phenomena of a different nature. In particular, we take $\lambda \sim \mathcal{G}(a^{(\lambda)}, b^{(\lambda)})$. As $c$ varies inside $\{I, G, N\}$, we put $M_c \sim \mathcal{G}(a_c^{(M)}, b_c^{(M)})$, $\beta_c \sim \mathcal{G}(a_c^{(\beta)}, b_c^{(\beta)})$, and $\nu_c \sim \mathcal{G}(a_c^{(\nu)}, b_c^{(\nu)})$, where the superscripts identify which parameter the hyperparameters are to be referred to.

### 4.5. The Probabilities of Zone and of Type of Corrosion

A formal connection between this section and Section 3 can be seen immediately. Let us split $\nu_c$ into the sum of two parameters, for example $\nu_{Ac}$ and $\nu_{Bc}$, $c \in \{G, I, N\}$, and perform the same with the observed values of $n_{ic}$, and with $l_i$ for all $i = 1, \ldots, r$, supposing for the moment that the lengths of the subnetworks laid in zones A and B are available. From Section 4.3, $n_{zic}$ conditional on $\theta$ is Poisson with mean $l_{zi}\nu_{zc}D_{zic}$, with the subscript $z$ indicating the zone. Then, $n_{z\ldots}$ is Poisson with mean $\sum_i \sum_c l_{zi}\nu_{zc}D_{zic}$, so, conditioning to $n_{\ldots} \equiv n$, $n_{z\ldots}$ has a binomial distribution with number of trials $n_{\ldots}$ and probability of "success"

$$p = \frac{\sum_i \sum_c l_{Ai}\nu_{Ac} D_{Aic}}{\sum_i \sum_c l_{Ai}\nu_{Ac} D_{Aic} + \sum_i \sum_c l_{Bi}\nu_{Bc} D_{Bic}}$$

where $p$ is the same parameter that appears in Section 3.3.1. The same property, yielding a multinomial distribution as in Section 3.4, holds for $n_{\ldots c}$ conditional on $n_{\ldots}$.

## 5. Elicitation of the Experts' Opinions and Results

Unlike the zone probability, the parameters $\lambda$, $M_c$, and $\beta_c$ ($c \in \{I, G, N\}$) are not easily related to an observable event whose probability can be assessed by an expert without difficulty.

As regards $M_c$ and $\beta_c$, following [19], the experts were asked to select an interval from a given list for the duration of the corrosion until failure (that is, an interval for $v$ as defined in Section 4.2) and an attached degree of belief $100\alpha\%$ to be chosen among 95%, 85%, and

75%. From each interval, a pair $(M_c, \beta_c)$ was found by assigning a value of $(1-\alpha)/2$ to the tail probabilities. The averages over the experts gave the prior means and standard deviations of $M_c$ and $\beta_c$, as $c$ varies within $\{I, G, N\}$, are presented in Table 6. The choice of the size of the intervals and the probabilities to be attached was dictated by the need to provide the experts, not acquainted with quantitative methods and prior elicitation, a time period sufficiently large to allow them to think about possible failures and three levels of probabilities ranging from a good chance of event (75%) to a great one (95%).

**Table 6.** Prior assessment of $M_c$ and $\beta_c$, $c \in \{I, G, N\}$.

| Type of Corrosion | Parameter | Prior Mean | Prior Std. Dev. |
|---|---|---|---|
| Natural | $M$ | $0.305 \times 10^{-3}$ | $0.209 \times 10^{-3}$ |
| | $\beta$ | 2.96 | 0.79 |
| Galvanic | $M$ | $0.229 \times 10^{-2}$ | $0.203 \times 10^{-2}$ |
| | $\beta$ | 2.79 | 0.95 |
| By interference | $M$ | $0.210 \times 10^{-1}$ | $0.381 \times 10^{-1}$ |
| | $\beta$ | 3.48 | 2.01 |

As for $\lambda$, where $1/\lambda$ is the mean time to damage of the protection of one kilometer of pipeline, the experts were asked to provide the probability that the protection of 5 km of pipeline is not damaged after 6, 15, 30, and 90 years. The value of $\lambda$ for each expert was then found as the one that gave the best fit of $\exp(-5\lambda y)$, where $y \in \{6, 15, 30, 90\}$, to the elicited probabilities. The average of $\lambda$ over the experts is $0.621 \times 10^{-2}$, with a standard deviation of $0.182 \times 10^{-2}$.

From the a priori means and variances, we can derive the hyperparameters of the Gamma prior densities, so we have $a^{(\lambda)} = 11.6$ and $b^{(\lambda)} = 1867$, $a_I^{(M)} = 0.30$ and $b_I^{(M)} = 14.5$, $a_G^{(M)} = 1.28$ and $b_G^{(M)} = 556$, $a_N^{(M)} = 2.13$ and $b_N^{(M)} = 6982$, $a_I^{(\beta)} = 3.00$ and $b_I^{(\beta)} = 0.86$, $a_G^{(\beta)} = 8.63$ and $b_G^{(\beta)} = 3.09$, and $a_N^{(\beta)} = 14.04$ and $b_N^{(\beta)} = 4.74$. The distributions of the $M_c$'s are concentrated on different parts of the real line, whereas the distributions of the $\beta_c$'s have approximately the same location, but are not equally dispersed. In particular, the experts seem to less clearly perceive the duration of the corrosion by interference.

The estimation of the posterior mean and standard deviation of the unknown parameters were carried out by Markov Chain Monte Carlo using the *mcmc* package [20], with numerical integration by quadrature for the computation of the intractable factors in the likelihood function (6), which are those involving $D_{ic}$ (see also Appendix A) and the kernel of the lifetime density (2). Since parameters $\nu_c$ are nuisance parameters, they were integrated out analytically in the actual calculations, which depend only on $a_c^{(\nu)}$ and $b_c^{(\nu)}$. We set both these parameters to 1 for all $c$, so that $\mathrm{E}(\nu_c) = 1$; other values had very little influence on the results. The factors in the likelihood depending on parameters $\nu_c$ are replaced by $1/(1 + \sum_i l_i D_{ic})^{n_{\cdot c}+1}$.

The posterior means and standard deviations of the parameters appear in Table 7. The main change with respect to the prior summaries of Table 6 is that galvanic corrosion and corrosion by interference have swapped places, a result which we comment on at the end of this section. Posterior standard deviations mostly show a small reduction in uncertainty. A further reduction could be obtained using more specific corrosion models and improving the method for type classification by the operators. We also remark that the failure observation period is one third of the network-lifetime.

The advantage of using the lifetime distribution (7) can be appreciated when a maintenance decision must be made. Suppose that priority for substitution must be assigned to two parts of the network of equal length $l$ laid in zone A and B, respectively, and let the lay year of the two parts be $s_1 > s_2$. A decision based on the posterior zone probability derived in Section 3.3.1 would be to substitute the part in zone A irrespective of $s_1$ and $s_2$. Alternatively, one can consider the hazard functions associated with the mixture densities

$$\sum_c P(c|A) f(t|\lambda, M_c, \beta_c, l, s_1) \quad \text{and} \quad \sum_c P(c|B) f(t|\lambda, M_c, \beta_c, l, s_2)$$

where $P(c|A)$ and $P(c|B)$ are the probabilities of corrosion conditioned to the zone derived in Section 3. These mixtures can be seen as an approximation to

$$\sum_c \frac{\nu_{Ac}}{\nu_{A\cdot}} f(t|\lambda, M_c, \beta_c, l, s_1) \quad \text{and} \quad \sum_c \frac{\nu_{Bc}}{\nu_{B\cdot}} f(t|\lambda, M_c, \beta_c, l, s_2)$$

that is, the lifetime distributions of the time to failure of a part of network that fails exactly once. In this way we avoid estimating the parameters $\nu_{zc}$.

**Table 7.** Posterior means and standard deviations of $\lambda$, $M_c$, and $\beta_c$, $c \in \{I, G, N\}$.

| Type of Corrosion | Parameter | Posterior Mean | Posterior Std. Dev. |
| --- | --- | --- | --- |
| All | $\lambda$ | $0.619 \times 10^{-2}$ | $0.181 \times 10^{-2}$ |
| Natural | $M$ | $0.338 \times 10^{-3}$ | $0.202 \times 10^{-3}$ |
| | $\beta$ | 2.21 | 0.42 |
| Galvanic | $M$ | $0.235 \times 10^{-2}$ | $0.163 \times 10^{-2}$ |
| | $\beta$ | 3.44 | 0.70 |
| By interference | $M$ | $0.266 \times 10^{-2}$ | $0.417 \times 10^{-2}$ |
| | $\beta$ | 2.68 | 1.19 |

A posteriori estimates of the mixing coefficients $P(c|z)$ are available from Section 3, whereas the pointwise estimate of the density functions is obtained by averaging the sequence $f(t|\lambda^{(i)}, M_c^{(i)}, \beta_c^{(i)}, l, s)$ across MCMC iterations, indexed by $i$. The comparison of the hazard functions might result in the substitution of the part in zone B instead of that in zone A.

The typical reliability profile of the network might be represented by the hazard function associated with the mixture density

$$g(t) = \sum_c P(c) f(t|\lambda, M_c, \beta_c, l, 0) \tag{7}$$

for some reference length $l$, where the unknown quantities are substituted by estimates as before, and again $P(c)$ approximates $\nu_{\cdot c}/\nu_{\cdot\cdot}$.

The plots of the hazard functions associated with $f(t|\lambda, M_c, \beta_c, 5, 0)$ for any $c$ appear in Figure 1. The difference between the two panels is mainly due to the asymmetry of the posterior distributions of the $M_c$ and $\beta_c$ parameters, which can be observed in the histograms of the MCMC simulations. Because of asymmetry, the sample averages of parameters used as plug in estimators are larger than the medians and select hazard functions that increase more rapidly.

The left panel of Figure 1 highlights that the tails of the lifetime distributions are exponential, so that the hazard functions stay constant after some years; besides, the hazard function of the natural corrosion increases less fast than the other two, as expected. This tail behavior has a straightforward interpretation: if, after installing a 5 km pipeline, we do not see any failure for a certain period (whose length depends on the type of corrosion), we may assume that the protection has not been damaged, so the risk of a failure is equal to that of damage. Another feature is that the hazard function of the corrosion by interference is closer to that for galvanic corrosion than the hazard function of the natural corrosion, so that the data confirm the experts' opinions (see beginning of Section 5). The less steep slope of the hazard function for the corrosion by interference with respect to the galvanic one reflects a longer mean time to failure; again, this might be imputed to failures by natural corrosion that happened in zone A and that were incorrectly classified as due to interference.

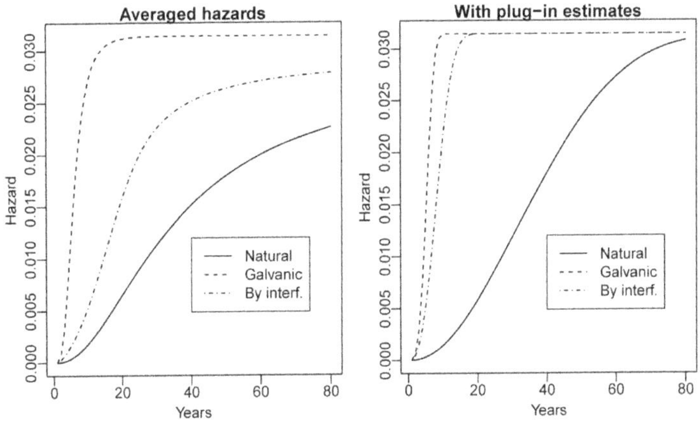


**Figure 1.** Hazard functions associated with $f(t|\lambda, M_c, \beta_c, 5, 0)$ for any $c \in \{N, G, I\}$. Left panel: posterior means of hazard functions for each failure type obtained from the MCMC simulation; right panel: computed by inserting the posterior means of parameters (plug-in estimate).

## 6. Concluding Remarks

A methodology for the assessment of the probability of gas escape from steel pipelines has been presented to support the implementation of the maintenance and renewal policy of a urban gas distribution network. We identified the factors that influence reliability, and focused first on the type of corrosion and the lay location (for design purposes), and then also included the age of the pipe in the analysis (for maintenance purposes).

The developed methodology answered the requirement to combine, according to the Bayesian paradigm, scarce information derived from historical data with the experts' knowledge grown inside the company during the last running periods.

At the design stage, a simple beta-binomial model proved sufficient, showing that streetcar substations greatly increase the probability of a fast corrosion; therefore, considering that it is not easy to tell whether a corrosion by interference can take place in a given location, newly installed pipelines should be cathodically protected.

At a maintenance stage, because of the presence of corrosion, we estimated a non-homogeneous Poisson process that accounts for the age of the pipes. The type of corrosion proved influential on the shape of the intensity function of the process, so that it is reasonable to compare the hazard functions derived from it when a priority decision for substitution must be made in presence of information on the most likely type of corrosion. The computation required for the estimation of the parameters are intensive in this case, but perfectly feasible thanks to modern computer power.

The real case study presented emphasized the relevance of the practical solution, to be reused in other industrial cases.

**Author Contributions:** Conceptualization, F.R., E.C., F.C., M.M. and A.P.; methodology, F.R., E.C., F.C., M.M. and A.P.; software, A.P.; validation, E.C., F.C., M.M. and A.P.; formal analysis, F.R., E.C., F.C., M.M. and A.P.; data curation, E.C., F.C. and M.M.; writing—original draft preparation, F.R., M.M. and A.P.; writing—review and editing, F.R., E.C., F.C., M.M. and A.P. All authors have read and agreed to the published version of the manuscript.

**Funding:** This research received no external funding.

**Data Availability Statement:** Restrictions apply to the availability of these data.

**Acknowledgments:** The authors are grateful to Massimo Fumagalli who collected and arranged the data from the gas company archives and carried out the interviews with the experts.

**Conflicts of Interest:** The authors declare no conflicts of interest.

## Appendix A. Derivation of Expressions

We derive (3), and other expressions, by omitting all quantities and notation that are unnecessary for this purpose. Conditional on $N$, (3) represents the probability density of $n$ failures at $t_1, \ldots, t_n$ inside $(\max\{T_0, s\}, T_1)$, and of the remaining $N - n$ failures outside. This occurs if $n$ failures are first assigned to the interval with binomial probability with success probability $D$ and $N$ trials, where $D$ is the probability that a failure falls inside $(\max\{T_0, s\}, T_1)$, given by (4). Then, given $n$, the joint density of the failures is that of the order statistics from $f(t)$ restricted to the interval. Taking the product of these two factors, we have

$$\binom{N}{n} D^n (1-D)^{N-n} \times n! \prod_{k=1}^{n} \frac{f(t_k)}{D}$$

which coincides with (3) after simplifications.

We now consider $D$ at (4). After writing $f(t|\lambda, M, \beta, l, s)$ explicitly, we can interchange the order of integration and obtain the following expression:

$$\int_s^{T_1} \left[ \int_{\max\{z, T_0\}}^{T_1} M\beta (t-z)^{\beta-1} e^{-M(t-z)^{\beta}} \, dt \right] l\lambda e^{-l\lambda(z-s)} \, dz$$

where the inside integral can be solved explicitly, since the integrand is a Weibull density, so we have

$$\int_s^{T_1} \left[ e^{-M(\max\{z, T_0\}-z)^{\beta-1}} - e^{-M(T_1-z)^{\beta}} \right] l\lambda e^{-l\lambda(z-s)} \, dz$$

which we solve numerically by quadrature using the *integrate* routine from R [21].

## References


1. Teixeira, A.P.; Soares, C.G.; Netto, T.A.; Estefen, S.F. Reliability of pipelines with corrosion defects. *Int. J. Press. Vessel. Pip.* **2008**, *85*, 228–237. [CrossRef]
2. Amaya-Gómez, R.; Sánchez-Silva, M.; Bastidas-Arteaga, E.; Schoefs, F.; Muñoz, F. Reliability assessments of corroded pipelines based on internal pressure—A review. *Eng. Fail. Anal.* **2019**, *98*, 190–214. [CrossRef]
3. Bouledroua, O.; Zelmati, D.; Hassani, M. Inspections, statistical and reliability assessment study of corroded pipeline. *Eng. Fail. Anal.* **2019**, *100*, 1–10. [CrossRef]
4. Faroz, S.A.; Pujari, N.N.; Ghosh, S. Reliability of a corroded RC beam based on Bayesian updating of the corrosion model. *Eng. Struct.* **2016**, *126*, 457–468. [CrossRef]
5. Jia, S.; Akiyama, M.; Frangopol, D.M.; Xu, Z. Bayesian inference of the spatial distribution of steel corrosion in reinforced concrete structures using corrosion-induced crack width. *Struct. Saf.* **2024**, *111*, 102518. [CrossRef]
6. Xu, H.; Gardoni, P. Probabilistic capacity and seismic demand models and fragility estimates for reinforced concrete buildings based on three-dimensional analyses. *Eng. Struct.* **2016**, *112*, 200–214. [CrossRef]
7. Chen, D.G.; Lio, Y.; Ng, H.K.T.; Tsai, T.R. *Statistical Modeling for Degradation Data*; Springer: Singapore, 2017.
8. Hermann, S.; Ruggeri, F. Modeling wear in cylinder liners. *Qual. Reliab. Eng. Int.* **2017**, *33*, 839–851. [CrossRef]
9. Martz, H.F.; Waller R.A. *Bayesian Reliability Analysis*; Wiley: New York, NY, USA, 1982.
10. Hamada, M.S.; Wilson, A.G.; Reese, S.C.; Martz, H.F. *Bayesian Reliability*; Springer: New York, NY, USA, 2008.
11. Gelman, A.; Carlin, J.B.; Stern, H.S.; Dunson, D.B.; Vehtari, A.; Rubin, D.B. *Bayesian Data Analysis*, 3rd ed.; Chapman and Hall/CRC: New York, NY, USA, 2015.
12. Saaty, T.L. *Fundamentals of Decision Making and Priority Theory with the Analytic Hierarchy Process*; RWS Publications: Pittsburgh, PA, USA, 1994.
13. Saaty, T.L. *The Analytic Hierarchy Process*; McGraw-Hill: New York, NY, USA, 1980.
14. Saaty, T.L. Highlights and critical points in the theory and application of the Analytic Hierarchy Process. *Eur. J. Oper. Res.* **1994**, *74*, 426–447. [CrossRef]
15. Vaidya, O.S.; Kumar, S. Analytic hierarchy process: An overview of applications. *Eur. J. Oper. Res.* **2006**, *169*, 1–29. [CrossRef]
16. Cagno, E.; Caron, F.; Mancini, M.; Ruggeri, F. Using AHP in determining the prior distributions on gas pipeline failures in a robust Bayesian approach. *Reliab. Eng. Syst. Saf.* **2000**, *67*, 275–284. [CrossRef]
17. Kutoyants, Y. *Introduction to the Statistics of Poisson Processes and Applications*; Springer: New York, NY, USA, 2023.
18. Rios Insua, D.; Ruggeri, F.; Wiper, M.P. *Bayesian Analysis of Stochastic Processes Models*; Wiley: Chichester, UK, 2012.
19. Winkler, R.L. The assessment of prior distributions in Bayesian analysis. *J. Am. Stat. Assoc.* **1967**, *62*, 776–800. [CrossRef]

20. Geyer, C.J.; Johnson, L.T. *MCMC: Markov Chain Monte Carlo*. R Package Version 0.9-8. Available online: https://CRAN.R-project.org/package=mcmc (accessed on 1 December 2024).
21. R Core Team. *R: A Language and Environment for Statistical Computing*; R Foundation for Statistical Computing: Vienna, Austria, 2013. Available online: https://www.R-project.org/ (accessed on 1 December 2024).

MDPI AG
Grosspeteranlage 5
4052 Basel
Switzerland
Tel.: +41 61 683 77 34

*Entropy* Editorial Office
E-mail: entropy@mdpi.com
www.mdpi.com/journal/entropy

*9783725847914*